0001576
AF598552

ENDOLARYNGEAL SURGERY

To my wife, Nellie, for her ever present patience and support

ENDOLARYNGEAL SURGERY

Bruce Benjamin

OBE, DLO, FRACS, FAAP
Clinical Professor of Otorhinolaryngology
Sydney University
Australia

MARTIN DUNITZ

First published in the United Kingdom in 1998 by
Martin Dunitz Ltd
The Livery House
7–9 Pratt Street
London NW1 0AE

A CIP catalogue record for this book is available from the British Library.

ISBN 1–85317–323–1

Composition by Scribe Design, Gillingham, Kent
Printed and bound in Singapore by Imago

Contents

Acknowledgements

I wish to express an appreciation to the many expert anaesthetists with whom I have worked, with particular thanks to Laurie Gadd and Neroli Best who each made many helpful suggestions for the chapter on anaesthesia and laryngoscopy. Nancy Bauman of Iowa City contributed the section on gastro-oesophageal reflux and the larynx and Niell Boustred of Sydney the section on laryngeal trauma.

The typing, retyping and corrections of the manuscript were made by Crystal Lockhart, Toni Joyce and Caroline Jirvane, with a special debt of gratitude owing to Crystal Lockhart. Tom Kertesz proved to be an enthusiastic and accurate proof reader.

Permission was given by Mrs Susan A. Ruby on behalf of her mother Joan Jackson Bugbee, to reproduce Figure 22.2 from *Diseases and Injuries of the Larynx,* written by her father (Chevalier L. Jackson) and grandfather (Chevalier Jackson) and published by MacMillan and Company, New York, in 1942. Figure 22.1 is from *Essay on Growths in the Larynx* (1871) by Morell McKenzie. Permission to use Figures 11.2, 19.1, 20.10, 25.3, 25.9, 25.11, 26.1, 26.2, 26.3, 27.3 and 27.5 was given by the *Annals of Otology, Rhinology and Laryngology*; to use Figures 3.1, 3.2, 3.6, 3.9, 15.4, 15.5, 16.4 and 28.5 from *Atlas of Paediatric Endoscopy: Upper Respiratory Tract and Oesophagus* by Oxford University Press; and to use Figures 3.18, 6.11 (c–f), 6.13, 12.23, 12.33, 14.1, 14.9, 15.1 and 15.31 from *Diagnostic Laryngology: Adults and Children* by W.B. Saunders Company.

Unfailing co-operation and helpful assistance was always available from Robert Peden, Commissioning Editor, and his team from Martin Dunitz.

Lastly, I would like to acknowledge the assistance given over many years by the Karl Storz Company, Tuttlingen, Germany, especially the encouragement for development of new laryngoscopes and instruments provided by Mrs Sybill Storz-Reling. The accuracy and precision application of Karl Storz equipment is a tribute to their superb quality and workmanship.

Bruce Benjamin

Preface

Advances in all aspects of otorhinolaryngology and head and neck surgery have occurred so quickly since the early 1960s until the present that it has been difficult for the practising physician to keep informed. Microsurgical techniques, applied in otology, were rapidly adapted to diagnose and treat diseases of the larynx with greater exactness and opened a new and exciting era in laryngology. Use of the operating microscope, advances in anaesthesia, development of precision surgical instruments, application of the carbon dioxide laser together with the initiative and ingenuity of laryngeal surgeons have all led to many new techniques in microlaryngeal surgery, laser treatment and more recently phonosurgery.

A single author book on endolaryngeal surgery was an ambitious undertaking. The result is based not only on the variety of experience in adult and paediatric airway disease gained at the Royal Alexandra Hospital for Children, Sydney Hospital and Royal North Shore Hospital, but also on the encouragement and assistance offered by various former Registrars and Fellows. The book is written as a practical reference for otolaryngology and head and neck surgeons. The chapter on anaesthesia will be of interest to many anaesthetists and various chapters may attract specialists in other fields. Registrar candidates for the Fellowship and Residents for the Boards should find it a helpful resource. The contents are intended as a systematic exposition of laryngeal diseases and endolaryngeal surgical and microsurgical techniques, with emphasis on methods of teaching and documentation, enhanced by the colour photographs and artwork.

I CLINICAL FEATURES

1 Clinical evaluation

VOICE

Production

Production of the human voice is a complex function which requires fine neuromuscular control and co-ordination. The sound varies according to the mass, tension and length of the vocal fold body (vocal ligament and vocalis muscle), the elastic recoil of the laryngeal tissues and the subglottic pressure generated by the lungs, all of which determine vibration of the vocal fold mucosa to produce the sound of voice.

The voice of an individual is an expression of their personality and their physical and emotional well-being and is vital in communication, e.g. in emphasizing a viewpoint. Minor or major changes in anatomical structure, neuromuscular co-ordination and psychological status can interact when the voice undergoes alteration.

Presenting features

Most adults and older children with laryngeal disease present with a voice abnormality and most infants with stridor. However, there are many other symptoms which relate to abnormalities in the larynx. Adults may complain of:

- an abnormality of the voice
- irritation in the throat
- persistent cough to clear secretions
- a feeling of 'something' in the throat
- pain referred to the ear
- pain or soreness on swallowing
- difficulty swallowing
- a lump in the neck
- aspiration causing coughing or choking
- haemoptysis
- obstruction of breathing
- shortness of breath
- difficulty forming intelligible words.

Systematic history taking will reveal the duration and course of a voice disorder, the nature of other associated physical symptoms and whether there have been previous similar voice problems. Enquiries are made about environmental irritants such as cigarette smoke, dry or dirty atmosphere or possible contamination by chemical or volatile agents; exposure to smog, pollution or air-conditioning may be important. The patient may be a professional voice user such as a singer, entertainer, actor, politician, media presenter or clergyman. Overuse, misuse or abuse of the voice must be ascertained. Is the voice used in stressful situations? It is often useful to ask patients to rate themselves on a 'talkativeness scale' from 1 to 5, thus giving a better idea of daily voice use. A printed questionnaire may be helpful to assist in history taking.

What is a normal voice? There is great variability depending on an individual's personality, age, sex, intelligence, occupation and emotional state. Many patients with minor or moderate vocal disability live quite happily with their voice, but others who find their dysphonia an embarrassment, a handicap or a threat to their communication or livelihood will seek assistance.

Characteristics of change

The nature of the voice change sometimes suggests the cause.

The duration of voice abnormality might be only a few days with laryngitis following an upper respiratory tract infection or it might be many years where huskiness is caused by Reinke's oedema.

The onset of dysphonia might be sudden when shouting causes haemorrhage into a vocal fold or immediately following a thyroid operation with damage to the recurrent laryngeal nerve.

The progression of symptoms over weeks or months strongly suggests a neoplastic cause. Variability of huskiness is characteristic of vocal nodules, depending on the demands placed on the voice.

Variable and irregular voice production where words are difficult to understand might be the first manifestation of a neurological disorder.

Systemic or neurologic disease

The alert clinician will always be mindful of the possibility that laryngeal symptoms can be the initial presenting feature of generalized systemic disease or neurologic conditions. There are many examples:

Systemic disease	*Neurologic disease*
Hypothyroidism	Vocal cord paralysis from primary or secondary tumour of mediastinum, neck or skull base
Hyperparathyroidism	Multiple sclerosis
Acute thyroiditis	Motor neurone disease
Gastro-oesophageal reflux	Myasthenia gravis
AIDS-related diseases	Spasmodic dysphonia
Tuberculosis	Amyotrophic lateral sclerosis
Syphilis	Parkinson's disease
Leprosy	Cerebellar degeneration
Sarcoidosis	Pseudobulbar palsy
Amyloidosis	Various forms of dystonia
Wegener's granulomatosis	
Blastomycosis	
Histoplasmosis	

Voice disorders in adults

Various classifications of voice disorders have been proposed, but in many conditions there is uncertainty of the aetiology and/or the relationship between structure and function. No classification has been entirely satisfactory. The following listings provide a helpful overview.

Organic

Chronic laryngitis, vocal nodules, Reinke's oedema, vocal cord polyp, idiopathic vocal granuloma, contact pachydermia, vocal cord haemorrhage, laryngeal trauma from prolonged intubation, external laryngeal trauma, multiple respiratory papillomas, laryngeal cystic disease, hyperkeratosis, dysplasia, carcinoma or other laryngeal malignancy, congenital abnormalities, Wegener's granulomatosis, idiopathic subglottic stenosis, rheumatoid arthritis, etc.

Neurologic

Cerebrovascular disease, cerebral palsy, vocal cord paresis or paralysis, gastro-oesophageal reflux from neuromuscular incoordination, parkinsonism, essential tremor, spasmodic dysphonia, multiple sclerosis, myasthenia gravis, orofacial dyskinesia, etc.

Hyperfunctional (muscle tension dysphonia)
Conversion aphonia or dysphonia, inappropriate or mutational falsetto, relapsing aphonia or dysphonia, musculoskeletal tension dysphonia, postoperative dysphonia, dysphonia plica ventricularis, etc.

In psychogenic and psychosomatic voice disorders there is increased tension in the vocal folds, thus requiring a greater subglottic pressure of air to overcome glottic resistance and to force the vocal folds apart.

Professional voice users

The disorders of professional voice users are often similar to those listed above, but the demands on the voice and the expectations of the individual exceed the precision expected from others. A respiratory ailment which may be merely a nuisance to the average person can be disabling and a threat to the livelihood of a classical singer or an actor. A singer will seek advice because of the inability to sing a certain pitch to their satisfaction, the inability to control volume, fatiguability of the voice or the loss of resonance. A change in the singing voice may occur without noticeable alteration in the speaking voice either to the singer or to those about them.

Popular singers and rock singers are unlikely to have had good technical training from a singing teacher and amateur or semi-professional singers are usually reluctant to admit limitations in their vocal ability. They are likely to 'push' their voice past its capabilities so that voice misuse compounds their already existing problems.

The complaints of classically trained singers include 'hoarseness' (which may be used to describe various symptoms), the inability to sing loudly or softly, fatigue of the voice over extended periods, the inability to hold particular notes, breathiness, soreness or even pain on singing, a tickling or irritation in the throat and stiffness or soreness in the muscles of the head and neck. Sataloff and Speigel (1991) have listed certain factors to be considered in the care of the professional singer: date of the next important performance, professional voice status and goals, amount and nature of vocal training, type of voice performance and environment, rehearsals, abuse in singing, abuse in speaking, exposure to irritants, smoke exposure, use of drugs (such as alcohol, antihistamines, hormones), reactions to foods (such as dairy foods, chocolate, spiced foods, fluid containing caffeine) and reflux laryngitis.

Voice strain is likely to be most apparent in individuals who frequent discotheques, clubs and hotels where they are exposed to cigarette smoke, the dry air of air-conditioning and where they must overuse their voice or even shout to overcome the constant background noise.

ASSESSMENT OF THE VOICE

Initial general observations

The cause of a voice abnormality is sometimes suggested by certain features before examination of the larynx, for example:

- the smell of cigarette smoke or the sight of nicotine-stained fingers – possibility of malignancy;
- an obese, overclothed female with a hoarse voice – myxoedema;
- weak, somewhat breathy voice in an older person – presbyphonia;
- persistent, variable huskiness over many months or several years in childhood, especially in a boy – vocal nodules;
- relentlessly progressive huskiness and airway obstruction – malignancy;
- difficulty in articulating words and incoordination of swallowing fluids – neuromuscular disorder;
- tense, jerky, strained, effortful voice – spasmodic dysphonia;
- persistent, severe huskiness with slowly progressive stridor and airway obstruction – respiratory papillomas in the larynx;
- sudden onset of huskiness after a choking, spluttering, coughing attack in a child – inhaled laryngeal foreign body;

- intermittent mild dysphonia or episodes of complete aphonia or a voice that is a forced whisper in a female – psychogenic dysphonia;
- weak, breathy voice and inability to produce a sharp cough – vocal cord paralysis;
- sudden onset of dysphonia after shouting – haemorrhage into a vocal fold;
- hoarse, thin, high-pitched, immature voice in a young male – mutational falsetto;
- inability to sing a high note – superior laryngeal nerve palsy;
- muffled voice – caused by large mass or cyst above the larynx.

An accurate diagnosis is not possible without indirect laryngoscopy. This may be difficult or impossible in young children or in adults who are tense, anxious, have a strong gag reflex, an overhanging epiglottis, difficulty opening the mouth or abnormal anatomy of the mouth and pharynx. If flexible laryngoscopy also fails to provide a satisfactory view, a final diagnosis depends on direct laryngoscopy.

Subjective clinical evaluation

Perceptual evaluation of the patient's voice is a complex matter which begins when the patient first speaks to the clinician and which continues throughout the consultation. Subjective evaluation of the voice is open to observer judgement variability or bias. A listener may perceive alterations in three variables – loudness, quality (breathiness, harshness, roughness and diplophonia) and pitch. Although a number of 'check lists' to rate the voice have been developed, the lack of standardization makes comparison between groups of patients or institutions difficult.

Voice evaluation by subjective and/or objective means is important:

- for diagnosis of the pathology in the larynx
- prior to voice therapy by a speech pathologist
- to follow the natural history of disease
- to compare voice before and after treatment
- for clinical research
- for medico-legal reasons.

Objective evaluation

Instruments are available which quantify voice output and analyse voice according to acoustic or aerodynamic characteristics. They offer little assistance in diagnosis but are helpful with documentation.

Objective evaluation is mostly confined to scientific laboratories or voice clinics; specific baseline data can be provided, for example, pre- and postoperative measurements. It has not yet been shown that objective voice assessment has consistent, reliable, diagnostic value in identifying laryngeal abnormalities. There has been little standardization of the test protocols and there is a lack of comprehensive normal measurements.

Methods which have been used to assess vocal fold motion include video-recordings, videostroboscopy, high-speed photography (seldom performed because of the cost and the cumbersome equipment) and electroglottography (which has not earned universal recommendation).

As a comparison, voice testing is not as common and certainly not as useful as audiometry but, nevertheless, the objective study methods of adult voice disorders can be applied in a fully equipped laboratory. Tests which are used include recordings of the voice formed in a standard fashion, stroboscopy (Fig. 1.1) and strobovideolaryngoscopy, acoustic signal analysis (an indirect measure of the vibratory patterns

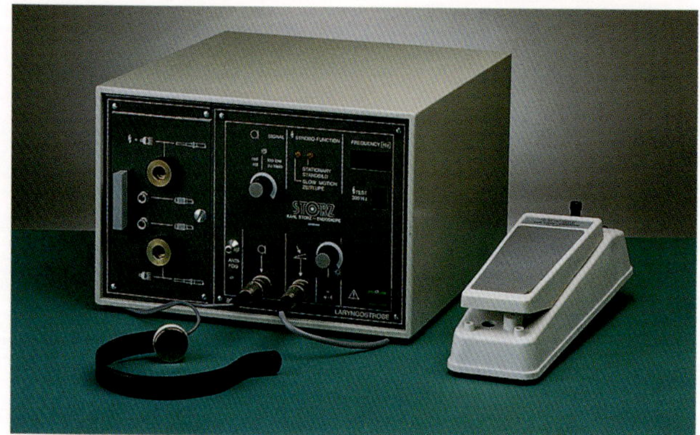

Figure **1.1**
Equipment for stroboscopic examination of the larynx includes sensitive throat microphone and footswitch.

of the vocal folds with measurement of frequency, intensity and time), aerodynamic frequency/intensity measurements, electromyography and electroglottography.

The success of videolaryngoscopy and videostroboscopy depends on good equipment, co-operation of the patient, an understanding of the principles of stroboscopy and an adequate illumination of the larynx by whichever technique of indirect laryngoscopy is used – mirror, flexible or rigid rod telescope.

GENERAL EXAMINATION

An alert clinician notes important features as the patient enters the room, e.g. ataxia, signs of unilateral paralysis from a stroke. During the consultation one may notice features of myxoedema, essential tremor, parkinsonism or undue nervousness. During history taking there might be a suspicion that some symptoms are hyperfunctional or psychosomatic. Patients with hypochondriasis often present a written or typed list of symptoms and some graphically describe sensational symptoms: 'like swallowing razor blades', 'my throat was on fire', 'I cannot swallow anything', 'it feels like red-hot needles'.

Evaluation of the patient's voice is vital, noting its character, variability and effectiveness. Does the patient complain of voice abnormality yet the voice sounds clear and normal at the time of examination? Is it harsh, husky, weak, breathy, tremulous, causing discomfort to the patient or accompanied by facial grimaces? As the patient describes severe or painful symptoms, do they seem to be enjoying the description? During the consultation it may be apparent that the patient is depressed, unduly anxious, aggressive, talkative, has a loud voice, or uses hard glottal attack with rapid speech.

Examination commences with the head and neck. Look, for example, for a scar indicating thyroidectomy, previous removal of a lateral neck mass or a tracheotomy. Note the presence and characteristics of a pathologically enlarged node or nodes in the neck. Check the framework of the larynx: the hyoid bone, thyroid and cricoid cartilages are palpated with reference to their position in the midline, evidence of previous injury, signs of a fullness or swelling, or lack of the normal crepitus moving the larynx. The thyroid gland, each lobe and the isthmus, is examined for localized or diffuse enlargement and for tenderness.

The oral cavity oropharynx, nasopharynx, nasal cavities and tympanic membranes are examined in the standard manner for signs of disease which may be related to the laryngeal condition.

INDIRECT LARYNGOSCOPY

The technique of indirect laryngoscopy is no longer taught to undergraduate students in many medical schools and, as most physicians in general practice have not been given sufficient training in the appropriate skills, they are unable to inspect the laryngopharynx satisfactorily. Thus, in many cases, patients are referred by the family practitioner to the specialist otolaryngologist because of symptoms which suggest pathology in the larynx or pharynx, e.g. husky voice, dysphagia, a lump in the throat but without an examination of the larynx.

The otolaryngologist has painstakingly acquired expertise in the art of indirect laryngoscopy and can visualize the larynx in most patients. The mouth and oropharynx can be inspected directly using a tongue depressor, but examination of the pharynx and larynx relies on visual access by indirect laryngoscopy performed by one or more of three different techniques.

One method is not used to the exclusion of the others, indeed some patients can be satisfactorily

Techniques of indirect laryngoscopy

Laryngeal mirror
Rigid rod lens angled telescope
Flexible fibreoptic laryngoscope

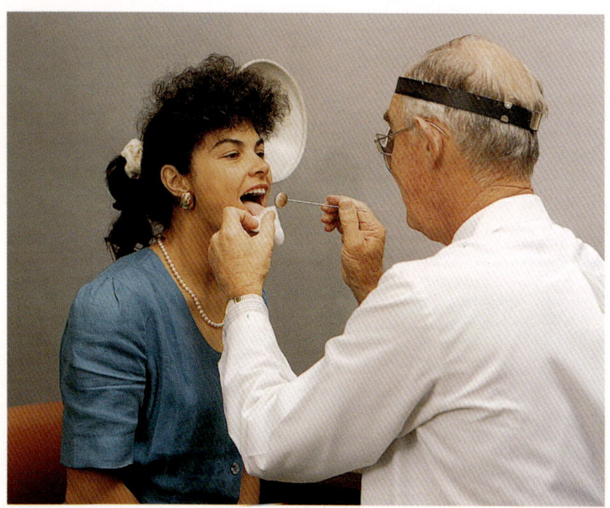

Figure **1.2**
Indirect laryngoscopy using a circular laryngeal mirror. This is the traditional method of laryngeal examination.

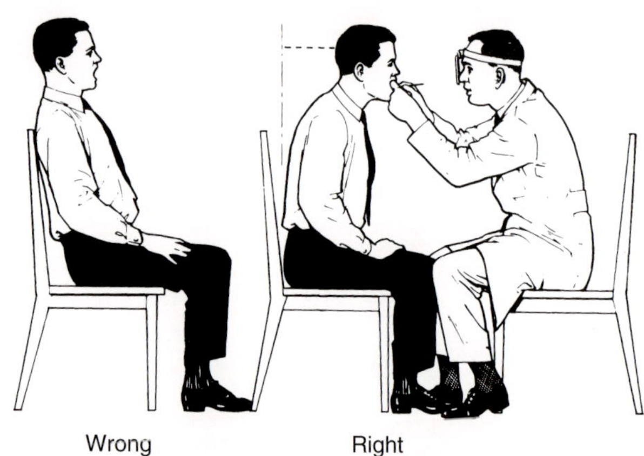

Figure **1.3**
Position of the patient's head and neck for indirect laryngoscopy to create the best angle for a comprehensive view of the laryngeal structures.

examined by one method only, e.g. pernasal flexible fibreoptic laryngoscopy can be used for patients who cannot open the mouth satisfactorily or for those with a very sensitive gag reflex. In some patients additional information is obtained by using more than one technique.

Most laryngeal mass lesions can be recognized on indirect laryngoscopy. Direct laryngoscopy is only occasionally required for diagnosis, but is essential for comprehensive examination, for biopsy and for microsurgical or laser treatment.

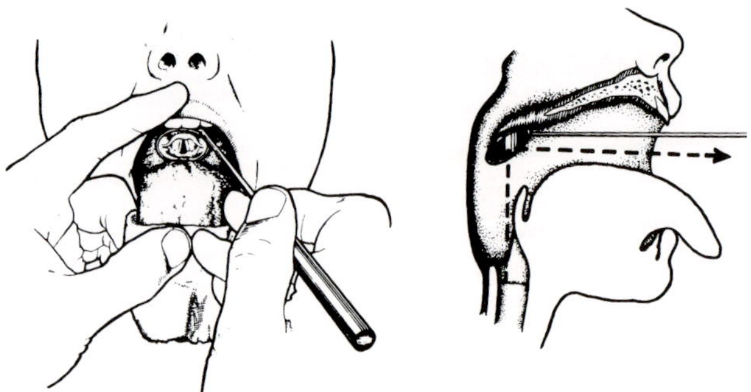

Figure **1.4**
Position of the mirror displacing the soft palate upwards and backwards, if possible without touching the posterior pharyngeal wall, to lessen the chance of gagging.

Laryngeal mirror

Indirect laryngoscopy requires light from an electric bulb reflected from a head mirror (or use of an electric headlight), a warmer for the mirror, gauze pads to grasp the patient's tongue and a choice between various sizes of laryngeal mirrors (Fig. 1.2). The head mirror and light source are adjusted for bright, sharply focused illumination. Skill in this examination will be attained with patience and practice. A confident yet gentle approach with prior explanation to the patient of the nature of the examination is helpful. If the patient is wearing dentures, they should be removed.

The patient sits opposite the examiner with the lower neck slightly flexed and the head slightly extended, a position which creates the best line of sight from the oropharynx to the larynx (Fig. 1.3). The patient is asked to remain relaxed, to breathe quietly and regularly through the mouth and to extend the

Laryngoscopy with a mirror

Head mirror and light
A mirror of suitable size
Patient breathes through the mouth
Examiner holds the tongue
Mirror gently pushes soft palate up
Slight rotation and movement of mirror
Patient phonates 'ee-ee-ee'
Local anaesthesia sometimes
Most common, cheapest technique

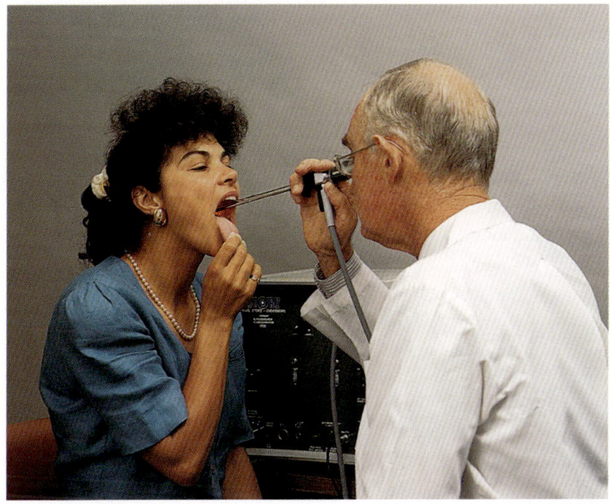

Figure **1.5**
Indirect laryngoscopy using a laryngeal telescope. A wide-diameter telescope with a 70° angle provides a clear, magnified image of the larynx, laryngopharynx and base of tongue.

tongue which is wrapped in gauze and grasped by the examiner's thumb and forefinger to hold it downwards and outwards. As the patient breathes through the mouth, the palate is elevated and the tonsillar pillars remain lateral, providing an opening to introduce the laryngeal mirror which is held in the right hand, much the same as a pen or pencil. The previously warmed mirror is slowly and smoothly placed in the mouth to contact only the soft palate and the uvula, both of which are displaced upwards and backwards, but without touching the posterior pharyngeal wall (Fig. 1.4). The examiner's grasp of the mirror can be steadied by resting the little finger against the patient's cheek once the mirror has been positioned for a view of the anatomical structures. The ease of examination varies from patient to patient. Some sensitive individuals require topical anaesthesia no matter which technique of indirect laryngoscopy is used. Local anaesthesia is often necessary for photography or stroboscopy and can be applied by spray, gel or by sucking a lozenge.

Although the view is two-dimensional, with experience, after moving the position of the mirror slightly, the concept of depth perception can be obtained. Some larynges are seen poorly with the laryngeal mirror and some are seen only during phonation. It is difficult to document pathology by photography with a laryngeal mirror; usually the clinician notes what has been seen in writing and draws a simple sketch.

Indirect mirror examination is the quickest, least expensive and most commonly used method for routine laryngeal examination, but it requires skill and cannot be used for small children.

Laryngoscopy with rigid telescope

90° or 70° telescope
Diameter 4–10 mm
Magnified, brilliant image
Ideal for documentation
Excellent for stroboscopy
Allows use of an observer tube

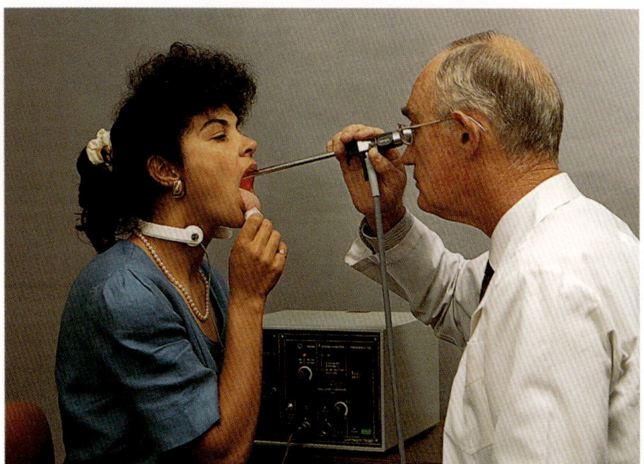

Figure **1.6**
Stroboscopic examination of the larynx. A neck microphone synchronizes the flashing strobe light during constant phonation so the vibrating edges of the vocal folds appear in slow motion.

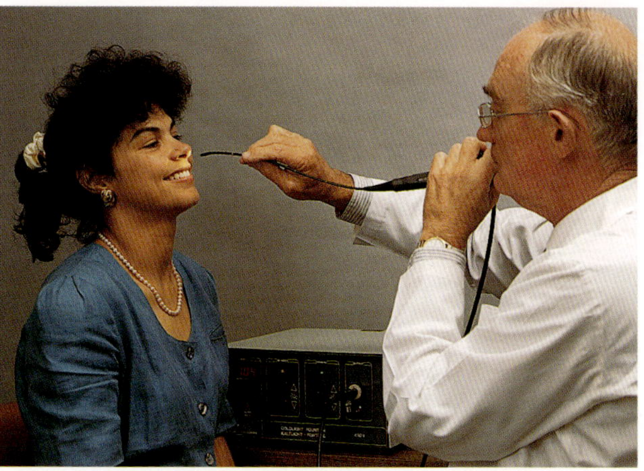

Figure **1.7**
Indirect laryngoscopy using a flexible laryngoscope 3.5 mm in diameter which is about to be passed through a nasal cavity which has had topical anaesthesia and vasoconstrictor spray applied.

Rigid telescope

A similar technique with the examiner sitting opposite the patient is employed (Fig. 1.5), but a rigid rod lens fibreoptic telescope with integral lighting is used. There are several different telescopes available with viewing angles of either 90° or 70° degrees (the latter is said to be better for visualizing the anterior commissure) and with external diameters from the smallest of 4 mm to the largest of 10 mm. The 4-mm external diameter, 70° telescope (Karl Storz 7200CK) is recommended for routine diagnostic indirect laryngoscopy as it provides an excellent view and is well tolerated by most patients. Although 35-mm photography and stroboscopy are possible with this 4-mm telescope, a brighter image is obtained with a larger telescope such as the Karl Storz 8706CJ which has a 7.2 × 9.3 mm oval sheath. The magnified, crystal-clear, wide-angle view of the larynx makes this telescope ideal for still photography, stroboscopy (Fig. 1.6) and video-recording. Topical anaesthesia is often required.

Indirect laryngoscopy with a rigid telescope allows use of an observer tube for teaching. A video-printer can quickly produce a colour print from the video image on a television monitor.

Flexible fibreoptic nasopharyngolaryngoscope

Flexible endoscopes of 3-, 4- or 5-mm diameter for adults are available; most are about 30 cm long (Fig. 1.7). The larger instruments may have a channel for suction or administration of oxygen. The proximal controls are capable of angling the distal tip through 180° in one direction, and the entire endoscope can be rotated in the examiner's hand, thus allowing manoeuvrability of the tip in any direction. A bright light source is necessary.

The patient sits opposite the examiner in the same position used for mirror or rigid telescope examination. The larger nasal cavity (if there is a nasal septal deflection the other side is used) is sprayed with a suitable mixture of decongestant and topical anaesthetic solution which is given a few minutes to take effect.

The tip of the instrument is passed along the floor of the nasal cavity into the nasopharynx – noting any abnormality – angled around the soft palate, passed downwards to reveal the base of the tongue and the valleculae, and worked behind the epiglottis to reveal the larynx and the piriform sinuses. Unless the glottis has been thoroughly anaesthetized and there are

Laryngoscopy with flexible laryngoscope

Usually 3–5 mm in diameter
Proximal steering controls
Anaesthesia for one nasal passage
Exposes nasal cavity, pharynx and larynx
Shows dynamics of supraglottis and glottis
Optical resolution less than rigid telescope
Expensive, needs special care

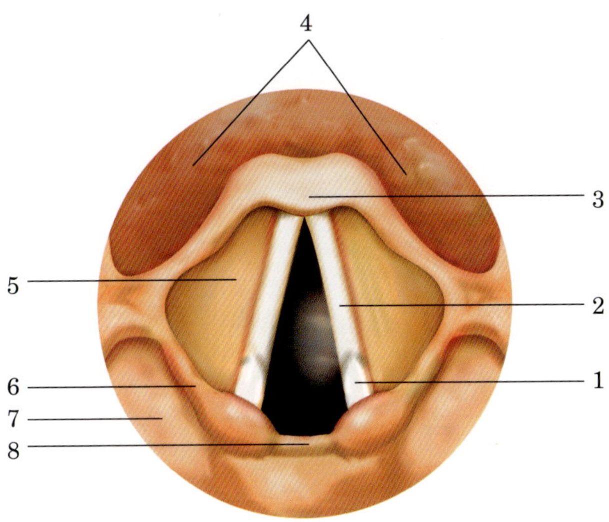

Figure **1.8**
Diagrammatic representation of structures in the normal larynx.

1 Vocal process of arytenoid
2 Vocal cord
3 Tubercle of epiglottis
4 Valleculae
5 False vocal cord
6 Aryepiglottic fold
7 Piriform fossa
8 Interarytenoid region

facilities for resuscitation, the glottis should not be touched for fear of precipitating laryngospasm. The dynamics of the supraglottic and glottic structures can now be examined, aided by stroboscopy if necessary.

A flexible laryngoscope is an expensive instrument needing special care to protect its delicate fibreoptic threads from damage, but it is easily portable and can be used in the consulting room, clinic, emergency department, intensive care unit or in the ward. The optical resolution is not as good as that provided by a laryngeal mirror or rigid telescope and, although subtle changes may be difficult to detect, it is in regular use by otolaryngologists for examination of the nasal cavities, nasopharynx, pharynx and larynx.

Smaller diameter, paediatric flexible laryngobronchoscopes are used by paediatric otolaryngologists and pulmonologists, in infants and children. The nasal cavities, nasopharynx and larynx can be examined in the consulting room or clinic with local anaesthesia.

If tracheobronchoscopy is necessary in paediatric patients, for safety reasons it is best performed in a fully equipped endoscopy room or operating theatre in co-operation with an anaesthetist and with the availability of suction, oxygen, pulse oximetry and resuscitation facilities in case of laryngospasm, hypoxia or bradycardia. Flexible instruments as small as 2.7 mm or ultrathin fibreoptic bronchoscopes which have neither a steering mechanism nor a suction channel can be passed via an indwelling endotracheal tube to examine the bronchi in the neonatal intensive care unit.

FINDINGS AT INDIRECT LARYNGOSCOPY

Routine examination

A routine of inspection should be followed in viewing the different anatomical structures: base of tongue, valleculae, anterior surface of the epiglottis, posterior pharyngeal wall, lateral pharyngeal walls, piriform fossae and postcricoid area. In the larynx itself the examiner looks for the tubercle of the epiglottis, the aryepiglottic folds and the cuneiform and corniculate cartilages which lie above the eminences of the arytenoid cartilages on each side with the interarytenoid area between them in the posterior glottis (Fig. 1.8).

Routine indirect laryngoscopy

Base of tongue and valleculae
Anterior and posterior surface epiglottis
Posterior and lateral pharyngeal walls
Piriform fossae
Aryepiglottic folds
Cuneiform, corniculate, arytenoid cartilages
Interarytenoid area and posterior glottis
Ventricular bands (false cords)
Vocal cord appearance and movement
Stroboscopy for vocal fold vibration

The ventricular folds (false cords) lie above the true vocal cords but the ventricles of the larynx cannot be seen. The vocal cords reflect a lot of light and appear as flat, pale, almost white, ribbon-like structures with straight edges. Vocal cord movements are observed in quiet respiration and during phonation. The anterior subglottic space and several arches of the trachea can often be seen.

The image of the larynx in the mirror is reversed with right-hand structures seen on the left and vice versa. The most difficult yet important structure to view is the anterior commissure – it is often seen more clearly as the larynx elevates and the epiglottis tilts anteriorly during phonation. In the past, in some European clinics, it was not uncommon to attempt removal of certain laryngeal lesions or obtain a biopsy at indirect laryngoscopy using curved laryngeal forceps, but this technique is now seldom, if ever, used.

The examiner notes and evaluates the significance of any abnormal appearance such as hyperaemia, oedema, ulceration, granulation tissue, vocal nodule or swelling and any cystic, solid or proliferative lesion. The dynamics of the supraglottic tissues and vocal cord movements are observed. Dynamic changes are, of course, best documented by a videotape.

Difficulties

1 It is better to remove full dentures, usually both but at least the upper denture, during examination.
2 Some patients are unable to open the mouth fully due to temporomandibular joint problems, others may elevate the tongue making examination difficult, but the most common problem is a sensitive gag reflex. The latter can usually be overcome by using topical anaesthesia.
3 The view varies with each patient: some tolerate the examination without discomfort and a leisurely view can be obtained, others become easily distressed and intolerant, permitting only an incomplete or fleeting view.
4 Although a more comprehensive view is obtained with a large laryngeal mirror, it may be better to use a smaller mirror which can be better tolerated. Slight rotation and movement of the mirror allows visualization of all accessible areas.
5 The mirror image is reversed and upside down, but an experienced examiner has no difficulty with correct orientation and interpretation.
6 A large and/or overhanging epiglottis may make visualization of the larynx difficult or even impossible. It can be 'hooked' forwards with a curved instrument in the examiner's left hand while the patient holds their own tongue. Successful use of this method requires liberal use of topical anaesthesia and manual dexterity.
7 Fogging of the rigid or flexible telescope is prevented by use of an anti-fog solution or by warming the instrument before use.
8 Indirect laryngoscopy with a slim flexible fibreoptic laryngoscope is useful for large lesions such as a cyst, neoplasm, mass of papillomas or the swelling of acute epiglottitis. Flexible laryngoscopy is especially helpful in vocal cord paralysis or laryngomalacia, but not all infants and children, or even all adults, can co-operate.

   Because the flexible instruments lack precise definition it may be difficult to be sure of small lesions such as early mucosal dysplasia, vocal nodules or an intracordal cyst. The anterior commissure, posterior glottic space and the subglottic region are especially difficult to examine.
9 The anterior commissure is often difficult to see; if it has not been visualized, the indirect laryngeal

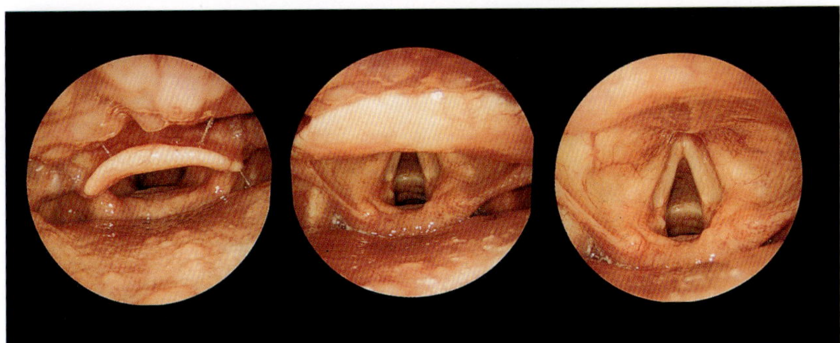

Figure **1.9**
Three photographs as a telescope is introduced and positioned. First, tongue base, valleculae, epiglottis and posterior pharyngeal wall but not the larynx. Second, most of the larynx but not the anterior commissure. Third, laryngoscope optimally placed to show an overall view of the larynx.

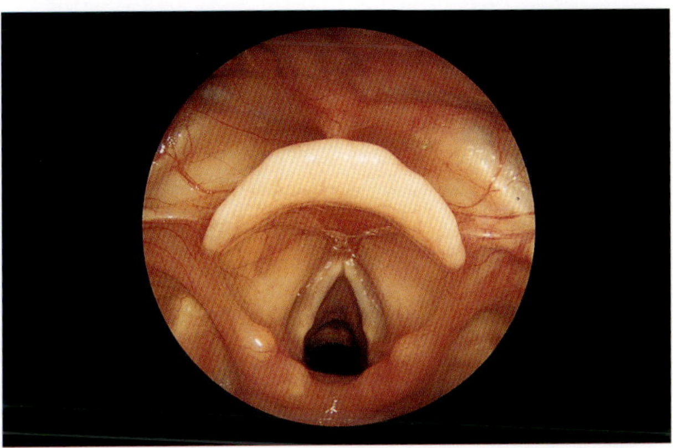

Figure **1.10**
A comprehensive view, seldom seen so well, where the normal valleculae, supraglottic and glottic structures are seen in a single view. Taken using a 4-mm telescope.

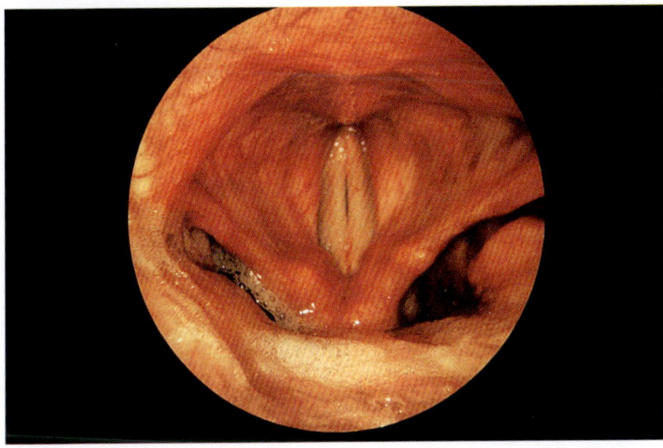

Figure **1.11**
Normal adult larynx with vocal cords in adduction. The aryepiglottic folds define the anteromedial border of the piriform fossae.

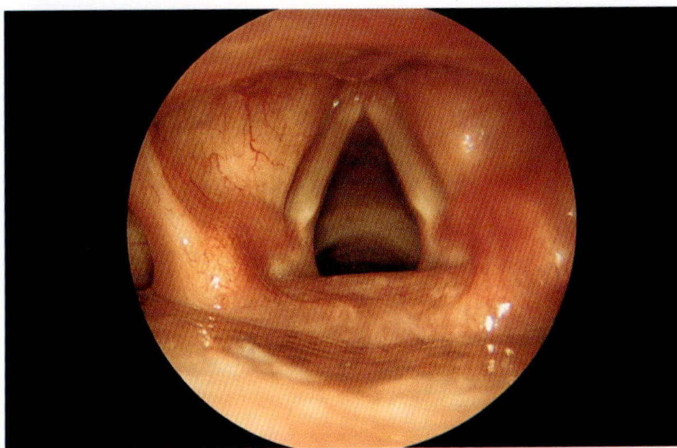

Figure **1.12**
Normal supraglottic and glottic structures during quiet respiration. Part of the subglottis can be seen.

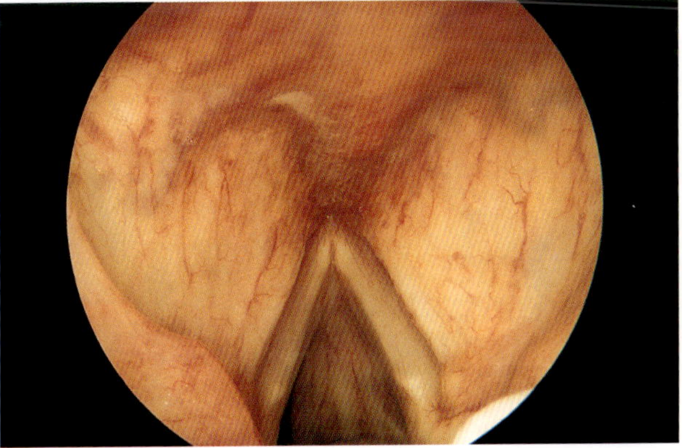

Figure **1.13**
The anterior larynx and tubercle (petiole) of the epiglottis. This anterior anatomy is the most difficult to visualize, irrespective of the indirect laryngoscopy technique used.

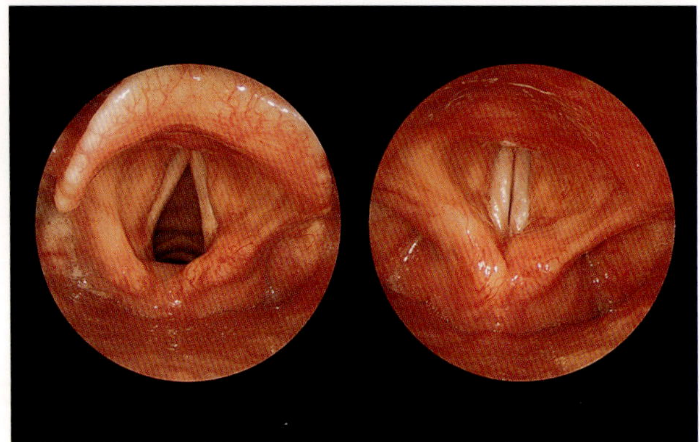

Figure **1.14**
Abduction and adduction with normal movement and normal appearance. In addition, the vocal folds, arytenoids and piriform fossae become more prominent on adduction. Taken using a 4-mm telescope.

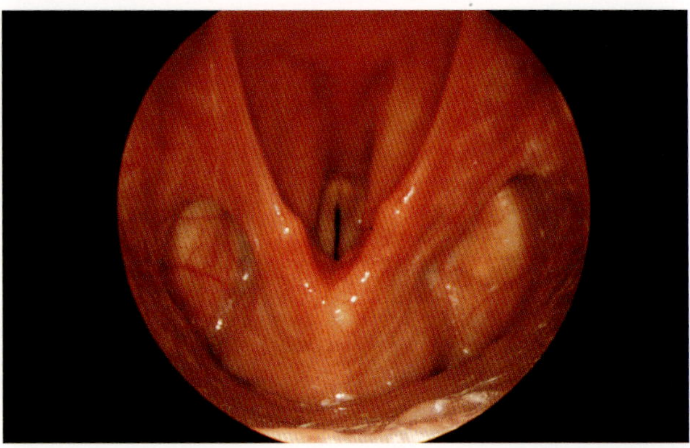

Figure **1.15**
The piriform fossae, aryepiglottic folds and part of the postcricoid area seen clearly during phonation.

examination is incomplete. It is often best seen during or just after the patient phonates 'ee-ee-ee-ee'.

10 The laryngeal ventricles and to some extent the posterior glottic space and the subglottic region are difficult to examine satisfactorily. The piriform fossae can be better seen in some individuals than others; a good view can often be obtained on phonation. All these areas can be better examined under general anaesthesia at direct laryngoscopy with rigid telescopes.

Normal appearances

The findings at indirect laryngoscopy are best demonstrated by photographs taken with rigid telescopes (Figs 1.9–1.15). The photographs in Figs 1.9–1.15 were taken with the 7.2 × 9.3 mm tele-laryngoscope, except when noted in the legend. At indirect laryngoscopy using a telescope, the view is upside down and a 'mirror image', thus placing the anterior commissure inferiorly, at the bottom of the image. For easier orientation, photographs taken at indirect laryngoscopy are shown with the same orientation as those taken at direct laryngoscopy, i.e. with the anterior commissure at the top.

BIBLIOGRAPHY

Sataloff RT, Speigel JR (1991) Care of the professional voice. *Otolaryng Clinics N Amer* **24**(5): 1093–1124.

2 Laryngeal and other airway problems in paediatrics

REFERRAL SOURCE

Patients with airway problems may be referred to the otolaryngologist from neonatology immediately after birth, from neonatal or paediatric intensive care, from a paediatric surgeon, from a paediatrician or a paediatric pulmonologist. Older children are often referred for voice abnormalities.

Thus paediatric patients, whether infants or children, have a variety of presenting symptoms with one or more of the following problems requiring diagnostic assessment.

PRESENTING FEATURES

These include:

- stridor, often present from birth or shortly after
- airway obstruction, partial or severe
- repeated aspiration
- cyanotic or apnoeic attacks
- husky, weak or absent cry in infants
- husky voice in older children
- acute airway obstruction due to inflammatory infection
- recurrent or atypical croup
- chronic progressive airway obstruction
- atypical 'pneumonia' or 'bronchitis'
- compression of the trachea or main bronchi
- mediastinal mass, cystic or solid
- inhaled or ingested foreign body.

In most newborns and infants the causes are congenital. Stridor is caused by laryngeal anomalies in about 65%, by tracheal or bronchial anomalies in 20% and by inflammatory, traumatic or other causes in the remaining 15%.

Discussion of upper airway obstruction in paediatric patients would be incomplete without at least a list of causes, as outlined below.

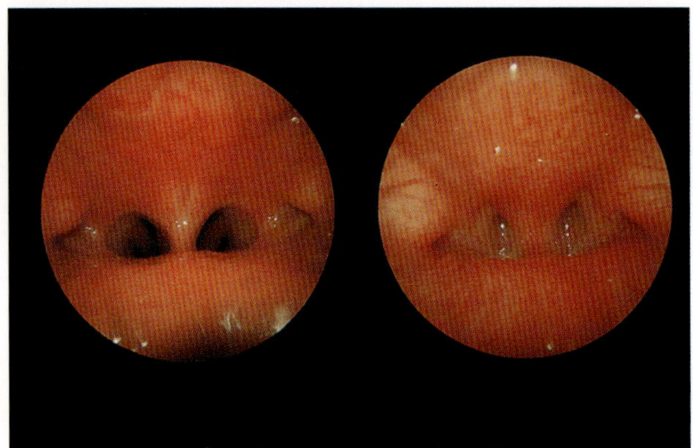

Figure **2.1**
Bilateral congenital posterior choanal atresia in a newborn infant. Normal anatomy (left) and bilateral atresia (right). Note that the obstructing bony partitions are several millimetres anterior to the plane of the posterior choanae.

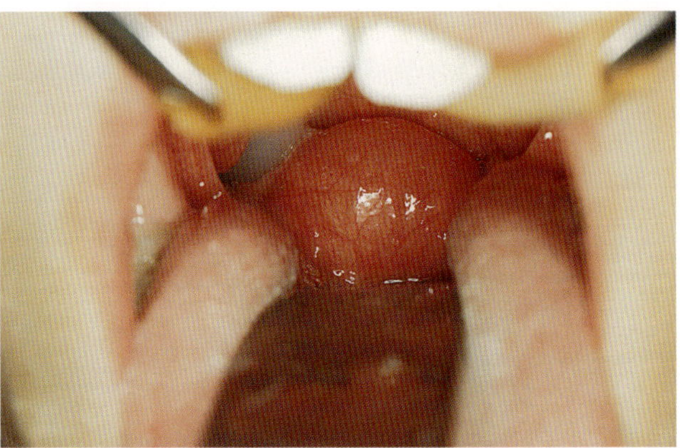

Figure **2.2**
Lingual thyroid tissue. A large, smooth, rounded mass at the base of the tongue, which can cause partial obstruction.

CAUSES OF AIRWAY OBSTRUCTION

The causative pathology is not confined to the larynx. Abnormalities may be identified in the nasal cavities (e.g. bilateral choanal atresia), in the pharynx (micrognathia and glossoptosis), in the larynx (laryngomalacia), in the trachea (external compression by a vessel, cyst or tumour) or occasionally in a main bronchus (congenital bronchial stenosis). A complete list of congenital causes of upper airway obstruction is lengthy; here the more common conditions are highlighted in bold type.

Nasopharyngeal

- **bilateral posterior choanal atresia** (Fig. 2.1)
- **turbinate hypertrophy** or 'stuffy nose syndrome'
- **traumatic nasal deformities** caused during birth – deviated nasal septum, fractured nasal bones, septal haematoma
- nasal or postnasal mass due to adenoids, encephalocoele, glioma, dermoid, chordoma, haematoma, etc.
- lachrymal duct cyst
- stenosis or atresia of the anterior choanae
- **craniofacial skeletal abnormalities**
  Treacher Collins' syndrome
  Apert's or Cruzon's syndrome

Oropharyngeal

- **enlarged tongue**
- **Pierre Robin sequence**
- **tumours or cysts in the pharynx** (e.g. cystic hygroma, haemangioma or dermoid)
- lingual thyroid tissue or lingual thyroglossal duct cyst (Fig. 2.2)

Laryngeal

- supraglottic
  laryngomalacia
  ductal mucous retention cyst
  cystic hygroma
  cyst of the saccule, lateral or anterior
  bifid or hypoplastic epiglottis
- glottic
  bilateral or unilateral vocal cord paralysis
  laryngeal web or atresia
  posterior laryngeal cleft
  other rare abnormalities
- subglottic
  congenital subglottic stenosis
  subglottic haemangioma
  membranous web
  ductal retention cysts

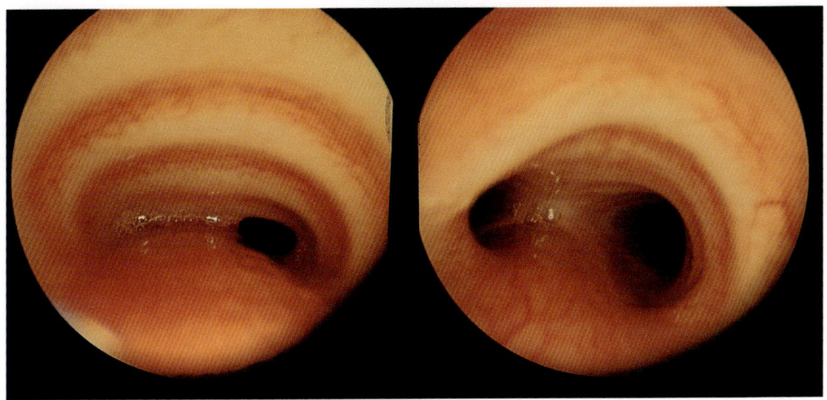

Figure **2.3**
Innominate artery compression of the trachea. Tracheomalacia and severe compression (left) at junction of upper two-thirds and lower third of the trachea. Larger lumen (right) below the narrowing.

Tracheal

- **tracheomalacia, bronchomalacia**
- **innominate artery compression** (Fig. 2.3)
- **compression by vascular ring**
- external compression from a mediastinal cyst or tumour
- congenital stenosis of the trachea
- haemangioma
- tracheal web.

Note that conditions outside the respiratory tract may cause respiratory distress, for instance, a large abdominal mass or a diaphragmatic hernia with eventration.

In older children, causes which are not of congenital origin become important, e.g. inflammatory conditions such as croup or acute supraglottitis and trauma which is either external or internal, iatrogenic or non-iatrogenic.

OBVIOUS CAUSES

Some conditions are easily recognized. A large neck mass due to cystic hygroma or haemangioma, a large thyroglossal duct cyst or a lateral neck mass can compress the pharyngeal or upper airway. Serious upper airway obstruction may be caused by oropharyngeal obstruction from micrognathia and retroposed tongue in a baby with Pierre Robin sequence. Similar features are seen with Treacher Collins' syndrome, Cruzon's syndrome, Apert's syndrome and macroglossia. The cause of the latter may be idiopathic, due to lymphangioma, haemangioma or associated with Down's syndrome, cretinism or Beckwith's syndrome.

HISTORY

The taking of an accurate and comprehensive history often begins with the laryngologist's involvement with the parents and provides an opportunity to discuss the clinical situation, the inevitable anxieties which are engendered, the need for various investigations, which may include endoscopy under general anaesthesia, and surgical procedures, e.g. laser treatment or tracheotomy. Possible alternatives can be explained, the pros and cons of treatment options explored and the possible need for consultation with other specialists outlined.

The history may reveal valuable information, e.g. a traumatic forceps delivery as the cause of nasal trauma with the dislocation of septal cartilage or the fracture of nasal bones.

As another example, polyhydramnios is associated with a higher incidence of oesophageal atresia and tracheo-oesophageal fistula.

OBSERVATION

Stridor caused by total nasal obstruction may be accompanied by periods of cyanosis, but when the infant cries and takes a breath through the mouth it will be observed that the airway obstruction is momentarily relieved – a reliable indication that the cause of obstruction is in the nasal cavities or nasopharynx and not in the larynx. Bilateral vocal cord paralysis is accompanied by stridor but the cry may be weak or normal. A supraglottic pharyngeal obstruction caused by a cyst or mass is accompanied by a muffled cry or even its absence. Tracheal obstruction caused by compression, stenosis or collapse is usually associated with biphasic inspiratory and expiratory stridor and a 'barking' cough.

STRIDOR

Stridor is a prominent, abnormal, audible manifestation of upper airway obstruction caused by turbulent airflow through a narrowed airway, usually the larynx or trachea. Stridor is most often inspiratory, sometimes expiratory and occasionally both. It is heard by listening beside the patient. **Wheeze**, such as the turbulent expiratory noise generated in small airways in asthma, is heard by auscultation with a stethoscope. **Stertor** is a term sometimes used to describe a low-pitched snoring sound usually produced by nasal or nasopharyngeal obstruction.

Stridor is a clinical feature but not a diagnosis. The term 'congenital laryngeal stridor' is unfortunate as not all causes of stridor in an infant are congenital, nor do they all arise from the larynx.

PHYSICAL SIGNS OF OBSTRUCTION

Obstruction of the major airways not only causes stridor but is also accompanied by rapid breathing, increased respiratory effort indicated by retraction of the chest, vigorous use of the accessory respiratory muscles and, when pulmonary ventilation is impaired, there may be bradycardia as hypoxia and hypercarbia increase.

ASPIRATION

Repeated aspiration into the tracheobronchial tree in infants requires radiological investigation for incoordinate swallowing or gastro-oesophageal reflux and endoscopy for H-type tracheo-oesophageal fistula, cleft larynx or vocal cord paralysis.

MONITORING

In intensive care, objective data measurement of patients with respiratory distress, stridor, cyanotic or apnoeic attacks may be helpful, e.g. pulse oximetry, transcutaneous carbon dioxide, apnoea and bradycardia monitoring.

ACUTE INFLAMMATORY AIRWAY OBSTRUCTION

A child with upper airway obstruction caused by acute infection will be usually toxic with characteristic clinical features which usually indicate the cause. Acute epiglottitis causes the most rapid and severe airway obstruction and must be differentiated from acute laryngotracheitis (croup) with subglottic oedema, gross enlargement of the tonsils and adenoids, an unsuspected foreign body in the larynx, subglottic region or upper oesophagus and diphtheria or one of the acute abscesses in the pharynx. When croup is persistent, recurrent or atypical, there may be an underlying pathology such as a congenital subglottic stenosis or conditions such as laryngeal papilloma, congenital subglottic haemangioma, tracheomalacia, tracheal stenosis or tracheal compression. See Chapter 28 for acute inflammatory airway obstruction.

DIAGNOSIS OF AIRWAY OBSTRUCTION

In infants and most children, because the larynx and hypopharynx cannot always be inspected by indirect examination, but only by direct laryngoscopy, the clinical features or combinations of features may suggest the possibility of the underlying pathologic cause. They are seldom absolutely diagnostic. In most cases examination of the nasal cavities, pharynx, larynx, tracheobronchial tree and oesophagus by flexible endoscopy and/or by direct endoscopy under general anaesthesia should be considered so that a final diagnosis can be made.

Laryngoscopy alone, whether with or without general anaesthesia and whether performed by indirect laryngoscopy using a flexible instrument or by direct laryngoscopy using rigid instruments, may be an incomplete examination – pathologic conditions in the tracheobronchial tree and in the oesophagus may remain undiagnosed. In over 10% of patients being investigated for stridor there are lesions at more than one anatomic site.

FLEXIBLE LARYNGOSCOPY

Small-diameter flexible fibreoptic nasopharyngolaryngoscopes are in regular use by paediatric otolaryngologists to examine the nasal cavities, nasopharynx and larynx in infants and children. Usually local anaesthesia is used but it can be a procedure done in the operating theatre.

Flexible fibreoptic bronchoscopy in infants and children is also undertaken by paediatric otolaryngologists and pulmonologists for examination of the trachea, bronchi and segmental openings, the examination being performed in the operating theatre with intravenous sedation, supplemental oxygen, monitoring of vital signs (including oximetry), facilities for resuscitation and a postoperative recovery ward. Therefore flexible fibreoptic laryngoscopy or tracheobronchoscopy in infants and children is performed as a diagnostic procedure and can be separate from or complementary to rigid laryngoscopy and tracheobronchoscopy. This largely depends upon whether otolaryngology or paediatric pulmonology becomes responsible for laryngeal and airway problems in the particular hospital and it depends upon the skill and experience of the individuals involved.

There are advantages and disadvantages to each method. Although rigid endoscopy has been the time-honoured mainstay over many decades and remains the 'gold standard', flexible fibreoptic endoscopy in selected cases is a safe and effective method. Specially manufactured paediatric instruments are used including endoscopes of 3.5- or 2.5-mm diameter which are steerable so that the tip can be extended and flexed. In addition there are ultra-thin fibreoptic instruments which have neither a steering mechanism nor a suction channel but are useful for bedside examination in the paediatric or neonatal intensive care wards.

The rigid endoscopes allow better and safer control of the airway, especially in patients with a pre-existing obstructive lesion. Solid or cystic masses can be biopsied and granulation tissue can be removed more satisfactorily than with a flexible instrument. Although a foreign body can be diagnosed by flexible endoscopy, removal should be performed under general anaesthesia with a rigid endoscope because of the added safety of anaesthesia through an open-tubed instrument. Optical foreign body forceps used through the lumen of the bronchoscope provide better control of the foreign body during removal. Thick secretions, impacted plugs or obstructing tenacious crusts (as in bacterial laryngotracheobronchitis) should be removed by rigid bronchoscopy. A rigid endoscope allows use of the carbon dioxide laser by providing a safe, straight lumen through which the beam can be directed.

The complication rate for either rigid or flexible endoscopy is very small with careful technique and skilled, experienced personnel. The use of flexible fibreoptic instruments in infants or small children with pre-existing airway obstruction or hypoxia is fraught with danger as bradycardia and desaturation may occur rapidly. Facilities for intubation, via either an endotracheal tube or an open tube bronchoscope, must be ready for immediate, rapid and effective resuscitation.

INDICATIONS FOR ENDOSCOPY

Paediatric patients present with a variety of clinical features which require endoscopic assessment. The pathology is not always in the larynx and a broad view of the upper respiratory tract must be kept in mind for all patients. The patient may present with a symptom for investigation, with findings on X-ray requiring elucidation or with a known disease needing treatment:

- stridor of unknown cause
- atypical, recurrent or persistent croup
- weak or absent cry
- repeated aspiration
- endoscopic removal of an inhaled or ingested foreign body
- narrowing or compression of the tracheobronchial tree
- respiratory papillomas, haemangioma or lymphangioma
- laryngeal trauma caused by prolonged intubation
- laryngeal trauma from external, sharp or blunt neck trauma
- web or stenosis, congenital or acquired
- tracheo-oesophageal fistula and oesophageal atresia
- acute inflammatory airway obstruction requiring laryngoscopy and intubation
- husky voice in older children
- conditions requiring endoscopic surgical procedures such as arytenoidectomy, laser of subglottic haemangioma, operative repair of a minor posterior congenital laryngeal cleft.

Each individual patient must be separately evaluated, but in most patients diagnostic endoscopy includes examination of the larynx, tracheobronchial tree and usually the oesophagus, where symptoms relate both to the airway and the oesophagus. Examination of the nasal cavities and nasopharynx is indicated in certain cases.

INDICATIONS FOR ENDOSCOPY IN INFANTS

Specifically, infants with stridor that appears to be of a congenital nature, require endoscopic examination for:

- severe stridor and airway obstruction
- stridor which is progressive
- stridor associated with unusual features such as cyanotic or apnoeic attacks, dysphagia, aspiration or failure to thrive
- an unexplained radiologic abnormality
- undue parental anxiety.

3 Diagnostic imaging

Until recently imaging of the pharynx, larynx and upper trachea relied on lateral soft-tissue radiographs in infants and children and tomography in adults. There are now advanced techniques including computed tomography (CT) and magnetic resonance imaging (MRI) which can provide additional information.

Imaging methods will be discussed firstly with regard to infants and children and secondly with regard to adults.

INFANTS AND CHILDREN

In paediatric patients the clinical features usually suggest a provisional diagnosis, but as the laryngopharynx and subglottic region can be examined only by direct endoscopy under general anaesthesia, radiological imaging before endoscopy is invaluable to delineate cysts, tumours, foreign bodies and inflammatory swellings. Compression, collapse or stenosis of the trachea can be demonstrated on X-ray and CT reveals tumours or cysts in the lower neck or mediastinum.

Interpretation of pathological changes requires a knowledge of the anatomy and physiology of the upper respiratory tract, remembering that there is great variability in the normal airway in infants and children depending upon respiration, swallowing, crying, movement of the patient and neck position (Fig. 3.1). Ideally the film should be taken with the neck extended during deep inspiration.

On lateral films of the upper airway (Fig. 3.1) the natural contrast at the air–mucosal interface allows visualization of the palate, base of tongue, adenoids, tonsils, epiglottis, arytenoids, aryepiglottic folds, laryngeal ventricle, subglottic region, upper trachea and retropharyngeal soft tissues. An antero-posterior (AP) film (Fig. 3.2) may be helpful in some cases to show the laryngeal and tracheal airway, vocal cords, subglottic region and trachea. It is usual to obtain AP

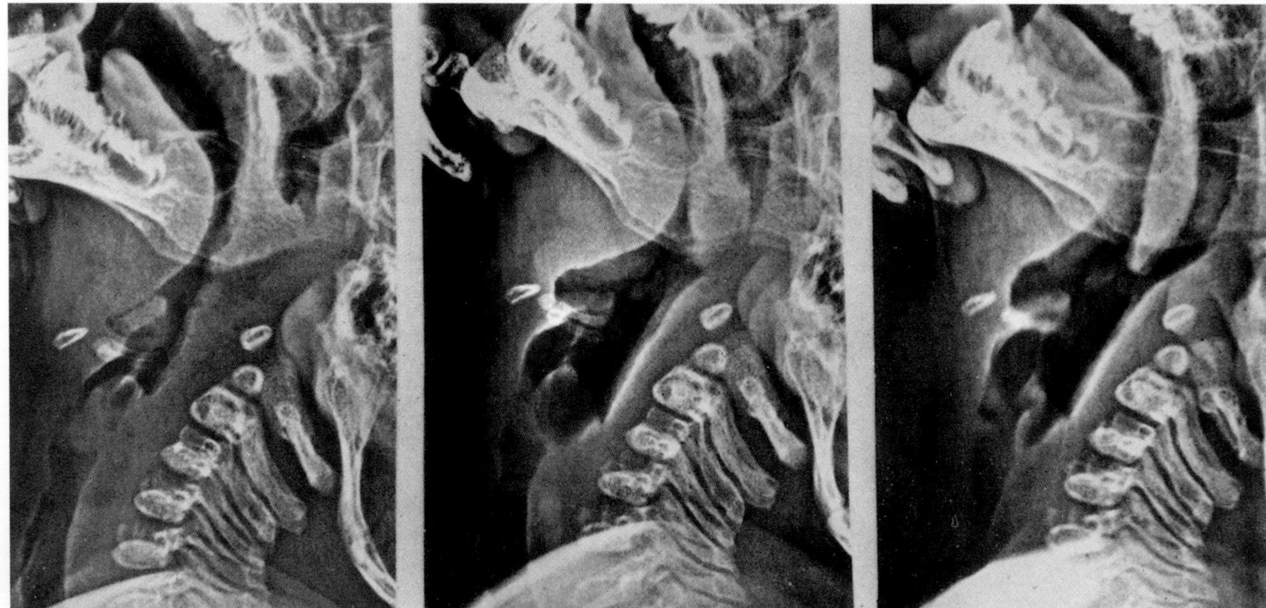

Figure **3.1**
Lateral xerograms of a child's larynx and pharynx at different times. The remarkable difference in appearance can be appreciated by studying the airway in different anatomical sites from one image to the other, e.g. the appearance of the trachea, the larynx with the supraglottic larynx and the nasopharynx.

and lateral chest X-rays when evaluating the paediatric airway, and with appropriate exposure the intrathoracic trachea can be seen to the level of the bifurcation.

Positioning and artefacts

Correct positioning with the patient upright, head and neck comfortably extended, and the film taken in full inspiration are important factors in minimizing confusing artefactual variations from the normal appearance. It must be remembered that, as a static study of dynamic structures, the pharynx, larynx and trachea (Fig. 3.1) may be visualized during any phase of respiration or deglutition so that the image may not truly represent the 'normal' in the resting state (Fig. 3.3). Although several films may be taken, they may not be representative as it is often difficult, especially in small children, to ensure an inspiratory film. Common artefacts at the glottic level include the appearance of a soft tissue mass due to 'bunching' of the vocal cords during crying; blurring of the vocal cords and laryngeal ventricles making features in the area difficult to distinguish; air in the piriform fossa giving the appearance of an air-containing cyst in the region of the arytenoids; a ridge in the posterior pharyngeal wall due to contraction of the pharyngeal constrictor muscles; and apparent thickening of retropharyngeal and prevertebral soft tissue. The distance between the posterior pharyngeal wall and the anterior portion of the third or fourth cervical vertebra should not normally exceed three-quarters of the diameter of a vertebral body.

Lateral and antero-posterior views

The plain lateral examination is fundamental in evaluating the upper airway in infants and young children. A soft-tissue film or a tightly coned, high-kilovoltage (Kv) magnified view is routine in most paediatric hospi-

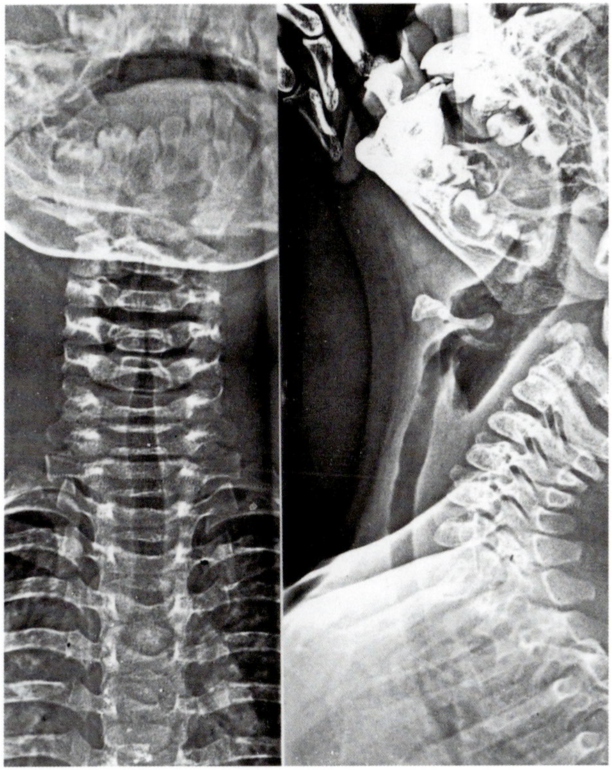

Figure **3.2**
Antero-posterior and lateral xerograms of normal upper airways. In the AP xerogram, the subglottic region, trachea, carina and main bronchi can be seen. In the lateral xerogram, both the intrathoracic and extrathoracic trachea are visible together with the soft tissue structures of the larynx and pharynx.

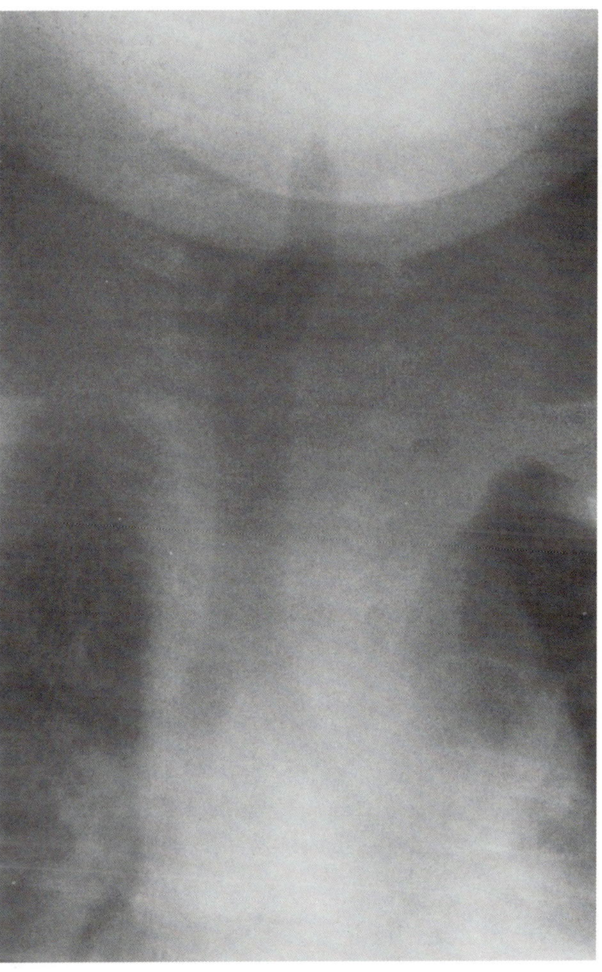

Figure **3.3**
Artefactual appearance on AP high KV of normal. If the head and neck are not extended, the upper trachea will 'buckle'.

tals. Antero-posterior frontal airway films (Figs 3.2, 3.3) are helpful in certain cases, e.g. subglottic haemangioma, compression of the trachea and tracheal stenosis. The high-Kv technique using a copper filter optimizes and enhances the air–soft tissue interface, minimizes bone shadows and can provide satisfactory views of the subglottic larynx, intrathoracic trachea and main bronchi in the AP plane.

Xeroradiographic studies can show the upper airway from the nasal cavity to the carina on one film (Fig. 3.2), but are now of historical interest as they are no longer performed due to the high radiation dosage. However, for many years they gave useful

Imaging technique for the paediatric larynx

Normal or high Kv lateral and AP films
Contrast oesophagography
Computed tomography
Magnetic resonance imaging

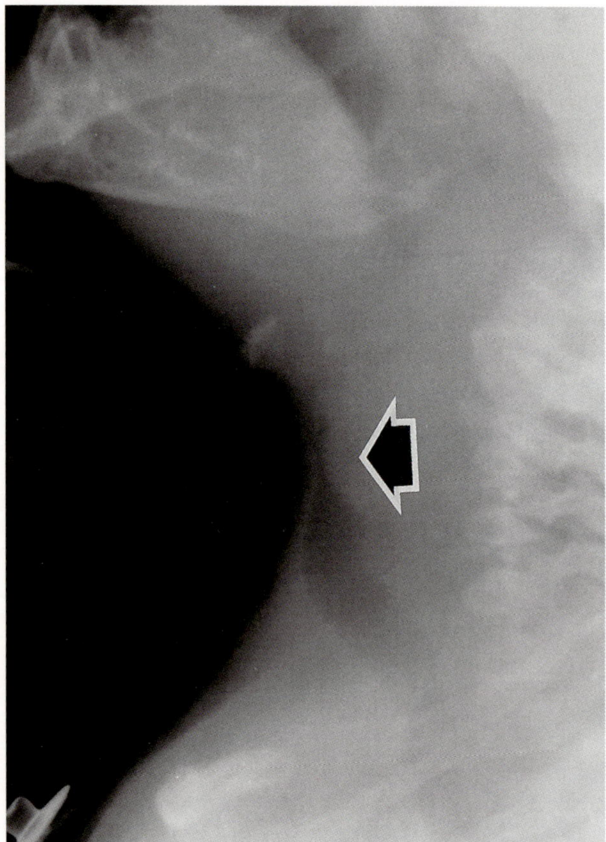

Figure **3.4**
Lateral high-kilovoltage film showing congenital subglottic haemangioma. The bulge on the posterior wall (arrow) of the subglottic region identifies the typical appearance of a subglottic haemangioma in an infant.

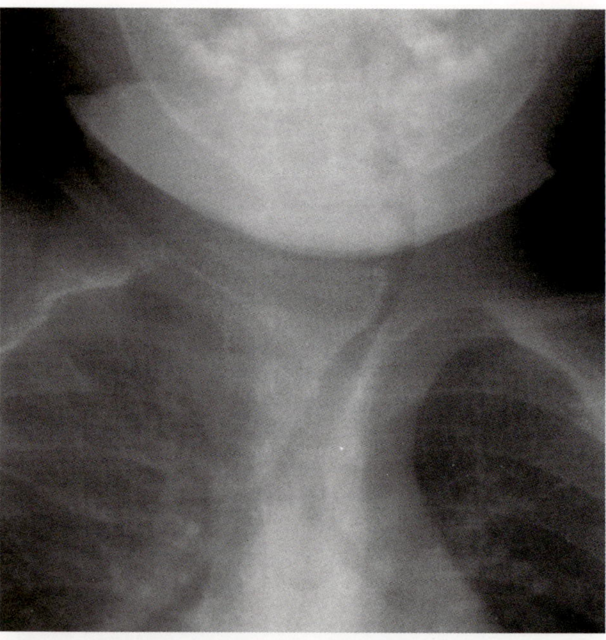

(a)

(b)

Figure **3.5**
Large reduplication cyst causing compression of the trachea. On the AP view (a) the trachea is grossly deviated to the left and extremely narrow. The CT scan (b) shows a large, oval cyst in the upper mediastinum and neck.

information to the otolaryngologist; the sharp contrast made xerograms easy to read, excellent for teaching and for reproduction in print – the reason why examples (Figs 3.1 and 3.2) are in this chapter.

In infants these radiographic imaging techniques are applied to demonstrate congenital abnormalities such as subglottic stenosis, subglottic haemangioma (Fig. 3.4), cystic hygroma, ectopic thyroid tissue, thyroglossal duct cyst, ductal retention cysts and saccular cysts and to show tracheal narrowing due to compression by vascular anomaly, tumour, cyst (Fig. 3.5), tracheomalacia or tracheal stenosis.

A large congenital laryngeal web is often associated with a substantial anterior subglottic stenosis, the thickness of which needs to be demonstrated on lateral films before corrective surgery is considered. Neither laryngomalacia nor vocal cord paralysis are well delineated by plain films but may sometimes be suspected at fluoroscopy.

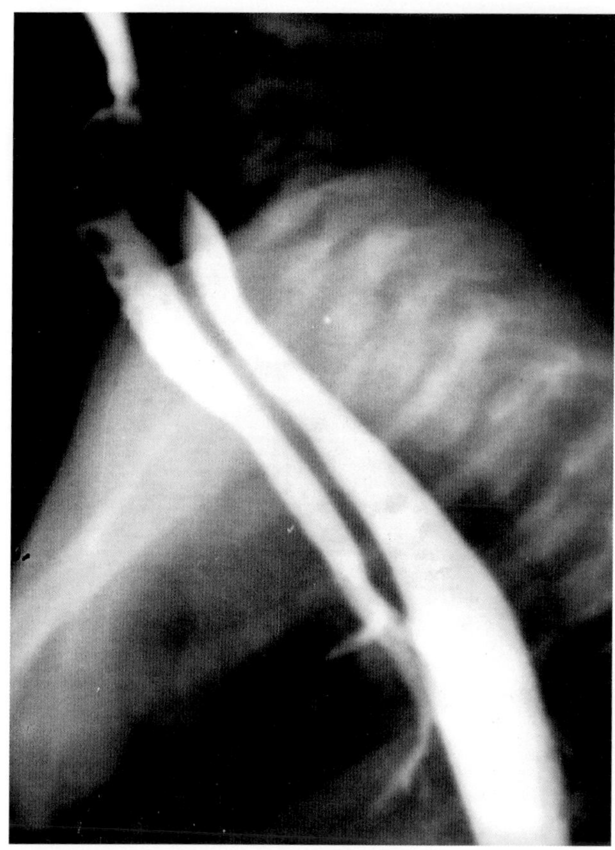

Figure **3.6**
Contrast oesophagram in cleft larynx. There is gross spillover and aspiration. Diagnosis should be confirmed by endoscopy, not by contrast swallow.

Contrast oesophagography

Barium swallow performed under fluoroscopic control, often at the same time as airway fluoroscopy, may identify conditions affecting the airway such as congenital vascular ring or sling, mediastinal cyst or mass, gastro-oesophageal reflux and aspiration into the tracheobronchial tree (Fig. 3.6).

Computed tomography and magnetic resonance imaging

These studies provide information about lesions in the tissues surrounding and compressing the airway. Thin-slice axial scans show retention cysts, cystic hygroma, duplication cysts (Fig. 3.5) and mediastinal tumours; when a vascular mass or inflammatory lesion is suspected intravenous contrast is used. These studies require general anaesthesia in infants and small children, but older children can co-operate by holding their breath so that scans can be performed in one phase of respiration.

Specific conditions requiring imaging

Except in an emergency, radiographic examination of the laryngeal and tracheal airways should be undertaken in infants and children before endoscopic assessment under general anaesthesia. The study may reveal a previously unsuspected obstructive lesion such as a cyst, tumour or mass of papillomas and alert the endoscopist and anaesthetist to possible obstruction during induction of anaesthesia; appropriate instrumentation to relieve the obstruction can then be made ready.

Abscesses of the pharyngeal spaces

Although peritonsillar abscess can be demonstrated by imaging, it is usually unnecessary as the clinical features indicate if surgical drainage is necessary. If spread from a peritonsillar abscess with an associated parapharyngeal space cellulitis or abscess occurs, contrast-enhanced CT shows distortion of the normal structures in the parapharyngeal space, increased fat density, postero-lateral displacement of the carotid sheath and soft-tissue displacement towards the midline impinging on the airway. An abscess shows as a low-density central collection with peripheral enhancement (Fig. 3.7).

Parapharyngeal or retropharyngeal abscesses in children are usually secondary to suppuration in lymph nodes, themselves secondary to upper respiratory tract infection. The lateral plain film shows widening of the prevertebral soft tissues and CT or MRI may delineate enlarged lymph nodes with a low-density centre. Phlegmonous cellulitis shows as fullness and distortion of soft tissues in the lateral and retropharyngeal spaces. It may be difficult to determine whether there is oedematous cellulitis or pus in the retropharyngeal space.

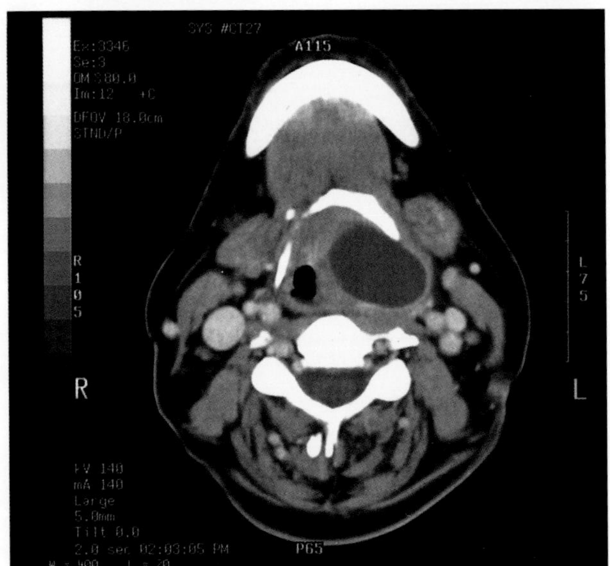

Figure **3.7**
Large abscess in the left neck. Oval-shaped low-density collection causing some compression of the airway.

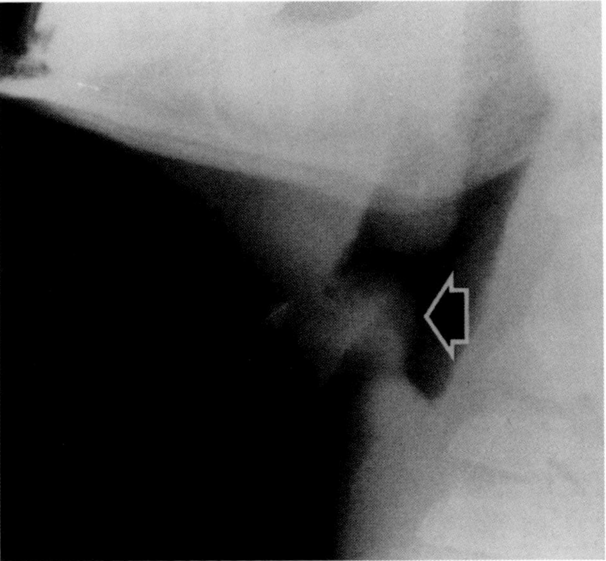

Figure **3.8**
Lateral film in acute epiglottitis. The so-called 'thumb sign' (arrow) due to suppurative swelling of the epiglottis and aryepiglottic fold.

Acute supraglottitis

There is considerable controversy concerning the safety of radiographic studies used to confirm the diagnosis of acute supraglottitis. Lateral X-ray should be performed when there is substantial doubt about the diagnosis, but only if the X-ray can be taken in or near the intensive care unit or operating theatre. Medical personnel capable of applying positive pressure-assisted ventilation or performing intubation to support the airway should accompany the child during the radiologic procedure. The 'thumb sign' may be seen (Fig. 3.8) representing the rounded swelling of the epiglottis. Doubt has been expressed about the sensitivity of lateral films for diagnosing supraglottitis. If interpretation is made by an experienced person, the appearance is diagnostic but films taken out of hours by a junior or unskilled physician may be erroneously interpreted.

Croup (acute laryngotracheobronchitis)

Radiographs are seldom necessary as the diagnosis of this common condition should be obvious clinically. As the X-ray appearance depends upon the degree of subglottic oedema and the phase of respiration, the reliability of specific radiographic signs is low. The most consistent appearance on the lateral film is diffuse narrowing of the subglottic region. On AP examination the so-called 'steeple sign' may be seen with a long segment of airway narrowing in the subglottic region.

Pseudomembranous bacterial tracheitis is a severe, atypical, uncommon, potentially lethal form of croup where staphylococcal infection forms obstructing crust-like membranes in the tracheobronchial tree. Lateral X-ray may show one or more of these membranes and narrowing of the subglottic airway.

Foreign bodies

Radio-opaque foreign bodies in the laryngopharynx, such as bones, pins, screws, safety pins, eggshell (Fig. 3.9) and small plastic radio-opaque foreign bodies will show on AP or lateral X-ray. Small plastic

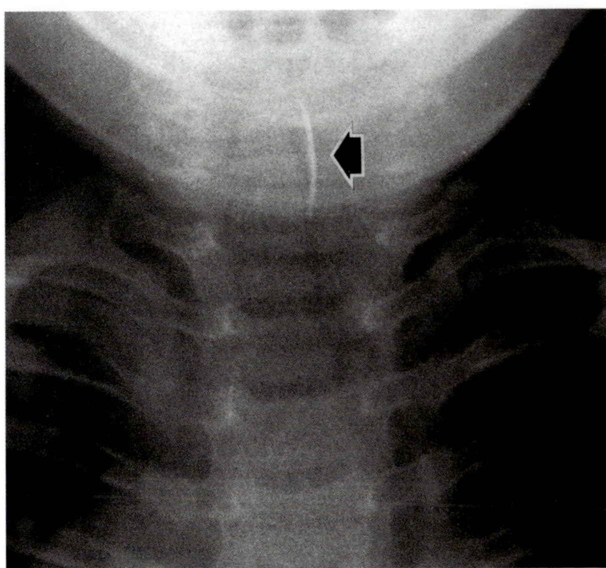

Figure **3.9**
Foreign body (egg shell) in the larynx. The infant had been diagnosed as having 'recurrent croup' for two months. The egg shell in the larynx (arrow) shows clearly on the AP film.

toys and radio-lucent foreign bodies such as meat or vegetable pieces might be suspected if they are large or there is surrounding soft-tissue swelling.

Foreign bodies in the tonsils, pharynx and base of tongue such as fishbones or pieces of wood should be seen at clinical examination but, in children, X-rays should be taken in every case of suspected foreign body in the pharynx, laryngopharynx, subglottis or tracheobronchial tree.

About 10–15% of inhaled foreign bodies lodge in the larynx, mostly in the subglottic region. The 85–90% of foreign bodies that localize in a bronchus (or sometimes in the trachea) are outside the scope of this discussion.

A foreign body impacted in the upper oesophagus for some days may present with airway obstruction secondary to pressure and soft-tissue oedema of the posterior wall of the upper trachea and should therefore be suspected on plain films if swelling narrows the airway. A sharp foreign body which perforates the oesophagus may cause surgical emphysema which will be obvious on X-ray or CT.

ADULTS

Available techniques

In adults the otolaryngologist will be reasonably confident from clinical features and findings at indirect laryngoscopy of the site and size of a lesion in the oropharynx, laryngopharynx, glottis and the subglottis. Usually the nature of the lesion will be known or strongly suspected, e.g. cyst, malignancy, subglottic stenosis. Imaging confirms the known features and identifies subglottic and upper tracheal changes not detected by indirect laryngoscopy. This additional information assists with assessment of deep soft-tissue involvement such as size and spread of benign and malignant tumours, presence of regional nodal metastases and identification of the size and nature of undiagnosed lesions in the neck and upper mediastinum.

Where possible, imaging should be done before examination and biopsy under general anaesthesia.

Image quality in the pharynx, larynx and subglottic region has been greatly improved by CT and MRI. The otolaryngologist will have evaluated the upper airway by indirect laryngoscopy – mucosal pathology such as vocal nodules, laryngeal polyp, intracordal cysts and granulomas do not need radiographic imaging.

Imaging techniques for the adult larynx

Lateral plain film or high-Kv soft-tissue film
Computed tomography
Magnetic resonance imaging
Barium swallow
Ultrasonography
Angiography
Radionuclide scanning
Helical (spiral) computed tomography
Fluoroscopy/cine studies

The surface appearance of a moderate-sized or large malignant lesion, although defining the tumour and its margins in the airway, cannot define spread into deeper tissues. CT and MRI have excellent application in laryngeal cancer, not only for the primary tumour but also for defining regional lymph node metastases which may or may not be detectable by physical examination.

Lateral films

Soft-tissue films are useful for a general survey as air in the laryngopharynx contrasts with the mucosal surface showing structures such as the epiglottis, aryepiglottic folds and laryngeal ventricle; the lower margin of the ventricle is the edge of the membranous vocal fold. Interpretation of pathological changes on the plain film is made difficult by the variability of calcification (ossification) in the laryngeal cartilages, especially when examining for foreign bodies.

High-Kv filtered radiographs improve imaging of the airway but the cervical spine often makes interpretation of AP views difficult.

Computed tomography and magnetic resonance imaging

CT has now virtually eliminated the need for conventional linear or multidirectional tomography. Coronal tomograms were valuable for assessing the degree of subglottic spread of a tumour, but only the surface mass, not the deep extent of tumour, could be visualized.

CT provides an assessment of lesions which are deep to the mucosa using rapid scans to decrease respiratory and swallowing artefacts. The patient should breathe quietly to minimize movement. Scanning should be from the epiglottis to the upper tracheal arches or, in larger lesions, to below the level of the pathological change and should include the neck where nodal metastases might occur.

The technique for the larynx usually consists of serial axial sections 3, 4 or 5 mm apart, but a particular level of interest can be imaged with adjacent 1- or 2-mm sections. The axial scans can be reformatted into coronal and sagittal images but they are unsatisfactory compared to MRI scans.

CT and MRI are the methods of choice for defining malignancy with or without metastases, solid or cystic mass lesions and traumatic disruption of the airway. They provide vital assessment of deep soft tissues including the pre-epiglottic space, paraglottic space, regional lymph nodes and cartilagenous skeleton. A bolus of intravenous contrast will enhance vascular structures and assist differentiation from nearby lymph nodes.

CT is valuable for imaging soft tissues but it is limited to the axial plane and exposes the patient to radiation. MRI gives excellent soft-tissue contrast having an ability which is superior to CT to separate various soft tissues. MRI uses no ionizing radiation and can provide coronal, transverse and sagittal plane images. MRI takes more time than CT and movement from respiration, cardiac pulsation or blood flow in the carotid arteries can be a problem. MRI does not image cortical bone or calcification well and is contraindicated in patients with cardiac pacemakers, aneurysm clips, cochlear implant and other magnetic metals in the field of interest.

Anatomy

The sections show epiglottis, fat-filled pre-epiglottic space, aryepiglottic folds, arytenoid, thyroid and cricoid cartilages, with their varying degrees of calcification or marrow fat. The paraglottic space (also known as the paralaryngeal space) starts above at the level of the false cord where there is predominantly fat density, changes to muscle density below the level of the vocal cord and ends at the upper margin of cricoid cartilage. On MRI, a bright signal on T1-weighted sequences is elicited by pre-epiglottic fat, hyaline cartilage and submucosal fascial planes such as in the paraglottic space and the false cords (Figs 3.10–3.11).

The arytenoid cartilages are usually clearly seen and are important anatomical landmarks in relationship to the vocal cords. The vocal process is the anterior projection which identifies the level of the vocal fold.

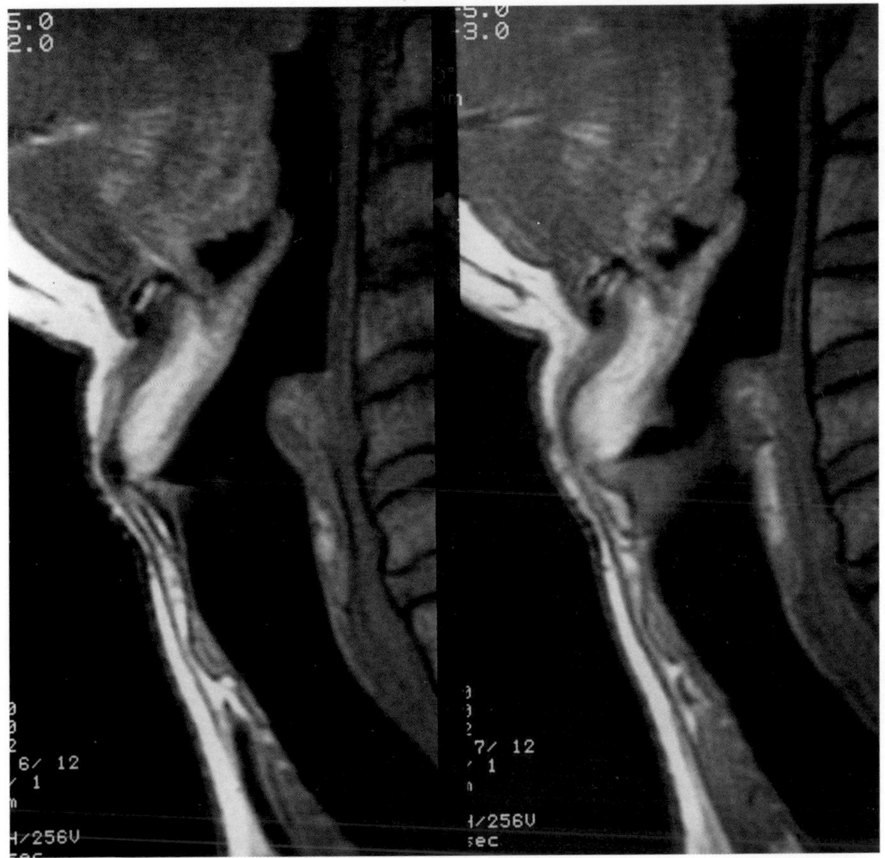

Figure **3.10**
Sagittal MRI of normal larynx. The two planes demonstrate the structures from the base of the tongue to the upper trachea. The true vocal cord, ventricle and arytenoid eminence are clearly seen.

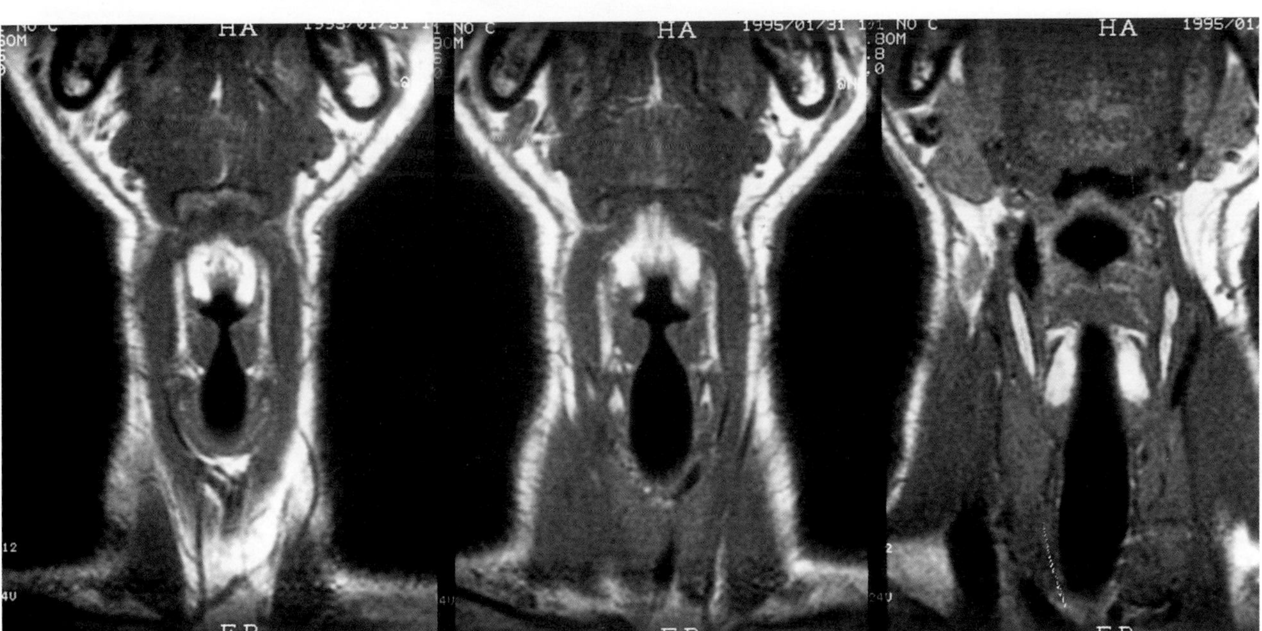

Figure **3.11**
Coronal MRI views of the normal larynx. Three selected planes from anterior to posterior are very useful to delineate the subglottic region, vocal cords, ventricles, false vocal cords and posterior glottic area.

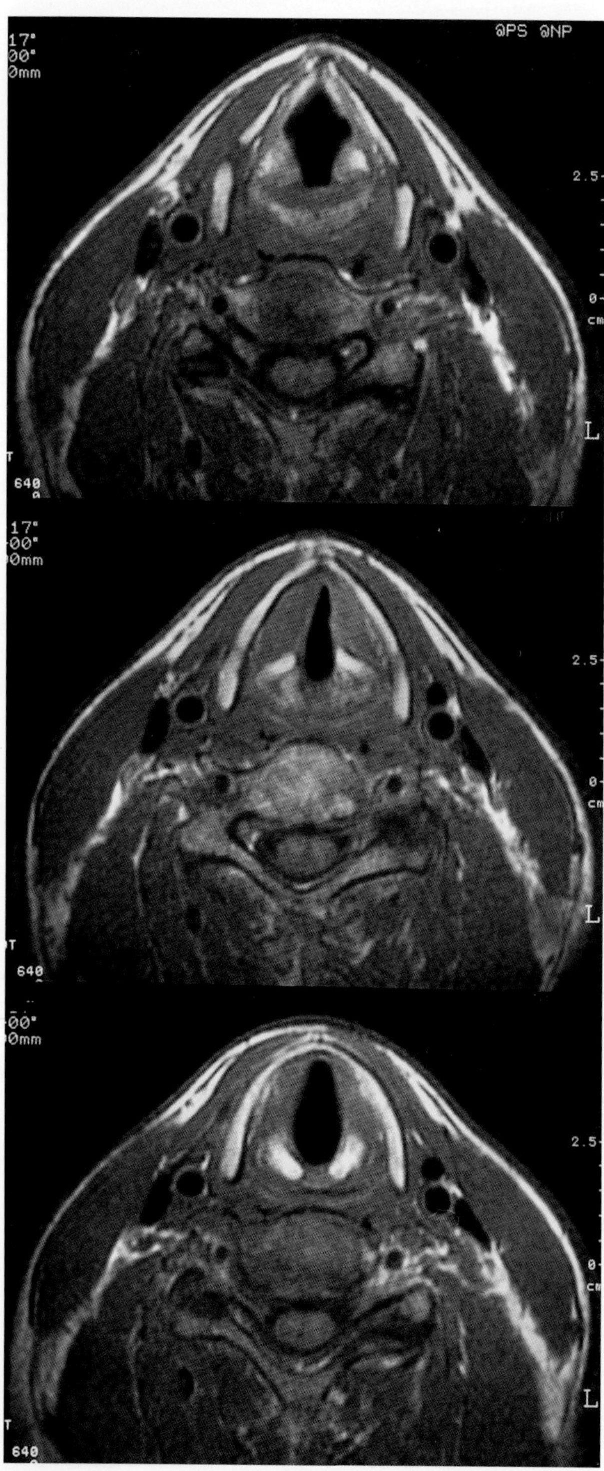

Figure **3.12**
Axial MRI of the larynx. Three selected views from above down show normal appearance. Malignant invasion in the deeper tissues, especially the paraglottic space, can be detected in these views.

Ossification or marrow fat in cartilage is common but usually irregular and incomplete in both thyroid and cricoid. Ossification not only occurs with increasing age but also in association with chronic infection (e.g. perichondritis), chronic irritation or inflammation (e.g. vocal granuloma) and tumour (e.g. squamous cell carcinoma). Allowance for variation in ossification must be made in interpretation of films, especially when destruction of the thyroid or the cricoid is important in assessing the spread of tumours into deep tissues.

The piriform fossae are recesses on each side of the larynx between the aryepiglottic fold and the mucosa covering the lamina of the thyroid cartilage and are vital areas in assessing the spread of malignant tumours. The postcricoid area in the inferior part of the laryngopharynx is often not only difficult to visualize endoscopically but also difficult to image.

In the sagittal plane (Fig. 3.10), MRI images show the base of the tongue, valleculae, epiglottis and its laryngeal surface, postcricoid region and arytenoid cartilages posterior to the laryngeal ventricle with false cords above the true cords. In the coronal plane (Fig. 3.11), views are usually displayed from anterior to posterior. They show thyro-arytenoid muscle in the vocal cord, the ventricle (and sometimes the saccule), paraglottic space, pre-epiglottic space containing fat, epiglottis, interarytenoid muscle, cricoid and piriform fossae. Axial images (Fig. 3.12) are helpful in evaluation of erosion of cartilage, depending upon the degree of ossification and the presence of fat in the medullary spaces. In the neck, the vascular contents of the carotid sheath and the upper and lower deep cervical lymph nodes can usually be differentiated. Therefore with multiplanar formatting in coronal, sagittal and axial views, MRI can give excellent definition of cartilage, muscle, fat and soft tissues in and around the larynx. CT techniques using the Valsalva manoeuvre, the modified Valsalva or reverse 'ee-ee-ee' phonation show the laryngeal ventricles and the piriform fossae to best advantage by distending them with air.

The choice of using CT and/or MRI is made according to the problem in the individual patient. In general, both modalities are complementary to endoscopy but cannot replace either indirect or direct laryngoscopy.

Laryngeal carcinoma

Almost all laryngeal malignancies are squamous cell carcinomas. The laryngologist can detect most of them as surface mucosal lesions at indirect laryngoscopy. Small lesions seen at laryngoscopy may be undetectable on CT or MRI – cancer of the larynx cannot be excluded by imaging. Direct laryngoscopy at the time of biopsy allows more accurate delineation of the appearance, size and distribution over the mucosal surface. CT and MRI have their best application in the evaluation of submucosal extension into soft tissue and are somewhat more reliable than palpation in the detection of regional nodal metastases in the neck. The laryngologist relies on comprehensive imaging to outline deep infiltration of the primary tumour and to detect lymph node involvement. Information from such imaging assists in the decision for treatment whether by radiotherapy, partial or total laryngectomy with or without neck dissection, chemotherapy or a combination of these methods.

The clinical appearance of mucosal or submucosal transglottic spread above and below the ventricle is associated with a high incidence of extra laryngeal spread and thyroid cartilage destruction. Involvement of the pre-epiglottic, paraglottic and subglottic spaces shown by CT and/or MRI provides vital information in determining treatment.

Sites of carcinoma of laryngopharynx

- Larynx
  - Supraglottic
  - Glottic
  - Subglottic
  - Transglottic
- Hypopharynx
  - Postcricoid
  - Piriform sinus
  - Posterior pharyngeal wall

Staging and anatomic classification. The tumour-node-metastasis (TNM) staging system (see page 303) is a convenient method for description of malignant lesions providing a concise description which is used for comparing outcomes of treatment, but the TNM classification does not allow for the findings on CT or MRI imaging.

Squamous cell carcinoma of the larynx and pharynx has been divided, on the basis of anatomy, embryology and lymphatic drainage, into compartments. Tumours are separated into those originating from the larynx and those from the hypopharynx.

As this book concerns the endolarynx, hypopharyngeal cancer will not be discussed.

Cartilage involvement. Malignant tumours of the larynx invade cartilage (Fig. 3.13) and when imaging demonstrates cartilage destruction, total laryngectomy is usually preferred to radiation therapy or partial laryngectomy. Gross destruction can be easily determined. Because thyroid cartilage may have an irregular pattern of calcification, minimal involvement by malignancy, even by comparison of the two sides, makes assessment difficult with either CT or MRI, although the latter appears to be more reliable.

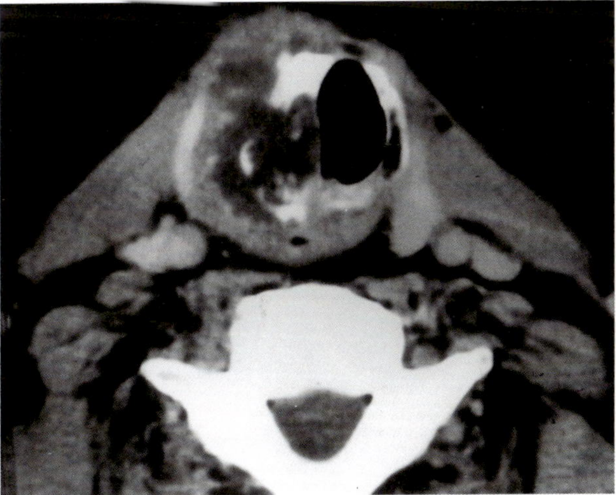

Figure **3.13**
Chondrosarcoma. Axial CT of a large chondrosarcoma of the right side of the cricoid cartilage.

Interpretation is difficult because the normal, ageing cartilage undergoes irregular calcification.

Supraglottic tumours. Approximately 30–35% of laryngeal malignancies are supraglottic. They tend to present later, to be larger than glottic lesions, to remain supraglottic and not to invade thyroid cartilage unless downward extension occurs. Nodal metastases are common.

Both CT and MRI show the supraglottic larynx well in the axial plane, but extension into the tongue base is best seen on sagittal MRI views. The epiglottis is a poor barrier to spread and either CT or MRI can identify deep extension as tumour replaces fat density in the pre-epiglottic space. Inferior extension into the paraglottic space is best seen in the coronal plane as the tumour extends towards the ventricle through the false cord (which is predominantly fat) and towards the true cord (which is mostly thyroarytenoid muscle). The lesion can cross the ventricle by mucosal extension which is recognizable at endoscopy; it then becomes transglottic. Cancer can also become transglottic by spread in the paraglottic space, detectable only by imaging. If the vocal cord and hemilarynx become fixed, the clinician will suspect invasion of thyroarytenoid muscle or recurrent nerve. MRI gives the best cross-sectional picture of the false cord, true cord and thyroarytenoid muscle because T2-weighted images give the tumour a higher signal intensity than normal thyroarytenoid muscle.

Glottic tumours. Approximately 60–70% of laryngeal malignancies are glottic (Fig. 3.14). Metastases to lymph nodes occur in less than 5%. Most tumours are limited to the vocal cords, very few invade the supraglottic larynx, but inferior spread to the subglottis is not uncommon. Spread can occur across the anterior commissure, by penetration of the thyroid cartilage or posteriorly by invasion around the arytenoid cartilage. Extension into the paraglottic space may be associated with cartilage invasion. The thick, ligamentous conus elasticus (or cricovocal membrane) is the lower boundary of the paraglottic space and a barrier to inferior extension. A total laryngectomy is usually necessary if the cricoid cartilage is involved.

Vertical hemilaryngectomy preserves speech and is applicable to some glottic malignancies, but cannot be safely performed if there is deep tumour extension, extension to the upper margin of the cricoid, involvement of the cricoarytenoid joint or in cases where there is invasion sufficient to cause fixation of the hemilarynx.

Anterior extension to or past the anterior commissure to the contralateral vocal fold is best assessed by laryngoscopy, but if air can be seen against the inner lamina of the thyroid cartilage on a scan, tumour extension can be excluded. Tumour seen anterior or lateral to the thyroid cartilage is reliable evidence of cartilage invasion; involvement of the Delphian node occurs either by lymphatic spread or direct extension. This deeper or anterior extension cannot be detected clinically, but may be identified by CT or MRI.

Transglottic tumours which involve structures above and below the ventricle have a tendency to spread deeply and to invade cartilage, and are often understaged. Many require total laryngectomy if CT or MRI reveal extension in the paraglottic space.

Although involvement in the region of the arytenoid cartilage is usually assessed endoscopically, deep para-arytenoid infiltration through or around the cricoarytenoid joint may be seen on CT or MRI.

Subglottic tumours. Subglottic tumours are rare, approximately 5% of all laryngeal carcinomas. Lymph node metastases, including to the paratracheal nodes occur in about 20% of subglottic tumours. Subglottic tumours tend to be advanced and frequently invade

Spread of glottic carcinoma

Metastases are uncommon
Subglottic extension is not uncommon
Anterior commissure to other cord
Penetration of thyroid cartilage
Paraglottic extension ± cartilage
Para-arytenoid infiltration
Transglottic spread

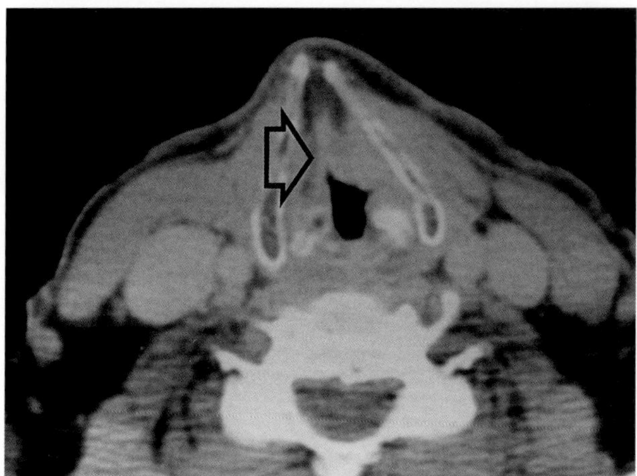

Figure **3.14**
Axial CT at the vocal cord level. Tumour (arrow) involving the left vocal fold and bulging into the glottic opening.

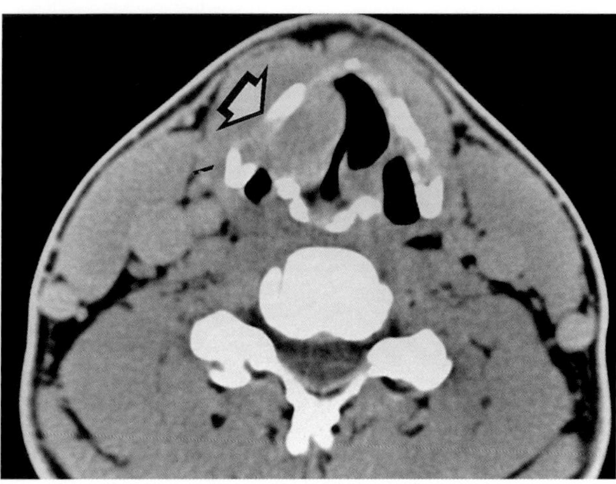

Figure **3.15**
Axial CT of the larynx at arytenoid level. Tumour extension beyond the arytenoid (arrow) and through the lamina of the thyroid cartilage. Lymphoma.

the thyroid and cricoid cartilages, the cricothyroid membrane and even the thyroid gland. They usually require total laryngectomy, although some small tumours may be suitable for irradiation or conservative surgery.

Recurrence. Recurrent malignancy after previous treatment may be detected on imaging by the presence of a subglottic mass, a tumour outside the laryngeal framework, involvement of the contralateral vocal cord and by demonstrating progression of the tumour compared to previous studies.

Nodal metastases. Metastases in the neck nodes occur most often with supraglottic tumours, less frequently with subglottic tumours, and are uncommon with glottic tumours. They are more frequent in large and poorly differentiated tumours. Both CT and MRI can detect clinically occult nodal neck metastases. CT with intravenous contrast is helpful in differentiating nodes from blood vessels, but contrast is unnecessary with MRI. Nodal metastases tend to have fascial planes obliterated around the enlarged nodes, at least in non-operated or non-irradiated necks. They tend to be spherical rather than ovoid and the occurrence of three or more adjacent ill-defined nodes appears to be significant. However, neither CT nor MRI can reliably distinguish between an enlarged matted group of hyperplastic lymph nodes and direct extension of the tumour. Spread outside the capsule of a node or fixation to surrounding structures such as the carotid sheath is impossible to image with certainty. A combination of physical findings, especially in a thin neck, and precise CT and MRI scans, which are more sensitive than palpation (although they may not detect small nodes), gives the best evaluation. Lymph node metastases show low signal intensity on T1- and high signal intensity on T2-weighted images. The precise place of CT and MRI in the detection of regional lymph node metastases has not yet been determined, mainly because of both false negative and false positive results found after correlation with histopathologic examination.

Additional studies. There is approximately a 15% chance of synchronous or metachronous second primary malignancy of the oral cavity, pharynx, lung or oesophagus, and physical examination, chest X-ray, barium swallow and CT scans of these areas may be indicated.

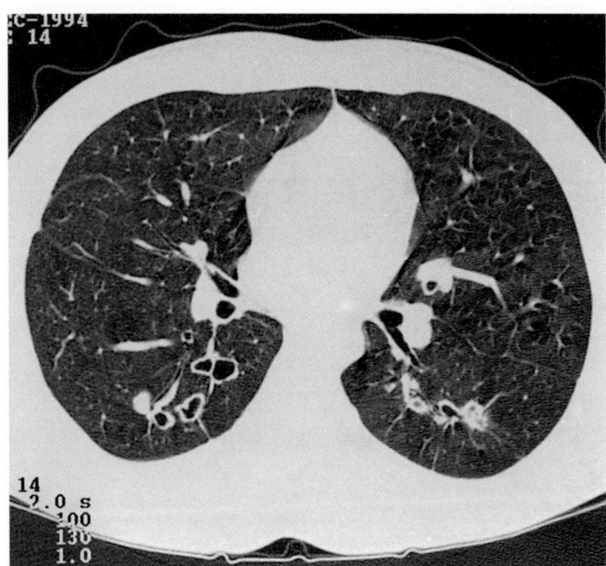

Figure **3.16**
CT of the chest showing papillomas. Patient with long-standing papillomas in the larynx and trachea. The CT scan shows solid nodules and cystic spaces indicating involvement of the lung parenchyma with papillomas.

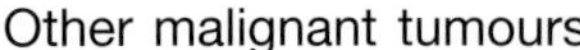

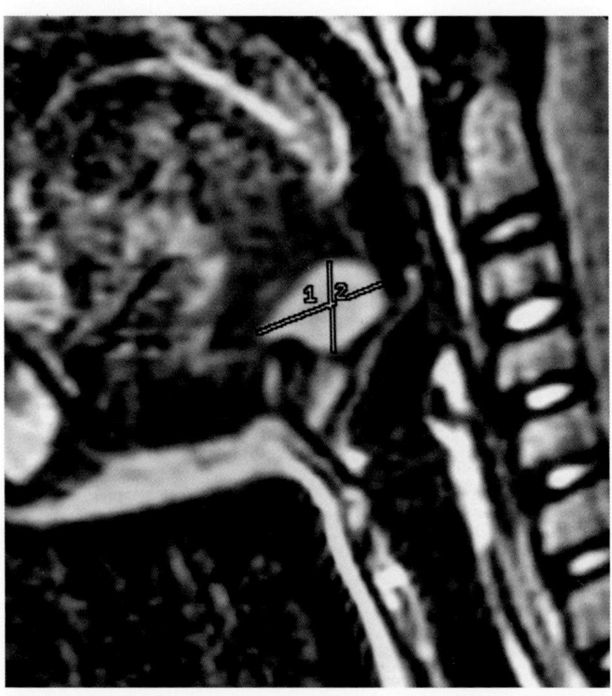

(a)

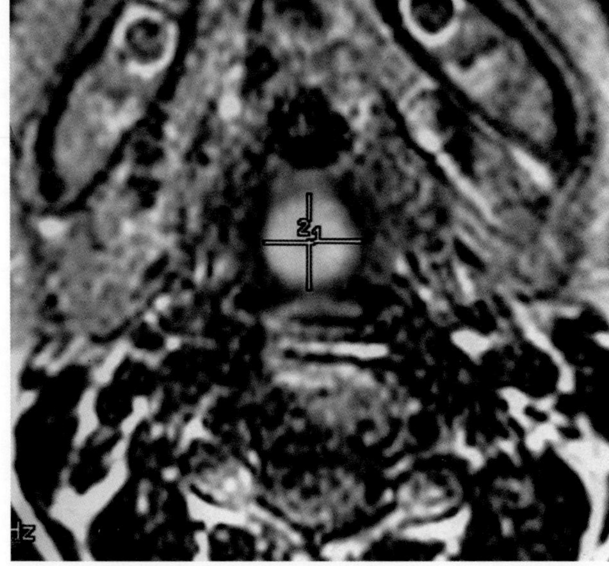

(b)

Figure **3.17**
Lateral (a) and axial (b) MRI of a cyst at the base of the tongue. A mucous retention cyst was removed with the carbon dioxide laser at endoscopy. No recurrence. The differential diagnosis included lingual thyroid.

Other malignant tumours

Non-squamous cell malignant tumours are represented by adenocarcinomas which arise from ectopic minor salivary glands, anaplastic carcinomas or verrucous carcinomas. Very occasionally there are other primary (Fig. 3.13) or secondary malignant tumours such as liposarcoma, other sarcomas, lymphomas (Fig. 3.15), myelomas and spindle cell carcinoma. CT and MRI scans are vital in the imaging of these tumours.

Benign tumours

The commonest benign tumours are respiratory papillomas, then haemangiomas followed by other rarer tumours such as neurogenic tumours, chondromas, lipomas, glomus tumours (paragangliomas), neurofibromas and granular cell tumours.

Papillomas will show on a plain lateral film or on tomography as multiple small or large scattered nodules or as one large mass. Lung parenchymal involvement is rare and is detected on a chest film or

CT scan (Fig. 3.16) as solid nodules associated with cavitation.

Subglottic haemangiomas in infants can usually be seen on imaging (Fig. 3.4); the lateral high-Kv film may show a posterior subglottic bulge or a unilateral bulge may be seen in the AP projection. Conventional tomography shows the same changes and the lesion enhances with contrast on CT or MRI.

Adult haemangiomas are usually supraglottic or glottic, enhance on CT and have a high T2-weighted intensity on MRI.

Cysts and laryngocoeles

Subglottic ductal retention cysts are usually too small to be seen on radiography and must be diagnosed at direct endoscopic examination. A vallecular mucous retention cyst anterior to the epiglottis can be seen at indirect laryngoscopy but may need to be distinguished from a thyroglossal duct cyst at the base of the tongue (Fig. 3.17). On CT and MRI the latter will be shown to have a deeper extension into soft tissues, an indication of their origin from the embryological thyroglossal duct.

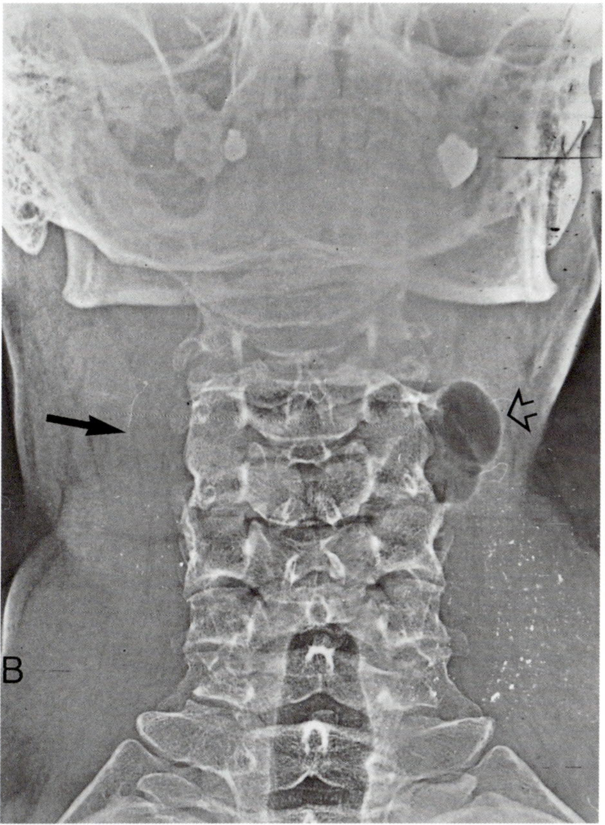

Figure **3.18**
Antero-posterior xerogram of laryngocoeles. Fluid-filled laryngomucocoele (solid arrow) and air-filled laryngocoele (open arrow).

Laryngeal cysts

- Thyroglossal duct cysts
- Ductal mucous retention cysts
  - Vallecular
  - Subglottic
- Laryngocoele
  - Air-filled
  - Mucus-filled
  - Pus-filled

A distinction needs to be made (Fig. 3.18) between an air-filled laryngocoele, a fluid-filled laryngocoele (also known as a saccular cyst or a laryngomucocoele) and a laryngopyocoele (which is an infected laryngocoele). A laryngocoele is an abnormal elongation and expansion of the normal saccule, which itself is an out-pouching of the anterior part of the ventricle lined by mucous membrane containing mucous glands whose secretions assist in the lubrication of the vocal folds. Obstruction of the saccular duct can be followed by formation of an air-containing laryngocoele. An internal laryngocoele extends into the adjacent aryepiglottic fold and enlarges in the substance of the false cord, but it is confined inside the larynx by the thyrohyoid membrane. An external laryngocoele extends into the neck through a weakness in the thyrohyoid membrane, thus forming a combined or mixed internal and external laryngocoele.

An air-containing laryngocoele can be diagnosed on plain films, tomography, CT or MRI, but fluid-filled laryngocoeles or laryngomucocoeles are seen only on CT or MRI which outline the extent of the mass in the paraglottic area. A mixed laryngomucocoele with both internal and external parts can be identified with CT or MRI.

Occasionally these derivatives of a laryngocoele are secondary to a primary lesion in the anterior ventricle, possibly an unsuspected malignancy or a benign lesion such as a mass of papilloma which obstructs the saccular duct thus causing a distension of the saccule.

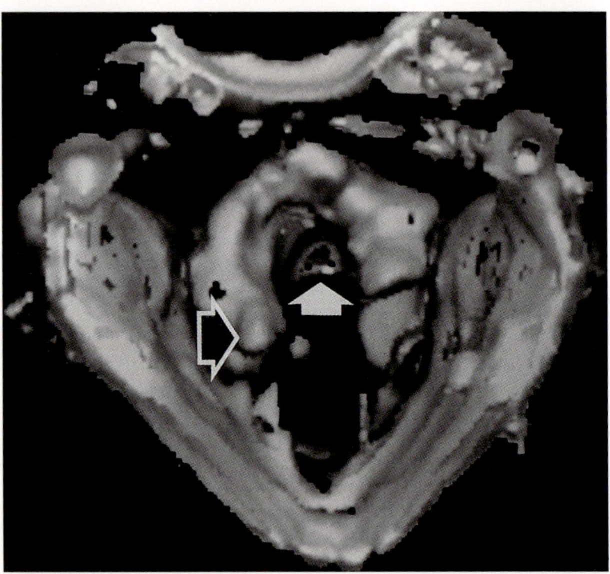

Figure **3.19**
Helical CT scan in the axial plane. There is forward dislocation of one arytenoid (black arrow with white edge) and posterior glottic stenosis (white arrow).

Laryngeal trauma

Laryngeal trauma caused by blunt injuries is characterized by soft tissue swelling, laceration of mucosa, bleeding and haematoma formation, surgical emphysema in the soft tissues of the neck and mediastinum and by fracture and/or dislocation of the cartilages of the laryngeal framework.

If there is acute airway obstruction requiring relief, radiologic imaging cannot be performed immediately, but should be done as soon as possible. CT is the modality of choice. Oedema fluid and blood can distend the paralaryngeal and parapharyngeal spaces causing various degrees of airway narrowing.

Thyroid cartilage fractures may be horizontal or vertical. A horizontal fracture usually involves both thyroid alae, the thyro-epiglottic ligament may be torn with dislocation of the epiglottis, and there is usually surrounding supraglottic soft-tissue swelling. Horizontal fractures are difficult to see on axial CT scans. Vertical fractures of the thyroid cartilage occur when the larynx is suddenly displaced backwards against the spine, and shows as a defect in the thyroid ala on axial CT, often with narrowing of the airway caused by soft-tissue swelling within the thyroid cartilage.

Cricoid fractures are usually vertical and often multiple with disruption of the ring and consequent subglottic airway obstruction, a situation which usually requires surgical intervention and stabilization.

Tracheal transection by avulsion of the trachea from the lower border of the cricoid cartilage can be rapidly fatal, but it is curious that the airway remains life-sustaining in some patients and in others perlaryngeal intubation is successful, the tube somehow passing into the separated tracheal stump. This serious injury can be accompanied by damage to both recurrent laryngeal nerves causing bilateral vocal cord paralysis, spreading surgical emphysema and extensive bleeding and oedema in the soft tissues. Urgent evaluation by axial CT scanning after stabilization of the airway is required before surgical repair of the separated segments.

Arytenoid dislocation or subluxation occurs in isolation when caused by passage of an endotracheal tube. When caused by external trauma, it is usually associated with trauma of the other cartilages. Complete dislocation and malalignment on the cricoid facet together with thyroid cartilage fracture and accompanying haematoma will impair vocal cord movement and contribute to airway obstruction. These changes are best seen on axial or spiral CT (Fig. 3.19).

The cricothyroid joint can be dislocated when the thyroid and cricoid cartilages are injured. CT scan may show rotation of the thyroid cartilage with a widening of the space between the thyroid and the cricoid.

These changes are more difficult to detect in paediatric patients because there is seldom calcification of the cartilages. Nevertheless, CT is the definitive radiographic imaging method for evaluating the traumatized larynx.

Thermal or caustic injuries

Paediatric patients are more likely than adults to have supraglottic oedema and airway obstruction from accidental inhalation of steam, the ash products of combustion, very hot liquids or ingestion of caustic or acid substances. Large volumes of strong alkali cause the most severe injury with laryngeal spasm initially, followed by supraglottic oedema and swelling. Plain X-ray shows thickening of the epiglottis and aryepiglottic folds, an appearance similar to that seen in acute epiglottitis.

The chronic sequelae of severe laryngeal injuries include different degrees of supraglottic, glottic or, more often, subglottic stenosis. The disrupted laryngeal framework may heal in a distorted configuration with arytenoid dislocation and cricothyroid joint dysfunction; although plain films or conventional tomograms are satisfactory methods for assessing the site and severity of the stenoses, axial CT reveals the cross-section of the airway and displacement or injury to the cartilages.

Barium swallow and fluoroscopy

Fluoroscopy to assess laryngeal dynamics supplements other studies. Motion recording techniques such as video recording and cineradiography are important for studying the functional dynamics of the larynx, mainly for detection of paralysis or fixation of a vocal cord. The ventricles can be seen by having the patient phonate 'ee-ee-ee' during inspiration to distend them with air. The Valsalva manoeuvre will fill the piriform fossae with air or they can be distended with barium to give an air contrast study of the barium-coated mucosa. A lateral view of the postcricoid region distended with barium may detect the presence or spread of tumours. Lateral fluoroscopy demonstrates tracheomalacia with collapse on expiration and increased calibre on inspiration.

These studies and the CT scan make contrast laryngography of historical interest only.

Angiography, radioactive scanning and ultrasonography

Vocal cord mobility in adults can be assessed in a limited way by ultrasonography but the study may be more useful in children whose vocal cords cannot always be readily seen at indirect laryngoscopy. Prenatal ultrasound studies have been used to detect cystic hygroma and tracheo-oesophageal fistula with atresia.

Ultrasonography shows the cystic nature of a laryngocoele.

Radionuclide studies are occasionally used to detect uptake in inflammatory arthropathies or relapsing polychondritis.

Arteriography can demonstrate the blood supply to laryngeal conditions such as haemangioma or arterio-venous fistula, and in some of these vascular catheterization will define an arterio-venous malformation or cavernous haemangioma and indicate that intra-arterial embolization can be employed for treatment of selected cases.

Helical (spiral) computed tomography

This new technology allows the neck to be imaged in a reasonably short time and is especially valuable in demonstrating the piriform fossae, the laryngeal ventricles and the subglottic region. Helical CT differs from conventional CT because the patient is moved continuously through the scanner during a prolonged X-ray exposure so that the entire neck is scanned within a single breath-hold in most patients. The technique was first introduced to evaluate vascular structures but can now be applied to produce high-quality, three-dimensional 'airway casts' (see Fig. 3.19).

Positron emission tomography (PET)

This imaging technique is based on demonstrating a difference in tissue metabolism using a radioisotope fixed to a glucose analogue. Areas of increased glucose uptake and increased metabolism can be seen on the PET images and the method has been applied to head and neck carcinoma and regional metastases. Resolution is limited with the current equipment to about 6 mm and there is some lack of definition at the anatomical site.

Which imaging technique?

The most appropriate radiological technique depends on the clinical problem under investigation. The otolaryngologist requesting image studies does so on the basis of the history, physical examination and, most importantly, on the findings at indirect laryngoscopy. A provisional diagnosis has usually been made, but there may be uncertainty which can be resolved by a particular imaging study or a series of studies. There is no necessity for imaging patients who have easily diagnosable conditions such as vocal nodules, a vocal cord polyp and vocal cord paralysis. In certain cases of multiple respiratory papillomas, although papillomas may be seen in the glottis or supraglottic areas, a lateral study may define small subglottic or upper tracheal papillomas preoperatively alerting the laryngologist to their presence.

Cysts are readily seen on CT scans. A bronchogenic or other duplication cyst or a mediastinal mass causing airway compression in an infant requires not only plain or high-Kv films but also CT scans.

The most important application of imaging is CT and MRI for outlining the deep extent of mass lesions of malignant or benign origin and detecting the presence of nodal metastases. Indirect and direct laryngoscopy are more reliable in detecting the presence of primary tumours in the larynx than CT or MRI. The latter, however, are more sensitive in delineating deep invasion and the spread of tumours to evaluate the most appropriate form of treatment. They appear to be slightly superior to palpation in detecting the presence of regional nodal metastases especially in the obese patient with a thick neck or in the post-irradiated patient.

BIBLIOGRAPHY

Castelijns JA, Gerritsen GJ, Kaiser MC et al (1987) Invasion of laryngeal cartilage by cancer: comparison of CT and MR imaging. *Radiology* **166**: 199–206.

Curtin HD (1996) Larynx. In: Curtin HD, ed., *Head and neck imaging* (St Louis: CV Mosby Year Book); 630–71.

Garel C, Contencin P, Polonovski JM et al (1992) Laryngeal ultrasonography in infants and children: a new way of investigating: normal and pathological findings. *Int J Pediatr Otorhinolaryngol* **23**: 107–15.

Hudgins PA, Jacobs IN, Castillo M (1996) Pediatric airway disease. In: Curtin UD, ed., *Head and neck imaging* (St Louis: Mosby Year Book); 585–98.

McGuirt WF, Greven KA, Keys JW et al (1995) Positron emission tomography in the evaluation of laryngeal carcinoma. *Ann Otol Rhinol Laryngol* **104**: 274–8.

Maffee MF, Schild JA, Valvassori GE et al (1983) Computed tomography of the larynx: correlation with anatomical and pathologic studies in cases of laryngeal carcinomas. *Radiology* **147**: 123–7.

Schaefer SD (1991) Use of CT scanning in the management of the acutely injured larynx. *Otolaryngol Clin North Am* **24** (1): 31–6.

Weber AL (1966) Radiology of the larynx. In: Fried MP, ed., *The larynx* (St Louis: Mosby); 101–14.

4 Gastro-oesophageal reflux and the larynx

CLINICAL FEATURES

Gastro-oesophageal reflux occurs when the stomach contents regurgitate through the lower oesophageal sphincter into the oesophagus. Brief episodes of reflux are common physiological phenomena in infants and toddlers. Most adults have about one episode of acid reflux per month. In some patients persistent reflux is severe enough to induce symptoms or cause histologic changes in the lower oesophagus; the symptomatic situation is then referred to as gastro-oesophageal reflux disease (GORD). During some episodes of reflux the acid contents of the stomach can reach the laryngopharynx.

The manifestations of GORD are diverse, especially in paediatric patients. Gastrointestinal symptoms occur most commonly and include recurrent vomiting, weight loss, failure to thrive, haematemesis and, in advanced cases, oesophageal stricture. In adult patients the common symptoms are indigestion, 'waterbrash' and retrosternal discomfort. In severe cases there may be chest pain and haematemesis.

Laryngeal and/or respiratory manifestations are the second most common feature of paediatric patients with GORD and are of the greatest interest to otolaryngologists.

Symptoms include apnoea/bradycardia spells, chronic cough, laryngeal dyskinesia, hoarseness, bronchitis and recurrent pneumonia. An estimated one-third of paediatric patients with GORD present with laryngeal/respiratory symptoms which often occur in the absence of gastrointestinal symptoms. These symptoms may arise through one of several mechanisms:

- aspiration during swallowing (primary aspiration) from reflux-induced oesophageal dysmotility;
- aspiration of refluxate (secondary aspiration) eliciting reflex responses or histologic injury;
- stimulation of distal oesophageal sensory neurones inducing reflex vagal responses, causing bronchospasm, apnoea or bradycardia.

Neurobehavioural symptoms are the least common manifestation of reflux but are often the most striking. Sandifer's syndrome is manifested by the triad of oesophagitis, irritability and extreme back arching. Such posturing was often attributed to severe neurological compromise prior to the recognition of its association with GORD.

DIAGNOSIS

Acid reflux in the adult larynx has been implicated in chronic laryngitis, vocal granuloma, in failure of laryngoplasty surgery, and as a cause of dysplastic changes in the laryngeal mucosa. However, no convincing proof to relate the finding of acidity in the laryngopharynx to these diseases has been offered.

Multiple diagnostic studies are available to evaluate patients with suspected GORD. Knowledge of the advantages and limitations of each study allows the clinician to tailor appropriately those necessary for each patient's evaluation.

The **barium oesophagogram** detects reflux in approximately two-thirds of paediatric and adult cases. Despite its relatively low sensitivity, the barium oesophagogram is an important screening study for infants with suspected GORD as together with a small bowel series it excludes congenital causes of vomiting such as malrotation, duodenal web or atresia, and pyloric stenosis. A **barium videoswallow** should be obtained concomitantly to detect primary aspiration as a cause of the patient's presenting respiratory symptoms.

The **extended pH probe study** (16–24 hours) is the gold standard for reflux diagnosis due to its relatively high sensitivity and specificity. The study is performed by placing a pH probe in the distal oesophagus to detect the number of times or percentage of time that the distal oesophageal pH is less than or equal to 4. It is at or below this pH value that most pepsinogen is converted to pepsin, the primary injurious agent.

Because all infants, many children and some adults normally have brief episodes of reflux, particularly postprandially, grading schemes have been established to determine what degree of reflux should be considered pathologic. Although controversial, reflux is considered excessive if the percentage of time that the pH is less than 4 is greater than 5%. For newborn infants in whom reflux is even more common, the reflux score is considered abnormal if the pH is less than 4 for 10% of the time.

GORD events reaching the hypopharynx may be detected by **dual pH probe monitoring** where a second pH probe is placed approximately 1 cm above the upper oesophageal sphincter. Because of the proximity to the upper airway, reflux events reaching this superior probe are thought to play a significant role in causing respiratory symptoms. The frequency and duration of events to this level which are considered pathologic has not yet been established. It is postulated, however, that the mucosa of the upper aerodigestive tract lacks the same protective factors of the lower oesophagus, thus rendering it more prone to injury by refluxate.

Oesophagoscopy with biopsy is less sensitive in diagnosing acid reflux than the pH probe. However, it often detects pathologic mucosal changes when the extended pH probe study is falsely negative. During oesophagoscopy, a biopsy of the distal oesophageal mucosa should be obtained even if it is normal in appearance as histologic evidence of excessive reflux may be present. Hyperplasia of the basal zone of the epithelium, elongated papillae, chronic inflammatory cells and intraepidermal eosinophils are pathologic evidence of chronic gastroesophageal reflux in addition to Barrett's oesophagitis.

Direct laryngoscopy and bronchoscopy are helpful diagnostic studies to perform in association with oesophagoscopy. Laryngeal oedema or erythema, particularly of the posterior glottic mucosa, may suggest gastro-oesophageal reflux. During direct laryngoscopy, the interarytenoid region should be carefully examined to identify a congenital laryngeal cleft which may render the glottis incompetent if hypopharyngeal reflux occurs. During bronchoscopy, the bronchial tree can be lavaged with sterile saline and the effluent examined histologically for **lipid-laden macrophages**. An elevated index is suggestive of aspiration, although it does not distinguish primary from secondary aspiration.

Technetium scintigraphy is performed by scanning patients who have ingested milk with technetium-labelled sulphur colloid. In addition to detecting reflux events, oesophageal motility and gastric emptying may also be assessed. Serial scanning up to 24 hours after the start of the study may be instrumental in detecting delayed aspiration. The barium swallow with an oesophagogram offers better resolution of the upper gastrointestinal tract although technetium scintigraphy exposes the child to less radiation.

The **modified Bernstein** or **distal oesophageal acidification test**, is an insensitive but highly specific study that is performed by alternating 10-minute infusions of 0.1 N hydrochloric acid with normal saline into the distal oesophagus. The appearance of the respiratory symptom (e.g. bronchial spasm) thought due to reflux and its resolution with normal saline infusion establishes a link between distal oesophageal acidification and respiratory symptoms. Although the modified Bernstein test is a rather time-consuming study, its ability to establish a cause and effect relationship between reflux events and symptoms is a unique advantage.

TREATMENT

The management of patients with reflux includes conservative pharmacological and surgical therapy and should be tailored to the severity and chronicity of the patient's presenting symptoms.

Conservative management of paediatric patients entails thickening feeds, administering small, frequent feeds to reduce gastric volume, limiting intake of foods that decrease lower oesophageal sphincter tone, and, for infants, raising the head of the bed approximately 30°. Conservative therapy is used in the management of patients with mild symptoms that are not life-threatening. Adults should receive dietary advice (such as frequent small meals avoiding spices, pepper, curries, chocolate and liquorice), sleep on a raised bed and stop smoking.

Pharmacological therapy is directed at reducing the acidity of gastric contents – or hastening gastric emptying – and improving lower oesophageal sphincter tone. Approval for use of these medications varies between countries. H_2-receptor antagonists reduce acid production by approximately two-thirds and include cimetidine, ranitidine, famotidine and nizatidine. Omeprazole and iansoprazole are proton pump inhibitors that eliminate all gastric acid production but are generally not prescribed for more than several consecutive months. Omeprazole is now available in a suspension form which improves the convenience of administration, particularly to paediatric patients with gastrostomy tubes or feeding jejunostomies. The most commonly prescribed promotility agents, metoclopramide and cisapride, may be used independently or in conjunction with acid-reducing agents to improve lower oesophageal sphincter tone and gastric motility. Unlike metoclopramide, cisapride lacks antidopaminergic activity and is not associated with extrapyramidal side-effects, although reports of prolonged QT interval from its use do exist. Antacids are effective in treating oesophagitis, but their role in the management of GORD-related respiratory symptoms remains to be established.

Patients with life-threatening manifestations of GORD (e.g. pneumonia, severe bronchospasm, apnoea or bradycardia) or with symptoms that are unresponsive to conservative and pharmacological therapy, are candidates for surgical therapy. Such therapy may entail a fundoplication and/or feeding via the gastric/jejunal route.

II ANAESTHESIA AND LARYNGOSCOPY

5 Anaesthesia techniques

INTRODUCTION

With the advent of microlaryngoscopy in the 1960s and microlaryngeal laser surgery in the 1970s, many new, ingenious and inventive anaesthetic techniques were developed but no one technique has yet become generally favoured. The method of anaesthesia is critical as the surgeon and anaesthetist must safely share the upper airway and yet allow diagnostic evaluation and surgical treatment to proceed with optimal access. General anaesthesia is always preferred for direct laryngoscopy, laryngoscopy with telescopes, microlaryngoscopy and laryngeal laser surgery.

Theoretical requirements for the 'ideal' anaesthetic technique include: maximum safety, simplicity, rapid induction, full control of the airway and of ventilation, protection against undesirable autonomic or somatic reflexes, continuous monitoring of the patient's pulmonary and cardiovascular responses, an immobile larynx during microsurgery, completely unobstructed access to all parts of the upper airway, safe use of the laser, no restriction on operative time, good conditions for documentation, provision at the end of the procedure to allow assessment of the dynamics of the larynx, prevention of aspiration into the tracheobronchial tree, minimal contamination by anaesthetic gases of room air in the operating theatre, minimal patient discomfort and prompt recovery with return of cough and protective reflexes.

Induction and maintenance of anaesthesia must allow for problems such as partial airway obstruction or the need for a totally immobile larynx during microsurgery. The anaesthetist and laryngeal surgeon must co-operate closely to share access to the airway, sometimes a narrow, compromised airway with a variable degree of obstruction. Mutual understanding of the anaesthetic and surgical methods is needed to overcome problems which may present. Nevertheless, despite careful planning, unexpected life-threatening obstruction sometimes arises. Control of the airway must be quickly regained.

CLASSIFICATION OF ANAESTHETIC TECHNIQUES

There is no single universally accepted anaesthetic method, as evidenced by the many methods which are described. The technique will vary depending on the age of the patient, the site of the lesion and the degree of airway obstruction.

A practical classification of anaesthetic techniques depends upon whether respiration remains spontaneous or whether controlled intermittent positive pressure ventilation with a muscle relaxant is used.

Anaesthesia for patients with a tracheotomy can be with a spontaneous respiration or a relaxant technique and usually presents no special problems, although a laser-protected tube positioned through the stoma should be used for carbon dioxide laser surgery.

PROBLEMS DURING ANAESTHESIA

Many problems and complications can occur during anaesthesia for endolaryngeal surgery and the operating theatre team should be prepared to deal with them. They include laryngospasm, loss of, or poor control of, the airway, difficulty visualizing the larynx, awareness during the procedure, debris, blood or tumour cells contaminating the lower airways, risk of laser ignition if an endotracheal tube is being used, difficulty with ventilation because of a poorly compliant chest or chronic obstructive airways disease, unwanted effects from anaesthetic drugs (e.g. respiratory depression), stimulation of the autonomic and somatic reflexes causing hypertension, bradycardia or arrhythmia, complications of jet ventilation such as barotrauma (pneumomediastinum

Anaesthetic techniques

Spontaneous respiration techniques
- No endotracheal tube
- Small-diameter endotracheal tube

Relaxant techniques
- Jet ventilation: proximal or distal
- Small-diameter endotracheal tube
- No endotracheal tube

Problems with anaesthesia for laryngoscopy

Difficulty with ventilation
Loss of control of the airway
Laryngospasm
Contamination of lower airways
Unwanted effects of drugs
Stimulation of autonomic or somatic reflexes
Complications of jet ventilation
Difficulties with scavenging

and pneumothorax) or gastric distention (by forcing gas into the stomach) and contamination of room air by anaesthetic gases when using an 'open' anaesthetic system.

It should be noted that oxygen, nitrogen and helium are non-toxic to the personnel in the operating theatre and can therefore be used safely in 'open' systems. A 'closed' system with a cuffed endotracheal tube and a means of effective scavenging protects staff in the operating theatre from possible side-effects of volatile anaesthetic agents.

PREFERRED TECHNIQUES

There are many techniques of anaesthesia available for endoscopy, depending on individual preferences. Our preferred anaesthetic techniques are based on wide experience over many years with varied types of procedures. In adults, for example, procedures to be performed include diagnostic endoscopy with or without biopsy, removal of laryngeal polyps and vocal nodules etc., laser removal of lesions such as papillomas, treatment of laryngeal and subglottic stenoses, assessment of prolonged intubation trauma, injection of Gelfoam or Teflon paste and endolaryngeal microsurgery such as removal of small or large cysts and arytenoidectomy. In infants and children procedures include the investigation of stridor, evaluation of prolonged intubation trauma, laser treatment of multiple papillomas, treatment of congenital or acquired cysts, vocal nodules and management of acute inflammatory upper airway obstruction.

The choice of anaesthetic technique depends on the experience of the anaesthetist and surgeon, the age of the patient, the site of the lesion, the degree of obstruction and the demands of endoscopy. For example, there are different requirements when performing diagnostic pan-endoscopy for a suspected but unproven upper respiratory tract tumour, biopsy of a mass causing airway obstruction, laser removal of respiratory papillomas and when examining an infant's larynx, tracheobronchial tree and oesophagus in the investigation of stridor. The problems and needs for each patient should be discussed before starting the procedure.

All procedures under general anaesthesia require constant vigilance by the anaesthetist and routine intra-operative monitoring of the patient's cardiorespiratory parameters including pulse oximetry, heart rate, blood pressure recording, electrocardiography, monitoring of neuromuscular blockade and, where practicable, capnography.

Preferred techniques of anaesthesia

Adults
- Relaxant technique with controlled ventilation using either jet ventilation or a modified endotracheal tube

Infants and children
- Spontaneous respiration with inhalational anaesthesia

SUPPLEMENTARY LOCAL ANAESTHESIA

In all patients general anaesthesia is supplemented by measured amounts of topical lignocaine (Lidocaine) applied to the mucous membranes when the depth of anaesthesia is adequate. Application can be achieved by:

- using a pre-packaged delivery bottle which delivers 10 mg of 10% lignocaine (Xylocaine) per spray;
- using a Cass needle on a syringe containing a measured total amount of 4% lignocaine solution (Fig. 5.1);
- having the patient inhale a mist of nebulized local anaesthetic solution before general anaesthesia is commenced (Fig. 5.2).

With any method the measured amount is limited to a maximum dose of 5 mg of lignocaine per kg body

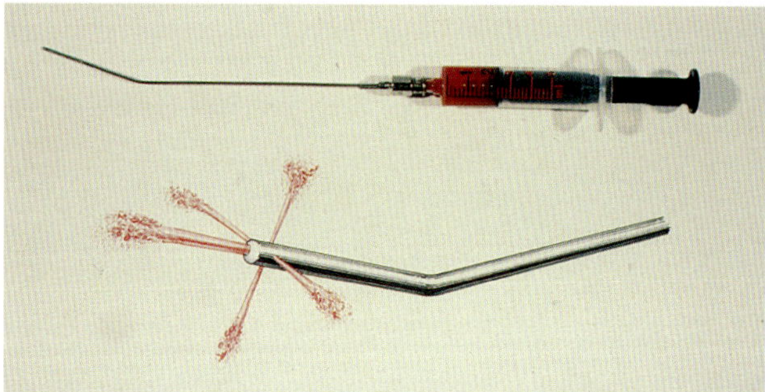

Figure **5.1**
Local anaesthetic spray. A Cass needle has four side openings and one forward opening at the distal end to spray topical anaesthetic solution in the larynx. Alternatively, a pre-packaged delivery bottle with an integral spray can be used.

weight. In infants the 4% solution can be diluted to 2% or even 1% to make sufficient volume for delivery.

PREPARATION FOR ANAESTHESIA

Before commencing the procedure the surgeon and the anaesthetist should plan their respective roles guided by their understanding of the requirements. Preoperative assessment by the anaesthetist includes history taking, physical examination and checking the results of investigations. Care in the selection of patients should be exercised, especially for those having day-only procedures. It is often possible to anticipate possible problems such as those caused by large, projecting or loose teeth, a large tongue, micrognathia, temporomandibular joint problems limiting opening of the mouth, lack of extension of the head and neck and, of course, cardiac or respiratory insufficiency.

The range of anaesthetic laryngoscopes, endotracheal tubes, anaesthetic equipment and emergency instrumentation requires thorough checking before commencing. An experienced anaesthetic assistant should always be readily available.

Baseline physiologic parameters need to be measured before initiating anaesthesia, and the surgical and anaesthetic team should be aware of any abnormalities.

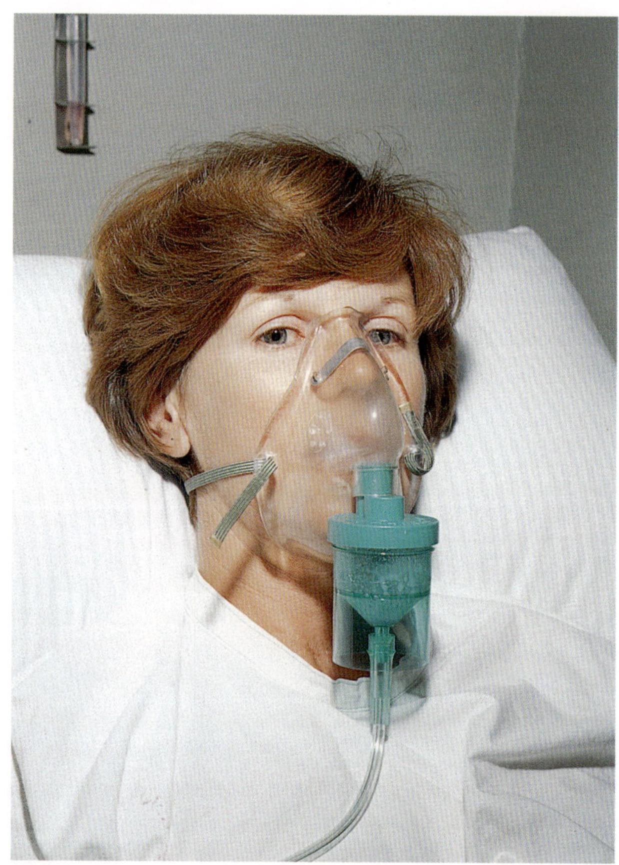

Figure **5.2**
Inhalation of nebulized local anaesthetic solution. Before the commencement of general anaesthesia local anaesthetic solution is inhaled as a nebulized mist to distribute it in the laryngopharynx and upper respiratory tract.

Lastly, but of great importance, the proposed procedure should be outlined to the patient with an explanation of what they can expect, i.e. the method of induction of anaesthesia, how long the procedure will take, information on possible complications, the location and nature of the recovery ward and the presence of an intravenous cannula.

ANAESTHESIA FOR ADULTS

In adults the technique using a muscle relaxant with jet ventilation depends on regular bursts of high-pressure air, oxygen, oxygen/nitrous oxide mixture or

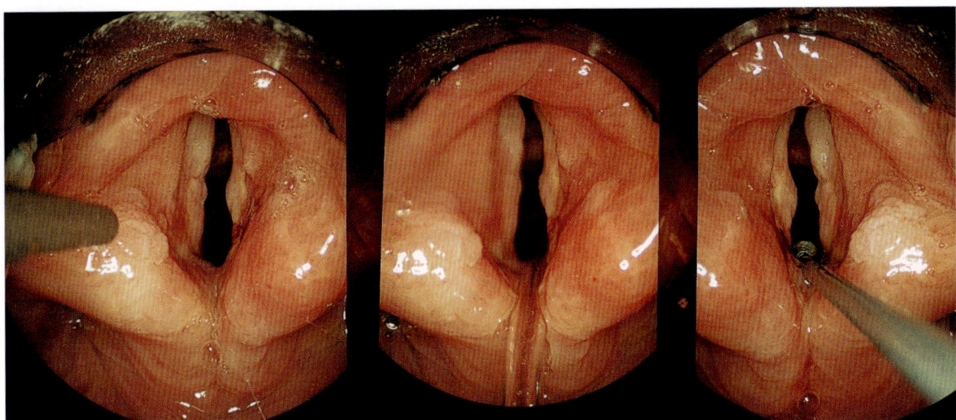

Figure **5.3**
Jet ventilation during anaesthesia. Left: the distal tip of a malleable metal cannula fixed inside the laryngoscope is directed at the glottic opening. Centre: a Benjet tube lies in the posterior glottic space for distal jetting in the tracheal lumen. Right: a longer metal cannula with a rounded head on the distal tip (to prevent laceration of the tracheal mucosa) is positioned through the glottic opening for jetting in the upper trachea.

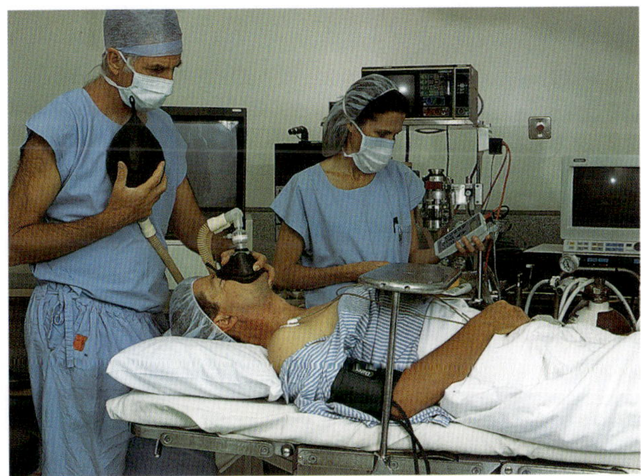

Figure **5.4**
Face mask ventilation. Anaesthesia has been induced and muscle paralysis established by the intravenous route. Face-mask ventilation is continued until muscle relaxation has been achieved.

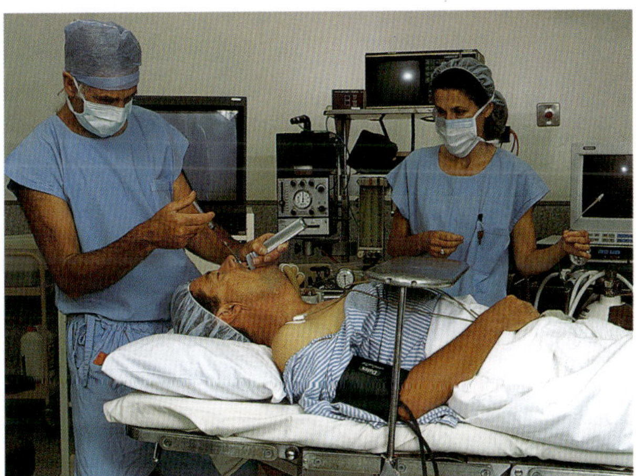

Figure **5.5**
Application of local anaesthesia. A measured amount, calculated on body weight, of local anaesthetic solution is sprayed on the larynx and subglottic region by the anaesthetist.

oxygen/helium mixture. During jet ventilation, according to the surgeon's preference and the laryngeal pathology, the jetting device can be positioned distally below the subglottic region, or mid-trachea, or proximally using a slim metal cannula in the lumen of the laryngoscope (Fig. 5.3).

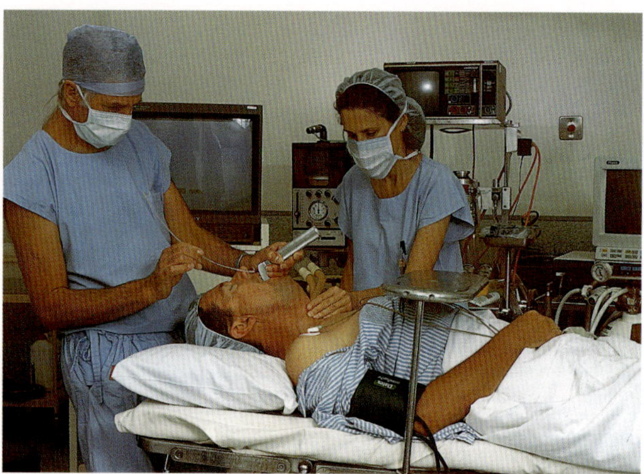

Figure **5.6**
Placement of the Benjet tube. A Benjet tube is about to be passed through the larynx into the trachea. The anaesthetic assistant depresses the larynx to assist visualization. Thereafter face-mask ventilation is continued prior to placement of the laryngoscope.

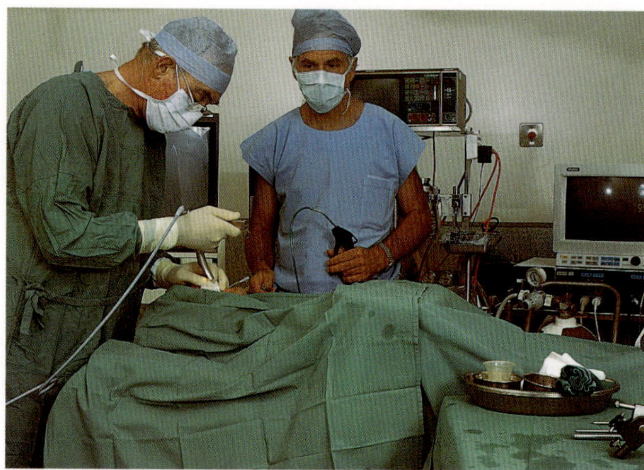

Figure **5.7**
Placement of the laryngoscope. A laryngoscope is inserted to visualize the glottic opening. When an unobstructed airway is assured, jet ventilation is commenced and the position of the tube in the trachea is adjusted to obtain optimal ventilation.

Distal intratracheal jetting

Anaesthesia is induced and maintained using an intravenous infusion. Muscle paralysis is established and maintained using either a short-acting or a longer-acting agent given intravenously. The infusion rates are varied according to requirements. Ventilation is assisted with 100% oxygen via a face mask (Fig. 5.4) and when muscle relaxation has been established the larynx is visualized, sprayed with topical anaesthetic solution (Fig. 5.5) and a Benjet tube, or similar tube, is inserted through the glottic opening into the trachea (Fig. 5.6). The anaesthetic laryngoscope is removed, the Benjet tube remains in place and once again ventilation is assisted with 100% oxygen via a face mask until the laryngologist is ready to position the laryngoscope.

The surgical drapes are placed and the apnoeic patient is then 'handed over' to the surgeon who introduces an appropriate laryngoscope to visualize the larynx (Fig. 5.7). Jet ventilation is not commenced until the endoscopist sees an unobstructed airway to ensure the expiratory phase. Jet insufflation with 100% oxygen (or with helium 60% : oxygen 40% for carbon dioxide laser surgery) is commenced. The placement and position of the tube in the trachea is adjusted up or down to obtain satisfactory chest movement and adequate ventilation. Each time the surgeon changes to another laryngoscope, jet ventilation ceases and is not recommenced until an unobstructed airway is again seen. Likewise, jet ventilation ceases whenever the expiratory phase of ventilation is occluded by instruments in the airway.

EXPIRATION MUST BE UNIMPAIRED DURING JETTING

Thus, distal intratracheal jetting is achieved with the Benjet tube (Fig. 5.8) positioned beyond the larynx in the mid-trachea. The tube is 2.8 mm in external diameter and sits unobtrusively in the posterior glottic space (Fig. 5.9). The tube can be easily displaced at the glottic level into the anterior larynx for an unrestricted view of the posterior glottis. Four soft plastic 'petals' stabilize the distal end of the Benjet tube in the trachea (Fig. 5.10) during jet ventilation to prevent the potential traumatic whipping effect of a free-lying tube.

Once successful jet ventilation has been achieved, it allows laryngoscopy with the naked eye (Fig. 5.11) or with a telescope (Fig. 5.12), photography (Fig. 5.13), video-laryngoscopy (Fig. 5.14), microsurgery or laser surgery (Fig. 5.15).

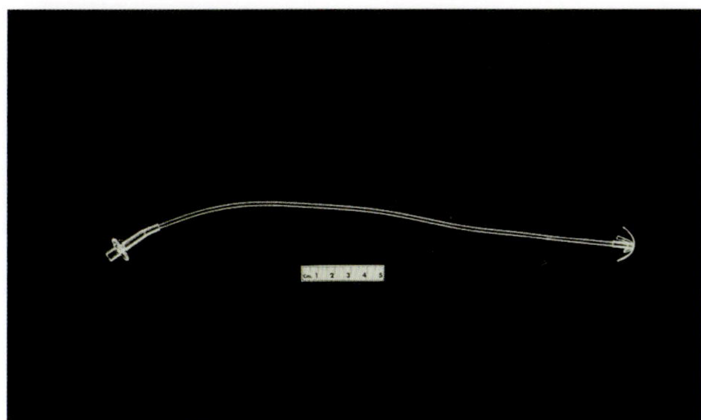

Figure **5.8**
The Benjet tube. This polyvinyl chloride tube is 2.8 mm in external diameter, 35 cm long and there are four plastic petals at the distal end to stabilize it in the trachea during jetting.

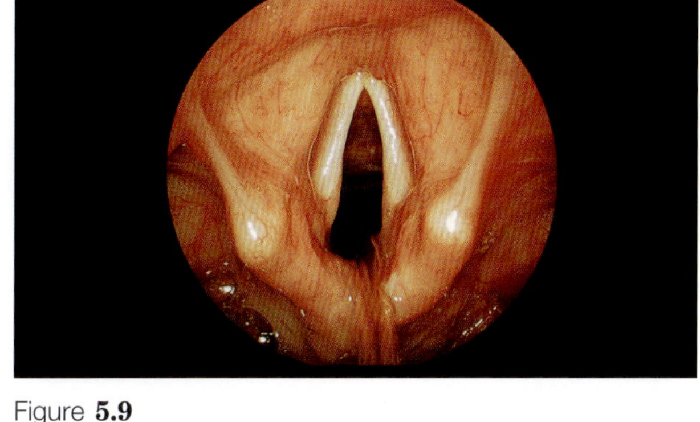

Figure **5.9**
Jet tube in larynx. The view of the larynx is unrestricted as the small-diameter tube sits, hardly noticeable, in the posterior glottic space. It can be positioned in the anterior commissure if necessary.

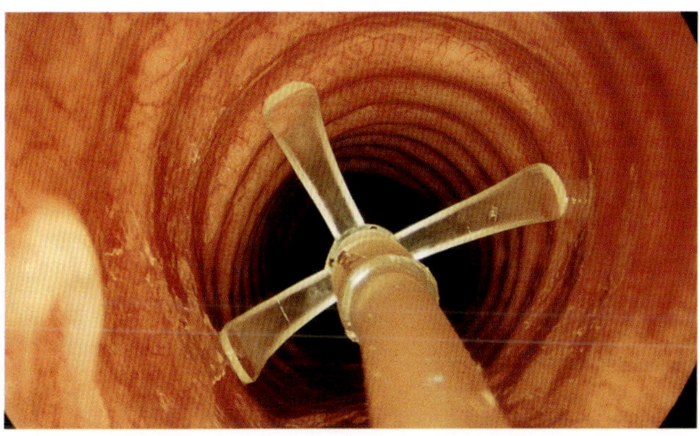

Figure **5.10**
Distal end of Benjet tube in trachea. The four soft plastic petals stabilize the distal end in the mid-trachea to prevent a 'whip' effect which might lacerate the mucosa.

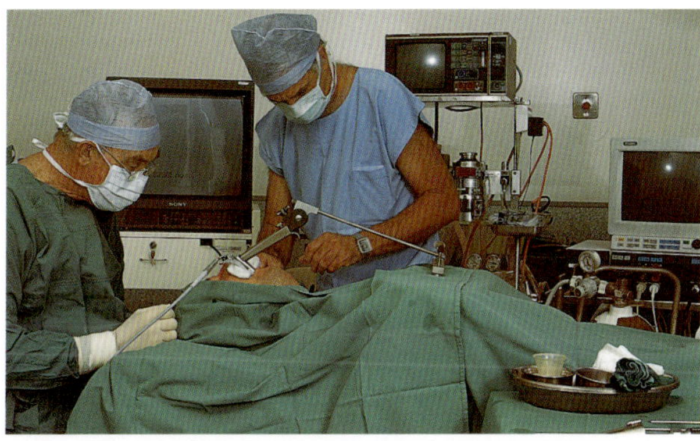

Figure **5.11**
Naked eye laryngoscopy; first stage of laryngoscopy. Preliminary naked-eye examination of the laryngopharynx is undertaken either with the laryngoscope held in the left hand or with it in suspension.

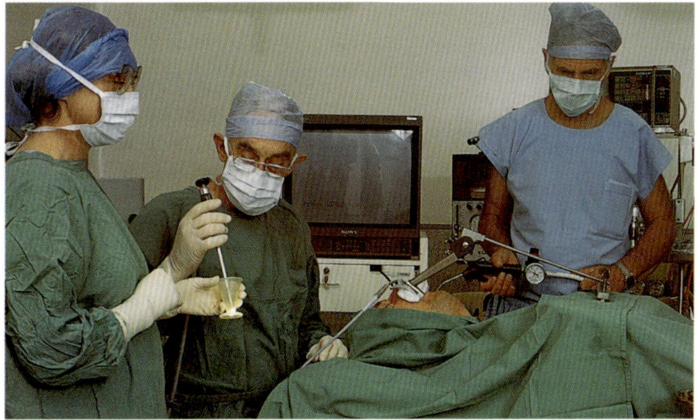

Figure **5.12**
Examination with a rigid telescope; second stage of laryngoscopy. A telescope is being dipped in anti-fog solution prior to image magnification laryngoscopy.

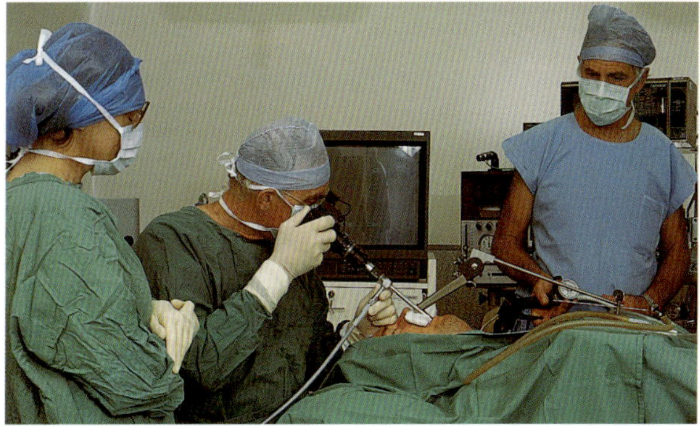

Figure **5.13**
Laryngeal photography. A 35-mm camera, with zoom lens and synchronization cable to the flash unit has been coupled to the telescope ready for photography.

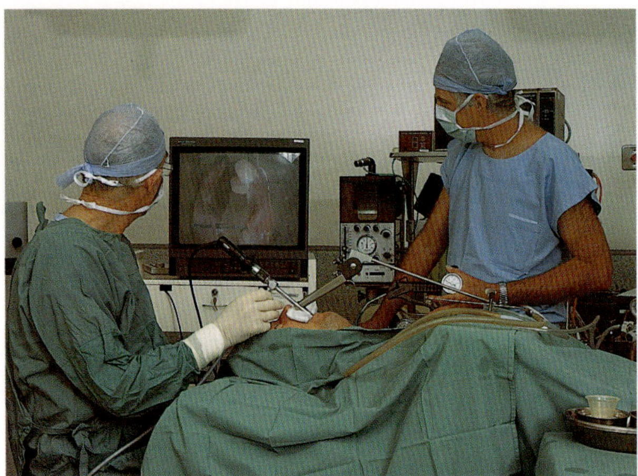

Figure **5.14**
Video-laryngoscopy. A miniature video-camera provides an image on the monitor screen for visualization by the theatre personnel, for video-recording or for instant prints.

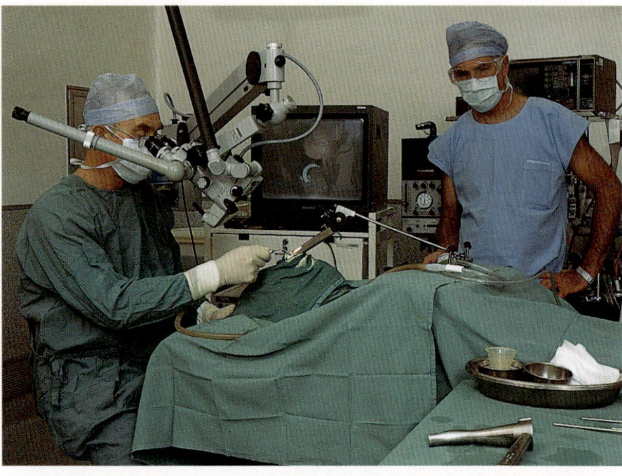

Figure **5.15**
Microlaryngeal surgery; third stage of laryngoscopy. Microsurgery is performed with miniature forceps, scissors etc., or with the carbon dioxide laser coupled to the micromanipulator on the operating microscope. A miniature video-camera is attached to the beam splitter of the microscope.

On completion of the procedure, the intravenous infusions are ceased, the muscle relaxant is reversed when necessary, the larynx receives a final spray of the remaining local anaesthetic solution (to minimize the chance of spasm), the Benjet tube is removed and the laryngopharynx is suctioned. Ventilation is assisted with 100% oxygen via a face mask until there is adequate reversal of muscle relaxant. The patient is placed in the lateral position and given supplemental oxygen during transport, and in the recovery room.

The advantages of this method are that the polyvinyl chloride jetting tube is sufficiently small and flexible for excellent surgical access to the entire larynx and subglottic region. The four soft distal petals assure that the tube will remain centred in the trachea preventing submucosal injection of the jetted gas. When used with due care, barotrauma does not occur. During the expiratory phase there is a rapid flow of gases outwards with expulsion of blood/smoke/secretions. There is minimal movement of the vocal cords, and if necessary ventilation can be interrupted for short intervals for delicate surgical procedures. The jet tube can be passed through a subglottic stenosis (Fig. 5.16) of 4- or 5-mm diameter and gently moved to one side so that the steno-

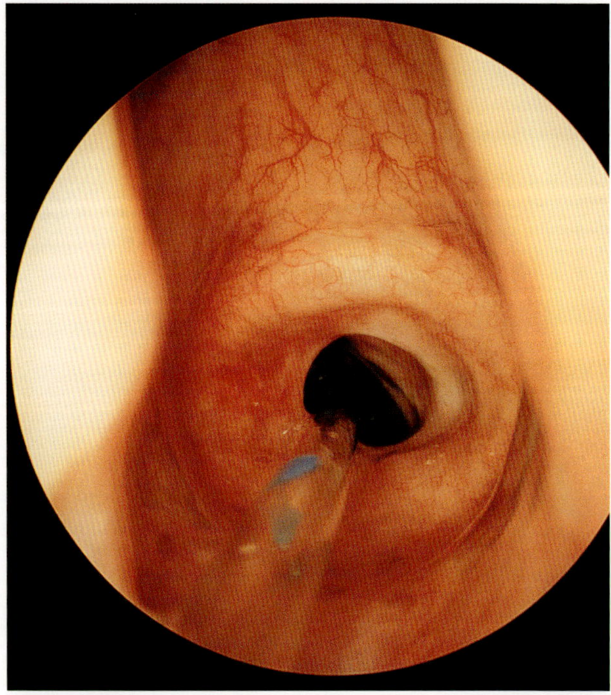

Figure **5.16**
Severe subglottic stenosis with jet tube. Anaesthesia is maintained and the surgical field is exposed without the need for tracheotomy, using a Benjet tube. Alternatively a proximal jet cannula can be used.

sis can be enlarged by laser vaporization. Biopsy or laser removal of tracheal or bronchial tumours can be conveniently performed through a bronchoscope while the jet tube continues ventilation in the trachea or even in one main bronchus. The technique allows accurate injection of Teflon or Gelfoam paste under general anaesthesia because the narrow tube causes no obstruction or distortion of the larynx. Temporary cessation of the intravenous muscle relaxant agent allows return of vocal cord movements so that placement of the paste can be precisely judged.

We have used the jet technique with the Benjet tube for laryngoscopy, microlaryngoscopy and microlaryngeal surgery for over 15 years without complication. No tube has been ignited and we have had no barotrauma complications. Safe jet insufflation requires careful patient selection, vigilant staff and adequate ventilation.

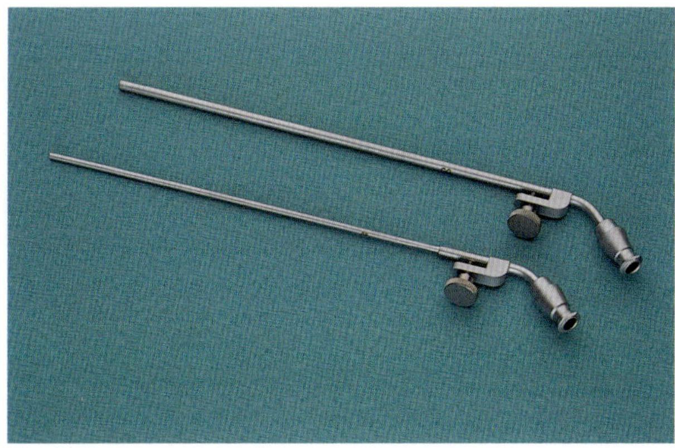

Figure **5.17**
Proximal jet cannulae. The cannulae have a working length of 13.5 cm. There is a choice of tubes with an outside diameter of 2 or 3 mm. The cannula is slightly malleable to permit adjustment of the direction of the jet to be aimed at the glottic opening.

Jetting technique

Intravenous anaesthesia
Muscle paralysis
Topical anaesthesia
Jet ventilation
- Distal – Benjet tube
- Proximal – malleable metal cannula

Minimize contamination of trachea

EXPIRATION MUST BE UNIMPAIRED

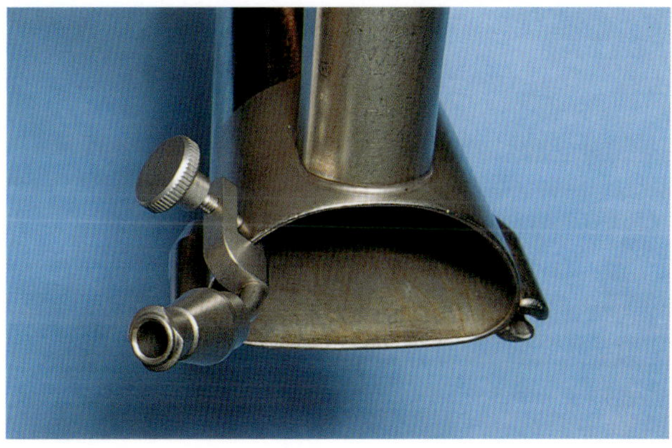

Figure **5.18**
Attachment of the proximal jet cannula. A small knurled knob allows firm attachment to the proximal end of any laryngoscope.

Proximal jetting

Anaesthesia is induced and maintained using the same intravenous method described above for distal intratracheal jetting, but with proximal jetting no endotracheal tube is used.

Following induction of anaesthesia, paralysis and ventilation, the endoscopist visualizes the larynx to ensure that the airway is unobstructed. A slim metal tube for jet ventilation (Fig. 5.17) is securely attached within the lumen of the laryngoscope (Fig. 5.18) and jet ventilation with 100% oxygen is commenced (Fig. 5.19). The use of a cannula which is slightly malleable allows bending to adjust the direction of the gas jet to be aimed at the glottis between the vocal cords (Fig. 5.20). In this way accurate directional placement of the metal cannula achieves optimal ventilation into the trachea for

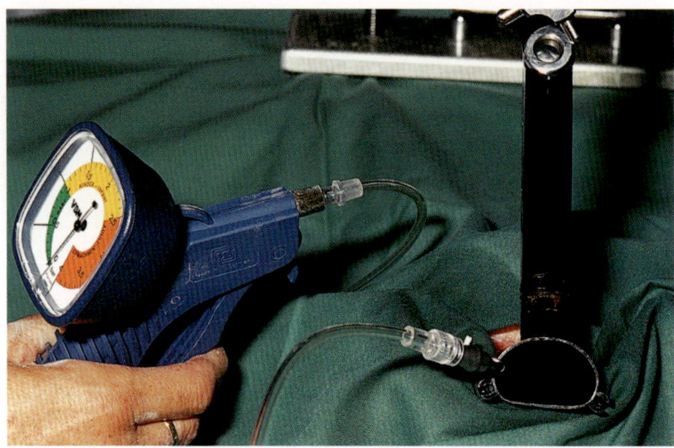

Figure **5.19**
Jet ventilation. The pressure used for jet ventilation can be adjusted. The anaesthetist triggers each jet ventilation by hand. We do not favour the use of an automatic ventilator.

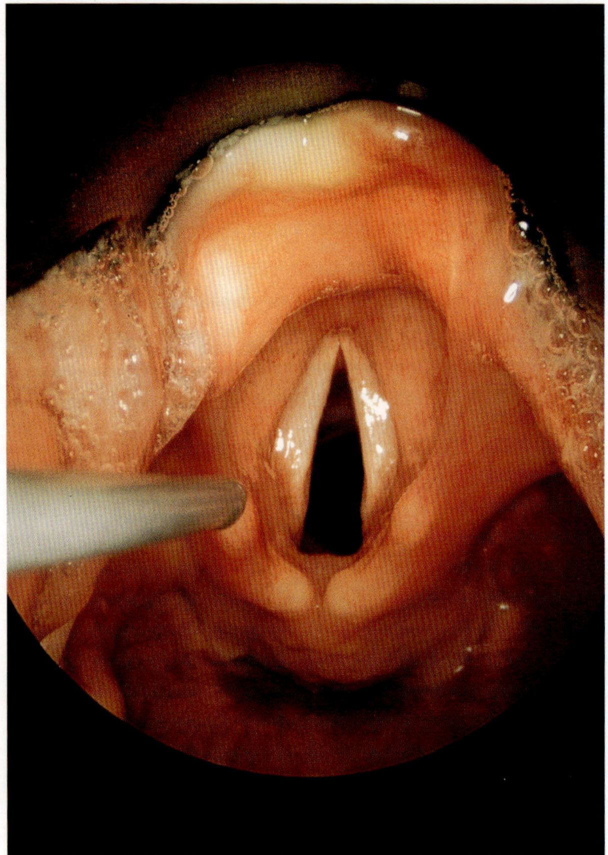

Figure **5.20**
Proximal jet ventilation. A Lindholm laryngoscope is in place and the metal cannula has been adjusted for ventilation directed at the glottic opening.

continued ventilation during suspension laryngoscopy.

The proximal jet ventilation technique has a number of advantages including absence of an endotracheal tube, an unobstructed view of the airway and a paralysed patient.

The laryngopharynx and subglottis are totally free of any anaesthesia tube leaving the field clear for the surgeon. As there is no potentially flammable endotracheal tube in the airway during laser surgery there is no risk of laser ignition. As the intermittent jets of gas may cause unwanted movements of the vocal folds, ventilation can be suspended at the surgeon's request during precise manipulations.

There are disadvantages: laryngeal mucosa becomes dry, and tissue, blood, other secretions, even fragments of papilloma or tumour, may be forced into the lower respiratory tract. The open nature of proximal jet ventilation may occasionally make ventilation impossible and accurate volume delivery uncertain and if gas is blown behind the larynx down the oesophagus, gastric distention may occur with a potential for gastric reflux and aspiration (Fig. 5.21). Jetting should cease while laser treatment is in progress because of the intense vibratory movements of the vocal cords which occur during jetting.

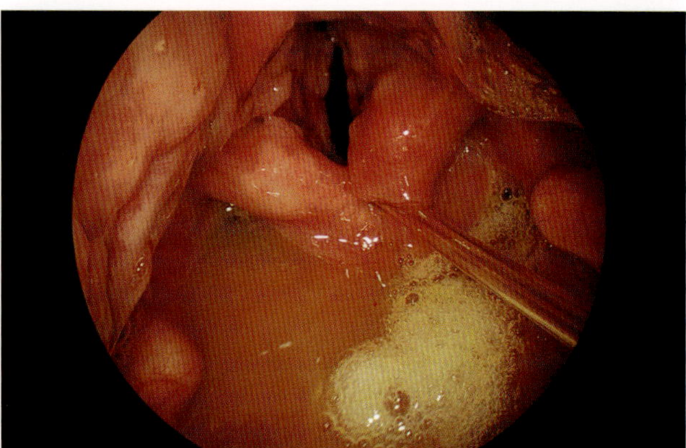

Figure **5.21**
Gastric reflux. Aspiration of regurgitated acid gastric contents is rarely a problem.

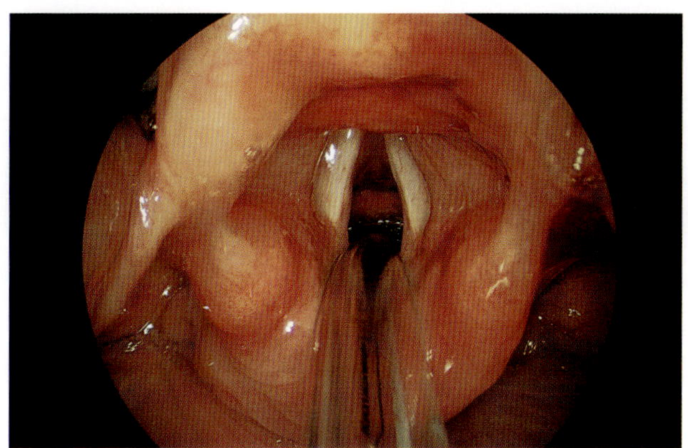

Figure **5.22**
Microlaryngoscopy tube. The larger outside diameter, even of a 5-mm microlaryngoscopy tube obscures the posterior glottic space and the subglottic region. The exposure is acceptable when the lesion is known to be supraglottic or in the anterior part of the larynx.

Microlaryngoscopy tube

This is the most commonly used modified endotracheal tube, a 4-, 5- or 6-mm internal diameter cuffed polyvinyl chloride microlaryngoscopy tube ensures a secure airway for ventilation when using an inhalational agent or a relaxant technique.

Anaesthesia is induced intravenously and the patient is paralysed either with a short-acting or a long-acting relaxant, the larynx is visualized and sprayed with local anaesthetic solution and the anaesthetist inserts the microlaryngoscopy tube into the trachea, the cuff is inflated and controlled ventilation is commenced and maintained. Use of a cuffed microlaryngoscopy tube allows standard use of inhalational agents and obviates the possible risk of barotrauma associated with a jetting technique. But this is at the expense of surgical access in the posterior glottis and the subglottic area (Fig. 5.22) which are difficult to expose despite the relatively small diameter of the microlaryngoscopy tube.

This technique is not appropriate for some lesions, e.g. posterior glottic or subglottic stenosis with a small-diameter lumen. The presence of the tube is a potential danger if laser treatment is required. Nevertheless, a small-diameter microlaryngoscopy tube might be preferred by the anaesthetist and is often acceptable to the endoscopist, particularly when the disease is known to be supraglottic or in the anterior part of the larynx.

Despite the small diameter of the cuffed tube, ventilation is predictable so this technique may be preferred when there is pre-existing upper airway obstruction, when bleeding is expected, where intubation is desired to secure safe ventilation in poor risk patients with pre-existing respiratory or cardiovascular disease and when an anaesthetist is working with an endoscopist whose technique is not known to him, perhaps in unfamiliar surroundings.

Anaesthesia through a tracheotomy

A tracheotomy allows use of relaxant or inhalational agents and provides ideal conditions for anaesthesia during endolaryngeal surgery.

ANAESTHESIA FOR INFANTS AND CHILDREN

Our preferred technique for infants and children is spontaneous respiration with inhalational general anaesthesia supplemented by topical anaesthetic solution applied as a spray to the mucous membranes. In small infants, direct laryngoscopy, for brief examination or intubation can be performed using no anaesthesia in certain selected cases.

Occasionally, for example, in a sick neonate or a baby with a difficult airway problem (such as occurs in Pierre Robin sequence) it may be safer to perform 'cold' laryngoscopy and orotracheal intubation without general anaesthesia.

In older children a relaxant technique with controlled ventilation, similar to the adult technique, may sometimes be preferable. We do not favour total intravenous anaesthesia or high-pressure jetting methods for infants or small children. The latter is reported to cause a high incidence of airway rupture.

Many paediatric patients require repeated procedures and a team approach to these patients gives them a feeling of security in their continuing management.

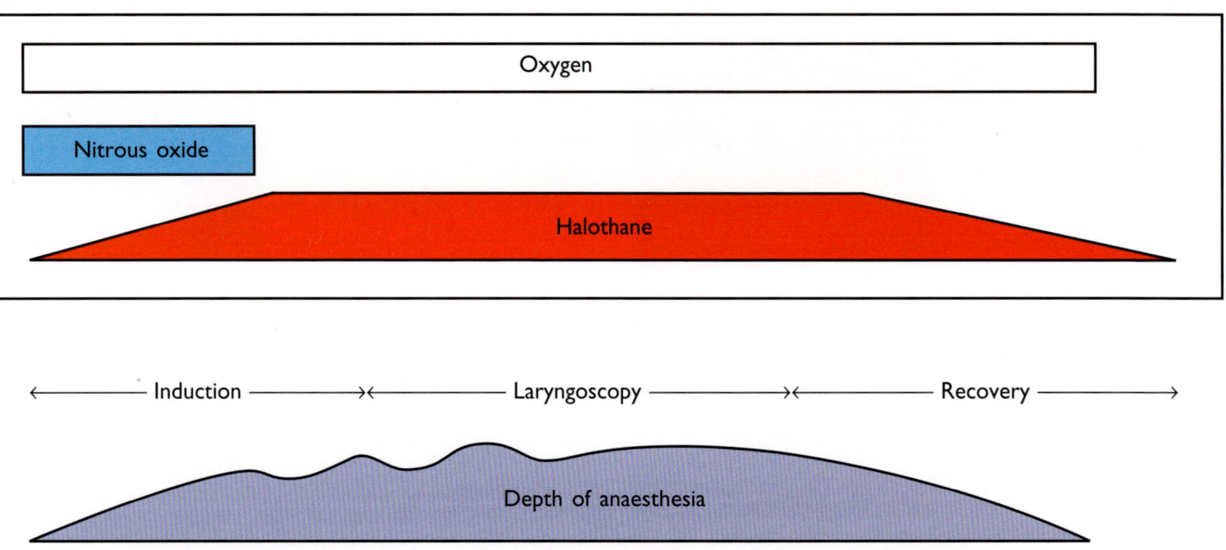

Figure **5.23**
Spontaneous respiration anaesthesia for children. For paediatric endoscopy induction may be either with an intravenous agent or by face-mask inhalation using nitrous oxide, oxygen and halothane. The depth of anaesthesia fluctuates as local anaesthetic solution is applied and as various endoscopes are introduced and withdrawn.

Spontaneous respiration inhalational technique

The most common anaesthetic technique for paediatric endoscopy relies on spontaneous respiration using oxygen, nitrous oxide and halothane (Fig. 5.23). Where it is available, some anaesthetists prefer to add methoxyflurane to the gaseous mixture regarding it as a supplement to provide additional analgesia that 'smoothes out' the procedure. In the case of an ill child with respiratory insufficiency or airway obstruction, oxygen and halothane without nitrous oxide is used. With this inhalational method no satisfactory technique for scavenging anaesthetic gases is currently available.

Premedication is seldom necessary for infants but may be beneficial in older children. A premedication should not be administered in the presence of respiratory obstruction. If atropine has not been given by intramuscular injection, it is usually administered after intravenous access has been achieved; atropine must always be drawn up for use since it affords protection against bradycardia and arrhythmia and helps minimize secretions in the respiratory tract.

A venipuncture is performed as early as possible to secure an intravenous route. A muscle relaxant is drawn up ready to be given if required, for example, for persistent or uncontrolled spasm or for a foreign body whose removal is made difficult by laryngeal spasm.

Anaesthesia is usually commenced in the anaesthetic bay or induction room, often with a parent present. Induction may be accomplished with an intravenous agent or by inhalation with a face mask (Fig. 5.24). With spontaneous ventilation, induction may be prolonged in the presence of airway obstruction. When the depth of anaesthesia is sufficient, topical lignocaine solution, up to a maximum of 5 mg/kg body weight, is used as a 4% solution in older children but in infants is usually diluted with saline to a 2% or even a 1% concentration to give sufficient volume to be handled conveniently. Using a syringe and a Cass needle (Fig. 5.1) or similar applicator it is sprayed onto the epiglottis, larynx and upper trachea (Fig. 5.25) to minimize unwanted reflex activity. This combination of general and local anaesthesia is most important as it virtually abolishes laryngeal spasm during and after endoscopy.

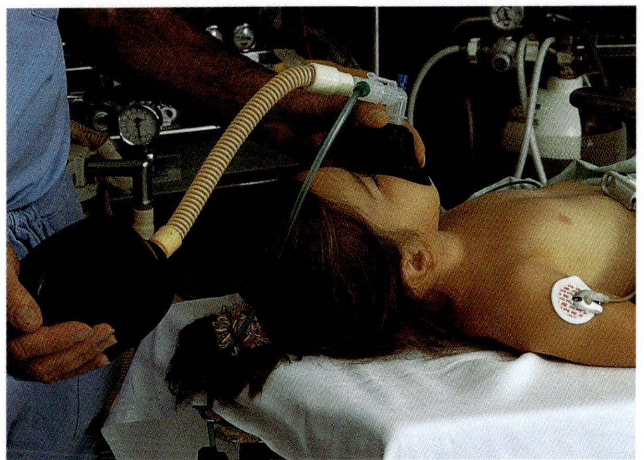

Figure **5.24**
Induction of anaesthesia in children. Induction may be with an intravenous agent or by inhalation with a face mask with the child continuing to breathe spontaneously.

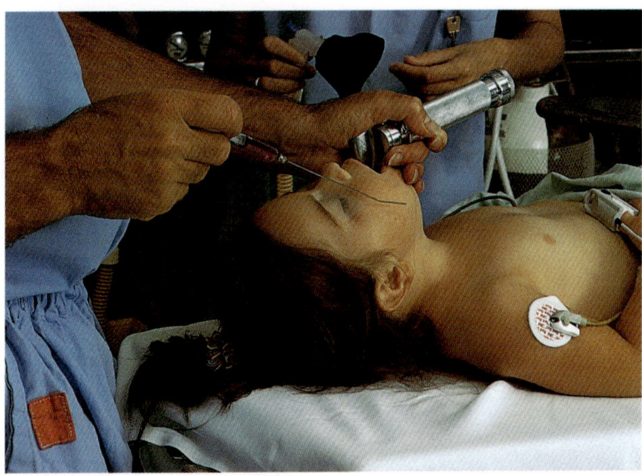

Figure **5.25**
Application of local anaesthesia. When anaesthesia reaches an appropriate depth, local anaesthetic solution is sprayed onto the larynx and upper trachea.

As anaesthesia begins to deepen during induction, the application of modest continuous positive pressure from the anaesthetic bag through the face mask may be of assistance in supporting the supraglottic and laryngopharyngeal airway. Before application of topical anaesthetic solution, anaesthesia should be continued to sufficient depth so that the airway is not manipulated during light anaesthesia;

Inhalational technique for children

- Seldom use premedication
- Atropine after IV access
- Oxygen/volatile agent by mask
- Topical anaesthesia
- Maintain by insufflation
- Ideal conditions for endoscopy
- Allows tracheobronchoscopy
- Laryngeal dynamics maintained

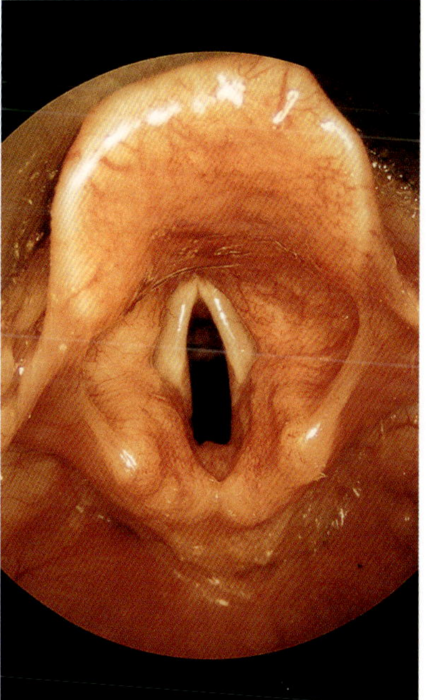

Figure **5.26**
Normal larynx. Child's larynx, using a Lindholm laryngoscope, under spontaneous ventilation general anaesthesia delivered through a metal cannula in the side of the laryngoscope.

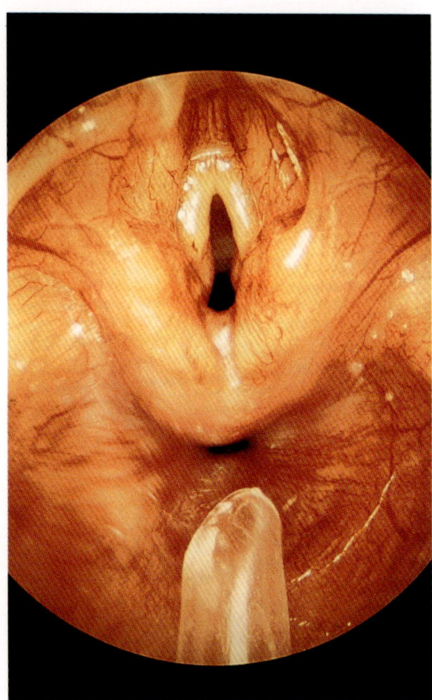

Figure **5.27**
Pernasal endopharyngeal insufflation. Anaesthetic gases are delivered into the oropharynx to maintain the depth of anaesthesia using a small-diameter tube passed through one nasal cavity.

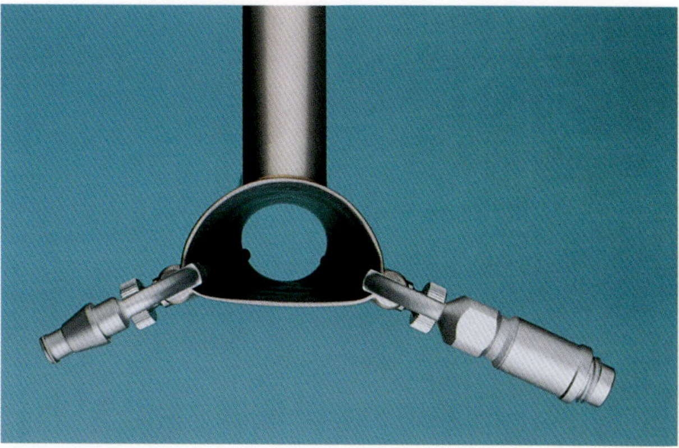

Figure **5.28**
Cannula for insufflation of anaesthetic gases. The metal cannula attached to the left side of the laryngoscope is for insufflation of anaesthetic gases during spontaneous respiration or for jet ventilation. It is not malleable and cannot be 'aimed'. A lighting rod is on the right.

this lessens the possibility of precipitating laryngospasm, breath holding or a coughing attack.

Thus, general anaesthesia without an endotracheal tube provides ideal conditions and unrestricted access to all parts of the airway for unhurried assessment (Fig. 5.26). During the endoscopic examination anaesthetic gases can be delivered through a metal cannula which is built into the side of some laryngoscopes (e.g. the Parson's laryngoscope) or alternatively through a small-diameter nasopharyngeal tube passed through one nasal cavity for insufflation into the oropharynx (Fig. 5.27).

Towards the end of the diagnostic procedure, oxygen alone is administered as the surgeon continues direct laryngeal observation to observe and record the dynamics of laryngeal movement as muscular tone returns. At this point the abnormality of the supraglottic structures in laryngomalacia can be appreciated and in other cases vocal cord paralysis can be observed.

For microlaryngoscopy, anaesthetic gases are delivered through a metal cannula in the left-hand side of the laryngoscope (Fig. 5.28) to ensure that insufflation is close to the glottic opening and to maintain a steady concentration. Absolutely clear access to the larynx without the obstruction of a tube is obtained; this method, with no endotracheal tube in the larynx, is especially useful for laser surgery.

A small-diameter standard uncuffed polyvinyl chloride translaryngeal anaesthetic tube may be preferred when the laser is not being used and when the disease is known to be supraglottic or in the anterior part of the larynx, e.g. vocal nodules.

Particular care should be taken in infants and children to maintain the airway during induction of anaesthesia for the initial examination in patients who have suspected or known papillomas even though airway obstruction may appear to be minimal at preoperative assessment. Progressive obstruction may occur as the depth of anaesthesia is increased, muscular tone decreases and the supraglottic airway narrows. It is safer to commence anaesthesia in the operating room with an endotracheal tube, laryngoscope and a bronchoscope readily available. Initial laryngoscopy may indicate severe laryngeal obstruc-

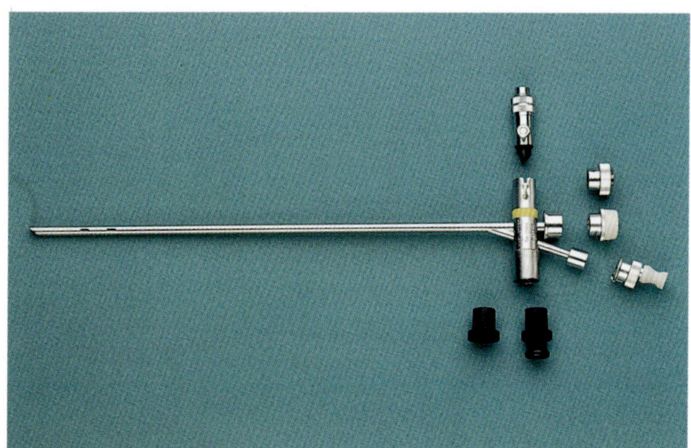

Figure **5.29**
Ventilating paediatric bronchoscope. 'Broken' view of a Karl Storz ventilating bronchoscope with various adaptors for lighting and anaesthesia.

tion so that repeated introduction and withdrawal of a small-diameter endotracheal tube (the so-called 'in-and-out' technique) may be necessary to maintain sufficient depth of anaesthesia between surgical manoeuvres to remove papillomas (see later section 'Anaesthesia for upper airway obstruction' in this chapter).

During tracheobronchoscopy, a ventilating bronchoscope is used with gaseous exchange taking place down the side port of the bronchoscope to maintain anaesthesia while it is in the tracheobronchial tree (Fig. 5.29).

No anaesthesia

This approach has very little application for thorough diagnostic endoscopy or where any form of laryngeal surgery is required and cannot be recommended. It may, however, occasionally be safest to intubate a very sick neonate 'cold' or to intubate a baby with a difficult airway problem without general anaesthesia using one of the special-purpose laryngoscopes such as the Holinger or Holinger–Benjamin.

Anaesthesia through a tracheotomy

As in adults, the presence of tracheotomy provides ideal conditions for anaesthesia with complete control of the airway during laryngoscopy.

Relaxant technique

Anaesthesia is usually easily maintained at an adequate depth by insufflation and spontaneous respiration in children up to approximately 10 or 12 years of age. Over this age the relaxant techniques as described above for adults may be necessary.

For persistent or uncontrolled laryngeal spasm or removal of a difficult foreign body, use of a muscle relaxant and intermittent ventilation using a face mask, an endotracheal tube or a ventilating bronchoscope may be the most satisfactory method.

Recovery Ward

The child must not leave the operating theatre until adequate spontaneous respiration is assured and there is return of the protective airway reflexes.

Observation and monitoring of vital signs, including the airway, are mandatory in the recovery ward. A doubtful airway sometimes needs temporary or even long-term support; children are remarkably tolerant of an indwelling nasotracheal tube.

Fluid and feeding are commenced within 1 or 2 hours.

ANAESTHESIA FOR UPPER AIRWAY OBSTRUCTION

Difficult visualization and attempted intubation for reasons of altered or unusual anatomy, but in the absence of laryngeal obstruction, is well known to anaesthesiologists and has recently been comprehensively reviewed by Cabley and Vaughn (1992). The many references to difficult laryngoscopy and intubation contrasts with the paucity of literature on the difficulties of airway management presented by acute or acute on chronic laryngeal and upper airway obstruction. Restoring the airway in a patient with severe laryngeal obstruction is a demanding responsibility for both the endoscopist and the anaesthetist.

The imperative of maximum patient safety during anaesthesia and endoscopic assessment cannot be over-emphasized. Nevertheless, the chosen anaesthetic technique for airway obstruction should not compromise diagnostic accuracy or subsequent definitive treatment.

General management techniques

There are many ways to manage the obstructed airway during diagnostic endoscopy.

In some situations tracheotomy may prove to be necessary to ensure a reliable airway or to allow subsequent treatment.

In all situations intravenous access is secured and facilities to establish an airway must be readily available, i.e. small-diameter endotracheal tubes with introducers, ventilating bronchoscopes and instruments for immediate tracheotomy.

Possible techniques for management of obstructed airway

- Direct endoscopy and/or intubation without general anaesthesia
- Tracheotomy with local anaesthesia followed by general anaesthesia for endoscopy
- Inhalational anaesthesia, intubation, then paralysis
- Inhalational induction of anaesthesia with assisted ventilation for performance of a tracheotomy followed by general anaesthesia through the tracheotomy during endoscopy
- Inhalational (or intravenous) induction and test ventilation to ensure an adequate airway before an intravenous relaxant for diagnostic endoscopy
- Intravenous anaesthesia incorporating initial paralysis, ventilation and establishment of an airway followed by diagnostic endoscopy

Illustrative cases

Case 1 Initial tracheotomy with local anaesthesia

A 38-year-old female fell from a horse, suffering direct injury to the neck with cricotracheal separation. Primary repair was achieved without tracheotomy but after some months progressive stridor developed and she was referred for further management. There was severe obstruction and any activity, including speech, was difficult. Induction of general anaesthesia was considered potentially hazardous and a tracheotomy was performed using local anaesthesia followed by general anaesthesia administered via the tracheotomy. Endoscopy confirmed not only a severe subglottic stenosis which was less than 4-mm diameter, but also a right vocal cord paralysis. Laryngotracheoplasty using a hyoid bone graft was performed a week later and remained successful at 5-year follow-up.

Comment. Severe obstruction indicated an undue risk for induction and maintenance of general anaesthesia. Tracheotomy under local anaesthesia, although not entirely without difficulty in a severely obstructed patient, was the safer technique.

Case 2 Endoscopy followed by tracheotomy

A 52-year-old male was intubated for 3 weeks following coronary artery grafting and had a tracheotomy for a further 2 weeks. Following decannulation he had exercise intolerance, inspiratory stridor at rest and a husky voice. Indirect laryngoscopy showed displacement of the right arytenoid and apparent loss of movement in both vocal cords. During spontaneous respiration inhalational induction with oxygen and halothane, test ventilation proved respiration could be satisfactorily assisted and paralysis was induced with an intravenous agent. A proximal jet cannula provided good ventilation and allowed unobstructed endoscopy. Both cricoarytenoid joints were fixed with anterior dislocation of the right arytenoid and a moderate posterior glottic fibrous stenosis. As definitive treatment would require a right arytenoidectomy, the tracheotomy was reopened. One week later laryngofissure and right arytenoidectomy with suture lateralization of the vocal fold was performed and decannulation was achieved in 3 weeks. The airway remained very good.

Comment. Obstruction was moderately severe and the precise diagnosis was in doubt. The airway was proven to be adequate with positive pressure ventilation through a face mask indicating that paralysis could be safely undertaken for endoscopy. Tracheotomy was necessary for corrective surgery.

Case 3 Management without tracheotomy

A 24-year-old female under treatment for Wegener's granulomatosis was referred with slowly progressive airway obstruction and mild stridor at rest. The lateral X-ray indicated a subglottic stenosis. Anaesthesia was induced with spontaneous ventilation via a face mask after infiltration of the neck in case an urgent tracheostomy became necessary. However, assisted test ventilation was easy, paralysis was induced and after introduction of the laryngoscope, ventilation was continued via a proximal jetting cannula. The subglottic stenosis was about 5-mm diameter and was vaporized with the carbon dioxide laser with immediate airway improvement. Further laser treatments were necessary and the airway remained satisfactory.

Comment. Obstruction was not severe and tracheotomy was not necessary either to relieve the airway obstruction or for subsequent treatment.

Case 4 Diagnostic endoscopy and nasotracheal intubation

A 3-year-old boy developed sudden fever, cough, increasing sore throat and progressive airway obstruction. In the emergency department he had inspiratory stridor. No X-ray or blood gas determinations were made. Acute epiglottitis was suspected, he was transferred to the operating theatre and within 30 minutes anaesthesia was being induced using gently assisted spontaneous respiration delivering 100% oxygen and halothane by face mask. When anaesthesia reached an adequate depth, brief endoscopy showed grossly swollen, red supraglottic tissues, confirming the diagnosis. An oral endotracheal tube, stiffened with an introducer was passed and replaced by a nasotracheal tube which was removed uneventfully 48 hours later in the intensive care unit where he was nursed and given appropriate intravenous antibiotics.

Comment. The diagnosis was likely to be acute epiglottitis, but in atypical cases endoscopy will rule out other possibilities such as subglottic swelling from croup, inhaled laryngeal foreign body, bacterial tracheitis or even diphtheria. Intubation for acute epiglottitis can be very difficult, requiring considerable skill and experience; an otolaryngologist with bronchoscopy and tracheotomy equipment should be present for the rare occasion when intubation fails.

General principles of management

The management of laryngeal obstruction requires an appreciation of the causes of airway restriction at a laryngeal level and an understanding of the principles of anaesthesia.

Preoperative evaluation

The nature, onset, progression and severity of dysphonia, stridor and exercise intolerance are important. Signs of obstruction include noisy or prolonged inspiration and/or expiration, tracheal tug, intercostal

Features of obstruction in children

- Stridor and respiratory distress
- Tracheal tug
- Intercostal recession
- May be reluctant to lie down
- Poor air entry to lungs
- Signs of hypoxaemia or hypercapnoea

The site of pathology is important to the anaesthetist

Supraglottic lesions

- may obstruct the view of the laryngeal opening
- may cause ball valve obstruction
- are occasionally vascular and bleed to touch

Glottic lesions

- usually small, present few problems
- a large mass, e.g. vocal granuloma may cause ball valve obstruction
- if posterior, a microlaryngoscopy tube is unsuitable
- bilateral cord paralysis may cause obstruction at the end of the procedure

Subglottic lesions

- may be 'fixed' – difficult to pass a tube
- require a range of smaller and uncuffed tubes
- jet insufflation may require a long expiratory phase

recession and the use of the accessory respiratory muscles. In severe cases the patient is anxious, reluctant to lie down, and has difficulty with even minimal exertion. There may be poor air entry on auscultation, pulsus paradoxus and signs of hypoxaemia and carbon dioxide retention. In acute cases the severity of obstruction is best judged on clinical features alone without the need for diagnostic preoperative flow studies or blood gases.

In all but the most urgent situations, indirect laryngoscopy with a laryngeal mirror, rigid 70° or 90° telescope or flexible nasopharyngoscope is essential with particular attention to supraglottic obstructive swelling, cyst or mass and vocal cord movement. Posterior glottic stenosis and subglottic narrowing are usually difficult to detect with certainty at indirect laryngoscopy.

A lateral X-ray may show a mass, cyst or inflammatory swelling (e.g. acute epiglottis). In non-urgent cases antero-posterior tomography may reveal the site and severity of a subglottic tumour or web, but horizontal computed tomographic scans are usually less helpful.

Therefore, in most cases, clinical and radiologic assessment suggests a provisional diagnosis for planning airway management. The laryngologist must understand the principles of the anaesthetic techniques and the action of the anaesthetic agents. Similarly the anaesthetist must be familiar with the instrumentation and methods of the laryngologist. Responsibility for control of the airway is shared but in an emergency it lies primarily with the laryngologist.

Initial airway management

From a practical point of view there are five broad possibilities:

1. Initial tracheotomy with local anaesthesia followed by general anaesthesia through the tracheotomy for direct endoscopy.
2. Spontaneous respiration using oxygen/volatile agent to achieve deep anaesthesia, laryngoscopy, topical anaesthesia, intubate and then paralyse.
3. Spontaneous respiration inhalational induction and test ventilation before administration of intravenous relaxant for endoscopic evaluation. Tracheotomy may prove to be necessary to ensure a reliable airway or to allow subsequent treatment.
4. Intravenous induction and test ventilation before administration of a muscle relaxant.
5. Intravenous induction, paralysis, ventilation, intubation and establishment of an airway for endoscopic assessment and treatment.

It is well recognized that preoxygenation and denitrogenation add a safety margin before induction of anaesthesia. To be effective the nitrogen in the functional residual volume of the lungs must be completely replaced by oxygen, a process that takes 6–8 minutes in a healthy adult but may take considerably longer in the presence of an obstructed airway. Prolonged preoxygenation is theoretically advanta-

Precautions for unexpected obstruction

Prepare for possible tracheotomy
- Infiltrate the neck
- Adjust overhead lights
- Tracheotomy tray ready to use

Prepare for 'crash' percutaneous tracheotomy

Prepare intubation equipment, tubes, bronchoscopes

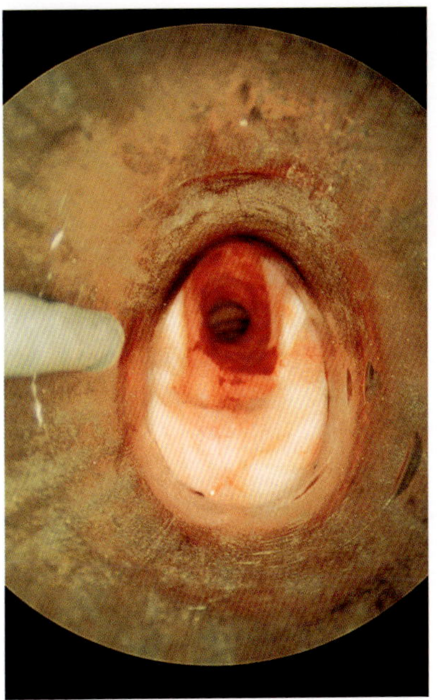

Figure **5.30**
Jet ventilation for subglottic stenosis. A subglottiscope retracts the vocal cords to display subglottic stenosis prior to laser treatment. A metal proximal jet cannula is in position for ventilation.

geous and, if it is not performed in all cases, a shortened period of preoxygenation should be considered for selected cases, where there is doubt that the airway can be secured in a reasonable time.

Patient safety must not be compromised for the sake of avoiding a tracheotomy; if there is serious doubt about effective airway control a tracheotomy should be performed under local anaesthesia. The anaesthetist provides supplemental oxygen via a face mask and secures intravenous access for additional safety and for anaesthesia once the airway is reliably established. In some cases a tracheotomy is required only after endoscopic assessment under general anaesthesia.

At all times, even when laryngeal obstruction is not severe and endoscopic assessment under general anaesthesia is considered reasonably safe, all precautions are taken to deal with sudden unexpected problems. The neck may be infiltrated with local anaesthesia, overhead lights are correctly positioned and a tracheotomy tray is made ready. Other equipment is prepared for immediate use: suction apparatus, light source with cables, laryngoscopes, various sizes of endotracheal tubes with introducers, a Benjet tube for jet ventilation, a proximal jetting cannula, a large-bore needle suitable for aspirating a cyst and, finally, bronchoscopes for forcible passage through an obstructed larynx or a subglottic stenosis. A short, large-bore needle passed through the cricothyroid membrane may be life saving in an acute emergency.

Intravenous access is always gained before any interference with the airway and monitoring equipment is connected before anaesthesia is commenced. Equipment is prepared to spray the larynx and upper trachea with topical lignocaine.

A good rule is never to abolish spontaneous respiration until it is certain that an airway can be established.

Which technique to use?

Initial laryngoscopy should confirm the most appropriate form of continuing ventilation, whether a proximal jetting cannula, a distal intratracheal jetting tube or repeated 'in-and-out' introduction (for ventilation) and withdrawal (for endoscopy) of a small-diameter endotracheal tube. The form of ventilation and anaesthesia chosen depends on the site and nature of the pathology, the chest wall compliance and the use of the carbon dioxide laser for endoscopic treatment. In some cases a combination of methods is useful, e.g. initial

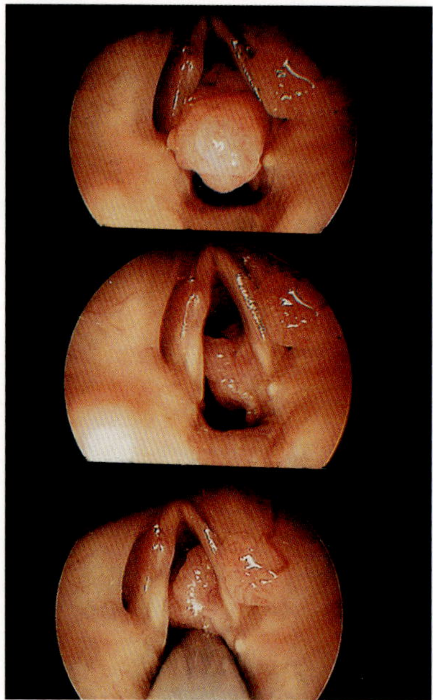

Figure **5.31**
Anaesthesia for obstructing papillomas. A 4-year-old with massive papillomas (top), the largest of which becomes subglottic on inspiration (middle). An endotracheal tube has been passed (bottom) to secure the airway while the large mass is removed.

intubation with later jet ventilation. If any form of jetting is used for ventilation, care is needed to guarantee the expiratory phase to avoid excessive intrathoracic pressure and the risk of airway rupture from barotrauma. Jetting is never commenced until a laryngoscope is in position to ensure an adequate airway, and intratracheal jetting must immediately cease if expiration is obstructed. An obstructed supraglottic or glottic airway makes ventilation by proximal jetting ineffective, but in subglottic stenosis successful ventilation can be achieved by distal jetting with a Benjet tube or by accurate aiming of the jet delivered by a proximal jet cannula with a subglottiscope in position (Fig. 5.30).

If control of the airway is lost at any time, a prompt and decisive response is needed. There are several options. Positive pressure ventilation with 100% oxygen can be applied using a face mask. A small-diameter, long endotracheal tube (4, 5, or even 6 mm) may be passed. A narrow-diameter ventilating bronchoscope can be forcibly introduced, e.g. past a mass of obstructing malignant tissue. Sometimes a tracheotomy is necessary once control has been regained. An emergency 'crash' tracheotomy can, in extremis, be life saving.

Other methods of airway management have been advocated. Although seldom required, awake intubation, usually pernasal, with topical anaesthesia, using an endotracheal tube guided over a flexible fibreoptic laryngoscope can be a valuable technique in experienced hands when dealing with extensive oropharyngeal and supraglottic tumours which do not permit adequate laryngeal visualization. Blind, awake intubation should be avoided because trauma might cause bleeding and precipitate complete obstruction. Percutaneous transtracheal jet ventilation is potentially hazardous and is not recommended as the needle is not introduced under visual control, expiration may be obstructed and there is a risk of surgical emphysema and pneumothorax.

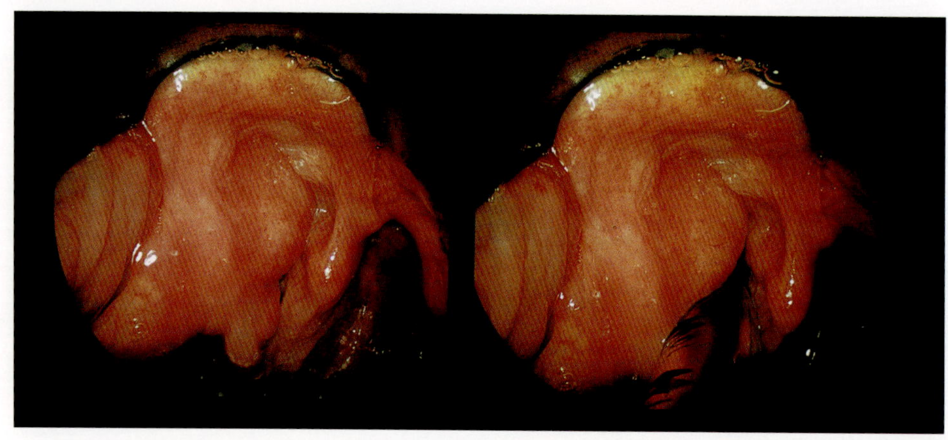

Figure **5.32**
Supraglottic obstruction and anaesthesia. A large left lateral saccular cyst in a 45-year-old woman (left) with progressive airway obstruction during induction of anaesthesia. An endotracheal tube has been positioned (right).

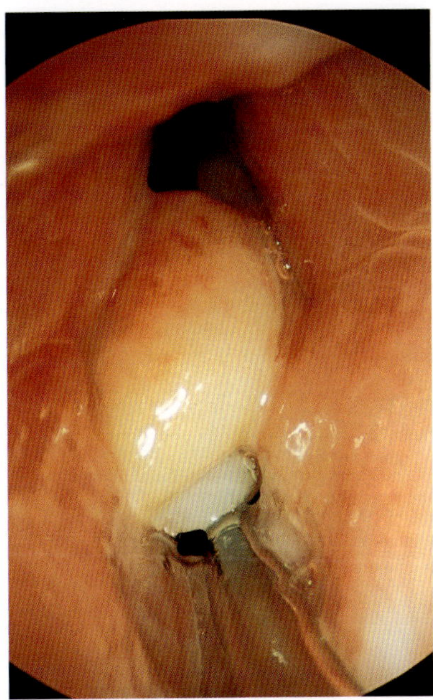

Figure **5.33**
Large granuloma causing obstruction. A very large left-sided vocal granuloma which acted as a 'ball-valve' making face-mask ventilation difficult. A small-diameter endotracheal tube was required to establish adequate ventilation.

Particular care should be taken to maintain the airway in patients with suspected or known glottic or supraglottic pathology such as a large mass of respiratory papillomas (Fig. 5.31), obstructing cyst (Fig. 5.32) or a large tumour such as a pedunculated vocal granuloma (Fig. 5.33) even when the obstruction may appear to be minimal at preoperative assessment. With an inhalational technique, progressive obstruction may occur as the depth of anaesthesia is increased. With a relaxant technique, assisted ventilation may be difficult or impossible if the mass acts as a ball valve; immediate intubation then becomes mandatory. In bilateral vocal cord paralysis or fixation of the cricoarytenoid joints, although inspiratory obstruction is present before induction of anaesthesia, neither face-mask ventilation nor intubation are difficult. An inhalational induction with gentle positive pressure is generally accepted as safest for acute epiglottis in adults – the same technique as advocated for use in children. In subglottic stenosis, satisfactory ventilation can usually be achieved by proximal jetting through a subglottiscope or distal jetting through a slim distal intratracheal tube.

Diagnostic assessment

The laryngoscopes we favour are the Lindholm, Benjamin slimline and Kleinsasser for adults and the Karl Storz, Benjamin–Lindholm and Holinger for infants and children. Various Hopkin's rod telescopes (0°, 30° and 70°) are used to examine the pharynx, larynx, subglottis and trachea in a systematic manner with careful attention given to the posterior glottic space, subglottic region, mobility of the cricoarytenoid joints and finally assessment of vocal cord movement as muscle tone returns at the end of the procedure. Biopsies are taken as necessary.

Subsequent management

The airway must be adequate to ensure safe recovery from anaesthesia allowing for residual respiratory depression and muscular weakness immediately following the procedure. In selected cases, pernasal endotracheal intubation for up to 1 or 2 hours permits return of muscle tone and a tracheotomy can be avoided. Postoperative monitoring in a fully staffed recovery unit with humidification of the inspired oxygen is a routine precaution.

Relief of airway obstruction is usually achieved at the time of initial diagnostic endoscopy, e.g. intubation for acute epiglottitis, removal of respiratory papillomas, vocal cord granulomas, polyps, laryngeal cysts, partial biopsy removal, laser removal of part of a tumour and treatment of a relatively 'thin' subglottic stenosis. However, if the airway has been made worse because surgical trauma has caused oedema or bleeding and the airway remains in jeopardy, a tracheotomy should be considered.

Summary

Endoscopic diagnostic assessment and treatment of upper airway obstruction is a difficult problem which can present unexpectedly. It requires a systematic and thoughtful approach to management with an understanding of the causes of airway obstruction and a knowledge of the principles of anaesthesia techniques and airway management.

A working diagnosis can usually be made from the history, the clinical features on examination, from

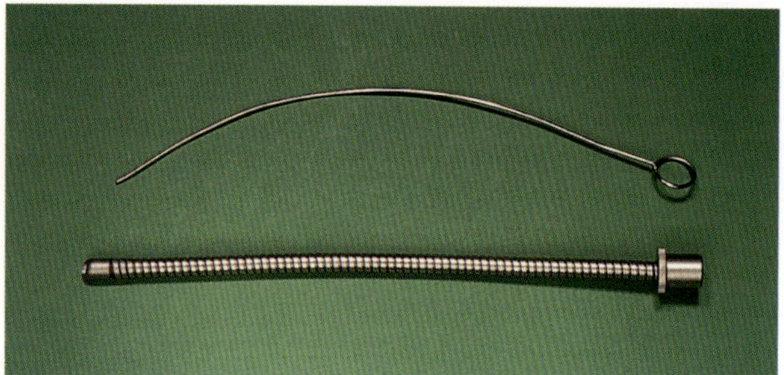

Figure **5.34**
Metal endotracheal tube. The tube is thick-walled, has a relatively small internal diameter and requires use of an introducer. (It is no longer manufactured.)

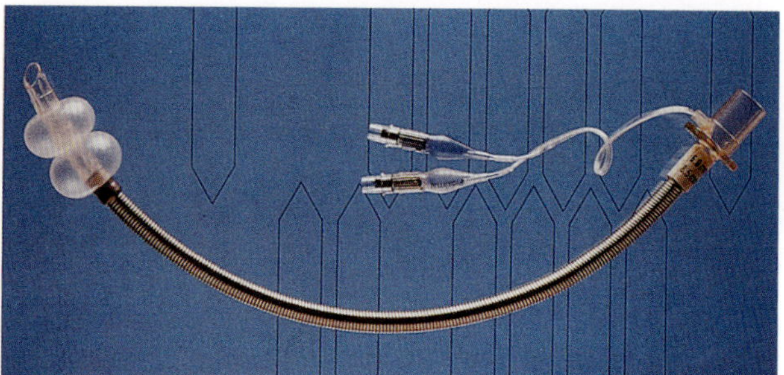

Figure **5.35**
Laser Flex tube. Constructed of flexible stainless steel with two distal polyvinyl chloride cuffs which are filled with saline. These tubes are useful to position through the stoma in a patient with a tracheotomy who is having laryngeal laser surgery.

indirect laryngoscopy and with assistance from the X-ray findings. It is then possible to plan the induction of anaesthesia for diagnostic endoscopy with maximum safety for the patient.

In most cases the safest and most controlled technique of general anaesthesia is a gaseous induction with assisted spontaneous respiration. When test ventilation indicates that the airway can be secured and maintained, administration of an intravenous relaxant provides the best conditions for endoscopy. Jet ventilation, either using a proximal jet cannula or a slim, distal intratracheal tube, usually offers the best conditions for the endoscopist. This approach permits accurate diagnosis and gives the best chance of avoiding a tracheotomy.

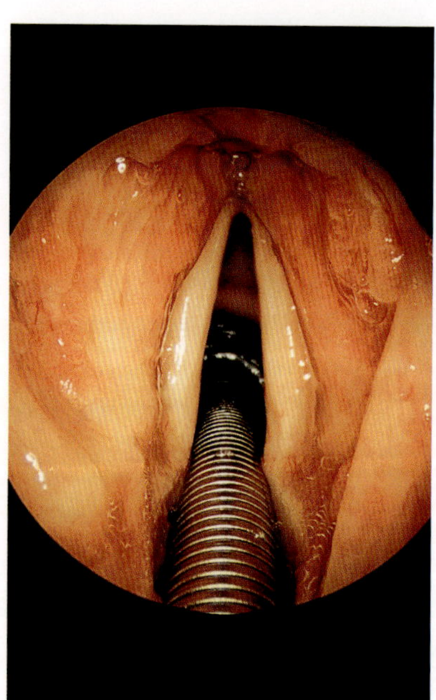

Figure **5.36**
Laser Flex tube in the larynx. Demonstrating good exposure of the supraglottis and vocal cords, but no view of the subglottis.

ANAESTHESIA FOR ENDOLARYNGEAL LASER SURGERY

Laser ignition of a combustible endotracheal tube positioned in the larynx during microlaryngeal surgery is a serious problem which has not been totally resolved. Tubes made of metal, red rubber, polyfluorotetraethylene and polyvinyl chloride have all been used. Tubes have been coated with so-called laser resistant material or covered with metal foil, but all are potentially flammable. Other important variables include the ambient oxygen concentration in the airway, the presence of body fluids, the presence of an opaque barium stripe on the tube itself, the power density of the laser strikes on the tube and the presence of helium to assist rapid dissipation of the heat.

Endotracheal tubes

The choice lies between laser-resistant tubes (made of metal, non-metal or a combination) and tubes with laser-resistant wrap (aluminium foil).

Metal

Metal endotracheal tubes cannot, of course, be ignited, but they are thick-walled, have a relatively small internal lumen, have no cuff, are cumbersome, may be traumatic during introduction, can become overheated and they severely limit exposure in the glottic and subglottic region (Fig. 5.34).

Red rubber

A red rubber endotracheal tube will ignite but burns with little smoke which is less damaging than the combustion products of a polyvinyl chloride tube because the latter produces very irritating smoke. Red rubber tubes are irritating to laryngeal mucosa and are no longer recommended for anaesthesia of any form.

Synthetic

Polyfluorotetraethylene or polyvinyl chloride tubes will ignite. A burning polyvinyl chloride tube produces poisonous gases such as hydrogen chloride. A siliconized rubber tube burns to an ash which is irritating to respiratory mucosa.

Attempts have been made to wrap a small-diameter plastic tube with aluminium foil to protect the tube or to coat it with a 'laser-proof' covering. Although this gives some protection, it is not always successful and cannot be given an unqualified recommendation. The foil may not adhere to the tube, it may become loose, kink or be dislodged so that the tube becomes relatively at risk. Superheating of the metal tape by repeated laser exposure or reflection from the metal tape may burn nearby tissue. The cuff and other unprotected parts of the tube may be at risk. If a cuffed tube is used the balloon should be filled with saline. Foil-wrapped or so-called laser-proofed tubes may give a false sense of security.

The Laser Flex endotracheal tube (Mallinckrodt, St Louis, Missouri) has two polyvinyl chloride cuffs which are filled with isotonic saline and a flexible stainless steel and polyvinyl chloride shaft (Figure 5.35). Ventilation requires careful monitoring because of the small bore of the tube. However, the presence of polyvinyl chloride cuffs means that ignition, although very unlikely, is still possible; the makers warn that exposure of the stainless steel to the laser beam can result in heating and damage to surrounding tissue. The tubes are made in a variety of adult and paediatric sizes (Fig. 5.36).

Anaesthesia and laser surgery

Avoid an endotracheal tube if possible
Use a small-diameter intratracheal jet tube
Otherwise use a laser-protected tube
Use 40% oxygen : 60% helium
Protect patient's eyes and face with a wet towel
Care by the laryngologist
Wide-diameter laryngoscope if possible
Be ready for a fire!

Acceptable techniques

In adults a proximal jetting technique with a metal cannula secured within the lumen of the laryngoscope avoids the presence of a combustible tube in the larynx, but ventilation may be unreliable, the mucosa becomes dry and secretions may be forced into the lower respiratory tract.

A distal intratracheal Benjet tube or a tube of similar design, whose external diameter is very small, is safe when used with reasonable care especially when the anaesthetic gas jetting mixture is helium and oxygen. Helium gas has a high thermal diffusivity and use of a 40% oxygen : 60% helium gas mixture has two advantages. Firstly, it reduces the oxygen concentration and secondly, due to the conductive qualities of helium, heat is rapidly dissipated minimizing the likelihood of endotracheal tube ignition. Using this gas mixture gives adequate and appropriate ventilation.

Care by the endoscopic surgeon using the laser remains the single most important safety factor. It is important to check the laser function, especially the alignment of the carbon dioxide and helium beams, before commencing an operation. The power switch of the laser is activated only immediately before use and it is turned off when the laser is no longer required. A laryngoscope with a wide proximal opening lessens the likelihood of inadvertent firing outside the lumen of the laryngoscope. Use of a dull metallic finish on the laryngoscope may reduce the chance of reflection of the laser causing indirect impact of the beam upon personnel in the operating theatre who must wear protective spectacles.

Fire in the airway

If an airway fire occurs or if there is any possibility that the tube has been burnt or is about to ignite, all laser treatment must be stopped and the tube removed immediately. Saline or water should always be available to inject into the airway or to douse an external fire. A plan of action should have been decided upon in advance and the operating room and ancillary personnel should be familiar with it.

If an endotracheal tube was in place, no ventilation should occur as it may spread the fire further down the tracheobronchial tree. The delivery of oxygen is stopped, the tube removed and ventilation by face mask resumed. Once the fire is under control, the airway should be carefully evaluated to determine the site and extent of any burns. There will be black carbon particles throughout the airway with coagulation of proteins in the mucosal surface epithelium. Loss of alveolar surfactant causes atelectasis and increased capillary permeability leads to frothy pulmonary oedema. The carbonaceous material should be removed by bronchoscopy together with any particulate foreign body or coagulated tissue. Further management includes chest X-ray to determine whether there is barotrauma, possible tracheotomy or long-term intubation, treatment of bronchospasm, and antibiotic therapy, but the use of corticosteroids is controversial.

Laser fire in the airway

HAVE A PLAN OF ACTION
Turn off the laser
Discontinue oxygen ventilation
Remove the endotracheal tube
Ventilate by face mask
Inject saline into the airway
Douse an external fire
Evaluate the burns
Remove carbonaceous coagulum

BIBLIOGRAPHY

Benjamin B (1984) Anesthesia for laryngoscopy. *Ann Otol Rhinol Laryngol* **93**: 338–42.

Benjamin B, Gronow D (1979) A new tube for microlaryngeal surgery. *Anaesth Intensive Care* **7**: 258–63.

Cabley M, Vaughn RS (1992) Recognition and management of difficult airway problems. *Brit J Anaesth* **68**: 90–7.

Hunsaker DH (1994) Anesthesia for microlaryngeal surgery: the case for subglottic jet ventilation. *Laryngoscope* **104** (Suppl 65): 1–30.

Kilham H, Gillis J, Benjamin B (1987) Severe upper airway obstruction. *Pediatr Clin North Am* **34**: 1–14.

Ossoff, RH (1989) Laser safety in otolaryngology head and neck surgery: anesthetic and educational considerations for laryngeal surgery. *Laryngoscope* **99**: 1–26.

Pashayan AC, Gravenstein JS, Cassise NJ, McLaughlin G (1988) The helium protocol for laryngo-tracheal operations with CO_2 laser: a retrospective review of 523 cases. *Anesthesiology* **68**: 801–4.

6 Direct laryngoscopy

BASICS

Direct endoscopy allows examination of the hypopharynx, larynx and trachea through an open laryngoscope which has been positioned through the mouth. Direct laryngoscopy is used routinely by anaesthetists for peroral and pernasal passage of an endotracheal tube for controlled ventilation during general anaesthesia. Anaesthetists' laryngoscopes, designed solely for intubation, are different to the laryngoscopes used by laryngologists. Direct laryngoscopy for intubation is also employed by anaesthetists and intensivists either in an emergency for resuscitation or, more often, for planned long-term assisted ventilation of a patient in an intensive care ward.

Laryngoscopy by laryngologists

Direct laryngoscopy has been used for many years by otolaryngologists for diagnostic inspection, biopsy, endoscopic microsurgery (e.g. removal of a vocal cord polyp, injection of Gelfoam or Teflon paste), or for carbon dioxide laser surgery of the larynx (e.g. removal of papillomas, treatment of early malignancy). Examination of the larynx under general anaesthesia is often combined with tracheobronchoscopy, oesophagoscopy and nasendoscopy in infants and children with suspected obstructive disease in the upper airways and in adults with suspected malignant disease.

Direct laryngoscopy is performed in a fully equipped operating theatre under general anaesthesia with monitoring of the patient's heart rate, electrocardiographic pattern, respiratory function, end-tidal carbon dioxide and oxygen saturation. Until recently, direct endoscopy was performed in some clinics in both children and adults using sedation and local anaesthesia but without general anaesthesia. Now with safer, more versatile techniques, general anaesthesia supplemented with local, topical anaesthesia is used. There are many techniques of general anaesthesia depending on the skill, experience and personal preference of the anaesthetist and endoscopist. When general anaesthesia was not used, procedures had to be performed quickly, but with modern, controlled conditions there is seldom a restraint on time, providing adequate opportunity for comprehensive evaluation, documentation and teaching.

The laryngoscope, which has many different designs, is fundamental to the laryngologist and is basically a modified open tube with illumination provided either at the proximal or the distal end. In adults the favoured laryngoscopes depend on the laryngologist's preferences in North America, Europe, Japan or other countries, while in infants and children the range of laryngoscopes and bronchoscopes manufactured in Germany by Karl Storz are generally favoured.

Laryngoscopes can be broadly classified as those:

- for general purpose and routine examination
- for special purposes, including microsurgical and laser procedures.

Many laryngoscopes are suitable for both purposes.

The personal preference of the laryngologist, the area to be examined, the procedure to be undertaken and the method of anaesthesia will influence which laryngoscope will be chosen.

The wide choice of purpose-designed instruments (e.g. an anterior commissure laryngoscope or a subglottiscope) often makes it necessary to change from one instrument to another to improve surgical exposure or gain optimal access to the anterior commissure or the subglottis and upper trachea. The advantage of a universal, quick change-over illumination attachment such as the Benjamin–Havas clip (Fig. 6.1) then becomes apparent.

For introduction of a bronchoscope or an endotracheal tube some older laryngoscopes have a removable slide to provide a side opening; others have a wide slot on the right hand side.

Laryngoscopes for adults

Those in common use include the Kleinsasser, Jako, Dedo, Jackson, Lindholm, Nagashima, Holinger and Benjamin laryngoscopes. Some are diagnostic, intubating or operative laryngoscopes. Others are special purpose laryngoscopes designed to facilitate exposure of particular anatomical areas. Some are advantageous for microsurgical or laser procedures.

General purpose

There are many all-purpose instruments of various sizes which are standard in many laryngology units.

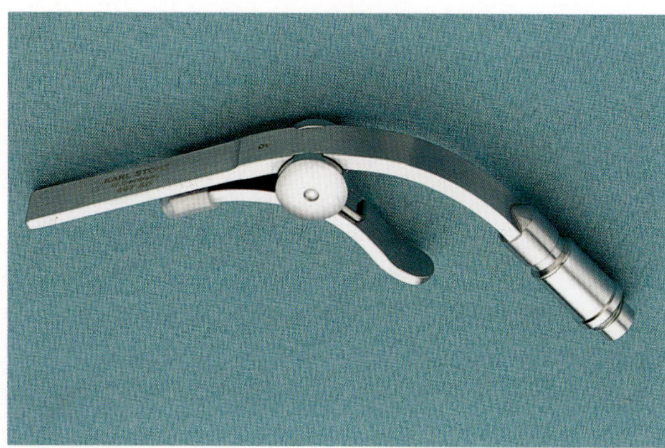

Figure **6.1**
Benjamin–Havas fibreoptic light clip which facilitates quick transfer from one laryngoscope to another. It can be used on almost all adult and many paediatric laryngoscopes.

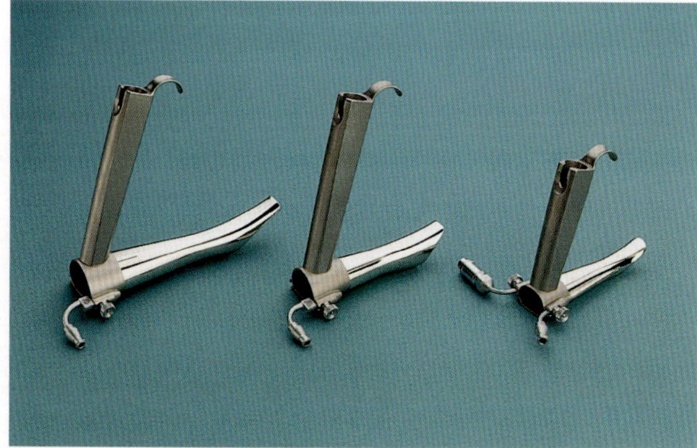

Figure **6.2**
Adult Lindholm (left) and the large and small paediatric Benjamin–Lindholm laryngoscopes. Each has its own metal cannula for anaesthetic gases.

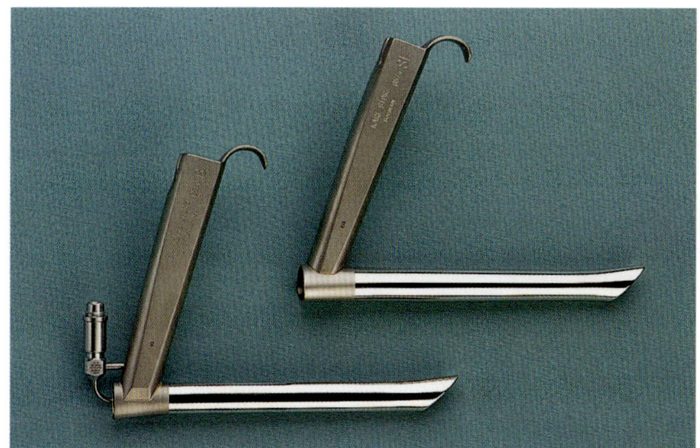

Figure **6.3**
Original monocular Holinger anterior commissure laryngoscope with distal lighting (below) and the Benjamin slimline laryngoscope and subglottiscope (above).

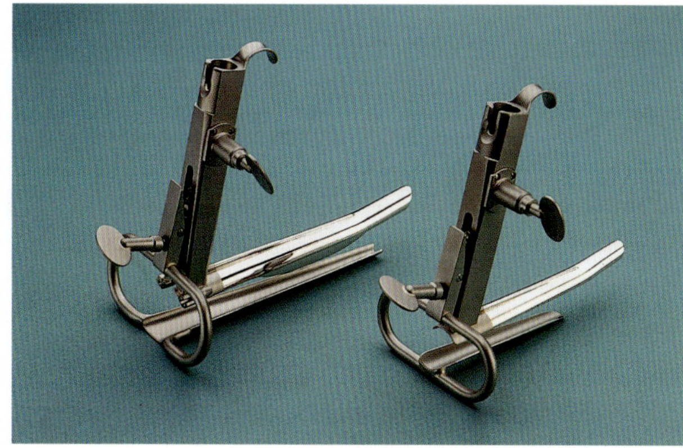

Figure **6.4**
Large and small Weerda distending operating laryngoscopes. Once in place, the blades are spread apart to enhance the working area.

The Lindholm laryngoscopes (Fig. 6.2) require special mention. They have a unique design which provides a wide view of the laryngopharynx when the distal beak is placed in the midline at the base of the tongue anterior to the epiglottis. The wide 20 × 40 mm proximal opening ensures binocular viewing with ample room for instrumentation.

Special purpose

The Holinger anterior commissure laryngoscope (Fig. 6.3) is a monocular instrument which has been in use for many years. It is usually hand-held but can be suspended and is especially useful in larynges which are difficult to see and where the anterior commissure requires exposure. As the proximal end is too narrow for a binocular view, it should not be used for laser surgery.

The Benjamin slimline binocular microlaryngoscope and subglottiscope (Fig. 6.3) is a modification of the Holinger laryngoscope with a wider proximal opening making it suitable for binocular viewing through the microscope and for laser surgery. It is designed for use in patients with anatomical abnormalities such as prominent teeth, large tongue or short neck which make the larynx difficult to expose with other laryngoscopes. When used as a subglottiscope, the distal tip spreads the vocal cords for examination or surgery in the subglottic region and upper trachea.

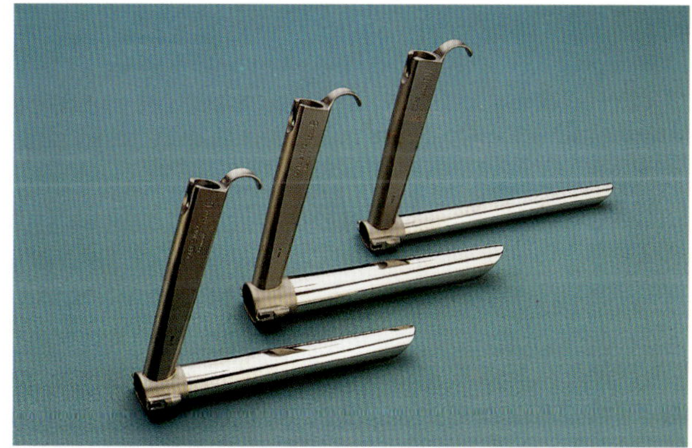

Figure **6.5**
Three of the complete set of seven well-known Kleinsasser laryngoscopes for adults and children.

The Weerda distending operating laryngoscopes (Fig. 6.4) are narrow and easy to introduce before expansion of the blades. Once in place, the blades can be spread in two directions, proximally and distally, for an improved view.

For regular routine use we prefer the Lindholm, Kleinsasser (Fig. 6.5) and Benjamin slimline laryngoscopes.

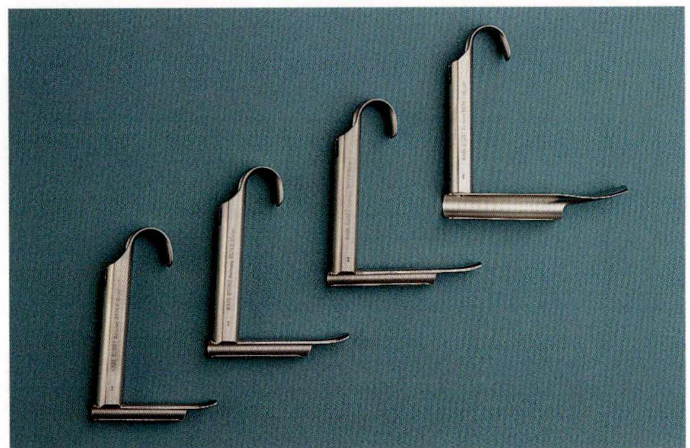

Figure **6.6**
Set of four Karl Storz open-sided laryngoscopes with proximal prismatic lighting for general purpose paediatric use.

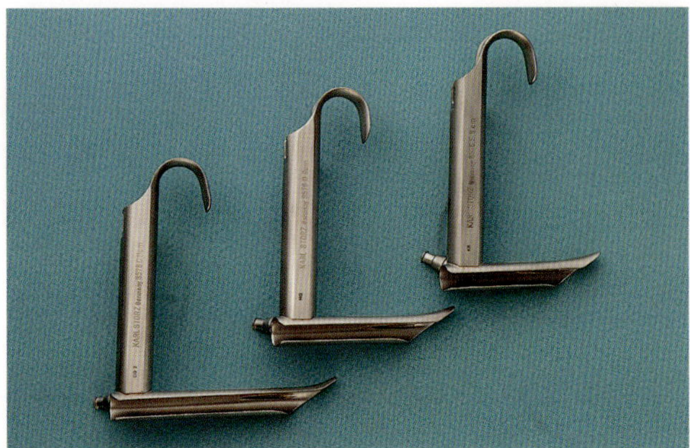

Figure **6.7**
Set of three Parsons operative and intubating paediatric laryngoscopes which can be positioned in front or behind the epiglottis.

Most of the adult instruments mentioned can be used for microsurgical operative procedures and for carbon dioxide laser surgery.

Laryngoscopes for infants and children

There are more laryngoscopes for paediatric than for adult use because they are required for both common and rare conditions in graduated sizes for patients of all ages. A direct view of the oropharynx, larynx and upper trachea allows investigation and treatment of the many congenital and acquired conditions of the upper aerodigestive tract in low birthweight or preterm babies, infants, toddlers and children.

The design of the Karl Storz paediatric laryngoscopes stands alone in providing a complete and innovative range. Standard paediatric laryngoscopes include the Karl Storz set and the Parson's set. Special purpose laryngoscopes include the Lindholm–Benjamin, the Holinger–Benjamin, the Kleinsasser, the Benjamin operating laryngoscope and the Benjamin subglottiscopes.

General purpose

Standard Karl Storz diagnostic and intubating laryngoscopes (Fig. 6.6) are made in four sizes: 8.0 cm for premature and newborns, 9.5 cm for infants, 11.0 cm for children and 13.5 cm for adolescents. The anterior beak can be positioned either in the valleculae (in front of the epiglottis) or in the larynx itself (behind the epiglottis). Lighting uses a proximal prismatic light deflector whose fibreoptic light-carrying cable is delivered inside the handle of the laryngoscope.

Parsons laryngoscopes (Fig. 6.7) are made in three sizes: 8.0 cm for premature and newborn, 9.5 cm for infants and 11.0 cm for toddlers and older children. They are suitable for general purpose diagnostic evaluation, passage of an endotracheal tube or bronchoscope and, after suspension, they can be used for some types of microlaryngeal surgery. A fixed channel on the left-hand side allows continuous insufflation of anaesthetic gases or oxygen.

A portable battery handle can be supplied for both the Parsons and Storz laryngoscopes and provides illumination for emergency situations.

Special purpose

Benjamin–Lindholm laryngoscopes (Fig. 6.2) are made in two paediatric sizes: 9.5 cm for premature babies from 1000 g to infants of a few months old, and 11.0 cm for children from 18 months to 8 years old. When positioned with the distal beak in the midline at the base of the tongue, a wide view of the

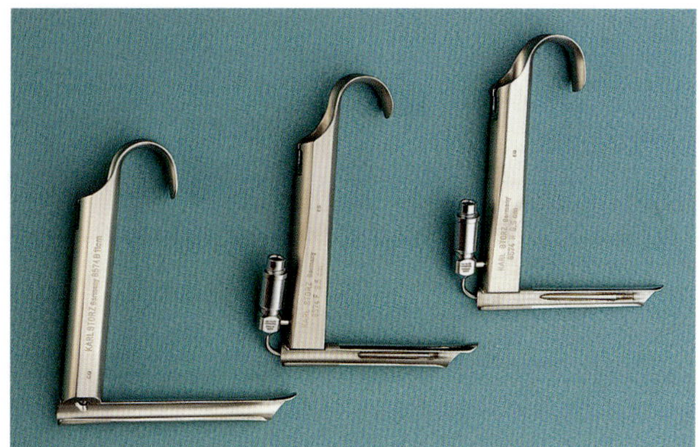

Figure **6.8**
Three different-sized Holinger–Benjamin slotted, small-diameter paediatric instruments for use when laryngoscopy and intubation is difficult or impossible with other laryngoscopes.

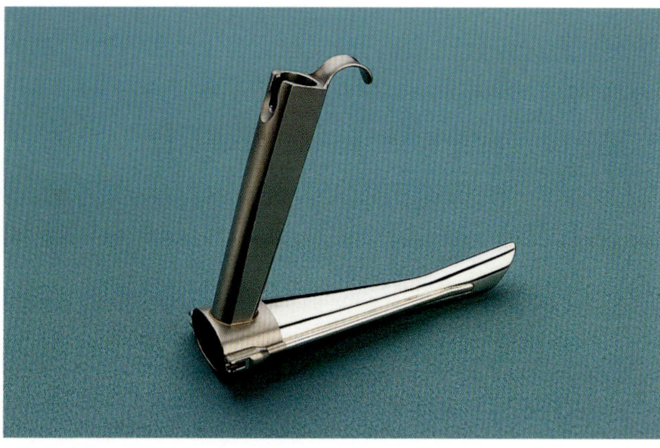

Figure **6.9**
Benjamin paediatric operating laryngoscope with a wide proximal end for microlaryngoscopy and laser surgery. There is a large and a small size.

laryngopharynx is readily available. Suspension not only facilitates precise diagnostic evaluation with telescopes, but in most patients provides a wide exposure for microlaryngeal or laser surgery. Anaesthetic gases are insufflated via a metal cannula which fixes in the left side of the laryngoscope.

Holinger–Benjamin laryngoscopes (Fig. 6.8) are made in three sizes: 9.5 cm with a very narrow distal end for very low birthweight and newborn babies, 9.5 cm with a larger distal end for newborn babies and 11.0 cm for older children. These laryngoscopes allow full evaluation of the anterior commissure, the posterior glottic space and the subglottis, and are essential for the introduction of an endotracheal tube or bronchoscope when the pharyngeal anatomy makes visualization of the glottis difficult or impossible with standard laryngoscopes. The slim blade and slightly upturned distal end allow laryngoscopy and intubation in patients with Pierre Robin sequence and other craniofacial abnormalities or where macroglossia or a large tumour obstructs the pharynx. They are especially useful for diagnosis of a congenital laryngeal web in the anterior glottis. In the posterior glottis they assist exposure in the diagnosis of a congenital interarytenoid web, congenital laryngeal cleft and acquired posterior glottic stenosis.

The Benjamin operating laryngoscopes (Fig. 6.9), now in two sizes, allow binocular vision during microlaryngoscopy and laser surgery and give an excellent view of the larynx because the wide proximal opening (20 × 40 mm for the larger and 15 × 28 mm for the smaller) provides stereoscopic viewing and easy introduction of instruments. Anaesthetic gases are introduced through a metal cannula which fixes into an external channel.

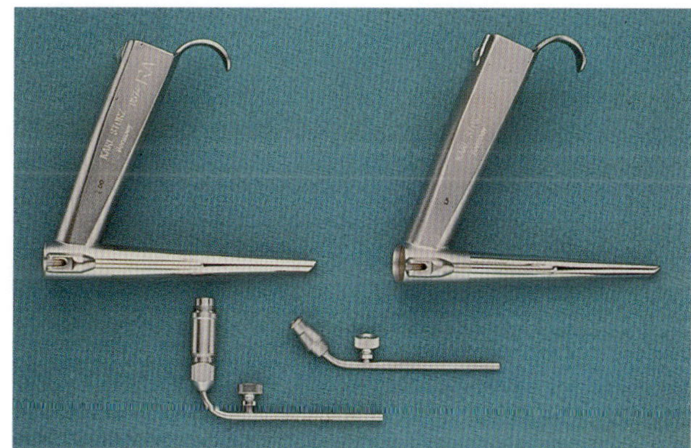

Figure **6.10**
Benjamin subglottiscopes, large and small, for diagnostic inspection, microsurgery and laser surgery in the subglottis and upper trachea in infants and newborn.

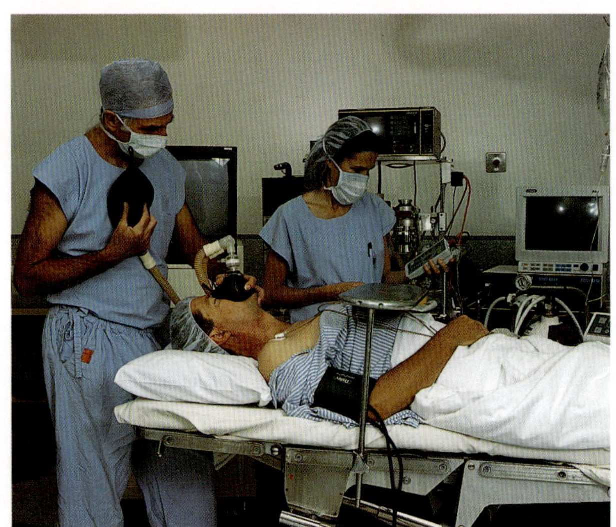

(a)

Figure **6.11a**
General view of an adult undergoing anaesthesia on a regular operating table prior to microlaryngeal surgery. Note the overtable to support the suspension apparatus. b. Suggested arrangement of personnel and equipment in the operating theatre. c. Diagnostic endoscopy in an infant under general anaesthesia. Note the overhead radiant heater, careful monitoring by the anaesthetist, the range of instruments available and the focus of attention on the procedure. d. Anaesthesia with spontaneous respiration has been induced using a face mask. Local anaesthetic solution will be sprayed on the larynx and into the subglottic region by the anaesthetist. e. The endoscopist sits at the head of the table; the face mask and Guedel airway are removed to allow direct laryngoscopy. f. While the laryngoscope is in place, the patient breathes room air for a short time as shown here. Alternatively gases can be administered continuously via either a nasopharyngeal tube or a metal cannula in the side of the laryngoscope.

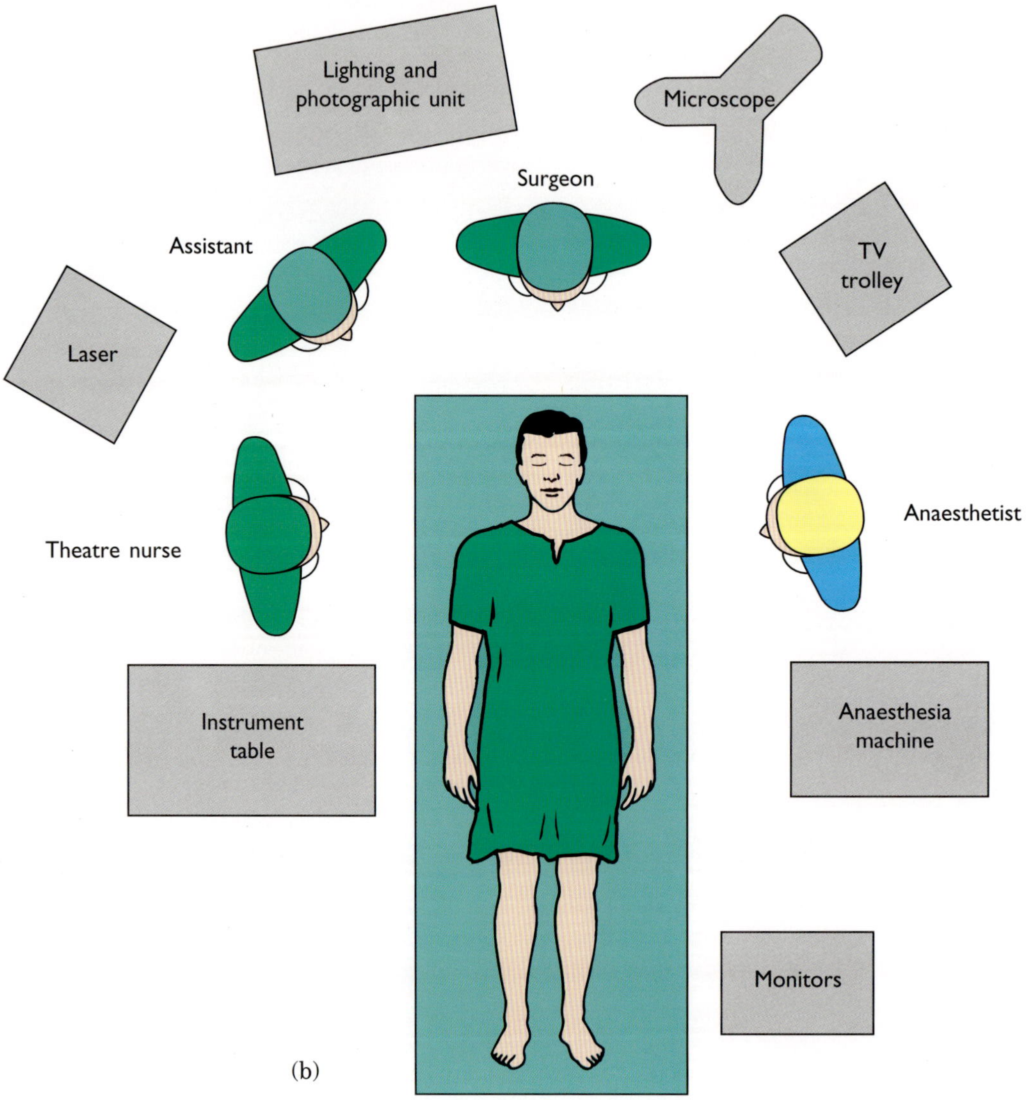

(b)

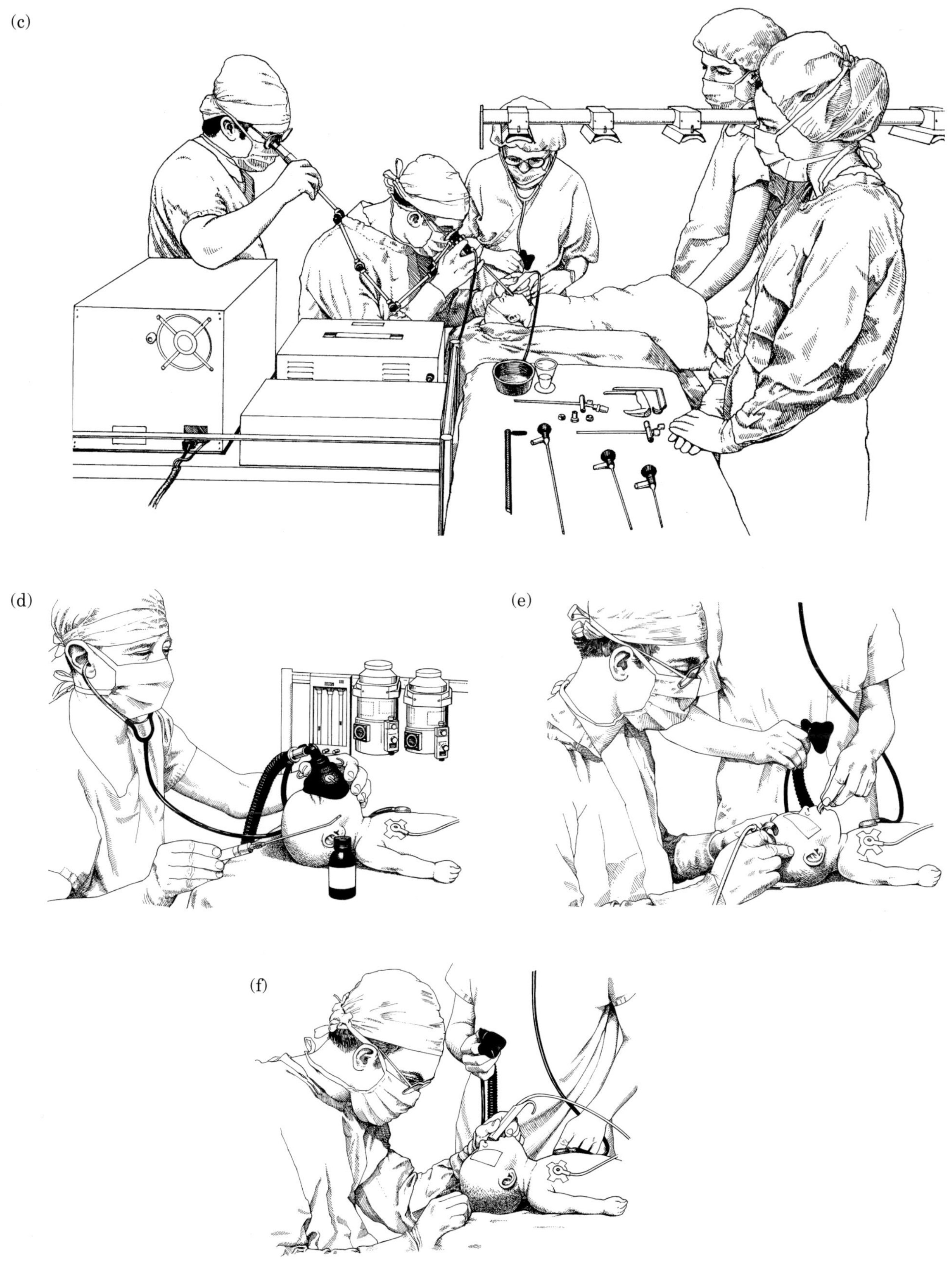
(c)
(d)
(e)
(f)

Paediatric laryngoscopes

General purpose
- Karl Storz (set of 4)
- Parsons (3)

Special purpose
- Benjamin–Lindholm (set of 2)
- Holinger–Benjamin (3)
- Benjamin operating (2)
- Benjamin subglottiscopes (2)

The Benjamin subglottiscope (Fig. 6.10) is available in two sizes, the larger with a distal opening of 4.7 mm, the smaller with a distal opening of 3.5 mm; both have a length of 11 cm, proximal opening 26 × 13 mm. They are designed for diagnostic inspection and surgical or laser treatment of subglottic or upper tracheal pathology in infants, e.g. congenital subglottic haemangioma, acquired subglottic stenosis, ductal retention cysts or granulations above the site of a tracheotomy.

TECHNIQUE OF DIRECT LARYNGOSCOPY

Positioning of patient

The patient, whether infant, child or adult, lies supine on a regular operating table (Fig. 6.11a); there is no need for a head support or for an assistant to hold the head. A small pillow under the head is optional. A suitably sized general purpose laryngoscope is chosen according to the circumstances and individual requirements.

Figure 6.11b shows an operating theatre 'set-up' which has been found suitable for both adults and children. Figure 6.11c shows a general view during endoscopy on a neonate.

In infants and small children anaesthesia is induced with a face mask (Fig. 6.11d) which is removed briefly and the administration of gases is temporarily suspended for application of local anaesthetic solution and thereafter, during each stage of the endoscopic procedure. An appropriate laryngoscope is selected, the face mask and Guedel airway temporarily removed (Fig. 6.11e) and the laryngoscope inserted for the initial naked-eye laryngoscopy (Fig. 6.11f).

Anaesthesia

The many techniques of anaesthesia are discussed in Chapter 5.

Introduction of laryngoscope

The barrel of the laryngoscope, smeared with lubricant, is passed into the right-hand side of the mouth alongside the tongue, taking care not to lacerate the lower lip or injure the teeth, gums or tongue. The anaesthetist will already have removed any dentures. Special care is required if there are sharp, protruding or irregular teeth, or dental crowns or caps. In some cases a dental protection device should be used, but in most instances careful technique and several layers of gauze will protect the edges of the upper teeth from trauma.

The laryngoscope is slid behind the base of the tongue in the midline to expose the epiglottis. The Lindholm laryngoscope is designed to be placed in the midline between the base of the tongue and the anterior surface of the epiglottis, positioned equally between the right and the left valleculae so that gentle lifting together with forward pressure against the midline glosso-epiglottic fold causes the epiglottis to lift, exposing the larynx and glottic opening. Most other laryngoscopes (e.g. Jako or Kleinsasser) are designed to be placed behind the epiglottis; they should be gently manoeuvred until an optimal view of the larynx is obtained. A lifting action is required; a lever action against the teeth should not be used. When the required visualization has been obtained the laryngoscope holder and chest support are fixed in position. If exposure of the anterior larynx is 'tight', further gentle extension after a few minutes, using the mechanical advantage provided by the laryngoscope holder mechanism can often improve access.

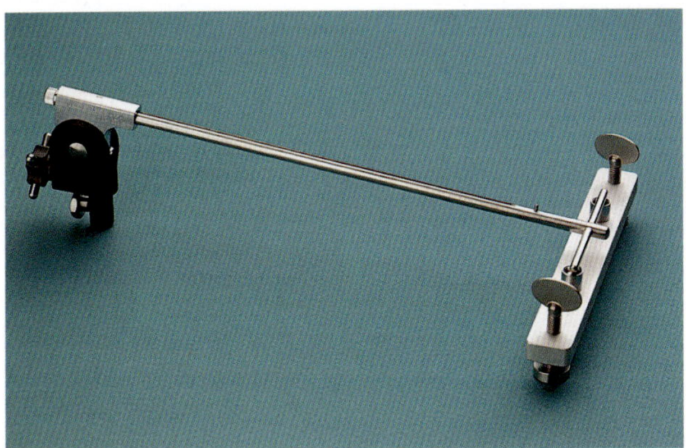

Figure **6.12**
Benjamin-Parsons suspension system with vertical adjustment by a single rotary knob on the handle. The crossbar (adjustable on each side) provides a wide, stable base resting on the metal overtable which itself is attached to the operating table.

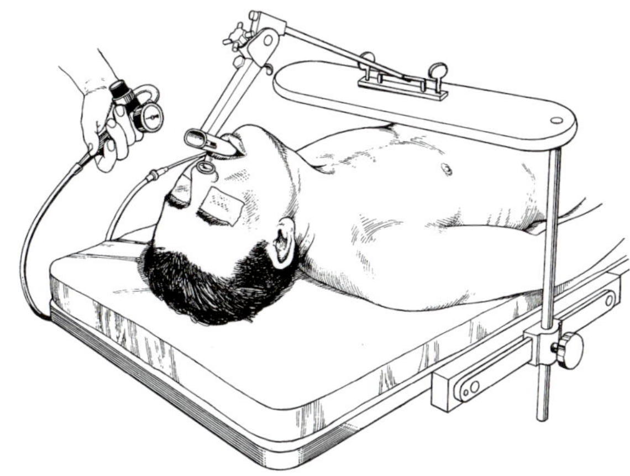

Figure **6.13**
A self-retaining laryngoscope holder is securely in position, supported free of the patient's chest by a Mustard table.

Laryngoscopy

During these positioning manoeuvres the head and neck are extended to improve exposure of the larynx by lifting the laryngoscope. External pressure on the neck over the larynx with gentle counter-pressure from the distal beak of the laryngoscope allows manipulation to give a better view of the larynx (Zeitels and Vaughan 1994).

When jet ventilation is in use for anaesthesia, ventilation *must not commence* until the glottic opening has been viewed to ensure unimpeded expiration.

The laryngoscope can be gently manipulated into as good a position as the individual patient's anatomy will allow. Endoscopic access to the larynx depends upon size of the teeth, degree of micrognathia, mobility of the temporomandibular joints, size and instability of the tongue, size and degree of overhang of the epiglottis, extension of the cervical spine and head and the nature of the pathology. A judgement is made whether to continue with the chosen laryngoscope or to change to a design which will give better exposure.

One of the Kleinsasser (or similar) laryngoscopes should be chosen for exposure of lesions on the vocal cords; the false cords are displaced out of the field by the beak of the laryngoscope which also partly abducts the vocal folds, widening the glottic opening.

While the laryngoscope is held in the left hand, all anatomical areas are checked including the posterior pharyngeal wall, the right and left piriform fossae, the epiglottis and its tubercle, the false cords, aryepiglottic folds, ventricles, vocal cords, anterior commissure, posterior glottic space and subglottic space. Particular attention is directed towards the membranous vocal folds, cricoarytenoid joints, general symmetry and, most importantly, the pathological lesion or lesions are carefully evaluated.

When access is extremely difficult the Benjamin slimline laryngoscope can be passed obliquely from the right-hand side of the mouth, at the same time turning the head to the left side as the laryngoscope is manipulated between the tongue and the wall of the pharynx.

Suspension

The Riecker–Kleinsasser, Benjamin–Parsons (Fig. 6.12) or Loewy laryngoscope holders are recommended. Suspension allows use of both hands and provides an unchanging view by maintaining the laryngoscope firmly in the airway.

The laryngoscope-holder is adjusted to rest firmly on an overtable (Fig. 6.13), which itself is clamped to the side of the operating table so that the whole assembly moves as a unit when the operating table is raised, lowered or tilted. Neither the transverse metal plate nor the rubber ring of the laryngoscope holder should lie directly on the patient's chest as respiration would be restricted.

Mucus is sucked from the surface of the larynx and the various structures examined with care. Palpation with a suction tube (preferably with a smooth beaded end) or a probe assists evaluation of the pliability of the vocal folds and the mobility of the cricoarytenoid joints. Examination with telescopes is undertaken, allowing an assistant and the operating room personnel to share the endoscopic view using a Wittmoser articulated optical arm or a beam splitter attached to a small television camera. Finally, the microscope is positioned for surgical procedures.

At the end of the procedure, as anaesthesia is discontinued, vocal cord movement can be observed. The adequacy and symmetry of vocal cord movement in adults and older children should, of course, have been fully assessed by indirect laryngoscopy prior to examination under anaesthesia.

Three-stage laryngoscopy

Under general anaesthesia there are three stages of direct laryngoscopy.

1 Hand-held laryngoscopy
- The first stage allows preliminary examination of the laryngopharynx with the naked eye or with a telescope. The airway for anaesthesia is secured and the site of pathology is localized.

2 Suspension laryngoscopy
- The second stage requires that a laryngoscope be placed in suspension facilitating detailed examination with rigid telescopes, both straight-ahead and angled. The laryngologist can use both hands for documentation either by still photography or tele-video.

In infants and children examination of the larynx is usually combined with tracheobronchoscopy (both with the naked eye and with telescopes) and sometimes with oesophagoscopy and nasendoscopy. These examinations are performed before microlaryngoscopy.

3 Microlaryngoscopy
- The third stage uses the unparalleled magnification provided by the operating microscope for precise microlaryngoscopy, microlaryngeal surgery or laser surgery.

During microlaryngoscopy or microlaryngeal surgery observation is confined to the larynx; there is not the flexibility of endoscopic visualization nor the ease of photographic or tele-video documentation that is available with telescopes.

Technique with telescopes

Difficult areas such as the valleculae, the piriform fossae, the laryngeal ventricles, the anterior commissure, the posterior glottic space and the subglottic region can be seen with the brightly illuminated magnified view obtained using Hopkins' telescopes. The full extent of malignancies can be accurately measured and mapped. Hidden pathology in the ventricle can be identified prior to biopsy or removal. The postcricoid region (and even the upper oesophagus) can sometimes be exposed while the Lindholm laryngoscope is in place (see Fig. 6.2), by lifting the thyroid cartilage through the soft tissues of the neck. Anatomy not visualized through the laryngoscope can be identified using an angled telescope. A selection of Hopkins' rigid rod lens optical telescopes should be available to provide superb resolution, contrast, natural colour and a wide viewing angle. They are produced in different lengths, different diameters and different angles of viewing including 0°, 30°, 70° and 120°. The diameters of the telescope range from 1.9, 2.8, 4.0, 5.0, 5.8 up to a 10.0 mm telescope which is designed especially for documentation.

Technique with microscope

After completion of hand-held laryngoscopy and suspension laryngoscopy, the microscope is moved into position for microsurgery or laser treatment. A 400-mm objective lens is used so that the working distance between the lens and the laryngoscope is approximately 200 mm. Magnification of 4, 6, 10, 16 or 25 times can be chosen, and some surgical microscopes have a zoom magnification system.

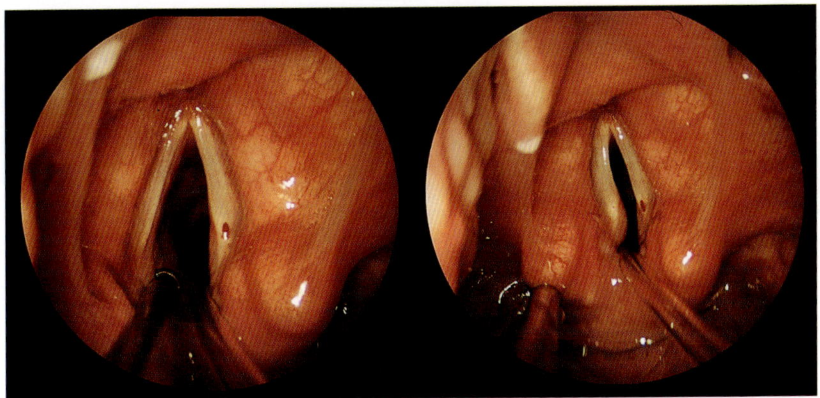

Figure **6.14**
Medial and lateral palpation using a sucker, to test mobility of the cricoarytenoid joint.

By lateral retraction of the ventricular fold with a suction tip or probe and with pressure on the external neck to rotate the larynx, most of the laryngeal ventricle can be evaluated through the microscope, but usually not as completely as with a 30° or 70° telescope.

The vocal cord can be 'rolled' to expose the subglottic surface by applying gentle pressure with a suction tip or blunt instrument just lateral to the edge of the vocal fold. The posterior surface of the epiglottis may be difficult to see using the microscope, but should already have been evaluated with telescopes. Mobility of the arytenoid cartilage on the articular facet of the cricoid cartilage on each side can be assessed only during direct laryngoscopy (Fig. 6.14). The operator must ensure that the position of the laryngoscope blade does not restrict joint movement or displace the arytenoid cartilage. A blunt probe or suction tip placed against the medial surface of the body of the arytenoid just behind the vocal process is used to move the arytenoid and test lateral displacement. The probe is then placed in the piriform fossa against the lateral surface of the arytenoid to move it medially. With experience accurate assessment of normal mobility, restricted mobility or fixation of the cricoarytenoid joint can be made.

Contact endoscopy

Andrea et al (1995) from Portugal advocate contact endoscopy during microlaryngoscopy using a Homau contact endoscope capable of 60 × 150 magnification, but the technique has not gained wide acceptance. After staining with methylene blue, the vocal cord epithelium is visualized to assess the cellular pattern and vasculature in vivo. Direct evaluation of the regularity of the epithelium, size and colour of the nuclei, ratio of nucleus to cytoplasm, presence of nucleoli and mitoses are assessed in an attempt to map cellular alterations and to observe the microvascular network.

INSTRUMENTS

There are many types and designs of instruments in various lengths available for endolaryngeal microsurgery.

The length of the shank can be from 18 to 23 cm, the shorter the length the less tremor is seen at the distal end during operative surgery. Most now have a reinforced and tapered shaft, so that the distal part is slim and does not obscure visualization.

The standard instruments consist of:

- scissors, straight-ahead, angled 45° upwards, curved left and right (Fig. 6.15);
- circular or oval cutting cupped forceps; various cup sizes; straight-ahead, curved upwards, curved left and right; the cups are from 1 to 5 mm in diameter (Fig. 6.16);

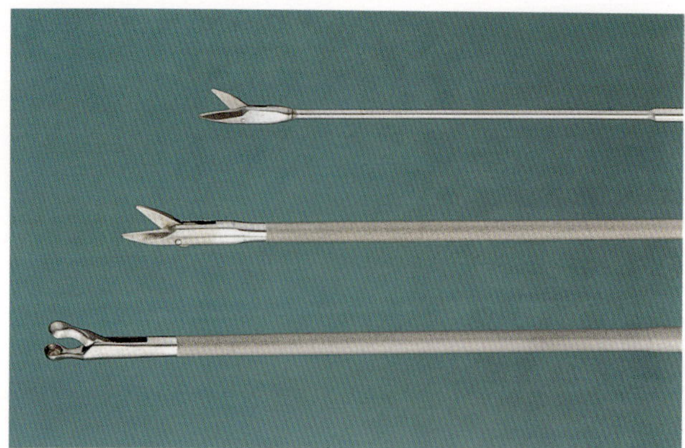

Figure **6.15**
Examples of microlaryngeal instruments. Fine scissors, medium scissors and fine cupped forceps.

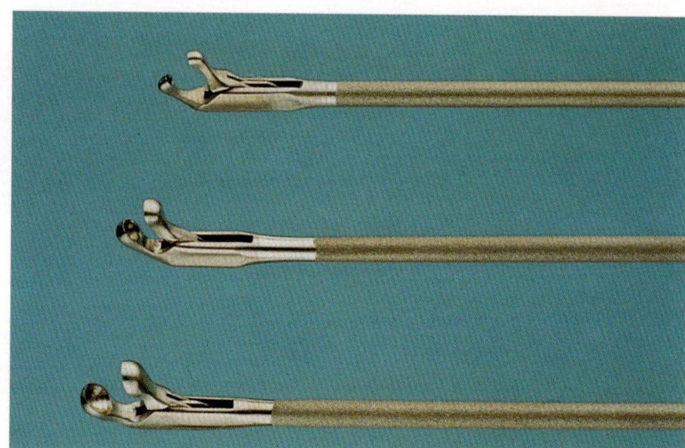

Figure **6.16**
Up-cupped forceps of different cup diameters, 1, 3 and 5 mm.

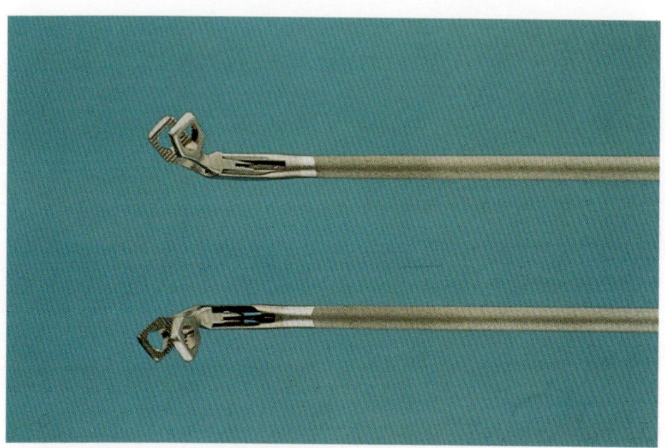

Figure **6.17**
Right- and left-sided Bouchayer grasping forceps.

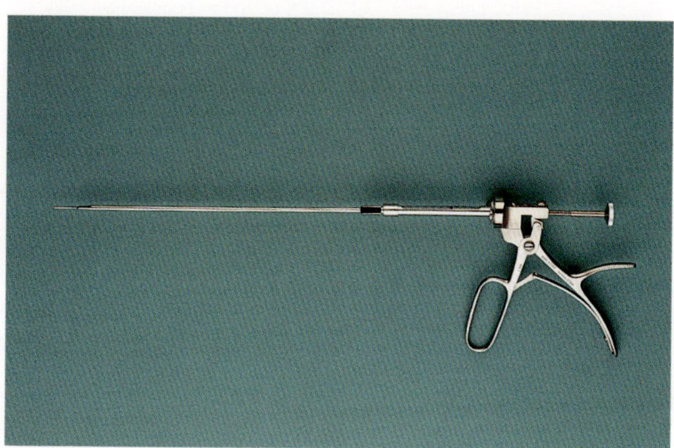

Figure **6.18**
High-pressure syringe for injection of Teflon paste or Gelfoam paste which is loaded in the barrel of a 1-ml plastic syringe before injection.

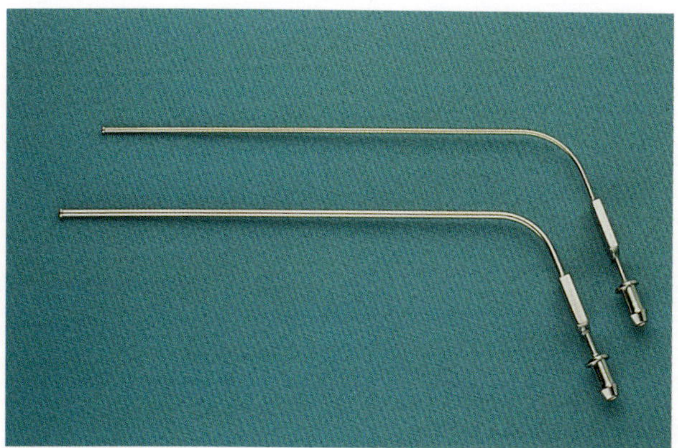

Figure **6.19**
Suction tubes, 2- and 3-mm diameter with beaded, atraumatic tips.

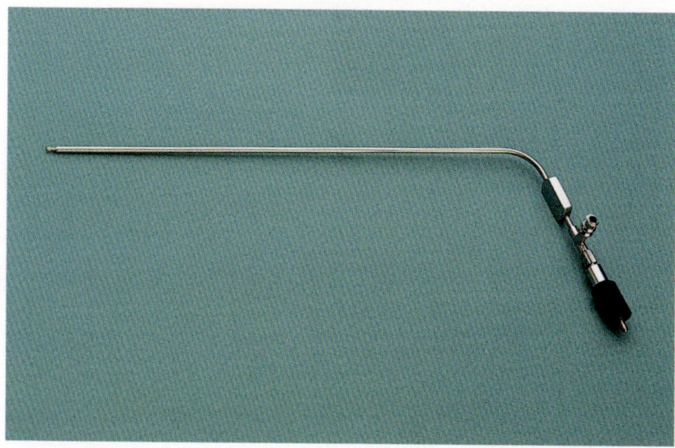

Figure **6.20**
Insulated suction for diathermy of bleeding points in the larynx.

- other specialized forceps include the Bouchayer and Jako forceps designed to grasp part or all of the edge of the vocal cord (Fig. 6.17);
- the mini-microlaryngeal instruments of Shapshay and Healy are very delicate, the shaft is reinforced by degrees from distal to proximal, working length 20 cm; the set consists of various scissors, alligator forceps, cupped forceps, grasping forceps, suckers and probes;
- a high-pressure syringe set for injection of Gelfoam paste or Teflon paste (Fig. 6.18) including an injection cannula of working length 18 cm, needle tip outside diameter 1.6 mm and a 45° bevel;
- suckers of various lengths and diameters with plain or beaded distal tip (Fig. 6.19);
- other optional instruments include the Kleinsasser telescopic gauge for measuring neoplasms or stenoses under optical control, the Glanz carcinoma gauge, the vocal and false cord retractor, combined laryngeal suction and diathermy (Fig. 6.20).

Details of endoscopic techniques such as biopsy of a mass, removal of vocal nodules or a vocal polyp, treatment of Reinke's oedema, and laser surgery will be discussed with reference to each disorder in following sections of the text.

BIBLIOGRAPHY

Andrea M, Dias O, Santos A (1995) Contact endoscopy during microlaryngeal surgery: a new technique for endoscopic examination of the larynx. *Ann Otol Rhinol Laryngol* **104**: 333–9.

Benjamin B (1987) Technique of laryngoscopy. *Int J Ped Otolaryngol* **13**: 299–313.

Zeitels SM, Vaughan CW (1994) 'External counterpressure' and 'internal distension' for optimal laryngoscopic exposure of the anterior glottal commissure. *Ann Otol Rhinol Laryngol* **103**: 669–75.

7 Observer techniques

Teaching students during indirect laryngoscopy performed using light from a head mirror reflected onto a laryngeal mirror is painstakingly slow and frustrating. One student after another looks over the shoulder of the examiner attempting to obtain a restricted view of the larynx; in addition each student sits opposite a patient to learn the indirect laryngoscopy examination technique by trial and error. Many students are overjoyed just to visualize the vocal cords – 'I can see them!'

Indirect laryngoscopy is difficult, often taking months of practice to become competent. Consequently, the art of indirect laryngoscopy is no longer taught to students in many medical schools – younger doctors are advised to refer patients to specialists when there are symptoms suggestive of disease in the larynx or pharynx.

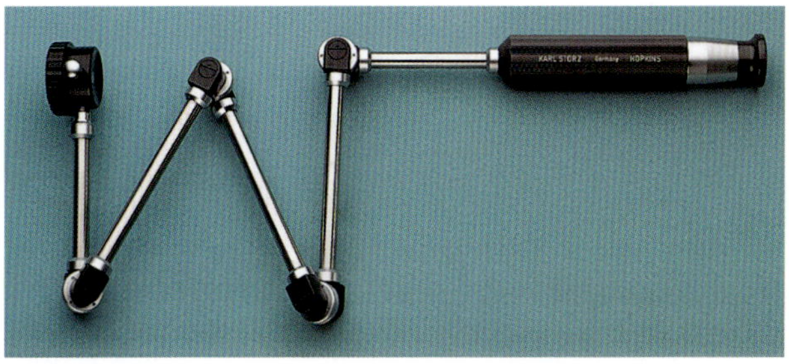

Figure **7.1**
Wittmoser articulated optical arm. This optical system has five Hopkins' rod lenses, and four joints, length 82 cm. Ideal for simultaneous observation by the operator and observer or optical connection of an endoscopic telescope to 35-mm camera, television camera or cine camera.

SIMULTANEOUS VIEWING

Fortunately modern optical and lighting systems allow simultaneous viewing of the laryngeal image both at indirect laryngoscopy and direct laryngoscopy:

1 Using rigid rod lens telescopes or a flexible laryngoscope:
   - an optical arm, such as the multi-articulated Wittmoser (Fig. 7.1);
   - a beam splitter for a television camera (Fig. 7.2);

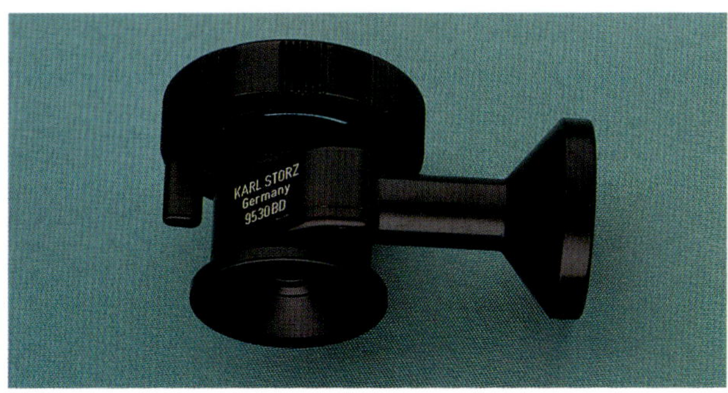

Figure **7.2**
Beam splitter. Integral rotating beam splitter for use during observation, television or cine-photography for simultaneous viewing by the surgeon and on the monitor screen.

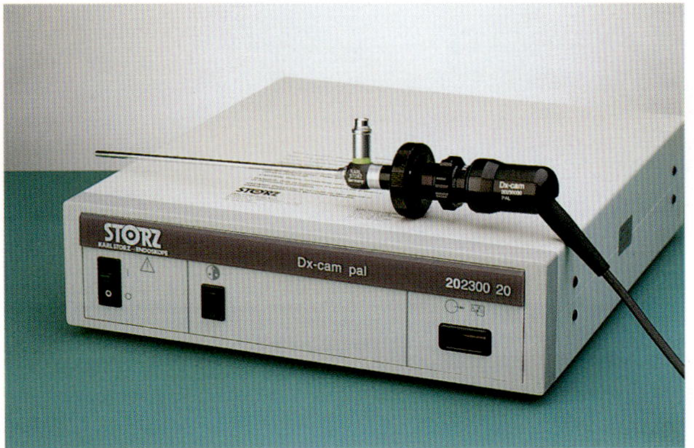

Figure **7.3**
Video camera. The camera control unit and telescope attached to the video camera. Alternatively, the camera can be attached to a flexible laryngoscope.

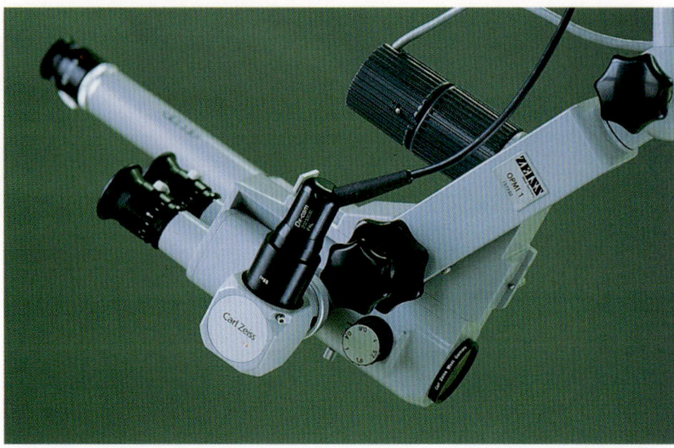

Figure **7.4**
Operating microscope with adaptors. A C-mount optical adaptor allows quick coupling of the video camera to the beam splitter of the microscope. There is an observer arm on the other side.

- a television camera attached directly to the proximal end of a telescope (Fig. 7.3) or flexible laryngoscope.

2 Using the microscope:
- an observer arm mounted on a beam splitter in the optics of the microscope (Fig. 7.4);
- a television camera mounted on a beam splitter (Fig. 7.4).

Telescopes

When using one of the teaching attachments, a student or an assistant can observe the exact image seen by the endoscopist through the telescope. The Hopkins' rigid rod lens optical system allows splitting of the reflected image into two images at the proximal end of the telescope while maintaining adequate brightness for each of two simultaneous observers.

Wittmoser optical arm

The Wittmoser optical arm (Fig. 7.5), which has four joints, is superb for either observation or documentation. The dual beam splitter can be switched to 50% of the light for the examiner and 50% for the observer

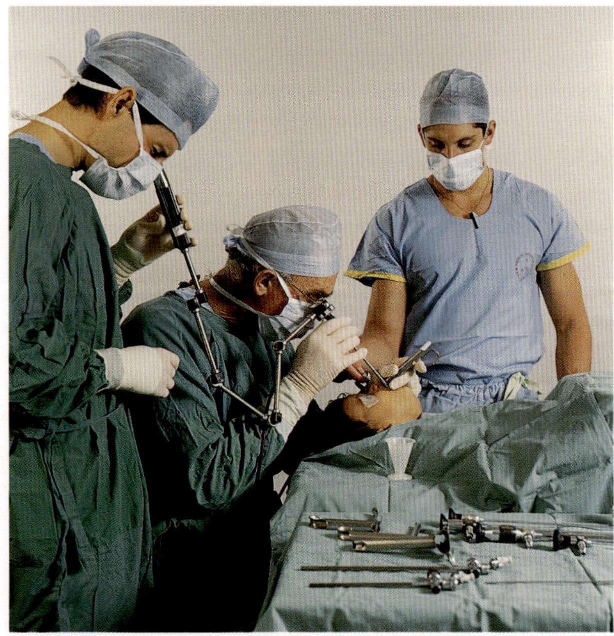

Figure **7.5**
Wittmoser optical arm during laryngoscopy. Detailed examination of the larynx with the telescope while an assistant observes through the optical arm.

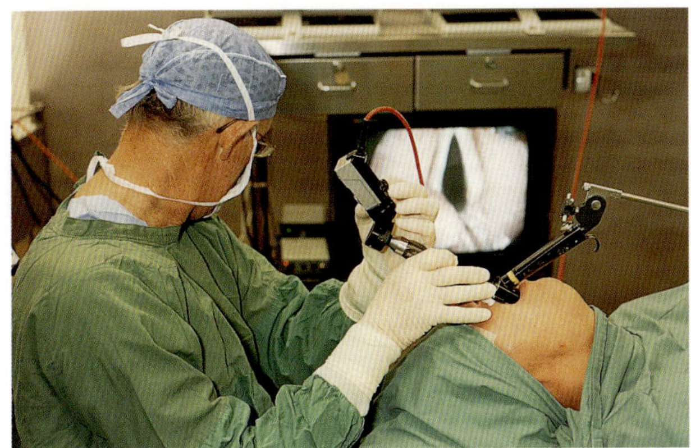

Figure **7.6**
Beam splitter in use with television camera. As the endoscopist performs image magnification examination with one eye to the proximal end of the apparatus, the beam splitter transmits an image to the video monitor.

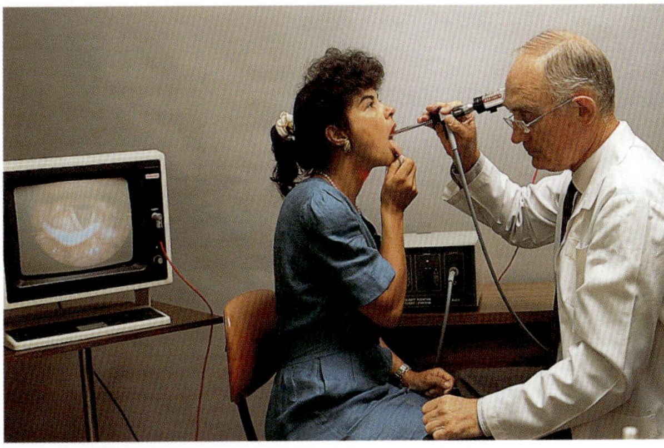

Figure **7.7**
Closed-circuit video laryngoscopy. Indirect laryngoscopy with a 70° telescope and a video camera provides an image on the television monitor. Video-recording, if desired with stroboscopy, through the rigid telescope or a flexible laryngoscope is possible.

or alternatively to 10% : 90%, so that the brighter image through the optical arm can be used for documentation with a 35-mm still camera, a television camera or a cine-camera. This excellent teaching aid provides a superb image with natural colour, complete safety for the patient and no interruption or interference to the examination.

Beam splitter

There are several other smaller rotating or fixed beam splitters which, when attached to the proximal eyepiece of a telescope (Fig. 7.6), function in the same way to allow the image to be delivered to the endoscopist's eye and another part of the light, carrying an identical image, to be diverted to a television camera. A beam splitter with a rotation system is designed to maintain correct orientation on the television monitor screen so that the image remains upright and always corresponds to the view of the surgeon.

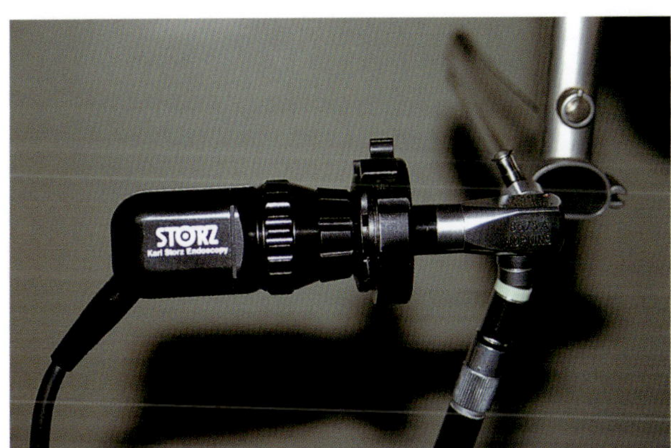

Figure **7.8**
Kantor–Berci video-laryngoscope Model I. A straightforward telescope, angled eyepiece, is used with the Kantor–Berci video-laryngoscope giving a consistent unchanging operative field.

Television camera

A television camera can be attached directly to the proximal eyepiece of a telescope (Fig. 7.7) during examination of the pharynx, larynx, subglottic region and trachea; both the surgeon, the assistant and other observers see the image on a television monitor. Similarly, when using the Kantor–Berci video-laryngoscope (Fig. 7.8) a video camera is attached to the telescope which is fixed in the side channel of the laryngoscope. In this case the surgeon can see the naked-eye view through the laryngoscope, use the operating microscope through the laryngoscope or perform surgical procedures by viewing the television monitor.

Microscope

A beam splitter in the optics of the operating microscope provides potential for an image on both the right and the left sides. For teaching it is customary to have an observer eyepiece on the beam splitter of one side (Fig. 7.4) and a television camera attached to a C-mount optical attachment on the beam splitter of the other side. The observer's view is monocular but the endoscopic surgeon obtains a binocular view with stereoscopic vision.

Observation using the microscope confines the view to the supraglottic and glottic larynx whereas the distal tip of a telescope can be placed in various positions to view the pharynx, larynx, ventricles, posterior glottic space, postcricoid region, subglottic region, trachea and bronchi.

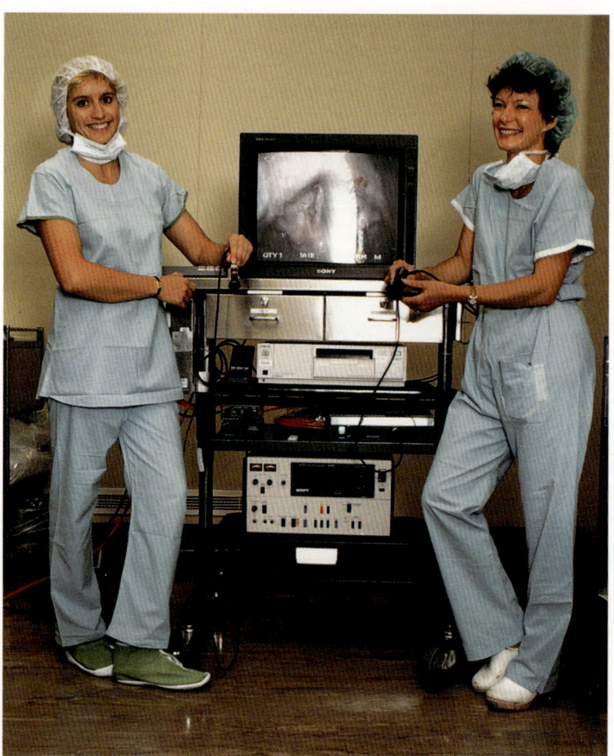

Figure **7.9**
Television trolley. From above down there is a monitor, drawers for storing video cameras, video printer, camera control units and a three-quarter inch video-recorder on the bottom shelf.

Television

While a larger, and not so expensive, television camera (often positioned on a tripod) can be used in many situations, it is more convenient to use one of the modern lightweight, miniaturized television cameras which provide high resolution even in low light situations. The image gathered by the camera, either from a telescope or the microscope, is shown on a high-resolution monitor. In the office or clinic, the patient or relatives can be shown the pathology in the larynx, while in the operating theatre the anaesthetist can observe the conditions of anaesthesia while monitoring the airway and the nursing staff can anticipate progress of the procedure. The operating room personnel become more involved in the operation.

The video monitor can be linked to a video-recorder or a video colour printer (Fig. 7.9).

Video-recorder

A recorder using U-matic 0.75 inch tape or VSH 0.5 inch tape can be employed. Tape in video cassettes is cheap and reusable and the operative procedure can be recorded to extract colour prints or be edited to demonstrate the steps in a surgical technique.

Video printer

A colour printer allows a selected image to be 'frozen' and stored ready for printing so that one or more hard-paper colour prints (Fig. 7.10) can be obtained within minutes. They are placed in the patient's record and are invaluable to show the patient or various consultants who might be involved in the patient's care, for instance a radiation therapist or an oncologist. The memory settings allow different printing methods, for example a single full size image or 4 (Fig. 7.11) smaller images. It is also possible to imprint a caption, the date or other information. It is increasingly important to have a permanent record for

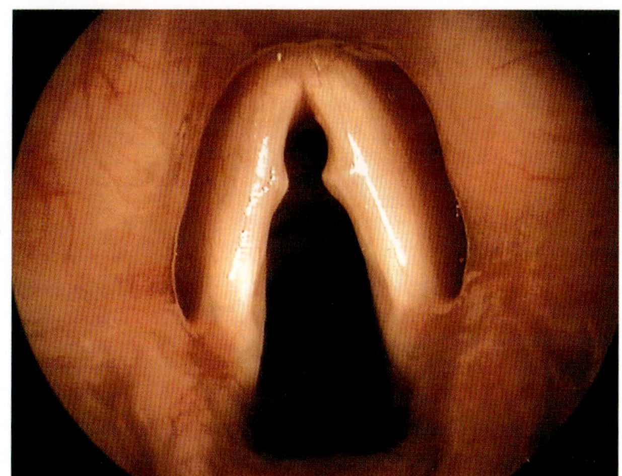

Figure **7.10**
Video print. Single frame video print of bilateral vocal nodules in a 10-year-old child. The quality of the print is almost as good as a 35-mm photograph.

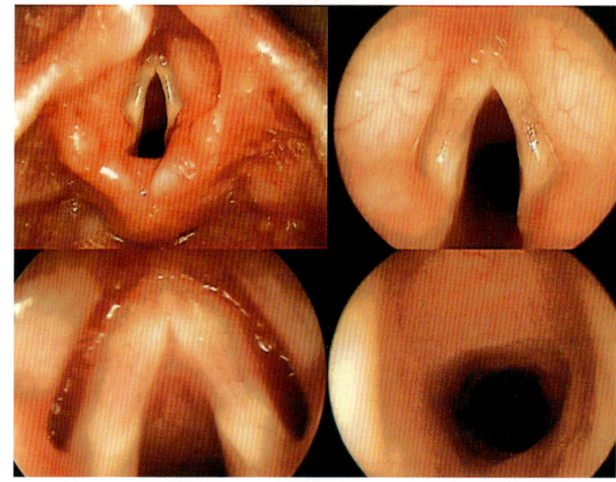

Figure **7.11**
Four images on a video print. Normal findings. The supraglottic and glottic larynx, vocal folds, 30° telescope view of the anterior commissure and the ventricles and the subglottic region.

documentation of disease. A permanent static 'single-frame' record can be most conveniently obtained with an instant print taken from the video monitor or captured by 35-mm photography. Cinephotography has largely been replaced by video recording on tape for documentation of dynamic changes. The video-recorder should have a still-frame feature, backward and forward search and playback facilities. It appears that in the future video-disc with digital technology may replace video-recording.

The cheapest and most convenient form of documentation of findings at laryngoscopy is a careful written description supplemented by suitable diagrams, but there are now various forms of permanent objective documentation which serve better for teaching, comparative study, clinical research and study of the natural history and results of treatment. A combination of radiological study, endoscopic colour photography and video-recording is currently the most practical method.

BIBLIOGRAPHY

Becker W, Buckingham RA, Holinger P et al (1969) *Atlas of otorhinolaryngology and bronchoesophagology* (Philadelphia: WB Saunders).

Benjamin B (1981) *Atlas of paediatric endoscopy: upper respiratory tract and oesophagus* (London: Oxford University Press).

Benjamin B (1984) Technique of laryngeal photography. *Ann Otol Rhinol Laryngol* **93** (Suppl): 1–11.

Benjamin B (1990) *Diagnostic laryngology: adults and children* (Philadelphia: WB Saunders).

Benjamin B (1993) Art and science of laryngeal photography. *Ann Otol Rhinol Laryngol* **102**: 271–82.

Benjamin B, Bingham B, Hawke M, Stammberger H (1995) *A colour atlas of otorhinolaryngology* (London: Martin Dunitz).

Holinger PA (1942) Photography of the larynx, trachea, bronchi and esophagus. *Trans Am Acad Ophthalmol Otolaryngol* **46**: 153–6.

Holinger PA, Brubaker JD, Brubaker JE (1975) Open tube proximal illumination, mirror and direct laryngeal photography. *Can J Otolaryngol* **4**: 781–5.

Kleinsasser O (1968) *Microlaryngoscopy and endolaryngeal microsurgery* (Philadelphia: WB Saunders).

Yanagisawa E (1997) *Color Atlas of diagnostic endoscopy in otorhinolaryngology* (New York: Igaku-Shoin).

Yanagisawa E, Walkier R (1987) Instantaneous 'video photography' with a low-cost black-and-white video printer – its value in otolaryngology and head and neck surgery. *Otolaryngol Head Neck Surg* **95**: 230.

Yanagisawa E, Yanagisawa R (1991) Laryngeal photography. *Otolaryngol Clin North Am* **24**: 999–1022.

Yanagisawa E, Yanagisawa K, Horowitz JB et al (1992) Comparison of new telescopic video microlaryngoscopic and standard microlaryngoscopic techniques. *Ann Otol Rhinol Laryngol* **101**: 51–60.

8 Documentation, teaching and normal endoscopic appearance

METHODS OF DOCUMENTATION

Endoscopists have searched for improved methods to permanently record their findings for over 100 years.

There are many ways to document laryngeal disease:

- written description
- free-hand drawing or sketch by the surgeon, resident or medical illustrator
- pre-printed diagram on which the pathology is hand-drawn
- photography at indirect and direct laryngoscopy
- hard copy black-and-white or colour prints from a video monitor
- video-cassette recording
- cinephotography
- imaging techniques as described in Chapter 3; plain lateral X-rays, CT and MRI studies are especially useful.

Laryngeal documentation

Written description
Drawing
Pre-printed diagram
Photograph
Video print
Video-recording
Cinephotography
X-ray, CT and MRI

Simple techniques such as a sketch are used most often; in general, the more sophisticated and accurate the documentation becomes the more it depends on complicated and expensive equipment.

In clinical practice the best documentation is a combination of a written description and a hand-drawn diagram supplemented by an 'instant' hard-copy colour print obtained from a video printer.

Photographic documentation is applied in all fields of medicine and surgery and is most important in endoscopic surgery where the view is often limited to the eye of the surgeon. Precision documentation in the upper respiratory tract, in particular the larynx, is of vital importance to the otolaryngologist/head and neck surgeon especially where the operative field is small, as in paediatric laryngology. Photographs are an essential record in the patient's notes.

Flexible fibreoptic transmission cables have provided bright light intensity, and the large variety of optical telescopes available facilitates the application not only of 35-mm photography but also of high-resolution miniature video cameras, 'instant' video prints and videotape recording. Documentation is more readily accessible, for both undergraduate and postgraduate teaching. As equipment has become more sophisticated, the problem of cost, the need for storage space, the cost of replacement and the responsibility for the maintenance of cameras and video equipment has assumed more importance.

Photography using a 35-mm camera gives excellent quality still colour photographs, but there is an expectation that digital images retrieved from a video disc may become the way of the future.

Video cassette recording is the most convenient means of representing dynamic changes, for illustrating an operative technique, for teaching or for presentation to a large audience. Cinephotography gives sharper images but is more expensive, and editing is very time consuming.

TECHNIQUES OF LARYNGEAL PHOTOGRAPHY

Photography has excited the interest of laryngologists since Thomas French of New York first photographed the larynx over 100 years ago using a laryngeal mirror and a primitive camera. Since then there have been many methods of still photography. The specially designed and developed Holinger–Brubaker endoscopic camera for laryngeal photography was heavy, cumbersome and awkward by today's standards and, although no longer in use, was the hallmark of the best in laryngeal photography for some 30 years.

Indirect laryngoscopic photography

For photography in the consulting room, office or clinic, one or other of the common methods for clinical examination of the larynx has been used.

- *Laryngeal mirror*. Photography at indirect mirror laryngeal examination is relatively inexpensive, but it is an awkward technique and the results are unpredictable with only a small success rate.
- *Flexible fibreoptic laryngoscope*. Photography can be successful but produces only a small image with a large surrounding area of black, often with resultant over-exposure.
- *Rigid rod lens telescope*. Telescopes designed for indirect laryngoscopy provide a brilliant, sharp, colour image and are recommended, not only for precise examination, but also for quality laryngeal photographs.

Indirect laryngoscopic photography

Laryngeal mirror
Flexible laryngoscope
Rigid telescope

Direct laryngoscopic photography

Many methods have been used:

- single-lens-reflex (SLR) camera with a close-up lens or macro-lens;

Direct laryngoscopic photography

Close-up or macro-lens
Close-up lens and ring flash
Beam splitter of microscope
Rigid telescope

Rigid telescope photography

Light unit for examination and photography
Light-conducting cable
Single-lens-reflex camera body
Synchronization cable
Zoom or fixed focus (80 or 100 mm) lens
Telescope

- SLR camera with close-up lens and a ring flash;
- photography through the operating microscope using a beam splitter or a photo-adaptor attached to the eyepiece;
- telescopic photography using a rigid rod lens Hopkin's telescope for both diagnostic inspection and for flash photography.

The technique to be described has been used by the author for many years and allows excellent visualization and consistent photography under all conditions. Employing Hopkin's telescopes this modern system relies on a 35-mm SLR camera and a remote computer-controlled, electronic flash generator with synchronized automatic exposure.

EQUIPMENT FOR PHOTOGRAPHY USING RIGID TELESCOPES

Laryngeal photographs are featured in many textbooks, atlases and scientific articles, but the details of the photographic techniques are seldom given.

The equipment for taking the photographs in this book was originslly designed in Germany by Dr Karl Storz thirty years ago. Since then it has been modified and improved. The most important component is the light unit which provides two types of lighting: constant illumination for diagnostic examination and momentary brilliant light for photographic exposure. There are two types of flexible light conducting cables: one with fibreglass threads and another which is filled with liquid. Either one is used to transmit light to a telescope attached to a lens (usually a zoom lens) on an SLR camera. Thus, in the consulting room, office, clinic or operating theatre, photographic documentation of the pharynx and larynx – and with appropriate telescopes, the nasal cavities, nasopharynx and tympanic membranes – can be undertaken. During endoscopy in the operating theatre, the technique can be applied not only to the larynx but also to the tracheobronchial tree and oesophagus. The instrumentation is versatile, easy to use and the image quality from colour 35-mm transparencies is excellent; the success rate is high in both adults and children making it the most reliable technique. In fact any anatomic area which can be seen by a telescope can be photographed.

Light unit

Many light sources are available and three are described here:

- The Karl Storz model 600 TTL-Computer Flash Unit (Fig. 8.1) has a 250 watt cold-light halogen lamp for continuous light, which is adjustable in four steps of intensity for routine examination. There is a built-in spare lamp which can be immediately switched on should the first lamp fail. A choice of two outlets for flash is available. This advanced TTL

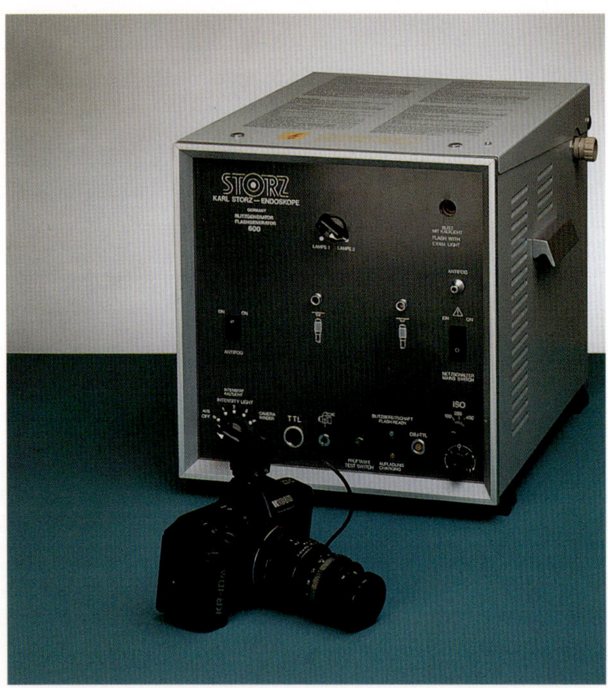

Figure **8.1**
Model 600TTL-Computer Flash Unit. The front panel has controls for the halogen lamp intensity, an anti-fog air pump, connections for the synchronization cable of the camera, a trigger button to test flash, a 'flash ready' lamp for flash function, a control for adjusting film speed and a control knob for exposure compensation. The Ricoh camera and zoom lens are also shown.

(through-the-lens) unit not only has continuous bright halogen light for viewing or use with a video camera but also has an integrated flash tube for electronic flash photography.

The light unit emits an audible 'beep' when the flash is fully charged ready for photography; after the photograph has been taken an automatic reminder of three audible 'beeps' indicates when optimal photographic conditions have been achieved and the exposure has been successful. The signal remains silent if the field is too distant for the light intensity to illuminate the area adequately. Thus this computerized unit with automatic TTL flash metering gives precise and accurate exposure. It is an expensive, sophisticated system which gives uniform picture quality.

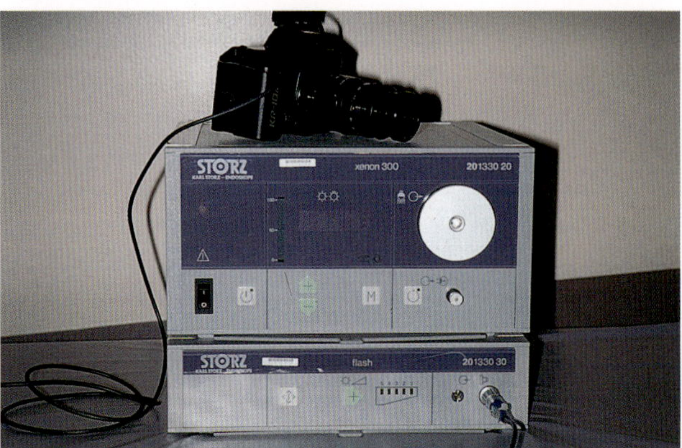

Figure **8.2**
Cold Light Fountain Xenon 300 and TTL Flash Module. The brightness from the 300-watt Xenon lamp can be controlled in steps. It can give high-intensity light and forms a highly efficient flash photography system when integrated with the TTL Flash Module.

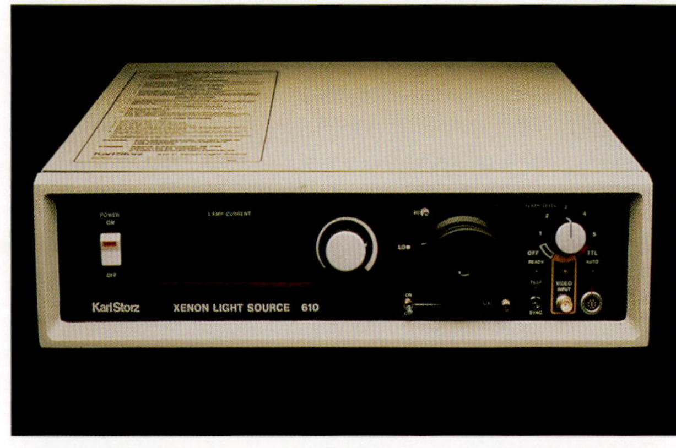

Figure **8.3**
Xenon Light Source 610. Provides Xenon light for diagnostic examination and television. The light can be boosted for still photography using manual or automatic TTL exposure control.

- The Cold Light Fountain Xenon 300 can be coupled with a TTL Flash Module (Fig. 8.2). The integrated, computer-controlled flash module automatically adjusts the flash and signals a successful exposure with a 'beep'. The 300-watt Xenon lamp and flash module are suitable for endoscopic work in any body cavity and produce excellent results for photographic and video documentation.

- The Xenon Light Source 610 (Fig. 8.3) is a unit which is in common use in North America. It provides continuous light for examination and boosted light with automatic exposure control for photography.

Camera

Although any 35-mm SLR camera body with light metering and motor wind can be used, best results are obtained using the camera body recommended by the manufacturer of the photographic equipment. The camera must have a modified, plain, clear focusing screen so that there is sufficient light for a brightly defined image to allow accurate focusing. The built-in motor drive for film advance allows repeat photography to be performed every 5–10 seconds, as soon as the capacitator has charged the flash, but to avoid overload it is recommended that no more than two to three photographs are taken in quick succession. A data back, interchangeable with the standard camera back, is an option for imprinting figures and letters, such as the date or the patient's name. An automatic light meter in the SLR camera body or a meter built into a newly developed zoom lens controls exposure.

Synchronization cable

A synchronization cable connects the electrical system from the hot shoe of the camera to a multi-pin plug on the front panel of the light unit for electronically synchronized opening of the shutter and flash illumination when the shutter button on the camera is depressed. There is a different cable for each light unit.

Lens

A conventional fixed 80- or 100-mm lens with an adaptor-mount can be used, but will not provide choice of image size which depends only on the diameter of the telescope.

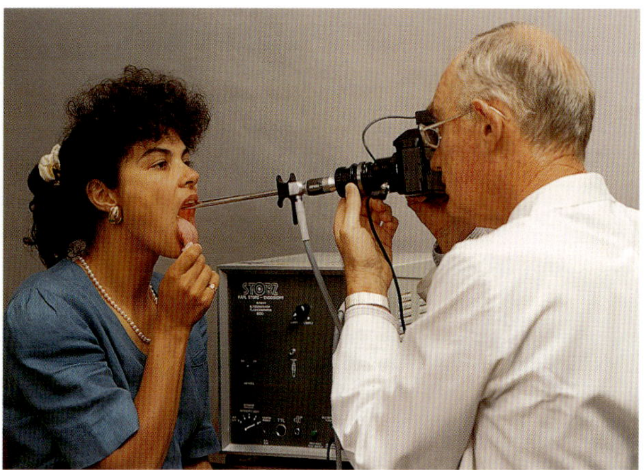

Figure **8.4**
Photography at indirect laryngoscopy. Using a 70°, wide-diameter telescope. The operator's left hand adjusts the focal length and the focus.

The special Karl Storz zoom lens (Fig. 8.11) which has a variable focal length from 70 to 140 mm permits variation of the size of the image which depends not only on the focal length chosen but also on the diameter and angle of view of the telescope. Choice of a longer focal length gives a larger image. A large-diameter telescope gives a larger image.

The telescope locks securely to an adaptor on the front of the lens. An improvement has been made in this well-known lens by integration of an electronic light meter for automatic exposure within the lens itself, providing the advantage that it can be used with any single SLR camera body.

Final focusing is achieved by turning the focusing ring on the lens (Fig. 8.4).

Film

Daylight film with fine grain and good colour tone should be used for transparencies. There is a considerable choice of film, each claiming differences in tone or quality of the colours: a film such as Ektachrome ISO 200 is satisfactory. Black-and-white film gives excellent results, but colour film is mostly used; black-

and-white prints made from colour transparencies are very satisfactory.

Telescopes

Hopkins of Reading University invented a rigid rod lens system composed of rods of glass with thin, air lenses thus creating an increase in light transmission compared to a conventional telescope which has small glass lenses. Many newer telescopes have a centrally placed viewing rod lens surrounded by symmetrically placed light-carrying segments which provide even illumination, ideal for photography. All glass surfaces are multi-coated.

A straight-ahead telescope achieves a viewing angle of 70° – approximately equivalent to a 28-mm lens on a 35-mm camera. There is a predictable brightness from one telescope to another except with slim telescopes of 2.8- or 1.9-mm diameter through which light transmission is limited.

There are telescopes purpose-designed for indirect laryngoscopy and others for direct laryngoscopy; selected telescopes will be described later in this section.

PHOTOGRAPHY AT INDIRECT LARYNGOSCOPY

Laryngeal examination

With the equipment described above, the co-operation of the patient and the use of topical anaesthesia, laryngeal examinations and telescopic photography can be accomplished in the consulting room or clinic. However, photography at indirect laryngoscopy is more difficult than at direct laryngoscopy.

The ease with which the larynx can be examined and photographed varies from patient to patient, but almost all adults and many older children can be examined or photographed using a slim 4-mm, 70° telescope (Karl Storz 7200CK). Even with this telescope a few patients are not sufficiently co-operative or have sensitive gag reflexes which require application of local anaesthesia. There remain a few individuals in whom neither laryngoscopy nor photography is possible with a rigid telescope. Pernasal flexible fibreoptic laryngoscopy allows a reasonable view of the larynx in many of these patients, but in exceptional cases general anaesthesia is necessary to properly visualize the larynx.

For the best photographic image a tele-laryngoscope of large diameter (8, 9 or 10 mm) should be chosen according to the laryngologist's personal preference. Karl Storz telescope 8706CJ (7.2 × 9.3 mm) is recommended as the best for general use, but other telescopes have features which may be advantageous, e.g. adjustable focusing and magnification.

Preparation

The nature of the planned examination and photography is explained to the patient, who sits opposite the examiner, is requested to remain relaxed and is asked to breathe through the mouth quietly and regularly. Any dentures they might be wearing are removed.

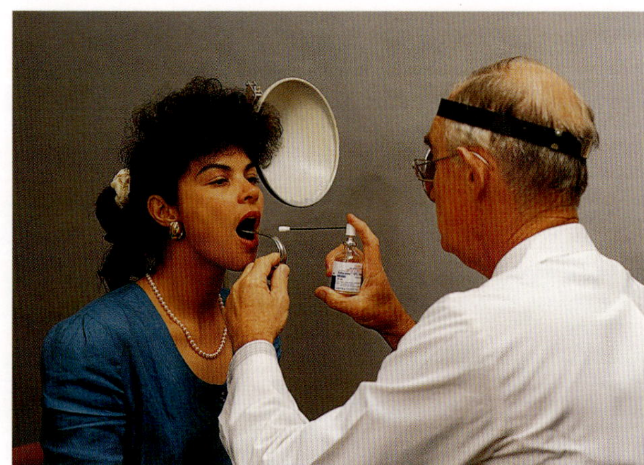

Figure **8.5**
Application of local anaesthesia. Topical lignocaine (Lidocaine) sprayed on the mucous membrane of the oropharynx facilitates patient acceptance of indirect laryngoscopy.

To comfortably tolerate the larger diameter telescopes most patients require topical anaesthesia (Fig. 8.5) applied with a spray or as a gel. The operator waits a few minutes for the full effect and prepares the equipment for photography.

Taking the photograph

The patient opens the mouth, extends the tongue, wraps it in gauze and pulls it outwards and downwards with the thumb and forefinger of their right hand, leaving both hands of the examiner free (Fig. 8.4). The telescope, having been dipped in anti-fog solution and already attached to the camera, is gently introduced into the oropharynx so that it is positioned in the midline, displacing the uvula and soft palate upwards and backwards, if possible without touching the posterior pharyngeal wall. A symmetrical view of the larynx should be obtained but the anterior commissure is sometimes difficult to see, especially when an overhanging epiglottis makes visualization difficult. The image is composed in the camera viewfinder to give a pleasing appearance and to display the pathological features clearly, preferably so that there is comparison of the normal side to the abnormal side. Symmetry and centring are important. Final focusing is achieved using either the focusing ring on the zoom lens or the appropriate lever on a telescope which has a focusing mechanism.

Photographs can be taken during quiet respiration and in phonation; often the best pictures are obtained as inspiration commences immediately after the patient has phonated 'ee-ee-ee'.

Photography at indirect laryngoscopy requires patience, practice and experience. The success rate, depending on the criteria for good photographs, is approximately 80%. Due to lack of co-operation, hypersensitive gag reflex or abnormal anatomy some patients cannot be photographed.

Orientation

Photographs taken at **direct** laryngoscopy show the anterior commissure at the superior aspect, but at **indirect** laryngoscopy the view is upside down so that the anterior commissure is placed inferiorly. For convenience and easier orientation, indirect laryngoscopy photographs in this text have been re-orientated to be the same as those taken at direct laryngoscopy with the anterior commissure at the top.

Indirect laryngoscopic method

Explain the procedure
Remove dentures
Patient holds own tongue
Shutter speed 1/15 second
Select focal length
Position the telescope
Focus and shoot

Telescopes

There are telescopes of various diameters and with different features; I prefer to use one of the following:

- Karl Storz 7200CK Slimline tele-laryngoscope (Fig. 8.6), 70° angle, diameter 4 mm, length 18 cm. No focusing required. Highly recommended for routine diagnostic indirect laryngoscopy, because it is well tolerated without the need for local anaesthesia. It can give excellent, small-diameter photographs (Fig. 8.7).
- Karl Storz 8700CK tele-laryngoscope, 70° angle, diameter 5.8 mm, length 20 cm, autoclavable. No focusing required. A new telescope which promises to be very useful for routine examination and photography.
- Karl Storz 8706CJ Strobo-laryngoscope (Fig. 8.8), 70° angle, diameter 7.2 × 9.3 mm, length 17 cm. No focusing required. Provides the best results not only for 35-mm and video documentation, but also

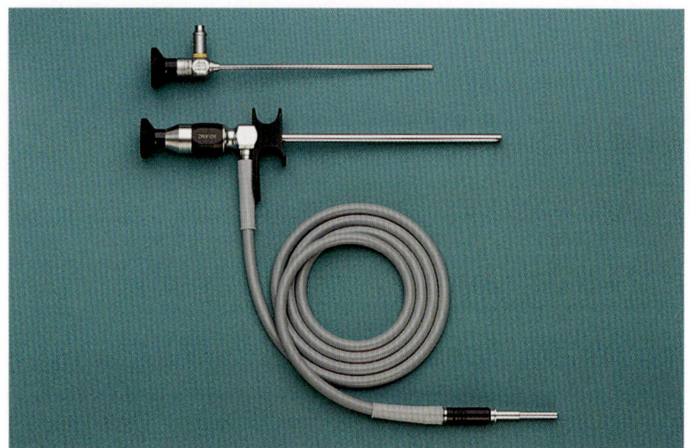

Figure **8.6**
Telescopes for indirect laryngeal photography. The smaller telescope is 4 mm in diameter (Karl Storz 7200CK). The larger telescope is 7.2 × 9.3 mm and has an integral light-conducting cable (Karl Storz 8706CJ). Both have a 70° angle.

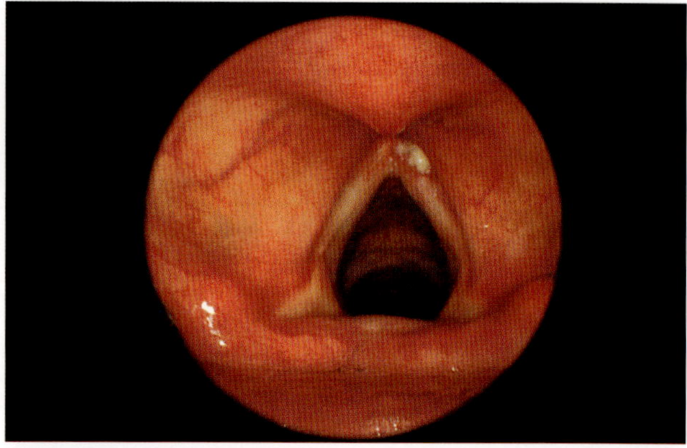

Figure **8.7**
Severe dysplasia of the anterior ventricle. Photographed at indirect laryngoscopy using the 4 mm, 70° telescope (7200CK).

for stroboscopy because it transmits more light for a brilliant image (Fig. 8.9). Many patients require topical anaesthesia.

PHOTOGRAPHY AT DIRECT LARYNGOSCOPY

Anaesthesia

Direct laryngoscopy under general anaesthesia offers the best opportunity for laryngeal photography. The field of view can be adjusted, using the most suitable laryngoscope, to obtain optimal surgical exposure and telescopes of different diameter can be used. Sometimes a 30° or a 70° angled telescope gives a better view than a straightforward 0° telescope.

There are several techniques. The method using an operating microscope has the camera attached to a beam splitter, but the depth of field is small, focusing is critical and the technique can be applied only in the larynx itself. Whereas supraglottic, postcricoid, and subglottic pathology is difficult to photograph with the microscope, these areas can be more easily captured with a rigid rod lens telescope.

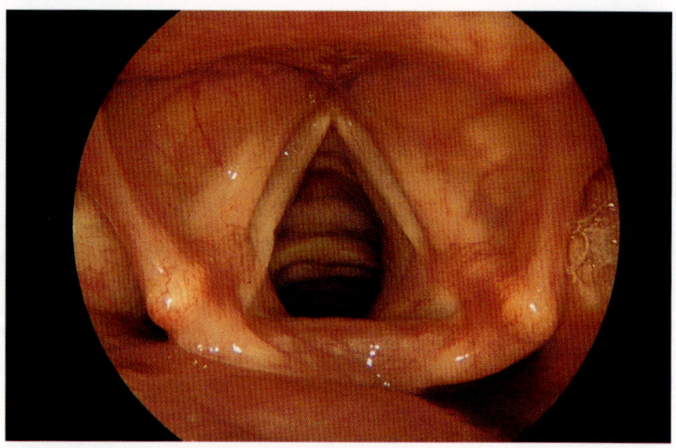

Figure **8.8**
Normal adult larynx. Photographed at indirect laryngoscopy using the 7.2 × 9.3 mm, 70° telescope (8706CJ).

A patient anaesthetist who understands the importance of photographic documentation is essential to success. The anaesthetist and surgeon must always co-operate to share access to a laryngeal airway which may be narrowed or partly obstructed and this principle remains important for laryngeal photography. Photography must never put the patient at risk. Where there is moderate or severe

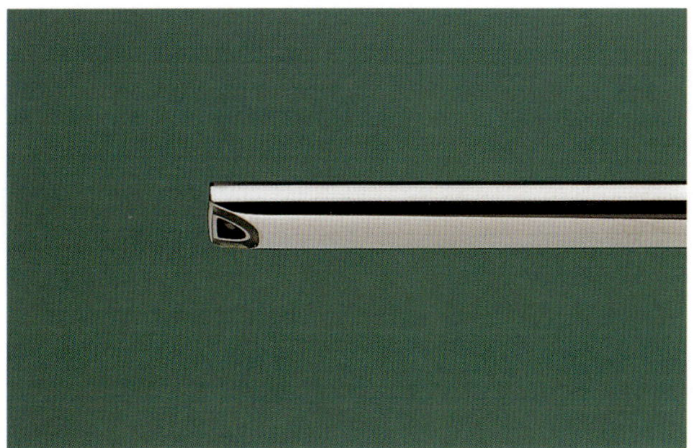

Figure **8.9**
Distal end of telescope 8706CJ. The central rod for the laryngeal image is placed as near the distal tip as possible – ideal for optimal visualization.

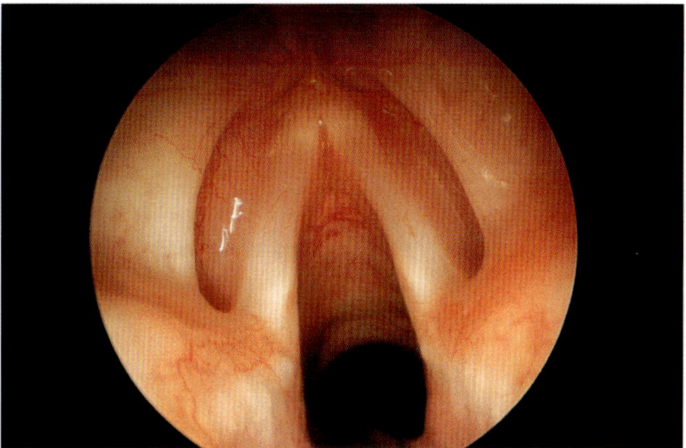

Figure **8.10**
Normal adult larynx with 30° telescope. Direct laryngoscopy. A 30° telescope angled forwards provides a comprehensive view of the true and false vocal cords, the ventricle and the anterior commissure.

airway obstruction, anaesthesia for photography in inexperienced hands could threaten the safety of the patient.

In infants and children it is preferable to perform photography under spontaneous respiration inhalational general anaesthesia because it does not require an anaesthetic tube. In adolescents and adults a small-diameter intratracheal tube for jet anaesthesia can be used, or even a small-diameter cuffed microlaryngoscopy endotracheal tube when there is supraglottic or anterior glottic pathology. A proximal metal jet cannula within the laryngoscope permits jet ventilation which can be momentarily suspended for photography so there is no movement of the larynx to blur the photograph.

Laryngoscopes

One of the Lindholm-designed laryngoscopes (adult, adolescent or infant) provides a remarkably wide panoramic exposure for documentation and, when placed in suspension, allows freedom of use of both hands not only for surgical manoeuvres but also for photography. To provide optimal exposure in each patient a laryngoscope is selected depending on the difficulty of insertion, prominent teeth, size of the tongue, pharyngeal anatomy, head and neck extension and the site and size of the laryngeal lesion.

The Kantor–Berci video-microlaryngoscope Model II is designed for documentation and for use with a video camera so that microsurgery can be performed by viewing the television monitor. It is claimed that the system can substitute for the binocular operating microscope, but it has disadvantages. The dimensions of the original laryngoscope made it difficult to insert in some patients. It exposed only the glottis and the telescope and smoke evacuator cannula interfered with the passage and manipulation of instruments. Nevertheless, this laryngoscope is advantageous for documentation because of the fixed, unchanged field of view – a series of photographs can be taken to show steps in a surgical procedure. A similar system, adapted for use in other laryngoscopes, would certainly assist in photographic documentation.

Telescopes

Telescopes vary in diameter, length and angle of view. The wider the diameter, the more detail seen in the photograph.

- Karl Storz telescope 8701AG 0°, 10 mm diameter, 20 cm long, developed for documentation at direct laryngoscopy, is highly recommended (Fig. 8.11).
- Karl Storz telescopes 8700A 0°, 8700B 30°, 8700C 70°, 5.8 mm diameter, 20 cm long for direct laryngoscopy in infants, children and adults. The 30° and 70° telescopes reveal the laryngeal ventricle (Fig. 8.10), posterior glottic space and the anterior subcommissure.
- Karl Storz telescopes 8712AA 0° and 8712BA 30°, 5 mm diameter, 24 cm long. Autoclavable.

Most documentation is performed with a 0°, straight-ahead telescope.

There are many suitable telescopes of similar design made by other manufacturers. A telescope is chosen according to the individual preference of the laryngologist for 35-mm photography, video documentation and stroboscopy.

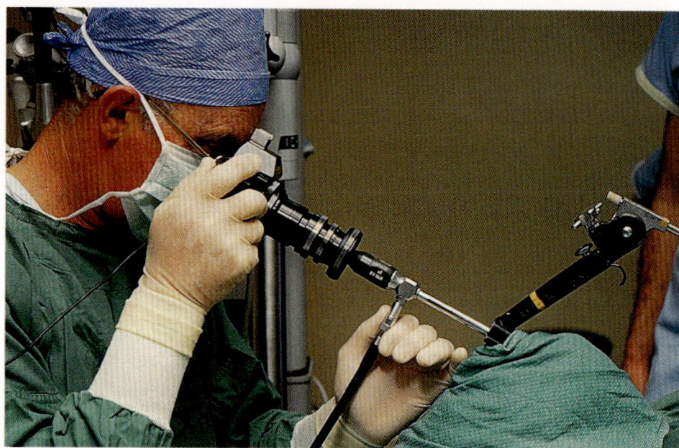

Figure **8.11**
Photography at direct laryngoscopy. The right hand holds the camera, the index finger ready to activate the shutter. The left hand positions and steadies the telescope (8701AG) with the laryngoscope.

Details of technique

Although it is possible to hold the laryngoscope in the left hand and the camera in the right hand, manipulation of the zoom lens and the focusing mechanism is awkward. Suspension laryngoscopy makes both hands available; the right hand holds the camera leaving the left hand free to adjust the focal length and the focus.

A telescope, selected for its length, diameter and angle of view, is fitted to the front of the zoom lens and connected by a light-conducting cable to the lighting unit for constant illumination and viewing through the eyepiece of the SLR camera. The telescope is passed into the laryngoscope (Fig. 8.11); viewing through the eyepiece of the camera shows the exact photographic field. External pressure on the anterior neck with a finger or fingers and gentle internal counterpressure from the beak of the laryngoscope allows manipulation of the larynx so that the pathological lesion is displayed in an optimal fashion.

All photographs are taken with the shutter speed set on 1/15th of a second. A focal length between 70 and 140 mm is chosen to adjust the size of the image. The choice of a longer focal length gives a larger, sometimes rectangular image that fills the screen; choice of a shorter focal length gives a smaller circular image with black surrounds. To avoid fogging of the cold telescope when it is first introduced, a demisting solution can be used or the tip of the telescope can be placed in warm water before use.

The composition is optimized, focus adjusted and finally the shutter is activated, a process usually taking 10–20 seconds.

Photography of the subglottic region, trachea and bronchi is an extension of laryngeal photography and

Direct laryngoscopic method

Children – no endotracheal tube
Adults – jet ventilation
Use the laryngoscope giving the best exposure
External neck pressure
Select focal length
Optimize composition
Focus and shoot

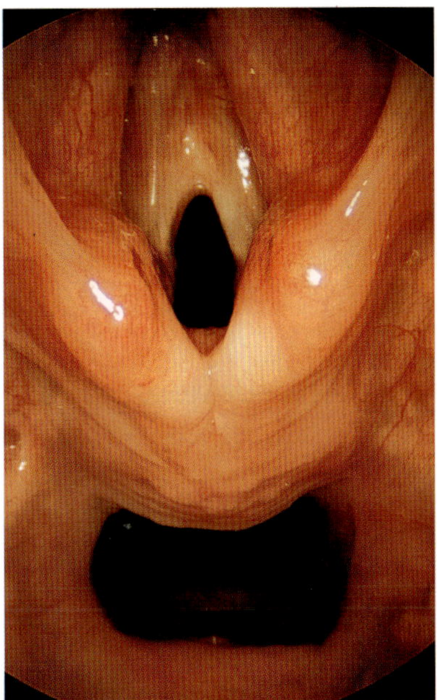

Figure **8.12**
Larynx and hypopharynx. The 'laryngeal lift' exposes the postcricoid region and the upper oesophagus, elevating the larynx by grasping it through the skin of the neck. Note the wide depth of focus and the even colour rendition.

is most easily accomplished while the laryngoscope is suspended. A longer, slim 30-cm telescope should be used.

Photography during endoscopy in the operating theatre has a success rate close to 100% in both adults and children and is without question the most reliable and simple technique. Rigid telescopes maintain a wide depth of field in focus (Fig. 8.12).

SUCCESS AND FAILURE

The overall appearance and impact of the photograph is affected by many variables; with more experience the endoscopic photographer will have more successes and fewer failures. The difference between a good and a bad photograph often needs only a small alteration in technique.

Good and bad photographs

Correct exposure
Sharp focus
Pleasing colours
Good composition
Easy orientation
Symmetry and centring
Consistency

Many questions arise. Is the exposure correct? Is the image in sharp focus? Are the colours pleasing? Can the viewer readily orient the picture and identify the salient features? The pathology should be easy to see without distortion of the larynx, there should be recognizable reference points, symmetry and centring are important and consistency from one photograph to the other is vital.

Various problems may be encountered by the dissatisfied and frustrated photographer, including blurring or difficulty with focusing, improper centring, restricted depth of focus, inadequate light, difficulty with exposure of the pathological anatomy, variability of colour rendition, inability to obtain consistent conditions for photography, inconvenience and time consumption during an operation, acquisition of only a small image and, lastly, unpredictability of success.

The photographic technique should not be so elaborate or complicated that it becomes difficult to use by an endoscopist who is not familiar with photography.

Success with 35-mm black-and-white or colour single frame laryngeal photography has been achieved with many methods. The most reliable and versatile state-of-the-art system for good-quality documentation has been described. This sophisticated system, although expensive, gives uniform picture quality and optimal exposure, and its operation has been dependable over years of regular use. Consistently reproducible photographs can be taken

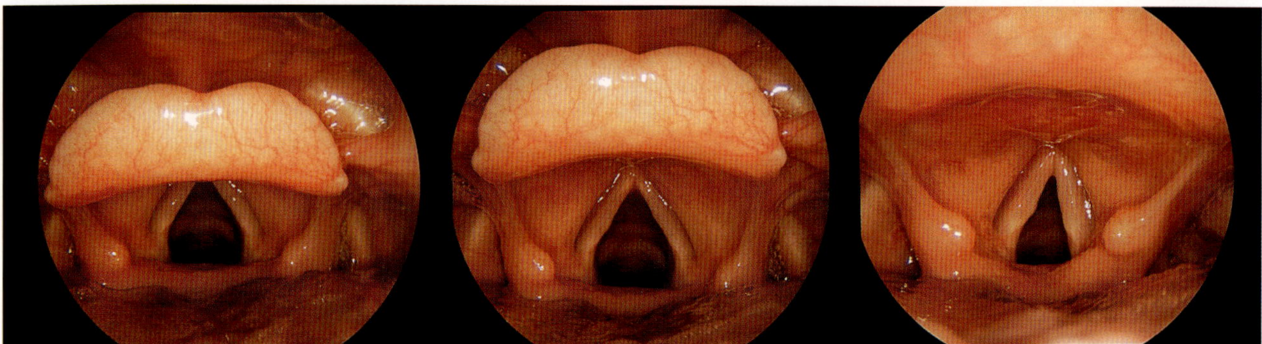

Figure **8.13**
Photographs taken as the telescope is introduced. The first shows the base of the tongue, valleculae, epiglottis and posterior pharyngeal wall; the larynx, however, cannot be seen. The second discloses more of the larynx, but not the anterior commissure. The third, when the telescope is optionally positioned, reveals the anterior larynx and some of the subglottis.

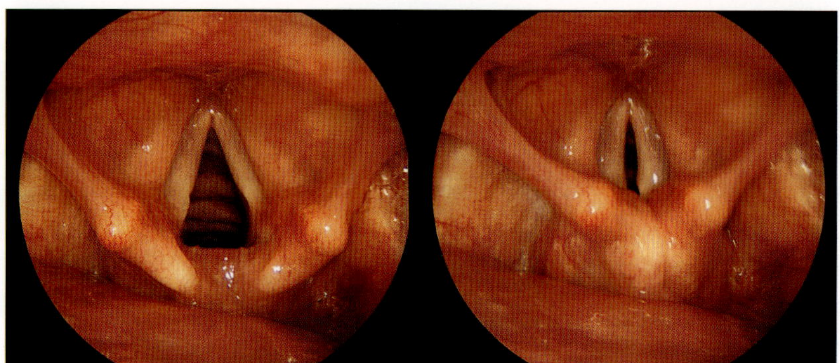

Figure **8.14**
Vocal cords in abduction [left] and just after adduction [right]. In the latter the piriform fossae are better seen. There is bilateral, equal vocal cord movement.

under both good and bad conditions by either the expert or the novice. In experienced hands the system is safe for the patient even in small infants or where there is partial airway obstruction. For best results the endoscopic photographer should have a good knowledge of the normal and pathological anatomy as well as the principles of the photographic system.

While the flexible fibreoptic instruments are versatile and have the great advantage of passing around corners, neither the visual nor the photographic image is as good as that obtained with rigid fibreoptic telescopes. Photography with a flexible instrument is not recommended when rigid telescopes are available.

The choice of photographic equipment for the individual laryngeal surgeon depends on their needs, their ability to use the equipment successfully and

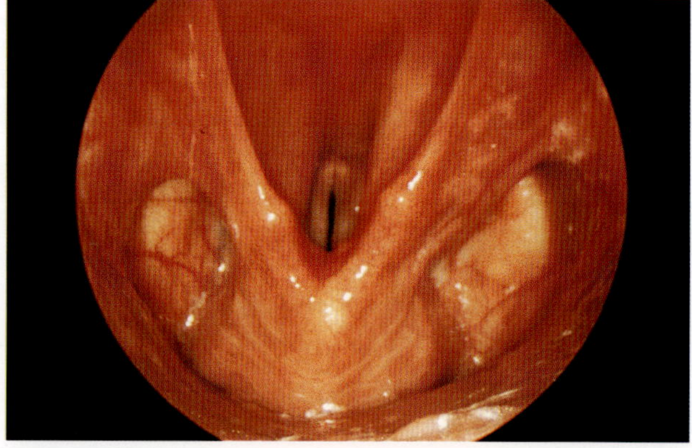

Figure **8.15**
During phonation in this larynx there is an excellent view of the piriform fossae and most of the postcricoid region. These areas are not always so well seen.

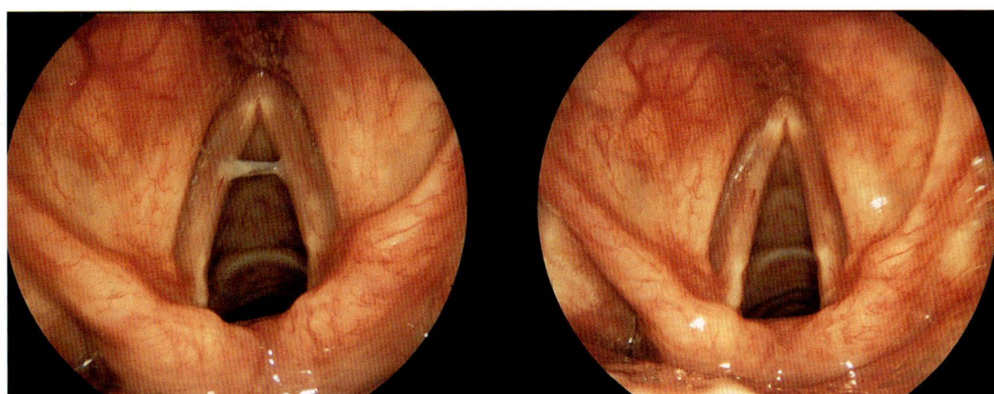

Figure **8.16**
The true and the false cords. Mucus has been cleared by asking the patient to cough.

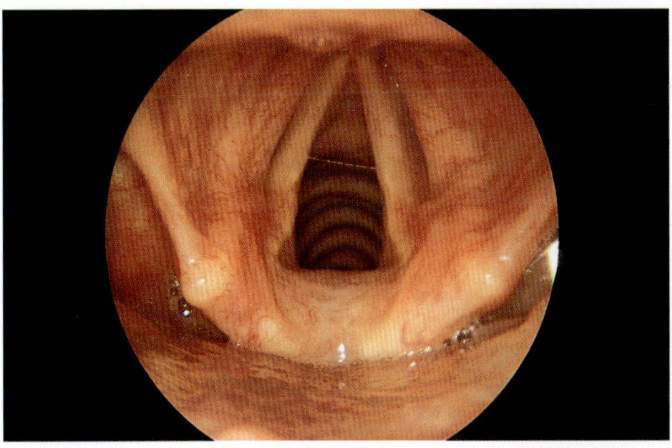

Figure **8.17**
Normal adult larynx during quiet respiration.

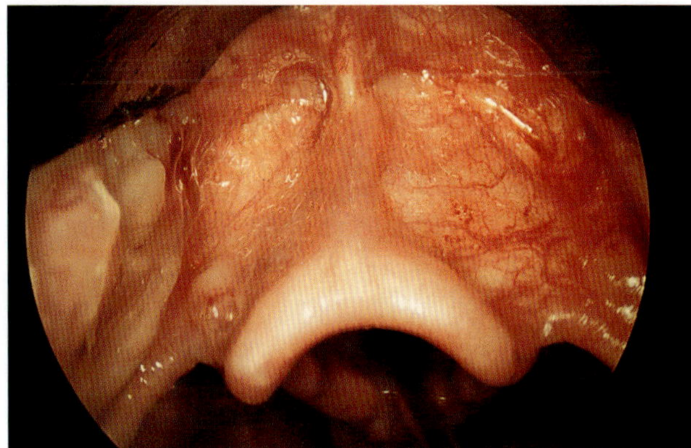

Figure **8.18**
Base of the tongue, valleculae, glosso-epiglottic fold, anterior surface and superior aspect of epiglottis.

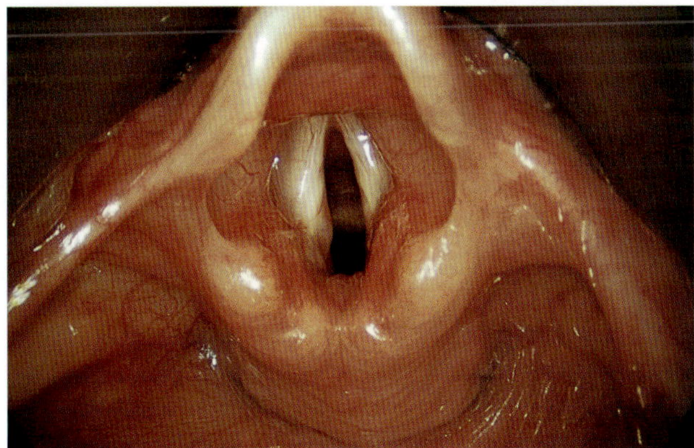

Figure **8.19**
Normal larynx and pharynx in a child under general anaesthesia.

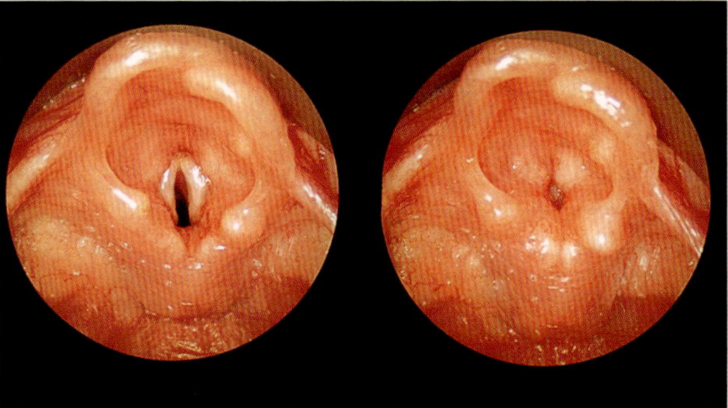

Figure **8.20**
Normal larynx during spontaneous respiration [left] and during temporary laryngospasm [right]. Use of topical anaesthesia markedly reduces the incidence and severity of laryngospasm.

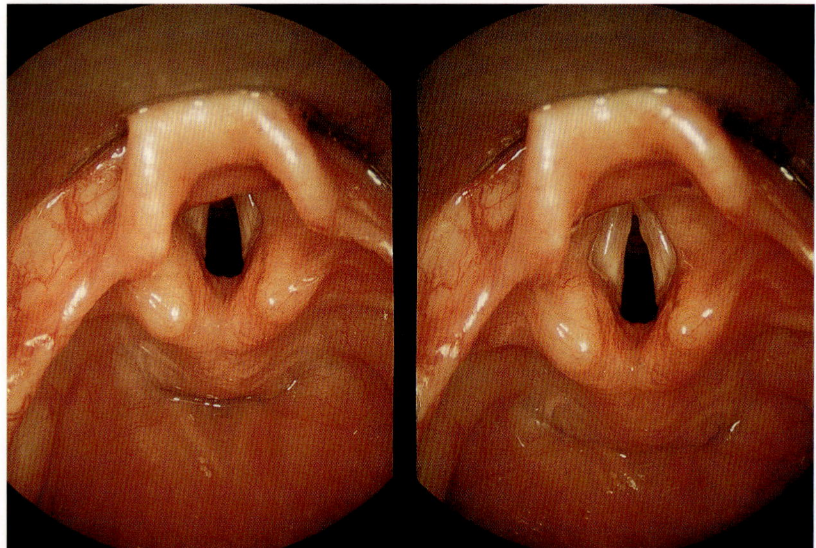

Figure **8.21**
Child's larynx exposed using a Lindholm laryngoscope. The anterior larynx is not seen [left] until the suspension angle is changed or the anterior neck is depressed [right].

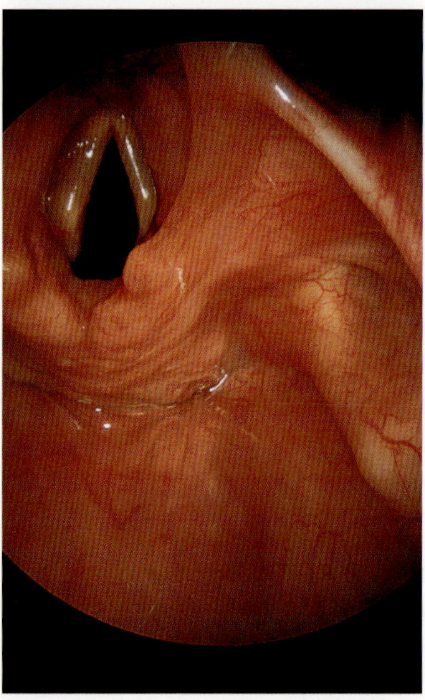

Figure **8.22**
The right piriform fossa, lateral and posterior pharyngeal walls and part of the postcricoid region exposed by angling the Lindholm laryngoscope.

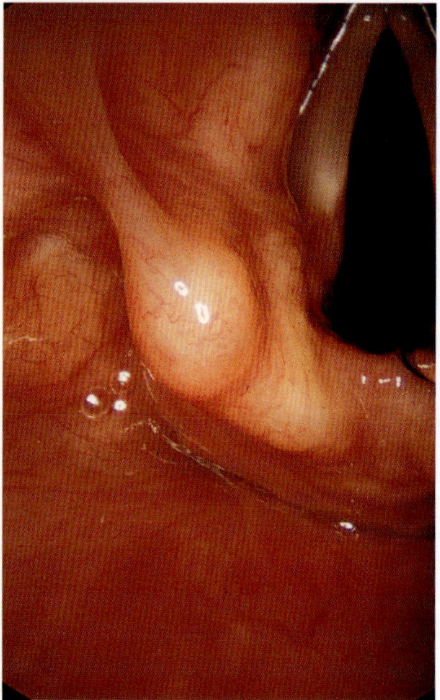

Figure **8.23**
Laryngoscope positioned to highlight the aryepiglottic fold, corniculate cartilage and left posterior glottis.

the costs. With the latest equipment, photographic documentation of any area accessible to a telescope is possible, exposure is automatic and close-up photography is feasible. Photographic documentation is positive proof of the extent and degree of pathology, and for teaching purposes image quality and natural colour reproduction cannot be equalled.

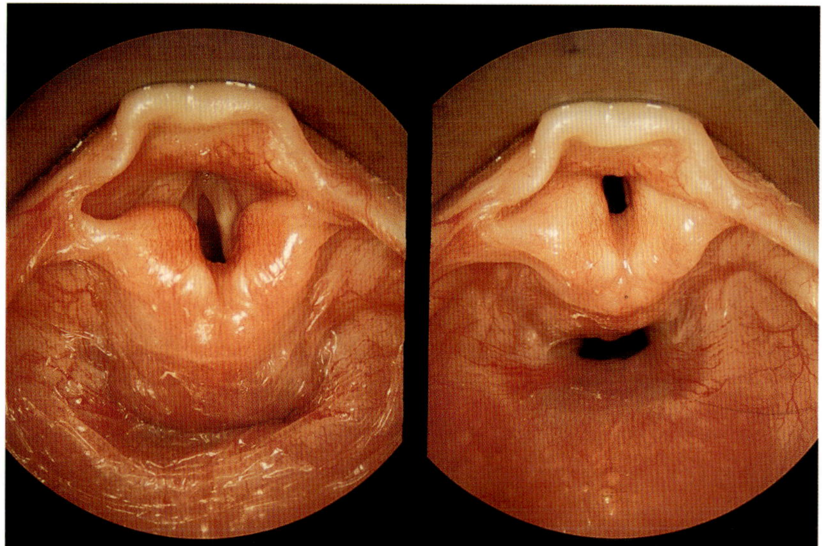

Figure **8.24**
'The Benjamin lift' often assists exposure of the postcricoid region – a telescope can often be passed to examine the upper part of the oesophagus.

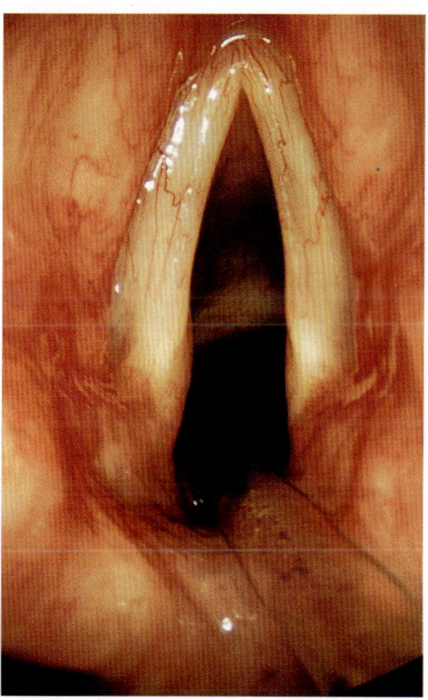

Figure **8.25**
Closer view of the glottis including true and false vocal cords, medial surface of arytenoids and anterior commissure. Note the Benjet anaesthesia tube in the posterior larynx.

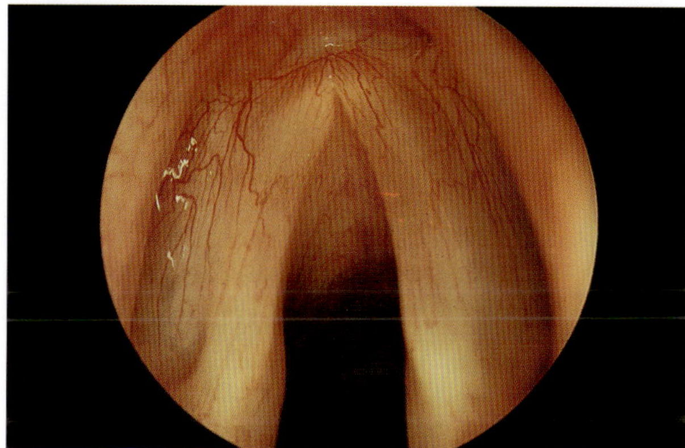

Figure **8.26**
Anterior commissure, ventricles and membranous vocal folds using a 30° telescope.

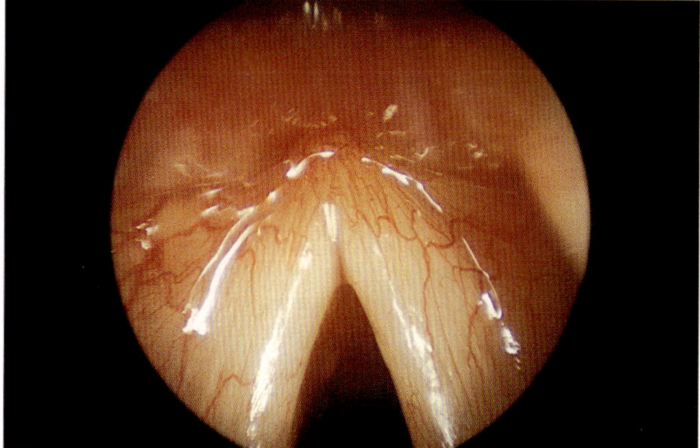

Figure **8.27**
Close-up showing details of anterior commissure and anterior ventricles using a 30° telescope.

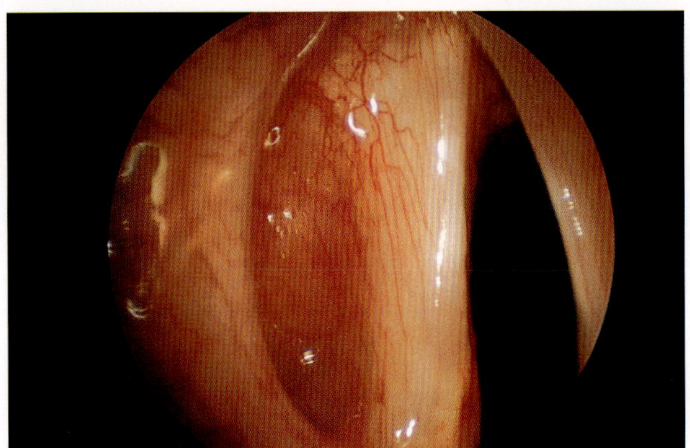

Figure **8.28**
Left ventricle, false cord and true cord seen with a 30° telescope.

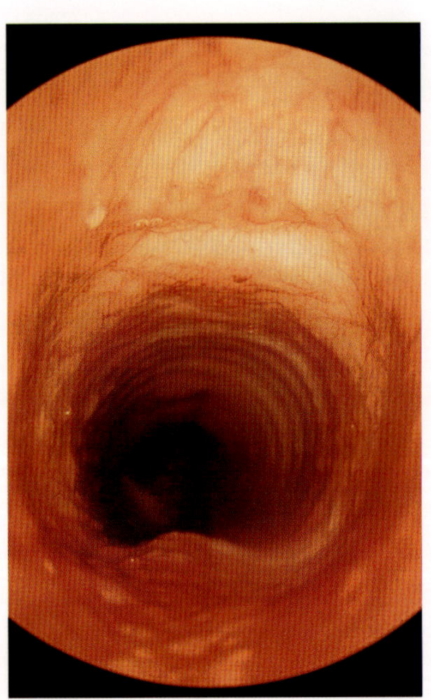

Figure **8.29**
Immediate subglottic region with tracheal arches in the distance.

NORMAL ENDOSCOPIC APPEARANCE

Familiarity with normal anatomy and its variations develops with experience and is essential for recognition of pathological change. To assist establishment of the normal, readers are referred to Figs 8.13–8.18, photographs taken at indirect laryngoscopy, and to Figs 8.19–8.29, taken at direct laryngoscopy.

BIBLIOGRAPHY

For publications on this topic, see the bibliography for chapter 7.

9 Carbon dioxide laser applications

FUNDAMENTAL LASER BIOPHYSICS

APPLICATIONS

COST

LASER SAFETY

A variety of lasers have been trialled for use in laryngeal surgery including the neodymium–yttrium aluminium garnet (Nd:YAG) laser and the potassium titanyl phosphate (KTP) laser, but the thermal damage to surrounding tissue is greater than with the carbon dioxide (CO_2) laser. The argon dye laser may possibly prove useful in treatment of early cancers using photodynamic therapy. The CO_2 laser has been used for over 20 years and is the treatment of choice for conditions such as papilloma, haemangiomas, dysplastic lesions, early carcinomas, cysts and some stenoses.

FUNDAMENTAL LASER BIOPHYSICS

A laser beam is generated when photons of energy are emitted from the atoms of an active medium (e.g. CO_2 gas) as radiant energy by exposure of the atoms to a high-energy electrical source. By increasing and amplifying the release of these photons, an intense coherent light energy beam is produced. The stream of photons are harnessed to travel in a parallel direction and accurately focused into a beam whose diameter can be varied within certain limits. The surgeon can vary the relation of power and spot size (power-density) by controlling the power (in watts), the exposure time (in fractions of a second) and the focal length of the lens (in millimetres). The higher the power-density the deeper the laser energy penetrates tissue.

The long wavelength (10.6 μm) of a CO_2 laser beam makes it invisible, so when using the laser a second low-power helium–neon beam, which *is* visible to the eye, is incorporated into the delivery

Lasers used in otolaryngology

Carbon dioxide
Nd:YAG
KTP/532
Argon

Variables to control laser energy

Power
Exposure time
Focal length of lens
Spot diameter

system to facilitate precise visual directional placement of the beam. Accurate alignment of the beams and the mirrors in the rigid tubes in the laser system arms is essential at all times.

Most of the energy of the CO_2 laser is absorbed by intracellular fluid in soft tissues with very little dissipation of heat to adjacent tissues. Thus the thermal energy causes disintegration and carbonization of the target biological tissue with generation of smoke, vapour and gas (the laser 'plume'). There is little damage to cells in the immediate surrounding tissue and little or no bleeding. This near bloodless, no touch, precise destruction of tissue makes the technique suitable for treatment of superficial lesions on delicate structures in the larynx which can be vaporized with minimal thermal damage to vital underlying tissues. With care there is little risk of undesirable scarring of mucosa, the underlying vocal ligament or vocalis muscle. There is little postoperative pain, minimal reactive oedema and less chance of the vibratory characteristics of the vocal cord being altered. The laser is not the instrument of choice for all endoscopic microlaryngeal surgery however; improper or ill-judged application can cause complications.

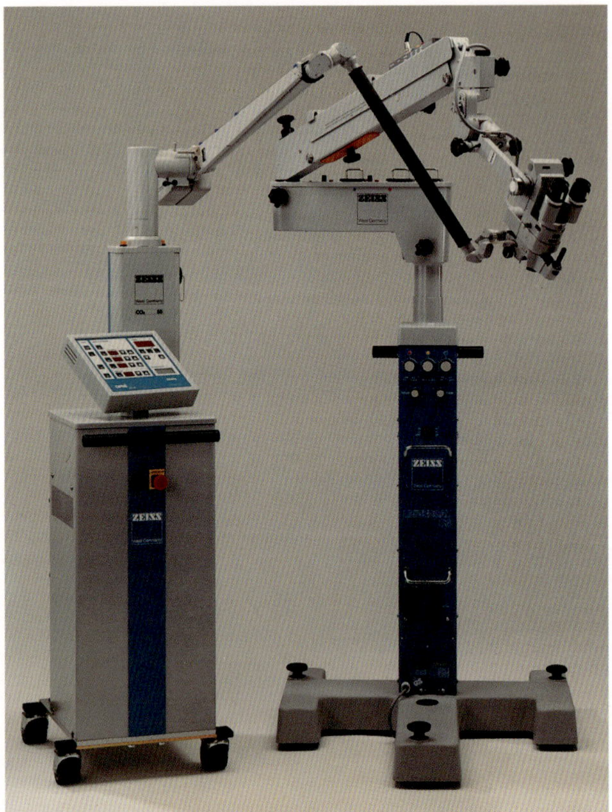

Figure **9.1**
Carbon dioxide laser for laryngology (Carl Zeiss, Germany).

Advantages of CO_2 laser in the larynx

Precision microsurgery
Little or no bleeding
Relatively painless
Little surrounding damage

For use in the larynx there are many commercial varieties of CO_2 laser units (Fig. 9.1) which deliver the beam by a coupling system to an operating microscope. Other lasers, e.g. the KTP/532 and the argon laser, have been adapted for transmission via a fibre system with consequent flexibility of delivery to the operative site. The CO_2 laser, however, cannot be delivered through flexible fibres, but its application for incision and photocoagulation during delicate microsurgery, excision of premalignant and malignant tumours and vaporization or excision of bulky obstructing lesions has stood the test of time.

There have been refinements and modifications. For example, microspot technology, engineered into the micro-manipulator has producd a smaller diameter beam for greater precision. The optics of a 'microspot' micro-manipulator reduce the diameter of the CO_2 laser spot to 0.3 mm (with a 400-mm focal length lens), but the consequent high power-density of the beam dictates that power of the laser should be reduced to 2 or 3 watts. New techniques such as endoscopic flap surgery and laser spot 'welding' methods appear to have promise but as yet are not universally employed.

Refinements for CO_2 laser surgery

Microspot micro-manipulator
Supra-pulse mode
Micro-flap surgery

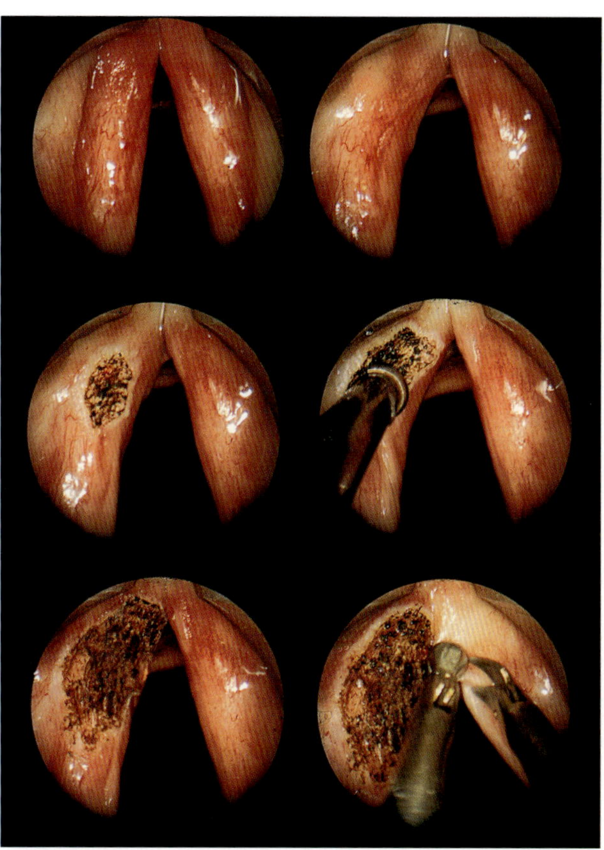

Figure **9.2**
Laser treatment of left vocal cord microinvasive carcinoma proven at previous biopsy. Appearance at laryngoscopy (top left). Improved exposure by advancing the laryngoscope (top right). Beginning laser treatment (centre left). Exposure of anterior aspect (centre right). Completion of wide-field laser vaporization (lower left). Biopsy of right side (lower right).

The supra-pulse modality with short duration of the pulse yet high intensity of the beam allows the laser to rapidly ablate abnormal tissue before the heat energy spreads by thermal diffusion.

The first wave of enthusiasm for laser use in otolaryngology has been tempered by the realization of certain limitations and the possibility of complications. When used inappropriately, e.g. by continuous exposure with a large spot size or at high power for delicate laryngeal work, deep scarring and fibrosis may result in a voice of poor quality. Thus, for safe and successful application the user should understand the basics of the genesis of the laser, the significance of its wavelength and its effect on tissues, the transmission by the delivery system and the use of intermittent and continuous modes.

APPLICATIONS

The laser should not be used indiscriminately for all lesions. There are relative indications and contraindications which have become more clearly defined in recent years.

CO_2 laser is advantageous for the treatment of laryngeal lesions such as multiple respiratory papillomas, premalignant conditions such as keratosis and dysplasia, carcinoma-in-situ, early carcinoma (Fig. 9.2) and verrucous carcinoma. Benign lesions such as granulomas (Fig. 9.3), lipomas and fibromas can be removed with minimal bleeding. Cysts, large or small, can be dissected, and selected congenital lesions such as laryngomalacia (Fig. 9.4), subglottic haemangioma or cystic hygroma are readily amenable to laser surgery. Congenital and acquired subglottic stenosis, up to a critical thickness (generally agreed as 5 mm in adults) can be successfully treated endoscopically and operations such as arytenoidectomy, aryepiglottoplasty or laser tenotomy (Fig. 9.5) can be performed. A metal 'paddle' may be necessary near the anterior commissure to protect nearby normal tisue (Fig. 9.6) On the other hand, use of the laser in the laryngopharynx has certain disadvantages. For instance, it is usually considered

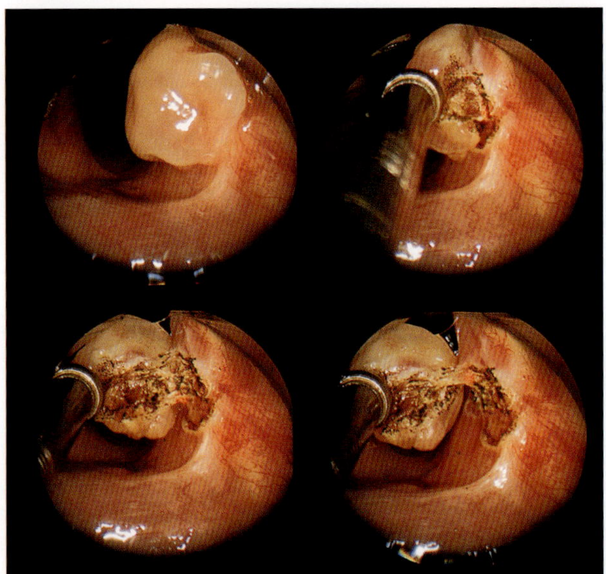

Figure **9.3**
Vocal granuloma arising from vocal process of right arytenoid. Showing the steps in laser removal, note suction is used to retract the granuloma medially and expose the pedicled base.

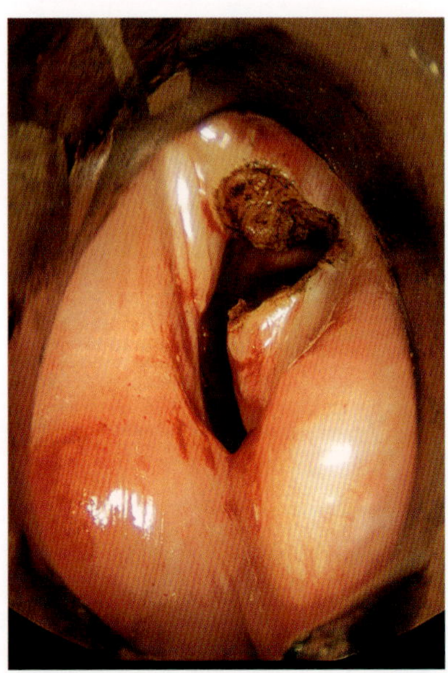

Figure **9.5**
Right laser tenotomy for vocal cord paralysis (see Fig. 11.19 for final result).

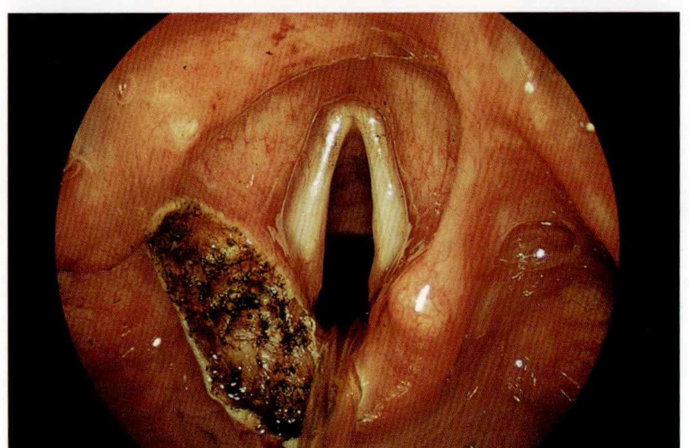

Figure **9.4**
Laser aryepiglottoplasty, removal of left cuneiform cartilage and aryepiglottic fold.

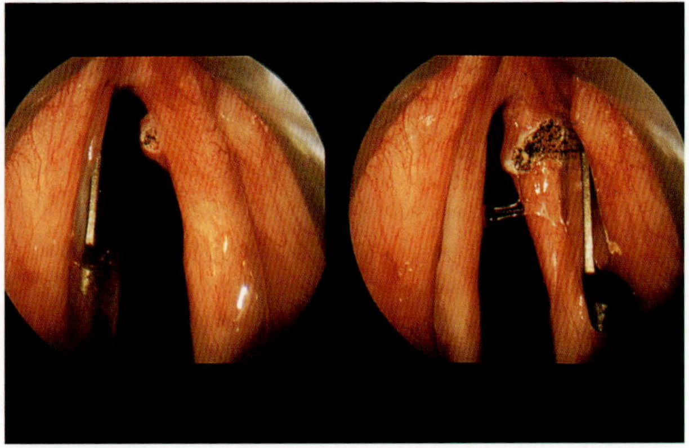

Figure **9.6**
Laser removal of a single remaining papilloma after seven previous treatments for widespread laryngeal papillomatosis. A metal 'paddle' protects the contralateral cord (left) and is used to roll the right vocal fold (right).

inappropriate to use the laser, whether with a conventional micro-manipulator or the microspot adaptation, for removal of vocal nodules. Most advocate that a vocal polyp should not be removed using laser but with 'cold' instruments including grasping forceps and appropriate scissors, stressing that surgical trauma must remain superficial to the intermediate layer of the lamina propria.

One of the major disadvantages of laser lies in the investigation of a patient with possible premalignancy

Applications

Laryngeal and tracheal papillomas
Epithelial dysplasias
Removal of benign and malignant tumours
Debulking of obstructive lesions
Granulomas, lipomas, fibromas
Cysts, haemangiomas
Subglottic stenoses
Arytenoidectomy
Aryepiglottoplasty

Laser safety precautions

Warnings on doors
Protect patient's face and eyes
Protect eyes of staff
Extraction of laser 'plume'
Moist cottonoids in airway
Avoid endotracheal tube if possible
Use 'laser-safe' tube
Oxygen 40%, helium 60% mixture

CONSTANT VIGILANCE

or malignancy. A small lesion cannot be removed by laser vaporization without tissue destruction, thus making histopathological evaluation impossible. It is wiser to take a conventional biopsy and await frozen section or routine haematoxylin and eosin preparation so that a histological diagnosis directs further treatment.

COST

Careful evaluation of the initial capital cost and the running expenses of laser technology is an important consideration; the advantage of laser surgery must be balanced against the expense. Most ear, nose and throat/head and neck surgery teaching institutions now have a CO_2 laser.

The most controversial and important factor involves safety of the laser, especially its use in the airway under general anaesthesia when the possibility of ignition of anaesthetic tubes can cause major morbidity.

LASER SAFETY

Laser ignition of a combustible anaesthetic tube resulting in an explosion burn in the respiratory tract during microlaryngeal surgery is a major potential hazard which has not yet been totally solved. Not only can the endotracheal tube ignite, but external anaesthetic tubing, packing and even surgical drapes have caught fire. There is also a potential hazard to the personnel in the operating theatre from 'stray' laser energy which might conceivably bounce off the metal of an instrument or the laryngoscope.

Users of the laser must be aware of the potential hazards and risks, especially those of fire in the airway. The safety procedures which must be put in place include:

- warnings on doors of the operating theatre that laser energy is in use to minimize people coming in and out of the operating theatre unnecessarily;
- protection of the patient's eyes, face and lips, usually by use of a moist towel;
- protection of the staff, especially their eyes, by the use of glass or plastic wrap-around spectacles with side guards to absorb the energy of the CO_2 laser; a laser strike may damage the cornea but will not reach the retina;
- use of an efficient vacuum extractor placed near the patient's mouth to remove the plume of laser smoke when it might be considered a hazard; analysis of smoke in the laser plume shows particulate matter, but it is doubtful if there are cells

which are viable. Special laser masks are available and are said to filter viral particles, but their efficacy is unproven;

- saline-soaked patties, cottonoids or pledgets in the airway to protect the endotracheal tube;
- avoidance of an endotracheal tube in the airway whenever possible;
- use of a laser-safe tube where an endotracheal tube is necessary or desirable;
- use of a metal or laser-protected anaesthetic tube to replace the usual plastic tube in a patient who has an existing tracheotomy;
- modification of anaesthetic gases to replace pure oxygen or oxygen/nitrous oxide with gases less likely to support combustion; a 40% oxygen : 60% helium mixture is recommended.

Anaesthetic methods for safe use of the CO_2 laser in the larynx and upper airways are discussed in chapter 5.

III CONDITIONS COMMON TO ADULTS AND CHILDREN

10 Vocal nodules

EPIDEMIOLOGY

PATHOPHYSIOLOGY

CLINICAL FEATURES

INDIRECT LARYNGOSCOPY

TREATMENT
- Medical
- Microlaryngoscopy
- Microsurgical removal

BIBLIOGRAPHY

Vocal nodules are chronic bilateral swellings on the edge and undersurface of the membranous vocal folds (Fig. 10.1). They interfere with voice production. This definition excludes acute swellings in the mucosa.

EPIDEMIOLOGY

Vocal nodules are common in school-age children. They are said to be the cause in up to 80% of children with voice disorders. They are commoner in boys (Fig. 10.2),

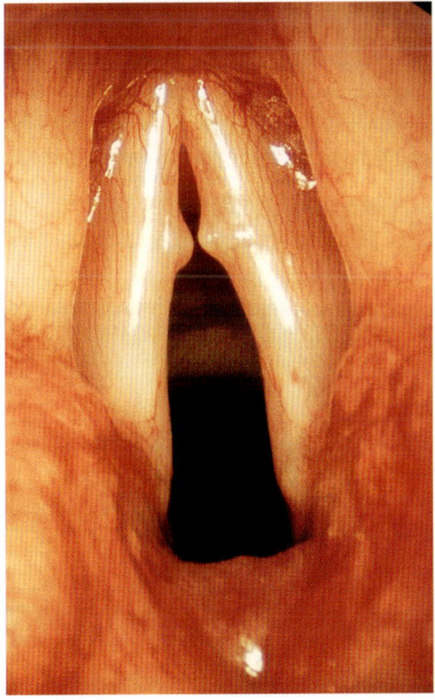

Figure **10.1**
Typical bilateral chronic vocal nodules with little surrounding oedema in a 12-year-old boy who presented with chronic intermittent huskiness which was unresponsive to speech therapy. The nodules were removed and his voice returned to normal.

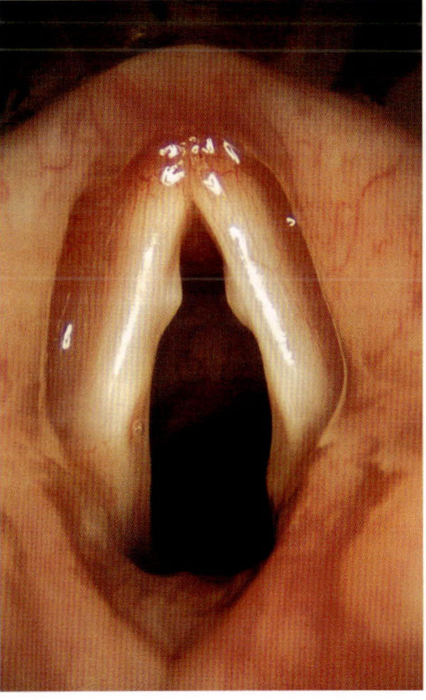

Figure **10.2**
Vocal nodules in a 10-year-old boy who shouted a lot. There are nodular thickenings and some surrounding perinodular oedematous swelling.

Vocal nodules
Commoner in boys than girls Commoner in women than men

Causes
Voice misuse or abuse Use of an unnaturally low voice

especially boisterous children who habitually misuse their voice during play or imitate sounds such as a racing car or a motor bike or the voice of their favourite cartoon character. Boys may yell excessively at sporting events. Not all children with nodules misuse their voice, nor are they excessively talkative. Children with repaired cleft palate sometimes develop nodules.

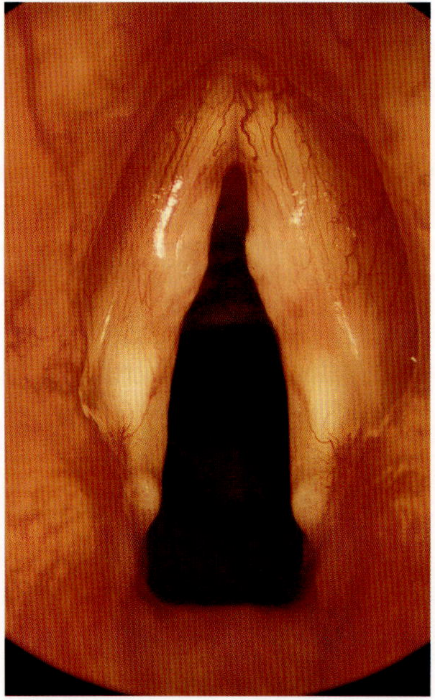

Figure **10.3**
Vocal nodules with surrounding subacute inflammatory changes including oedema and vascular dilatation in a 25-year-old singer who had been working in a stage show for many months. Voice rest for 6 weeks resulted in a marked improvement in the voice and in the appearance of the nodules.

In adults vocal nodules are more common in females than males. Those prone to form nodules include teachers, telephone operators, entertainers, singers (especially 'rock' singers) (Fig. 10.3), travel group leaders, high-pressure salespersons, stock traders, politicians, ministers of religion and others who make heavy demands on their vocal abilities from day to day.

Professional singers with vocal nodules may be straining to achieve special effects by harmful use of the voice. They often sing in an unnaturally low register even though they may have had adequate singing training. Vocal nodules are dreaded by classically trained singers.

PATHOPHYSIOLOGY

The cause of vocal nodules is usually related to overuse, misuse or abuse of the voice in conversation, shouting, yelling, attempting to create an impression by speaking in a lower register.

Use of an unnaturally low fundamental frequency and an excessively loud voice cause congestion and vascular dilatation in the lamina propria of the vocal cord submucosa, with oedema in Reinke's space and later hyalinization with organization and fibrosis in the submucosal connective tissue as vocal cord trauma persists. Specific histological observations show thickening of the basement membrane, absence of haemorrhages and absence of large areas of oedema. These changes occur at the junction of the anterior third and the posterior two-thirds of the vocal cord, that is in the middle of the membranous vocal

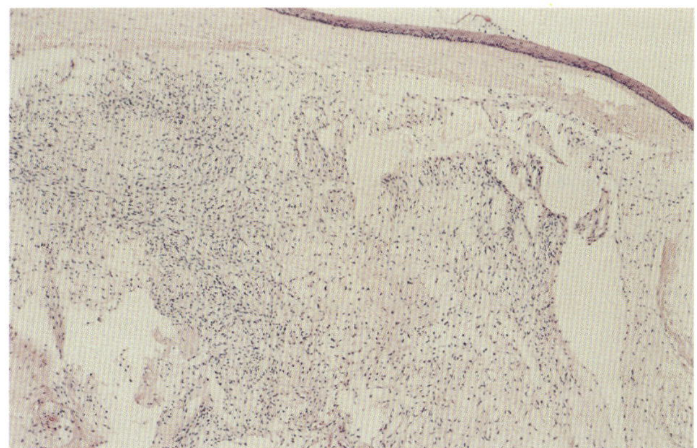

Figure **10.4**
Histopathology of vocal nodule. Section showing thin mucosa with thick basement membrane. The submucosa shows fibroblastic proliferation and oedema with cyst formation.

fold on each side, the site of maximum amplitude of vibration. Nodules interfere with normal vibration and cause hoarseness, breathiness and disruption of the frequency range, especially higher frequencies.

The histopathological findings (Fig. 10.4) in a chronic nodule include hyperplasia of the epithelial layer and thickening of the basement membrane with or without keratin formation, chronic surrounding Reinke's oedema, presence of fibroblasts, fibrous tissue, hyalinization, sometimes microcystic degeneration and minimal inflammatory changes.

Immunohistochemical techniques for protein identification in the lamina propria have shown intense fibronectin deposition in the superficial layer of the lamina propria, often coupled with basement membrane zone injury, indicated by thick collagen type IV bands. Fibronectin is a glycoprotein deposited by fibroblasts and therefore a precursor for scar formation; this pathologic response may explain why some nodules do not respond to voice therapy.

Oedema in the anterior subcommissure is often seen at microlaryngoscopy when using a 0° or a 30° telescope. It is a secondary change and does not alter treatment.

Histopathology of chronic nodule

Hyperplasia of epithelial layer ± keratin
Surrounding Reinke's oedema
Fibroblasts and fibrous tissue
Condensations of hyalinization
Microcystic degeneration
Thickening of basement membrane
Minimal inflammation

CLINICAL FEATURES

In adults there is variable huskiness, breathiness and the voice 'tires' after prolonged use. Teachers may find it difficult to continue – especially in a noisy classroom – telephone operators may be frustrated and

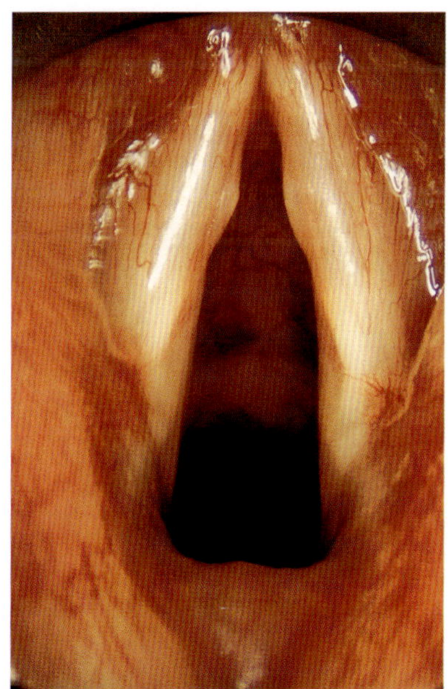

Figure **10.5**
Chronic nodules in an 8-year-old girl whose friends teased her about her voice, causing embarrassment. The nodules were removed.

Symptoms

Huskiness
Breathiness
Reduced vocal endurance
Loss of high singing frequencies
Worse with RTI

quizzed by their callers about their voice abnormality and professional singers notice loss of range, especially for high frequencies although their conversational voice may be normal.

Some children have periods of 'loss' of voice. Occasionally the voice will 'block' with delay of phonatory onset when talking or reading in class. Some children, especially girls (Fig. 10.5), may be teased or ridiculed because of a deep, unusual voice.

Children with vocal nodules are usually talkative, use a loud voice, may be emotionally labile, hyperactive and come from a dysfunctional family; some may manifest nervousness, muscle tension or aggressive behaviour.

Nodules can occur in small infants (Fig. 10.6) and cause a harsh unusual sound during vocalization in babies who cry and scream excessively – so called 'screamer's' nodules.

The symptoms of vocal nodules in adults and children are often made worse by an intercurrent upper or lower respiratory tract infection (RTI).

Subjective perception evaluation of voice quality is difficult, unreliable, is not comparable from one examiner to another and requires extensive experience. Nevertheless, huskiness in the adult or child is the single most important clue to the presence of vocal nodules.

Documentation of the speaking and singing voice using audiometric and video or video-stroboscopic recordings provide the best documentation of both voice abnormality and laryngeal appearance.

INDIRECT LARYNGOSCOPY

Examination of the larynx with a mirror, rigid telescope or flexible fibreoptic laryngoscope in adults, older children and co-operative younger children will confirm vocal nodules (Fig. 10.7). Mucus on the edge

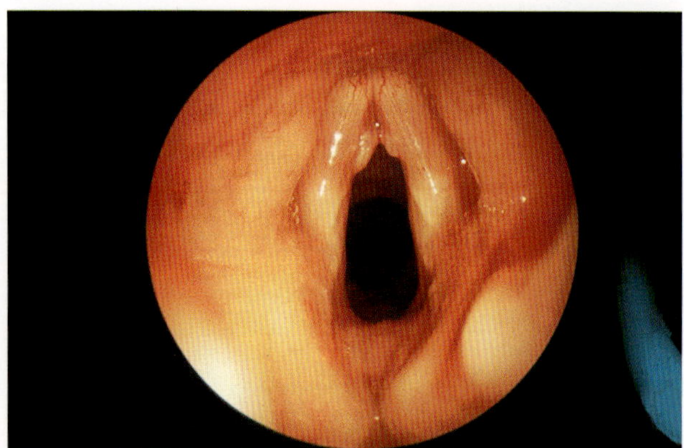

Figure **10.6**
An 8-month-old baby boy with large rounded bilateral nodules. They appear to be very anterior but they are actually in the central part of the membranous vocal fold. The vocal process of the arytenoid reaches to the centre of the vocal cord.

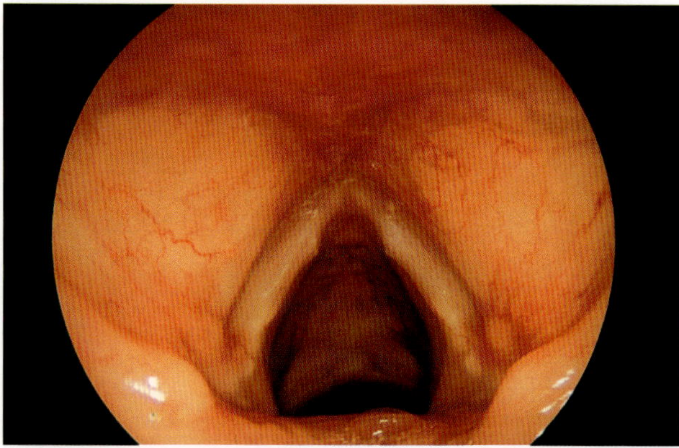

Figure **10.7**
Vocal nodules in a 20-year-old female photographed at indirect laryngoscopy. Less detail can be seen at indirect laryngoscopy than is visualized with telescopes at direct laryngoscopy.

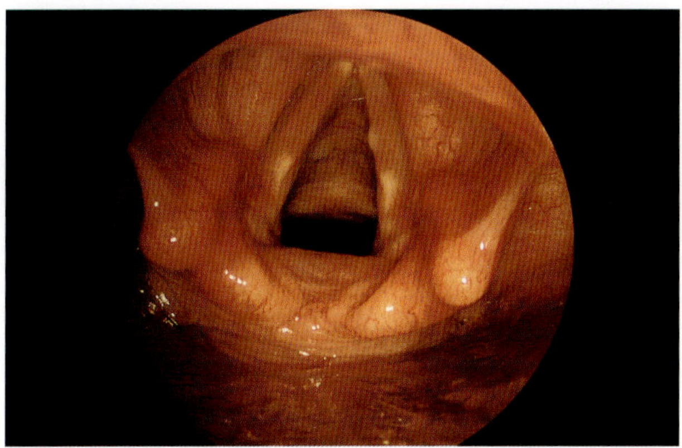

Figure **10.8**
Photograph at indirect laryngoscopy showing mucus in the centre of the right vocal fold mimicking pathology; when the patient coughed the appearance was normal.

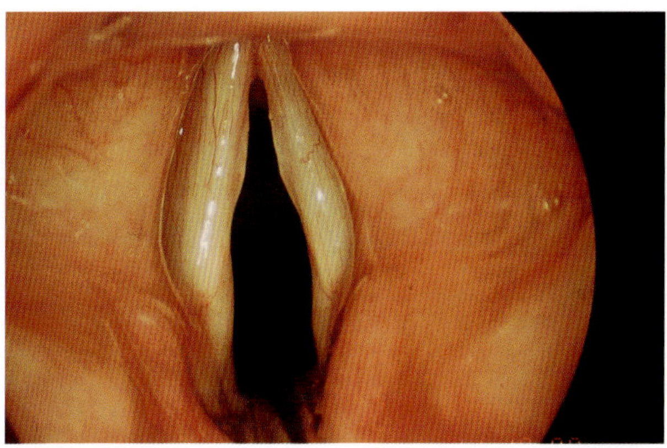

Figure **10.10**
Chronic vocal nodules in an adult. Note the long fusiform base. White patches on the surface may prove to be fibrin, keratin or even fungus.

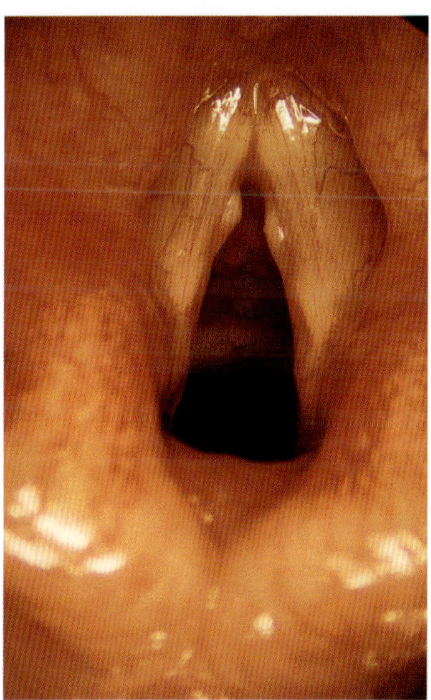

Figure **10.9**
Prominent vocal nodules at slightly different sites on the two vocal cords. There is surrounding oedema in the vocal fold and some minor oedema at the anterior subcommissure.

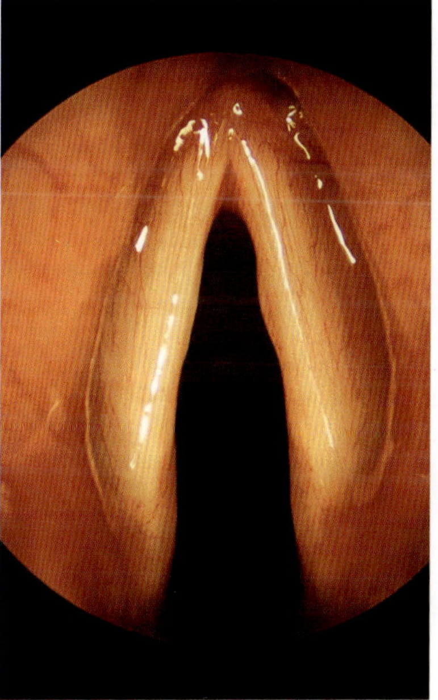

Figure **10.11**
Small area of vocal cord polyp on the edge of the right vocal fold, simulating a vocal nodule. There is surrounding oedema in the vocal fold and histopathological examination showed the lesion to be a polyp.

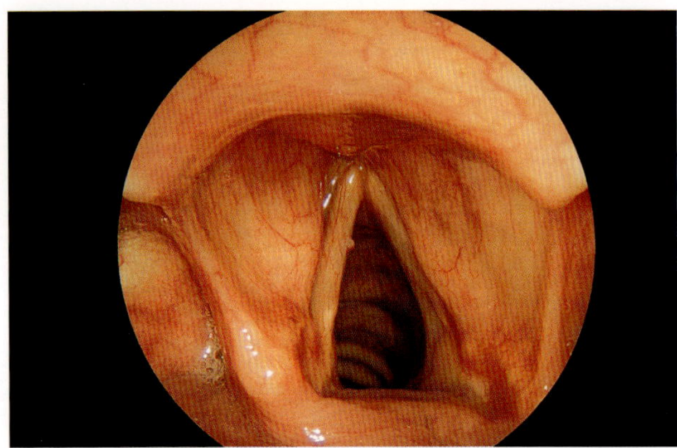

Figure **10.12**
Indirect laryngoscopic photograph of a tiny surface mucus retention cyst in the centre of the edge of the left vocal fold.

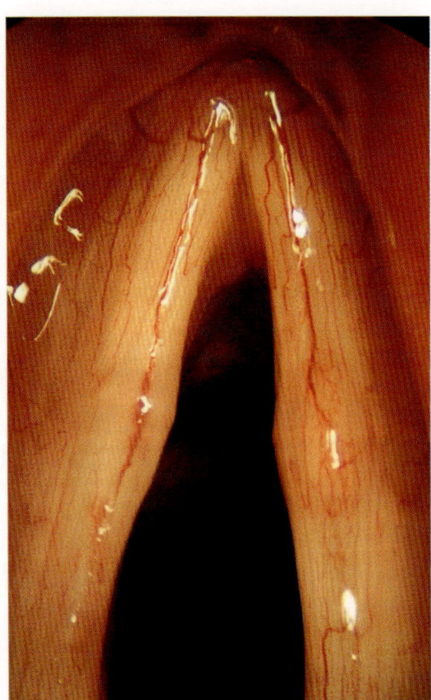

Figure **10.13**
Intracordal cyst in the right vocal fold in a young woman of 18 years. There is vascular dilatation, prominent capillaries on both sides with some reaction on the edge of the opposite cord. The cyst needs to be finally identified and then removed by microsurgery.

of a vocal fold can mimic the appearance of a nodule (Fig. 10.8) but the mucus clears after coughing; vocal nodules are always bilateral.

There is a spectrum of appearance. Most nodules appear as localized fusiform or nodular prominences (Fig. 10.1) of the mucosal surface on the edge of the membranous vocal fold. Larger nodules show prominent, irregular, focal nodularity (Fig. 10.9) with surrounding longitudinal oedema and sometimes secondary oedema in the anterior subcommissure. Thus the appearance of nodules depends on the length of time they have been present and whether excessive voice use or an upper respiratory tract infection has caused recent exacerbation. Nodules can vary in size, symmetry and colour. The surface may be inflamed, finely irregular or show areas of leukoplakia (Fig. 10.10) due to keratin. The appearance of the nodules and the surrounding oedema are visualized with greater clarity using the magnification provided by a large-diameter rigid telescope.

Occasionally patients are seen who have been evaluated elsewhere and told their vocal cords are 'normal'.

A diagnosis of 'unilateral nodule' must be questioned. There may be bilateral nodules, one of which is large so that the other appears insignificant. There may be a small unilateral vocal cord polyp (Fig. 10.11) or there may be a cyst near the surface (Fig. 10.12) or a cyst within the substance of the cord (Fig. 10.13) and each of the unilateral lesions may cause some reactionary swelling of the opposite vocal fold. An intracordal cyst can be diagnosed with confidence only at direct laryngoscopy; a diffuse, yellowish bulge is detected within

Causes of 'unilateral nodule'

One large, one small nodule
Small unilateral polyp
Vocal cord cyst
Mucus simulating a 'nodule'

the central part of the membranous vocal fold on one side.

In younger children indirect laryngoscopy may not be possible, either for anatomic reasons or owing to inability to tolerate the necessary instrumentation. Diagnostic direct laryngoscopy under general anaesthesia may be warranted when huskiness has been steadily progressive over a short time or when there are features of airway obstruction. The diagnosis usually rests between vocal nodules and respiratory papillomas affecting the vocal folds or even a vocal fold cyst. A diagnosis of vocal nodules is strongly supported by a history of several years of variable hoarseness which becomes worse following overuse of the voice and better with voice rest.

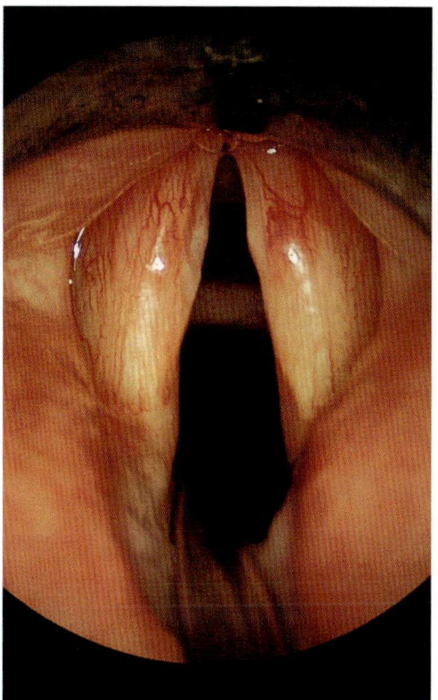

Figure **10.14**
Subacute inflammatory laryngitis from an intercurrent respiratory tract infection. The patient was a young female professional singer. After treatment with antibiotics and 4 weeks of voice rest the vocal folds returned almost to normal.

TREATMENT

Medical

Therapy from a speech pathologist encourages reduction of vocal abuse, more appropriate methods of voice production, modification of periods of loudness and voice rest. This treatment will sometimes bring about an improvement. Some so-called 'soft nodules' which have not been present for long (Fig. 10.14) may resolve with time or coincidentally with speech therapy.

It is common experience that large, firm-looking nodules in adults often fail to improve even when an experienced voice therapist skilled in behavioural therapy treats the patient for several months. Surgical removal should be considered in patients with chronic voice disability when medical management and voice rest have failed to eradicate the nodules.

Children with vocal nodules should be reviewed by indirect laryngoscopy at regular intervals (every 6–12 months) noting possible aggravating factors such as tonsillitis, rhino-sinusitis, bronchitis or asthma. The indications for removal of nodules include voice disability for several years, no improvement after voice therapy and severe hoarseness causing embarrassment during conversation or reading in class (Fig. 10.5). The symptoms may cause the child to be ridiculed. A recommendation for operation is seldom made before the age of 8 years. As most vocal nodules in older children are self-limiting, often resolving in teenage years, the possibility of natural remission should be considered by the prudent laryngologist when considering removal of vocal nodules from patients in their early teens.

Microlaryngoscopy

Using suspension laryngoscopy under general anaesthesia, the vocal folds are visualized and the edge and undersurface displayed using external finger pressure, first on one and then on the other side of the neck combined with gentle use of a suction tube or blunt instrument to roll and evert the vocal fold. A 30° telescope (Fig. 10.15) assists in accurate assessment. There is nodularity and focal thickening in the mid-part of the membranous vocal fold with surrounding longitudinal oedema in Reinke's space.

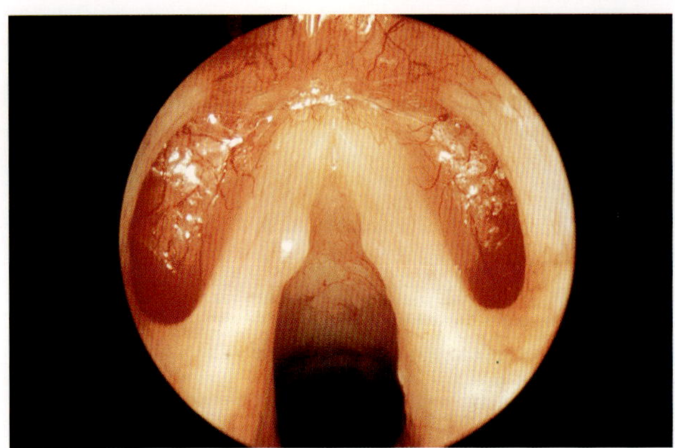

Figure **10.15**
Chronic vocal nodules seen with the 30° telescope confirming that the nodules are on the edge and undersurface of the mid-point of the membranous vocal fold.

The most prominent swelling is on the edge and undersurface of the vocal fold. The nodules are usually symmetrical but sometimes one nodule is larger.

There may be a difference in the appearance of nodules seen at indirect laryngoscopy compared to direct laryngoscopy under general anaesthesia using magnification with telescopes or the microscope. Nodules which are prominent at indirect laryngoscopy may be less obvious at direct laryngoscopy (Fig. 10.16), or vice versa.

Microsurgical removal

Precise and careful technique is necessary. Most laryngologists prefer use of cupped-shaped forceps and curved scissors for accurate removal. Use of the carbon dioxide laser, even with the microspot technique, remains controversial.

Use of conventional cupped forceps and scissors allows superficial removal of the prominent nodule together with surrounding oedema without injury to the underlying vocal ligament. The free-edge of the nodule is grasped with upturned cup-shaped forceps or Bouchayer forceps with due care not to include the lamina propria. The nodule is retracted medially to stretch and emphasize the wide base and separate it from the underlying structures. The mucosa near the anterior commissure should be kept intact; preservation of this mucosal edge allows both

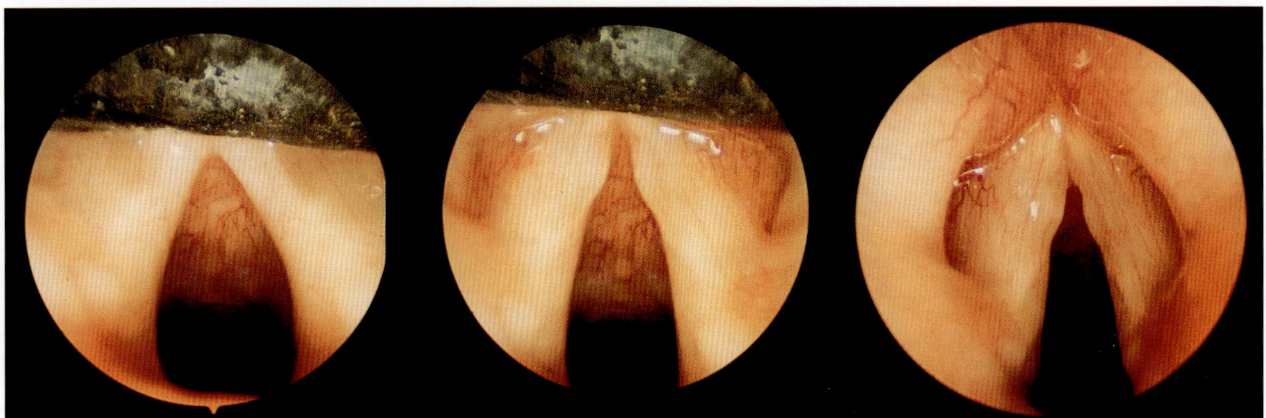

Figure **10.16**
Nodules seen at direct laryngoscopy under general anaesthesia. First picture: the tip of the laryngoscope has been introduced too far and shows the stretched undersurface of the vocal folds but not the nodules. Second picture: the laryngoscope has been withdrawn a little and the nodules are seen. Third picture: the laryngoscope has been further withdrawn to give a more natural, undistorted view.

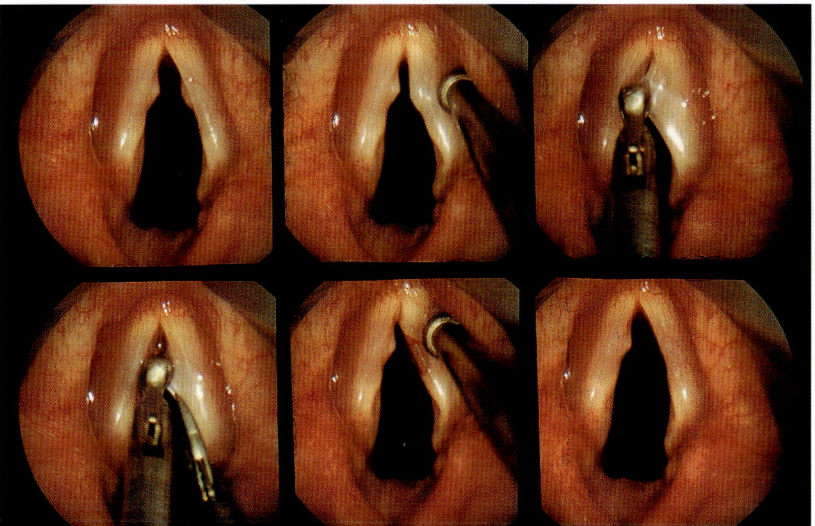

Figure **10.17**
Steps in the surgical removal of right-sided vocal nodule. The nodule is identified, rolled and everted with the tip of the sucker, cupped forceps grasp the mucosal edge of the nodule but not the underlying lamina propria and scissors remove the nodule and some surrounding oedema. The vocal fold is again rolled to show the elongated oval defect with an intact lamina propria. The last photograph shows the straight edge of the right side before removal of the other nodule.

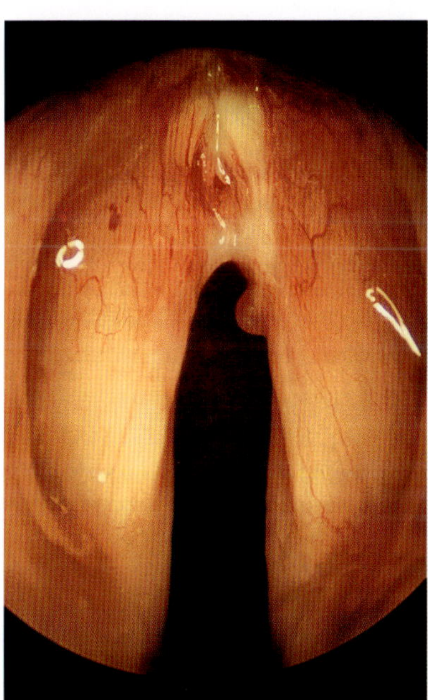

Figure **10.18**
Larynx of a 21-year-old woman who had both vocal nodules removed at the same operation by another surgeon 5 weeks before. An adhesion is forming and there is an area of granulation. Under general anaesthetic an attempt was made to divide the adhesion but it re-formed and the result is shown in Figure 10.19.

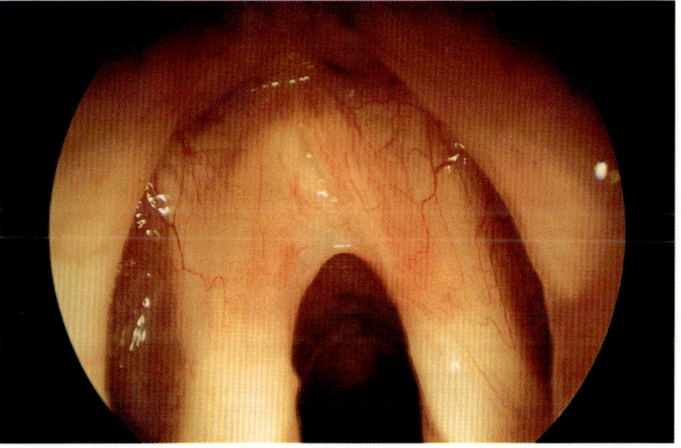

Figure **10.19**
Chronic mature anterior glottic web after simultaneous bilateral removal of vocal nodules many months before. The voice was poor, the web was divided with scissors with about 50% improvement. The patient did not wish to have any further surgery.

nodules to be removed at one operation. If, however, the excision extends towards the anterior commissure (Fig. 10.18), staged removal of the contralateral nodule some weeks later should be planned to eliminate the possibility of adhesion and web formation (Fig. 10.19). After removal, the resultant shallow surgical defect under the vocal cord edge has an elongated oval shape and the intact vocal ligament

Microsurgical removal

Cupped or Bouchayer forceps
Curved or up-turned scissors
Retract edge of vocal cord medially
Excise with scissors
Identify and preserve lamina propria
Staged operations if necessary

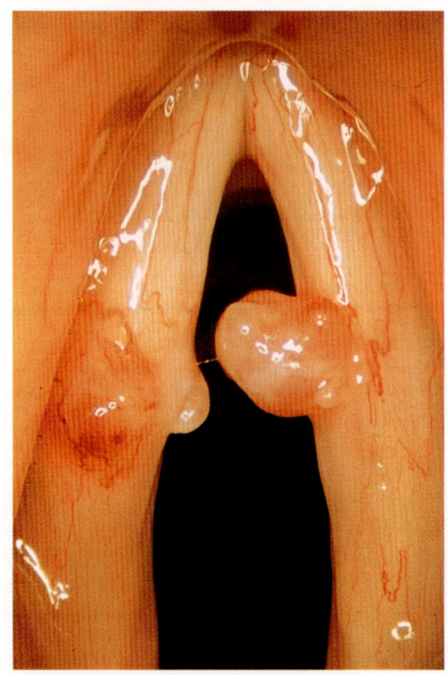

Figure **10.20**
Polypoidal degeneration with vascular dilatation and surrounding oedema. A woman in her 30s had refused treatment of her vocal nodules for many years. Eventual removal of these lesions produced a reasonably good voice.

can be seen lining the base. At the end of the procedure, the edge of the vocal fold should be smooth and straight; no depression should be visible.

Rarely, untreated nodules undergo hyalinization and/or polypoidal degeneration (Fig. 10.20), and operative removal is clearly necessary.

'Stripping' of the vocal cord is contraindicated in the treatment of vocal nodules. Nor is there any necessity to use a technique where a 'divot' might be removed from the tissues.

The same technique is used in children. A child's larynx is no more delicate than that of an adult when microscopic surgery is performed using gentle, precise technique. Some authorities have had a conviction that removal of nodules in children is harmful, difficult and unnecessary because they believed that the child's larynx is more easily traumatized than that of the adult; they warn that prompt recurrence of the nodules may occur. Most children find co-operation with speech therapy regimes difficult or impossible and it is time for a reappraisal of the treatment of vocal nodules in children. Removal of vocal nodules in adults is acknowledged as proper treatment. It is also safe, justifiable and effective in selected paediatric patients.

The result of removal should be a normal or near normal voice, although a few children continue to have fluctuations of symptoms with voice abuse. There is a recurrence rate of approximately 1 in 30. Appropriate preoperative and postoperative speech therapy may improve results.

Quiet use of the voice for 10 days is advised after removal of vocal nodules. No steroids or antibiotics are necessary. There is usually rapid healing, absence of complications and the voice returns to normal some weeks after removal.

BIBLIOGRAPHY

Bastian RW (1993) Benign mucosal and saccular disorders: benign laryngeal tumours. In: Cummings CW, Fredrickson JM, Harker LA, Krause CJ, Schuller DE, eds, *Otolaryngology – head and neck surgery* (St Louis: CV Mosby); 1905–6.

Benjamin B (1990) The vocal nodule: to remove? In: Healy GB, ed., *Common problems in paediatric otolaryngology* (Chicago: Yearbook Medical Publishers); 439–46.

Benjamin B, Croxson G (1987) Vocal nodules in children. *Ann Otol Rhinol Laryngol* **96**: 530–3.

Dikkers FG, Nikkels PGJ (1995) Benign lesions of the vocal folds; histopathology and phonotrauma. *Ann Otol Rhinol Laryngol* **104**: 698–703.

Gray SD, Hammond E, Hanson DF (1995) Benign pathologic responses of the larynx. *Ann Otol Rhinol Laryngol* **104**: 13–18.

Lehmann W, Pidoux J-M, Widmann J-J Pseudotumours–nodules. In: *Larynx. Microlaryngoscopie et histopathologie* (Geneva: Inpharzam Medical Publications); 68–75.

Von Leyden H (1985) Vocal nodules in children. *Ear Nose Throat J* **64**: 29–41.

11 Vocal cord paralysis

INTRODUCTION

Vocal cord paralysis can be due to central or peripheral pathology and may involve the central connections, the vagus nerve, the recurrent laryngeal nerve and/or the superior laryngeal nerve. It may affect one or both sides of the larynx. Paresis, or weakness without paralysis, sometimes occurs. As 'vocal cord paralysis' is not a diagnosis, thorough investigation is required in an effort to determine the cause. Many cases of unilateral paralysis, especially in adults, will finally be labelled 'viral' or 'idiopathic' and some cases of bilateral vocal cord paralysis in infants will also remain undiagnosed. In addition, the laryngologist must be assured that the lack of movement in the hemilarynx is not caused by cricoarytenoid joint arthritis, fixation or dislocation nor due to a nearby neoplasm.

Vocal cord paralysis in infants

	Unilateral	*Bilateral*
Stridor	uncommon	always present
Cry	weak	near normal
Usual cause	peripheral	central
Tracheotomy	seldom	almost always

Vocal cord paralysis may not be an isolated neurologic disorder but may be a manifestation of a broader pathology or of a multiple system problem.

Full neurological assessment, with intracranial studies, should exclude central neurological disease such as multiple sclerosis in adults or raised intracranial pressure in infants. This chapter looks at unilateral vocal cord paralysis and bilateral vocal cord paralysis. Within each of these divisions the condition is discussed for infants and children and for adults because the causes and treatment are different in the different age groups.

UNILATERAL VOCAL CORD PARALYSIS IN INFANTS AND CHILDREN

After laryngomalacia, vocal cord paralysis is the second commonest laryngeal anomaly, accounting for about 20% of all laryngeal lesions. Vocal cord paralysis in an infant may cause symptoms at birth or may not be recognized for some weeks. The neurological injury occurs somewhere along the course of the vagus nerve anywhere from the brainstem through the neck, chest and into the larynx, to the neuromuscular junction in the larynx. There may be involvement of the vagus nerve, the superior laryngeal nerve or, more often, the recurrent laryngeal nerve. In both children and adults unilateral vocal cord paralysis is seen more often on the left than the right side because the recurrent laryngeal nerve descends further into the chest, looping under the aorta before it returns to the neck to supply the laryngeal muscles, whereas the right recurrent nerve loops higher under the right subclavian artery before returning to the larynx.

Causes

It is probable that some cases of unilateral vocal cord paralysis in infants go undiagnosed, that there is later recovery of laryngeal function and that the problem is never documented. Left recurrent laryngeal nerve paralysis is often associated with congenital anomalies of the heart and great vessels. It occurs after intrathoracic surgery for mediastinal tumours or duplication cysts or for congenital cardiac anomalies including ventricular septal defect, tetralogy of Fallot, abnormalities of the great vessels and patent ductus arteriosis. Surgical damage to a nerve can occur after operation for an H-type tracheo-oesophageal fistula, cervical oesophagostomy and, in older children, after an anterior approach to the cervical spine. In other cases paralysis is caused by birth injury, presumably due to stretching of the nerve. Finally, the cause is not identified in some infants.

The lesion in the vagus nerve which is affecting the motor nerve supply of the larynx can be anywhere from the nucleus ambiguus to the distal branches of the recurrent laryngeal nerve and each case must be investigated individually in an attempt to locate the causal lesion.

Causes of unilateral vocal cord paralysis in infants and children

Traumatic birth injury – 'stretching' of vagus nerve
Congenital anomalies of heart and great vessels
Surgery for anomalies of heart and great vessels
Intrathoracic surgery for cysts and tumours
Repair of H-type tracheo-oesophageal fistula
Cervical oesophagostomy
External neck trauma
After endotracheal intubation
No cause found

More often affects the left side than the right side
The cause of unilateral paralysis is usually peripheral

Clinical features

In a new born baby, especially one who is ill with other congenital or acquired problems, the clinical features may be overlooked. There is a weak breathy cry, often with swallowing problems and inhalation of secretions. There may be choking and cyanotic attacks during feeding as the loss of sensation of the involved hemilarynx contributes to aspiration. Stridor is seldom a prominent feature but it can occur, and in the occasional patient consideration must be given to provision of an artificial airway.

Endoscopy

Laryngoscopic examination is necessary to confirm the suspected diagnosis of unilateral cord paralysis either by indirect flexible laryngoscopy in the office or clinic or by direct laryngoscopic examination in the operating theatre. The latter, performed under general anaesthesia, not only allows assessment of vocal cord function but also assists in ruling out other structural abnormalities as the cause of symptoms. Care must be taken not to cause interference with laryngeal movement during respiration or crying by pressure from the laryngoscope blade; improper positioning will distort assessment of vocal cord function and alter the shape and dynamics of the larynx. Placing the blade in the valleculae, in front of the epiglottis, as the patient recovers pharyngeal and laryngeal movements when anaesthesia is discontinued, allows sufficient time for reliable evaluation during inspiration and expiration. The mobility of the cricoarytenoid joints on each side are compared to be sure there is no fixation of the joints. The laryngologist can usually be confident with the diagnosis of unilateral cord paralysis in an infant but diagnosis of bilateral paralysis is more difficult.

Further assessment of vocal cord function as the weeks and months pass can usually be reliably assessed using a flexible fibreoptic laryngoscope in the unanaesthetized child.

Treatment

Tracheotomy is occasionally necessary, even in unilateral paralysis, not only for persistent airway obstruction but also for troublesome aspiration. The majority, well over 50%, of unilateral vocal cord paralyses in infants resolve spontaneously, usually by 6 or at most 12 months of age with corresponding improvement in the cry. If no improvement has occurred at a later age, consideration can be given to vocal cord medialization but there are few reports of treatment before teenage.

BILATERAL VOCAL CORD PARALYSIS IN INFANTS AND CHILDREN

Paralysis of both vocal cords is the cause of stridor in about 10% of infants with airway obstruction. A lesion above the ganglion nodosum may cause loss of laryngeal sensation, an ineffective cough, some weakness of the voice, and chronic aspiration may be a potential threat to life. However, most infants with bilateral vocal cord paralysis appear to have intact laryngeal sensation, a reasonable cough and, although there may be some aspiration, it is seldom serious.

Causes

Bilateral vocal cord paralysis seldom occurs in an otherwise normal child. Many infants with bilateral vocal cord paralysis have an anomaly of the central nervous system such as Arnold-Chiari malformation, myelomeningocoele, encephalocoele, cerebral dysgenesis, leukodystrophy or hydrocephalus with raised intracranial pressure. The causal relationship between these intracranial diseases and vocal cord paralysis has never been clearly defined. In other infants, bilateral cord paralysis occurs with birth trauma due to difficult, prolonged labour, forceps delivery or undue traction on the cervical spine; recovery in 6 months or so can be expected. Bilateral vocal cord paralysis can occur in otherwise normal infants and the cause may never be found.

Clinical features

Persistent stridor with each breath in a newborn infant may be due to bilateral vocal cord paralysis, especially in the presence of an obvious intracranial problem.

Causes of bilateral vocal cord paralysis in infants and children

Central nervous system disease
- Arnold–Chiari malformation
- Myelomeningocoele
- Encephalocoele
- Hydrocephalus
- Cerebral dysgenesis
- Leukodystrophy

Traumatic birth injury
External neck trauma
After endotracheal intubation
Post-infectious e.g. diphtheria
No cause found

The cause of bilateral paralysis is usually central

The cause must be distinguished from severe glottic web, tracheal compression or stenosis, bilateral posterior choanal atresia or a large cyst or mass in the laryngopharynx. Inability of the vocal cords to abduct results in consistent, severe stridor, cyanotic attacks, aspiration and recurrent chest infections with scattered small areas of atelectasis on the chest X-ray. The cry is usually normal because the cords are usually paralysed in the paramedian position. Deglutition problems and aspiration are common.

Every infant with bilateral vocal cord paralysis must have a neurological examination and a skull CT and brain MRI.

Endoscopy

In neonates in whom bilateral vocal cord paralysis is suspected, laryngoscopic and bronchoscopic examination under general anaesthesia is essential, but it is not uncommon that a confident diagnosis cannot be made at the first examination. When the diagnosis remains in doubt it is our practice to place a nasotracheal tube in situ for up to a week and perform re-examination. If bilateral vocal cord paralysis is confirmed a tracheotomy is usually necessary (see later).

Radiology

Examination of the skull base and intracranial contents with CT and MRI are important in evaluation of Arnold-Chiari malformation, herniation of the cerebellar tonsil, posterior fossa tumours, cerebral dysgenesis and hydrocephalus. Chest X-rays and contrast oesophagram may show abnormalities of the heart, great vessels or mediastinum.

Treatment

Tracheotomy is almost always necessary for bilateral cord paralysis. A small number of infants, although having persistent stridor, do not desaturate, are not noticeably handicapped and do not necessarily need an immediate tracheotomy; they certainly require continued close observation. Sometimes the patient's pulmonary condition, e.g. bronchopulmonary dysplasia, will be a factor in the decision to perform a tracheotomy. On the other hand, tracheotomy is sometimes necessary even in cases of unilateral vocal cord paralysis with stridor and partial airway obstruction or troublesome aspiration. After a tracheotomy has been performed for bilateral vocal cord paralysis, careful evaluation to detect central neurological abnormalities must be undertaken. Alleviation of raised intracranial pressure by a shunt procedure may be followed by improvement in cord movement.

If spontaneous resolution of the paralysis on one or both sides does not occur, correction of the airway obstruction in unremitting bilateral paralysis is a major problem; the best age for attempted alleviation with surgical procedures is difficult to judge. It seems reasonable that a nerve–muscle reinnervation could be considered for patients over 4 years old, although the results are not predictable. The operation is not performed within the larynx but within the soft tissues of the neck and should the operation be unsuccessful intralaryngeal procedures such as arytenoidectomy can be performed later. The results of arytenoidectomy with or without vocal cord lateralization are reasonably predictable in maintaining voice and providing a sufficiently improved airway for decannulation. Some of the patients continue to have stridulous breathing at night and limited exercise tolerance after the tracheotomy has been removed. Narcy (1995) has recommended arytenoidopexy by an external lateral approach, a variant of King's technique, adapted for children.

Surgery for bilateral paralysis will be discussed in more detail in the following section referring to adult patients.

Causes of unilateral vocal cord paralysis in adults

- 'Viral' or 'idiopathic'
- Postsurgical
  - Thyroidectomy
  - Coronary artery bypass
  - Other cardiac surgery
  - Anterior cervical fusion
  - Removal neck masses
- Malignancy in neck or mediastinum
- After endotracheal intubation
- Neck trauma
- Jugular foramen syndrome
- Thyroiditis

UNILATERAL VOCAL CORD PARALYSIS IN ADULTS

When indirect laryngoscopy in a patient with change in the voice shows vocal cord immobility, it cannot always be assumed that there is paralysis. Electromyography is useful in establishing denervation, and only palpation at direct laryngoscopy can detect cricoarytenoid joint fixation.

In adults it is uncommon for lesions of the corticobulbar pathways to affect laryngeal movement whereas lesions in the neural pathways between the medulla and the laryngeal muscles are the commonest cause of unilateral paralysis. Both motor and sensory losses can occur in patients who have had a focal stroke, multiple sclerosis, intracranial trauma or tumours in the medulla. Lesions at the skull base may also affect cranial nerves IX, X and XI, so there may be a vocal cord paralysis as well as pharyngeal paralysis; loss of sensation and aspiration of secretions may also be a feature.

Causes

Although it has been considered that 20 or 30% of cases are 'viral' or 'idiopathic', it now seems the proportion of cases where the cause is not discovered is higher than this.

Other causes of unilateral vocal cord paralysis in adults include an occult thyroid carcinoma, thyroiditis, penetrating trauma, following surgery for anterior cervical fusion, following coronary artery bypass surgery with trauma to the left recurrent nerve and compression injury of the anterior ramus of the recurrent nerve as a result of endotracheal intubation.

The commonest acquired cause of injury to the recurrent laryngeal nerve has been, and still is, as a complication of thyroid surgery. Unilateral paralysis or paresis is thought to occur in approximately 5% of thyroidectomy patients, even in experienced hands.

Superior laryngeal nerve damage

The external branch of the superior laryngeal nerve supplies only the cricothyroid muscle, which pulls the anterior cricoid ring upwards. Contraction of one muscle rotates the posterior cricoid to the contralateral paralysed side. It is damaged in up to 15% of thyroid operations, the main symptoms being a deep,

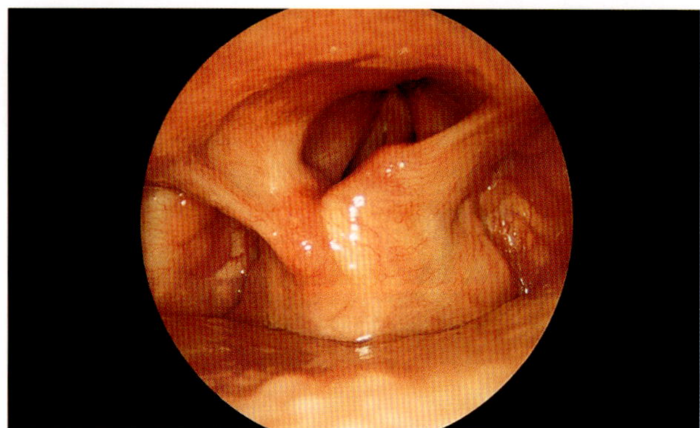

Figure **11.1**
Superior laryngeal nerve damage. Right vocal cord paralysis with rotation of the cricoid cartilage, tilting of the larynx and prolapse antero-medially of the posterior part of the aryepiglottic fold.

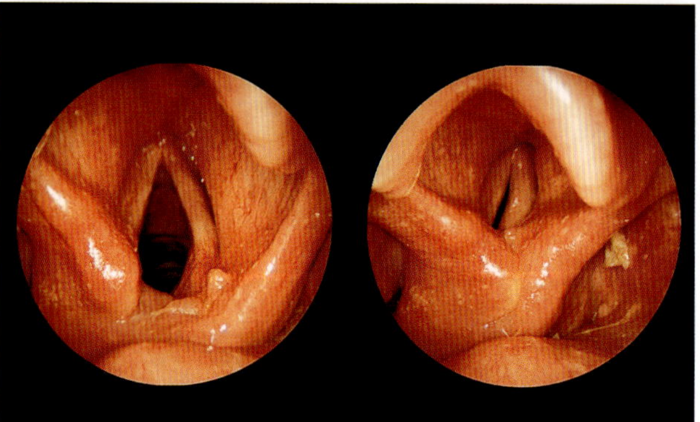

Figure **11.2**
Vocal cord paralysis at indirect laryngoscopy. Left cord paralysis seen with abduction (left) and adduction (right) of the contralateral cord. Video-recording is the best way to study dynamics of the larynx.

breathy, slightly husky voice which fatigues easily. The situation usually compensates in time but may continue to be a problem for professional singers who can no longer reach high notes. The initial presentation is usually with both loss of sensation of the supraglottic mucous membrane (the internal branch) and rotation of the larynx during phonation due to unilateral loss of activity of the cricothyroid muscle (external branch). Therefore the lesion should be suspected when the larynx is tilted and the affected vocal fold lags in adduction after repeated rapid phonation. The vocal folds are usually in the normal position during quiet respiration, although the affected side may be slightly flaccid and remain below the level of the normal side with some forward prolapse of the posterior aryepiglottic fold, the cuneiform and the arytenoid cartilage, so that the area droops forward over the posterior end of the vocal fold making it appear shorter than its fellow (Fig. 11.1).

Clinical features

Adults with uncompensated unilateral vocal cord paralysis have a breathy weak husky voice, ineffective cough and, at least for some time after the initial paralysis, aspiration. Because of air escape, some patients complain of shortness of breath when speaking. In many patients, given time, there is a return of function, especially in those presumed to be of a 'viral' or 'idiopathic' nature. In other patients, despite persisting paralysis, there is eventually functional compensation and the patient is little troubled by laryngeal symptoms. Each patient may require complete general and neurologic examination, blood tests and radiologic investigations, concentrating on the pathways of the vagus and recurrent laryngeal nerves.

Endoscopy

Paralysis is best diagnosed at indirect laryngoscopy (Fig. 11.2) where pooling of secretions in the paralysed side may be seen (Fig. 11.3). Direct laryngoscopy under general anaesthesia allows confirmation of the mobility at the cricoarytenoid joint – a fixed joint or a dislocated, fixed arytenoid cartilage is a contraindication to any medialization procedure. During direct examination local pathology such as an otherwise occult tumour in the ventricle, subglottis, piriform fossa or even the upper oesophagus can be

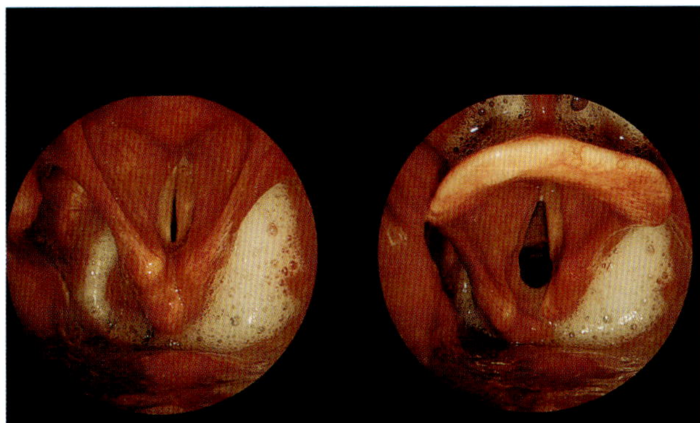

Figure **11.3**
Right vocal paralysis, after Teflon injection. Photographs at indirect laryngoscopy several months after injection of Teflon paste in the right hemilarynx. In this patient pooling of frothy secretions has persisted.

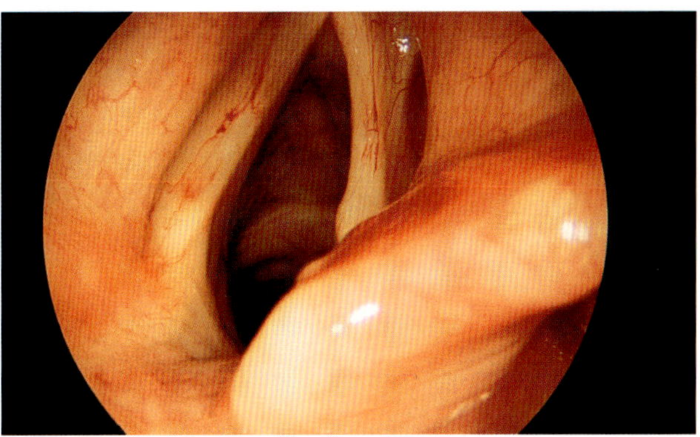

Figure **11.4**
Chronic vocal cord paralysis. Long-standing paralysis in a 28-year-old following cardiac surgery as a teenager. The right cord is thin, shortened and the posterior aryepiglottic fold has prolapsed medially.

excluded. In longstanding cases the vocal cord may be thin and atrophied (Fig. 11.4). In selected cases Gelfoam or Teflon paste is injected under the same general anaesthetic.

Treatment

Where there are persistent, troublesome symptoms, it is advisable to wait at least 9–12 months, during which time (in cases where no cause has been found) recovery of function is possible, before embarking on definite surgical treatment. There need be no delay in using Teflon paste for cases of recent onset with no hope of recovery, e.g. malignant mediastinal metastases involving the recurrent laryngeal nerve. On the other hand, Gelfoam paste, as advocated by Schramm et al (1978), may be used during the period when recovery is possible and temporary rehabilitation of glottic competence is desirable. The patient and the surgeon are able to observe the result of Gelfoam injection before proceeding to Teflon injection or some other form of phonosurgery. Gelfoam causes little tissue reaction, but its beneficial effects last only a few weeks as it is metabolized and absorbed leaving the hemilarynx in its pre-injection state.

Transcutaneous injection of Teflon paste with indirect laryngoscopic guidance is possible, but it is difficult to place the Teflon accurately, with the result that it may be left superficially and may even worsen voice quality.

Teflon has often been reported to cause an adverse reaction such as extrusion, migration, inflammatory granulomas, acute local inflammatory swelling or regional lymph node enlargement, hence the incentive to find other injectable substances such as collagen or fat.

Glutaraldehyde cross-linked collagen causes very little inflammatory reaction and, although partly resorbed in time, it is well tolerated. If over-injected by 20% or so, the long-term effect is very satisfactory; stability in the larynx is good compared to the use of collagen in cosmetic surgery of the face. Collagen can fill in tissues in the vocal ligament or deep part of the lamina propria (Fig. 11.5) without inflammatory reaction, and it is then colonized by fibroblasts and new vessels which stabilize it. It must be injected with precision using a very fine 27 gauge needle (Fig. 11.6).

Collagen is in a liquid form and is easy to inject with accuracy, can reduce scar tissue and can even be placed in adynamic segments. A skin test must be performed 6 weeks before to detect the possibility of

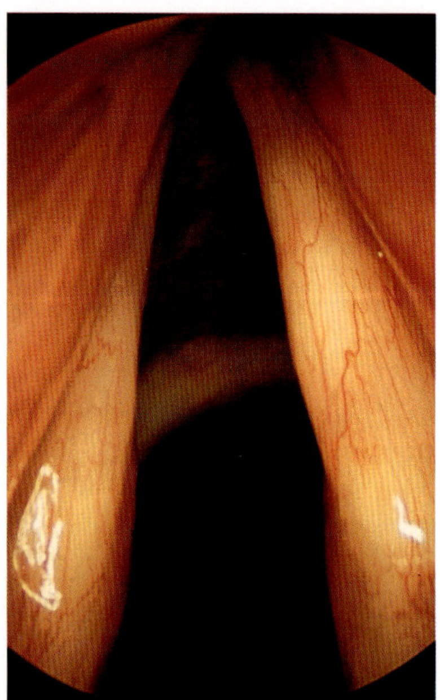

Figure **11.5**
Collagen as a filler. The right vocal fold has been injected to correct a defect following biopsy several years before.

an adverse reaction from collagen injection in an individual.

Injection of autologous fat has been reported in a few patients as having good results, but in practice accurate injection of a known volume of fat is difficult. Animal studies show that the fat graft resorption rates are related to the ability of the graft to establish vascularity. Variability in resorption is to be expected; it may be that this technique is suitable for patients whose paralysis is not considered 'permanent'.

It is clear that Teflon injection is not an ideal or perfect technique, but when carefully performed it remains a satisfactory procedure (Fig. 11.7) especially in patients with a poor prognosis for survival. The untoward results in some patients suggest that other, more physiological and more easily reversible surgical procedures which do not require injection of a foreign material should be considered, especially in younger patients.

Technique of injection of Teflon or Gelfoam paste

The aim is to augment the paralysed and abducted vocal cord by expansion of the hemilarynx to displace the vocal fold to the midline so that the contralateral, functioning vocal fold can adduct to meet its fellow. The injection technique is the same for Gelfoam or Teflon paste.

Although commonly referred to as 'vocal cord injection' or 'intracordal injection', both terms are inaccurate and misleading; the injection is 'paracordal' to augment the lateral hemilarynx so that vibration of the vocal folds becomes more effective. The paste

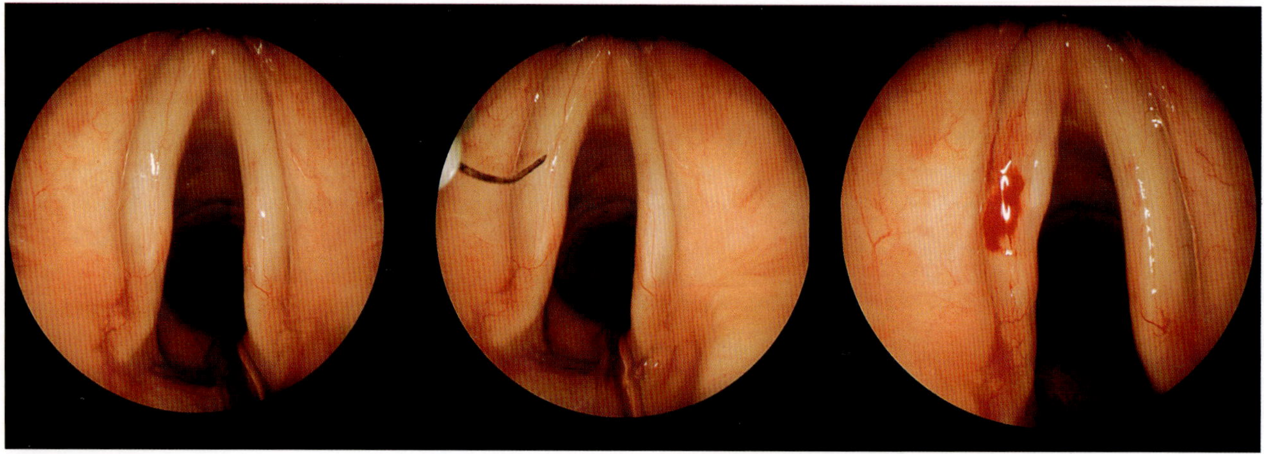

Figure **11.6**
Injection of collagen. Elderly man with bowed vocal cords (left). Fine 27 gauge needle (centre) about to inject the left vocal fold. Slight 'overinjection' with small mucosal haematoma. The right side can be treated later.

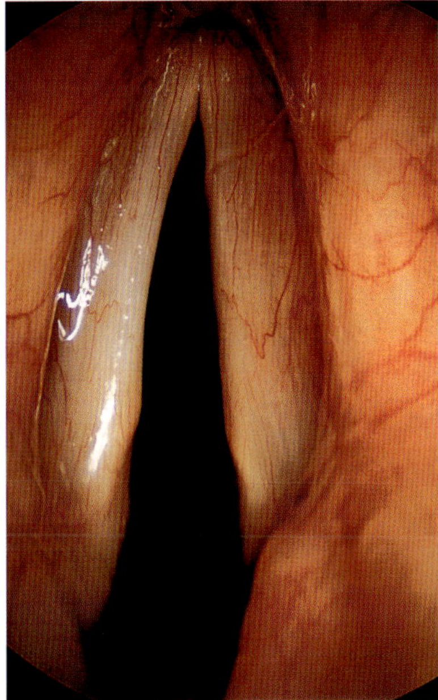

Figure **11.7**
Teflon injection. Satisfactory result following Teflon injection in the right hemilarynx 6 years previously.

Technique of Gelfoam or Teflon injection

Test cricoarytenoid joint mobility
Use 19 French gauge 20 cm needle
Expose floor of posterior ventricle
Inject lateral to vocal process
Avoid subglottic bulge
Judge adequate amount for medialization

must not be placed superficially or in the membranous vocal fold; injection is in the postero-lateral hemilarynx in the substance of the lateral part of the thyroarytenoid muscle, medial to the lamina of the thyroid cartilage and lateral to the vocal process of the arytenoid. This is the first and often the only site of injection, although sometimes a second or occasionally even a third smaller supplementary injection anterior to the first is needed to achieve adequate medialization. If paste is placed in the vocal fold itself vibration will be poor because of reduced compliance and cord stiffness. The volume and site of injection are critical; if there is any doubt, too little rather than too much is injected, not only to minimize the chance of untoward results but also to lessen the risk of postoperative respiratory obstruction. Later supplementary injection is an option should closure prove to be insufficient.

It has been advocated that local anaesthesia be used because the change in voice can be evaluated during the procedure to help determine the volume of injection. However, general anaesthesia is more comfortable for the patient and less stressful for the surgeon. For some years now we have used a relaxant general anaesthetic technique with a Benjet tube lying in the posterior larynx where it causes no distortion or interference with injection.

Certain important points should be considered in the technique of injection:

- the mobility of the cricoarytenoid joint must be tested and found to be normal before injection (Fig. 11.8);
- the laryngoscope should push the posterior part of the false cord laterally to expose the floor of the posterior laryngeal ventricle ready for injection (Fig. 11.9);
- the ideal needle has a 45° bevel is 19 French gauge and 20 cm long; it should be introduced laterally just inside the lamina of the thyroid cartilage and lateral to the vocal process of the arytenoid;
- paste is delivered, one click at a time, until the vocal fold reaches the midline; if a bulge appears in the subglottic region, injection is stopped and the needle is withdrawn a little;
- when enough paste appears to have been injected the paralysing anaesthetic agent is stopped, and, as spontaneous respiration begins, brisk vocal cord movement returns in the contralateral side and a judgement can be made whether further injection is necessary.

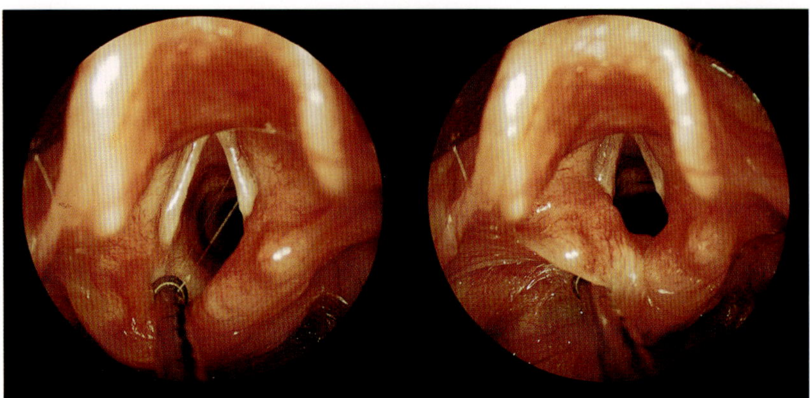

Figure **11.8**
Testing mobility of the left cricoarytenoid joint. Mobility of the joints must be tested both for lateral and medial movement prior to injection.

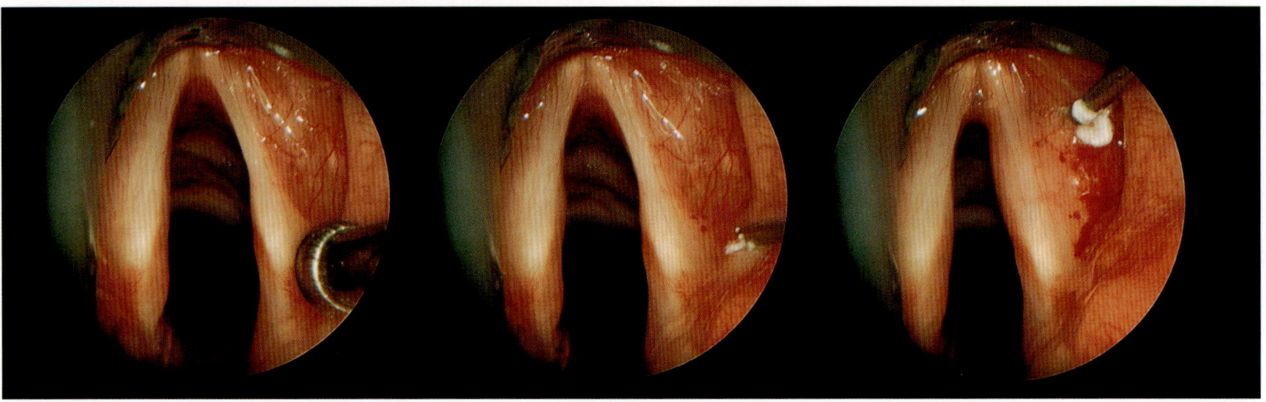

Figure **11.9**
Technique of Teflon injection. The false cord is pushed aside (left), injection is made in the lateral thyroarytenoid muscle lateral to the vocal process (centre) and sometimes a small anterior injection is necessary (right).

It must be noted that it is often not possible to close the posterior 'respiratory' part of the glottic opening between the arytenoid cartilages.

Errors in technique can occur. Often too much paste is injected (Fig. 11.10). Paste can be misplaced anterior to the vocal process with injection too close to the edge of the vocal fold, too deep in the subglottic region or too high in the false cord (Fig. 11.11) rather than at the glottic level. Troublesome granuloma formation is more likely when there is excess paste, it is too superficial or there is inappropriate placement. When Teflon paste has been injected incorrectly, stroboscopy will show an adynamic vibratory margin. This is sufficient evidence to advise against any further surgical procedure even if the edge of the vocal fold is straight and smooth. Over-injection and Teflon granuloma formation may not only cause the voice to be worse but may produce partial airway obstruction. Removal of the Teflon may sometimes be indicated.

Technique of Teflon removal

Evaluation by horizontal computed tomography of the larynx and endoscopy with telescopes is helpful in considering removal of the Teflon. Teflon is radiolucent on plain radiography or conventional laryngeal tomography, but high-resolution, narrow-slice unenhanced CT will give a clear high-density signal and provides information about the volume and site of the Teflon (Fig. 11.12).

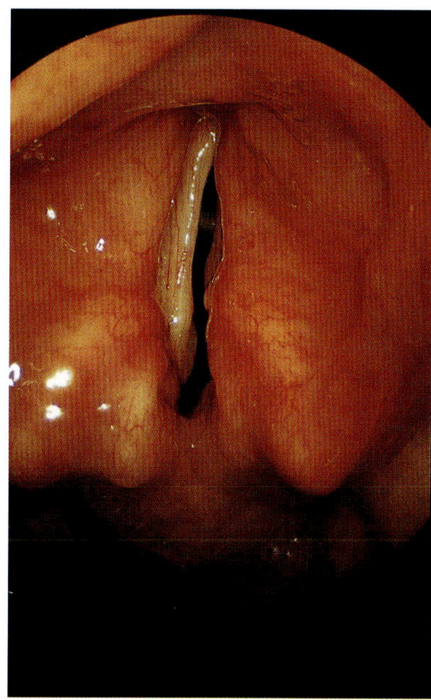

Figure **11.10**
Excessive injection of Teflon paste and granuloma formation. Misplaced, ill-judged excessive Teflon injection resulting in an irregular Teflon granuloma on the right side.

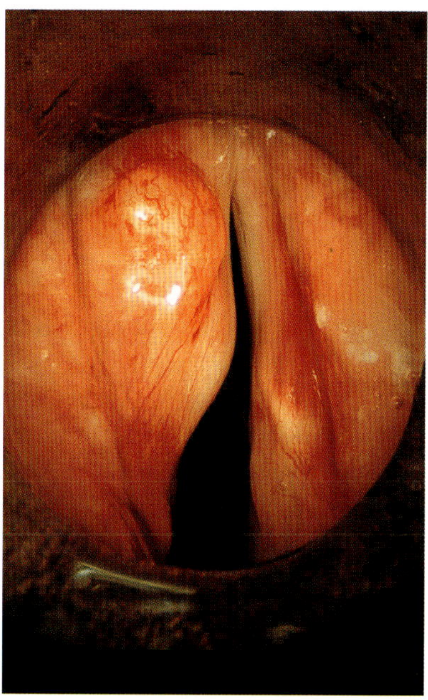

Figure **11.11**
Complication from Teflon injection. Large, rounded supraglottic mass. The voice was very poor and improved substantially after removal of most of the Teflon and surrounding granuloma.

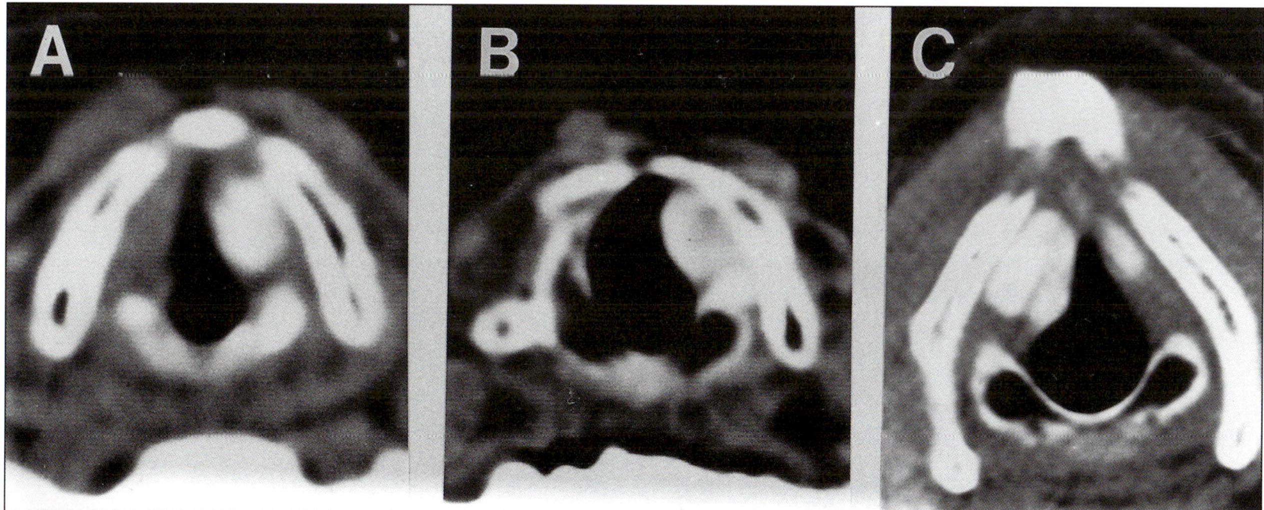

Figure **11.12**
CT scans of Teflon in the larynx of three different patients. A. A small amount placed superficially and centrally in the left vocal fold. B. Rounded mass distending and deforming the left subglottis. C. Large, irregular mass in right side, smaller mass in the left side, in a patient who was injected on both sides, a procedure which is contraindicated.

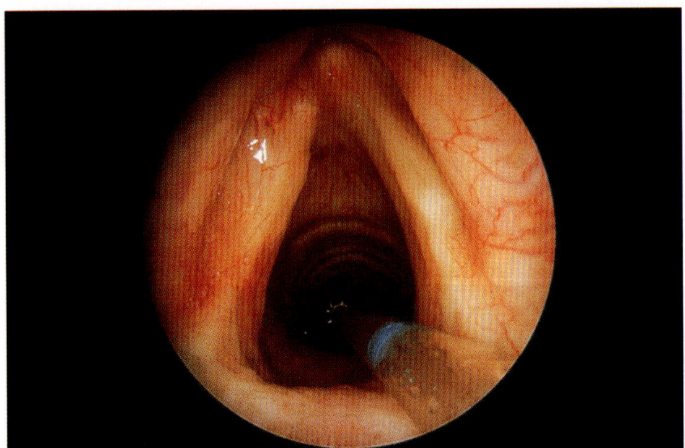

Figure **11.13**
Teflon granuloma, small. The left vocal fold is plump and at stroboscopy had no vibration. The voice remained hoarse. The Teflon was not removed.

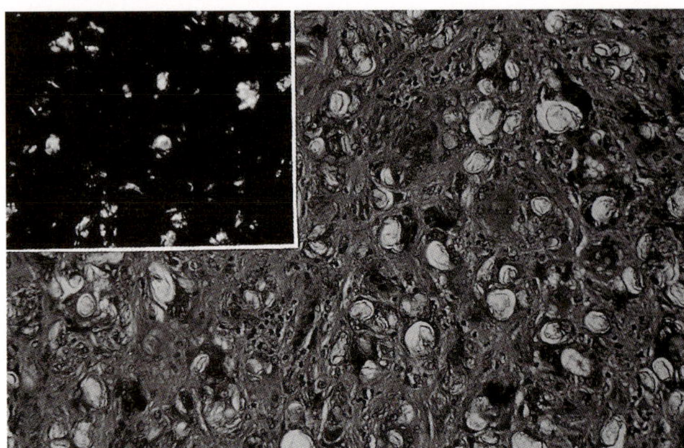

Figure **11.14**
Histologic appearance of Teflon granuloma. Teflon particles surrounded by giant cells and dense collagen tissue. Inset shows birefringement particles. There is no encapsulation of the granuloma.

Laryngoscopy with rigid rod lens telescopes (Fig. 11.13) provides additional precise information about the distribution of Teflon and the fixation and stiffness of the involved hemilarynx. Therefore, the combination of CT examination and telescopic evaluation enables the surgeon to get an almost 'three-dimensional' appreciation of the volume of Teflon to be removed.

Implanted Teflon causes local irritation with formation of multinucleated giant cells having Teflon particles within their cytoplasm. These cells are surrounded by dense collagenous tissue with minimal inflammatory cell infiltrate (Fig. 11.14). There is no capsule to surround the Teflon granuloma and particles may be disseminated through local lymphatics. Tracheotomy followed by removal of the Teflon granuloma via horizontal thyrotomy is one approach; most of the vocalis muscle is replaced by yellowish, gritty particles which are difficult to remove.

The endoscopic technique for removal of Teflon granuloma uses suspension laryngoscopy. An anteroposterior laser incision is made at the junction of vocal fold with the floor of the ventricle, a few millimetres from the edge of the fold. Deeper dissection using the laser and cupped forceps allows piecemeal dissection of fragments of the granuloma (Fig. 11.15) until satisfactory removal has been obtained. Total removal is neither possible nor desirable – the more dissection for removal, the more trauma to surrounding

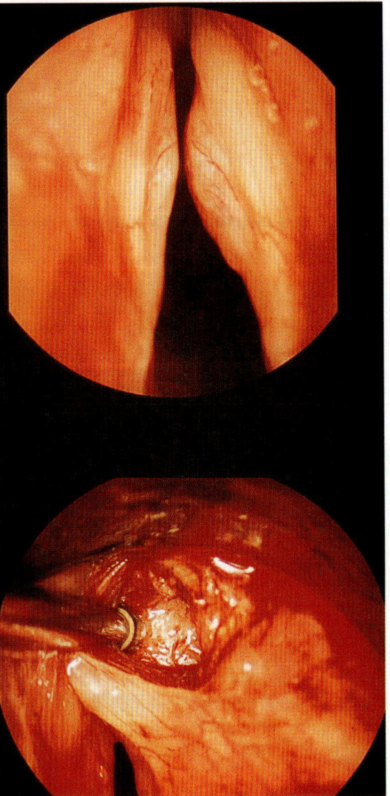

Figure **11.15**
Removal of Teflon granuloma. Bilateral swellings in a patient inexplicably injected on both sides (above). Sucker retracts the intact vocal fold edge during removal of the greyish-white mass of the granuloma.

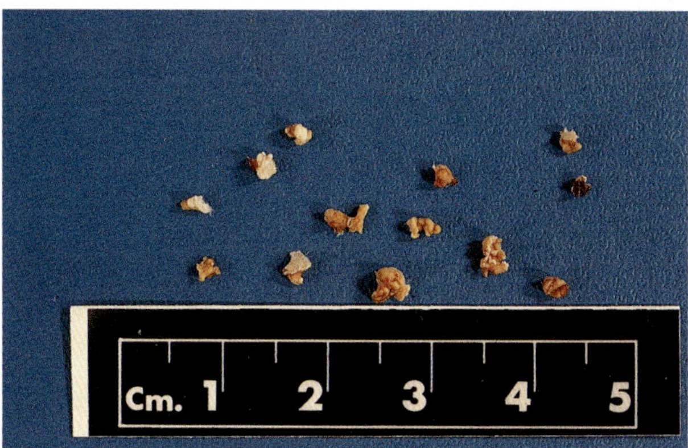

Figure **11.16**
Fragments of Teflon granuloma. Piecemeal dissection of fragments, using the carbon dioxide laser, blunt dissection and cupped forceps.

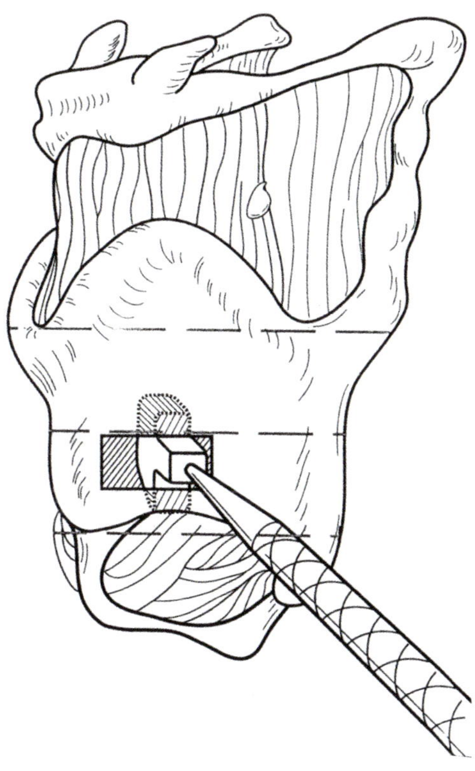

Figure **11.17**
Fitting of VoCoM hydroxyapatite implant. The appropriate-sized implant, selected with a sizing instrument, is positioned through a surgically created window. It is positioned and secured with a preformed locking mechanism also made of hydroxyapatite.

tissues. The free edge of the vocal fold should be kept as intact as possible to maintain vibratory characteristics. The Teflon particles glow white when impacted by the laser so low power settings of 5 watts or less and short exposure times are used because of a theoretical risk of ignition of the particles (Fig. 11.16).

About half the patients indicate they have a 'good' voice after granuloma removal, some have 'improvement' and some are no better. The results for voice improvement are therefore unpredictable.

Thyroplasty techniques

There are some patients with a permanent vocal cord paralysis who live happily with minor voice problems and do not need or wish to have a surgical procedure. The untoward results in some patients injected with Teflon paste suggest that other more physiological and more easily reversible procedures which do not require injection of foreign material should be considered, especially in younger patients.

Various external operations are available. For optimal results each patient with vocal cord paralysis in the paramedian and abducted positions requires individual selection for one of the techniques of treatment.

Surgical procedures through a skin incision in the neck include the original Type I thyroplasty proposed by Isshiki et al (1985) where a rectangle of thyroid cartilage is depressed inwards to move the paralysed vocal cord towards the midline; it is held in place by a wedge of silastic. Other thyroplasty techniques involve the use of autologous cartilage or synthetic prosthetic implants constructed from biocompatible medical grade polymer or hydroxyapatite. Graduated sizes of preformed implants are available to fit into the individual larynx through a precisely measured rectangular window cut into the lamina of the thyroid cartilage. We are currently using the VoCoM vocal cord medialization system (Flint and Cummings, 1993). The chosen size of hydroxyapatite prosthesis is positioned snuggly through the window, under the perichondrium, and held firmly in place by a prefabricated locking system which makes displacement most unlikely (Fig. 11.17).

A detailed description of these operations is outside the scope of this text on endolaryngeal surgery, but is available from sources in the bibliography.

BILATERAL VOCAL CORD PARALYSIS IN ADULTS

Causes

The commonest cause for bilateral vocal cord paralysis has always been thyroidectomy, although it is seen less frequently now, except after radical removal of the thyroid gland for malignancy. The results after attempts to re-anastomose a divided recurrent nerve at the time of surgery are mostly poor, and the outcome for voice is unsatisfactory. Other causes are malignant neoplasms of the cervical oesophagus, subglottic larynx, neck and upper mediastinum, bilateral neck dissection and external neck trauma such as blunt trauma causing distraction of the trachea from the larynx, gunshot wound or an open knife wound. In some cases the cause is undetermined. Bilateral paralysis is very occasionally seen after endotracheal intubation and is sometimes associated with neurological disorders such as cerebrovascular accidents, Parkinson's disease, amyotrophic lateral sclerosis, Guillain–Barré syndrome or cerebral tumour.

Causes of bilateral vocal cord paralysis in adults

Post-thyroidectomy
Malignancy in neck or mediastinum
Bilateral neck dissection
Neck trauma
After endotracheal intubation
Neurologic disease
No cause found

Clinical features

Bilateral vocal cord paralysis in an adult is sometimes not recognized because the speaking voice may be near normal, much better than the voice of a patient with unilateral paralysis. Speech can become monotonous with sentences or phrases said in a hurry and interrupted by loud stridulous inspiration as the patient draws breath in preparation for the next sentence. There may be a reluctance to laugh because the loss of air requires an immediate distressing inspiration. There is often some degree of aspiration at first, especially for liquids, but the patient usually learns to control the aspiration so that coughing and choking becomes minimal. The typical loud, high-pitched stridor is distressing to others in the room, but many patients learn to tolerate their problem, sometimes for many years. Occasionally patients are seen who have had bilateral vocal cord paralysis since thyroidectomy 10–20 years previously. Subsequently they have been treated for 'asthma' or 'emphysema', but their slowly increasing obstruction finally brings them to the notice of the otolaryngologist.

Aims of surgical treatment

Bilateral vocal cord paralysis is a difficult management problem. The many forms of surgical treatment available attest to the fact that not one of them is superior to the other, nor can the result be guaranteed with any procedure. The ideal result would be an unimpeded airway for everyday activity after removal of a tracheotomy, if one was present, together with preservation of a good voice. To some extent, the wider the laryngeal opening is made by surgery to improve the airway, the poorer the voice. The 'happy medium' is difficult to achieve and, although many patients have their tracheotomy removed after a surgical procedure, the airway may still be marginal with partial obstruction and noisy breathing during sleep.

Treatment options

Most patients require a tracheotomy but some manage without, often coping for years with limitation of their exercise tolerance. There are many treatment options:

1 no tracheotomy but continued regular observation;
2 tracheotomy with a speaking valve;
3 endoscopic surgery:
   - vocal cord lateralization; using a suture placed under endoscopic control;
   - arytenoidectomy, partial or total using microsurgical instruments and/or the carbon dioxide laser;
   - laryngeal muscular tenotomy (Rontal and Rontal, 1994);
   - transverse cordotomy (Kashima 1991);
   - laser cordectomy with or without arytenoidectomy (Eckel et al 1994).
4 external procedures, including operations performed using lateral neck incisions, midline neck incisions and reinnervation procedures:
   - the original Woodman arytenoidectomy, lateral external approach avoids not only division of the anterior commissure but also surgery in the larynx itself; it is combined with a suture to fix the vocal process of the arytenoid in the lateral position and it may be combined with submucosal cordectomy to increase the glottic aperture;
   - arytenoidectomy via midline laryngofissure with thyrotomy and open removal using transmucosal incisions, subperichondrial dissection; this is considered by many to be the most effective operation and is usually combined with a lateralization suture to fix the vocal process in the lateral position;
   - the success of reinnervation procedures is an unresolved question; they involve use of nerves such as the ansa hypoglossi, vagus nerve, or a split phrenic nerve graft. Results have been unpredictable;
   - reanimation of the denervated larynx by means of functional electrical stimulation (Zealear et al 1994); the feasibility of electrical pacing of the laryngeal muscles has yet to become a reliable reality.

None of these external procedures will be discussed in any further detail.

Endoscopic surgical procedures

Endoscopic arytenoidectomy can be achieved through a laryngoscope with or without the laser but is a difficult procedure requiring considerable experience. Removal of the cartilage generally improves the airway by a small amount, but excessive postoperative scarring may contract the vocal cord medially instead of laterally as intended. Crumley (1993) has reported endoscopic medial arytenoidectomy for improving the posterior glottic opening. The arytenoid cartilage is reduced on the medial side with the carbon dioxide laser, replacing complete ablation or removal of the cartilage; a concavity is created along all of the medial glottic surface leaving the vocal

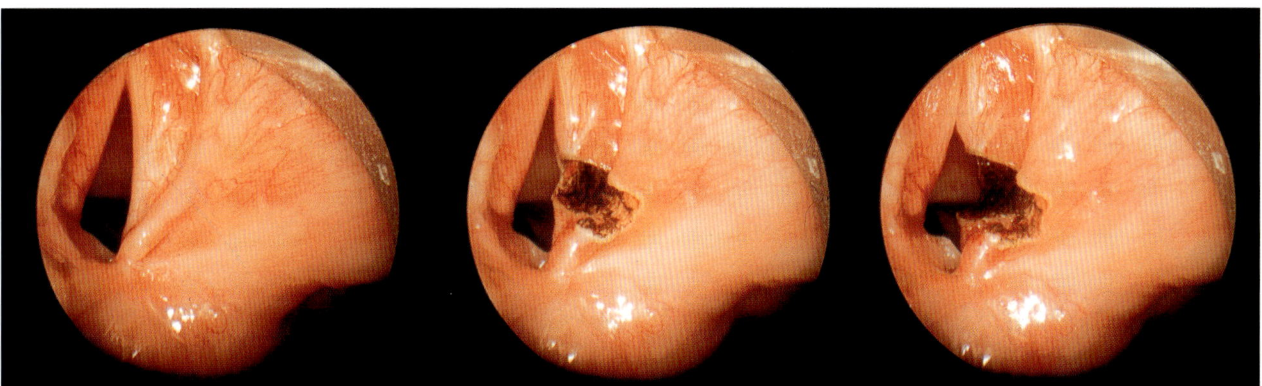

Figure **11.18**
Steps in right laser tenotomy. Exposure is improved by positioning the tip of the laryngoscope (left). The membranous vocal cord is then easily divided from the vocal process. In this larynx there is a band of scar tissue from a previous right arytenoidectomy.

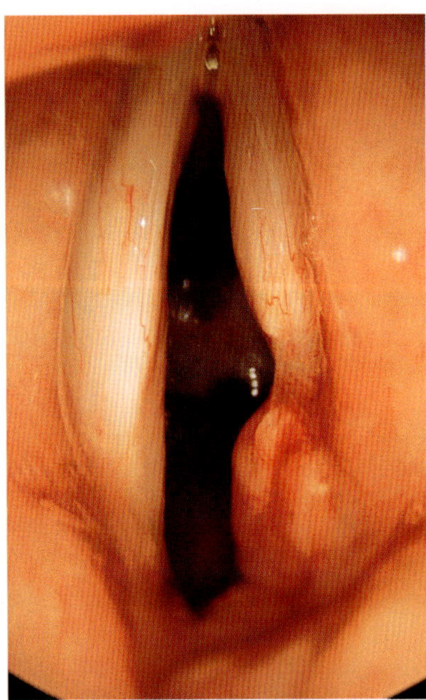

Figure **11.19**
Result of right laser tenotomy for bilateral vocal cord paralysis. The posterior glottis has been widened sufficiently to significantly improve the airway obstruction.

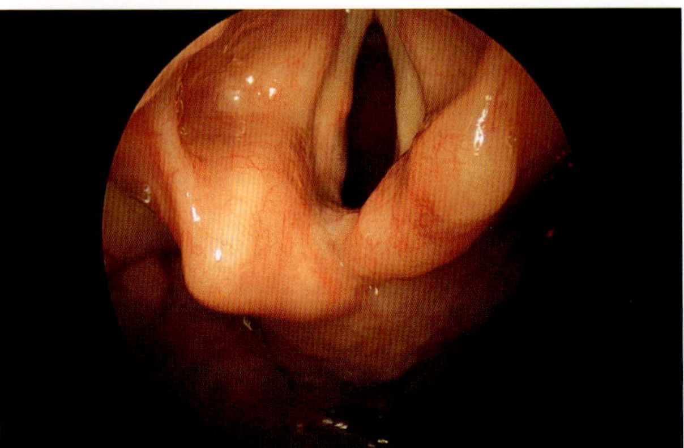

Figure **11.20**
Result of laryngeal muscular tenotomy for bilateral vocal cord paralysis. The left arytenoid has moved posteriorly and away from the midline with improvement of the glottic airway.

process and interarytenoid regions intact. The raw semi-lunar concavity becomes covered with thin regenerated epithelium; the airway is said to be improved by 1 or 2 mm.

Removal of an arytenoid cartilage to widen the posterior 'respiratory' glottic airway has been the most popular operation until recently when Kashima (1991) described transverse cordotomy, a relatively simple endoscopic carbon dioxide laser procedure which does not require removal of any tissue mass. The vocal ligament and vocalis muscle fibres are widely separated from the vocal process of the arytenoid by transverse incision which results in a wedge-shaped widening due to lateral retraction of the divided thyroarytenoid muscle (Fig. 11.18). The results of this operation have been good (Fig. 11.19).

Rontal and Rontal (1994) extended this idea to include treatment, not only of bilateral vocal cord paralysis, but also bilateral midline vocal cord fixation as a result of prolonged endotracheal intubation causing cricoarytenoid arthritis. Their concept involves not only laryngeal tenotomy but also muscular release using a laser incision curved from the midline of the interarytenoid area anteriorly to the vocal process. A postero-lateral flap of mucosa and periosteum is dissected to expose the medial surface of the arytenoid cartilage and to separate the interarytenoid muscle and fascia from it. Dissection is carried anteriorly to expose and transect the vocal process of the arytenoid to release the vocal ligament and thyroarytenoid ligament. This allows rotation of the arytenoid out of the airway and widening of the posterior glottis (Fig. 11.20). Our experience with this operation for bilateral vocal cord paralysis has been very satisfactory so far.

Each of these endoscopic procedures to widen the posterior glottis can be repeated on the opposite side if the airway is not satisfactory after some months.

BIBLIOGRAPHY

Blaugrund S, Varvares M (1993) Thyroplasty: a new approach. *Ann Otol Rhinol Laryngol* **102**: 571–9.

Crumley RL (1993) Endoscopic laser medial arytenoidectomy for airway management in bilateral laryngeal paralysis. *Ann Otol Rhinol Laryngol* **102**: 81–4.

Eckel HE, Thumfart M, Wassermann K et al. (1994) Cordectomy versus arytenoidectomy and the management of bilateral vocal cord paralysis. *Ann Otol Rhinol Laryngol* 852–7.

Flint P, Cummings C (1993) Phonosurgical procedures. In: Cummings C, Fredrickson J, Harker L, Krause C and Schuller D, eds, *Otolaryngology – head and neck surgery* (St Louis: CV Mosby) 2072–99.

Holinger LD, Holinger PC, Holinger PH (1976) Etiology of bilateral vocal cord paralysis. *Ann Otol Rhinol Laryngol* **85**: 428–37.

Isshiki N, Tanabe M, Ohkawa M, Kita M (1985) Laryngeal framework surgery for voice disorders. *Auris Nasus Larynx* **12** (Suppl 2): 217–20.

Kashima HK (1991) Bilateral vocal fold motion impairment: pathophysiology and management by transverse cordotomy. *Ann Otol Rhinol Laryngol* **100**: 717.

Kirchner F (1979) Endoscopic lateralisation of the vocal cord in abductor paralysis of the larynx. *Laryngoscope* **89**: 1179.

Levine BA, Jacobs IN, Wetmore RF, Hander SD (1995) Vocal cord injection in children with unilateral vocal cord paralysis. *Arch Otol Hand Neck Surg* **121**: 116–19.

Montgomery WW, Blaugrund SM, Vavares MA (1993) Thyroplasty: a new approach. *Ann Otol Rhinol Laryngol* **102**: 571–9.

Narcy P (1995) Arytenoidopexy for laryngeal paralysis in children. *Int J Ped Otolaryngol* **32** (Suppl): S101–S102.

Rontal M, Rontal E (1994) Use of laryngeal muscular tenotomy for bilateral midline vocal cord fixation. *Ann Otol Rhinol Laryngol* **103**: 583–9.

Schramm VL, May MM, Lavorato AS (1978) Gelfoam paste injection for vocal cord paralysis: temporary rehabilitation of glottic competence. *Laryngoscope* **88**: 1268–72.

Tucker H (1982) Nerve muscle pedicle reinnervation of the larynx: avoiding pitfalls and complications. *Ann Otol Rhinol Laryngol* **91**: 440.

Vavares MA, Montgomery WW, Hillman RE (1995) Teflon granuloma of the larynx: etiology, pathophysiology and management. *Ann Otol Rhinol Laryngol* **104**: 511–15.

Woodman D (1953) Bilateral adductor paralysis. *Arch Otolaryngol* **58**: 150.

Zaretsky LS, Shindo ML, Detar M, Rue DH (1995) Autologous fat injection for vocal fold paralysis: long-term histologic evaluation. *Ann Otol Rhinol Laryngol* **104**: 1–4.

Zealear DL, Lainey CL, Jerles ML et al (1994) Technical approach for reanimation of the chronically denervated larynx by means of functional electrical stimulation. *Ann Otol Rhinol Laryngol* **103**: 705–12.

12 Intubation injuries

INTUBATION AND TRACHEOTOMY

CAUSES
- Endotracheal tube factors
  - Size, composition, shape and texture
  - Movement
  - Duration of intubation
  - Physical trauma
- Patient factors
  - Abnormal larynx
  - Impaired mucociliary mechanism
  - Bacterial infection
  - Gastro-oesophageal reflux
  - Impaired wound healing
  - Acute or chronic disease states

PATHOGENESIS
- Pressure necrosis
- Healing
- Sites of injuries

ENDOSCOPIC ASSESSMENT
- Continue intubation
- Consider tracheotomy
- Duration of intubation
- Flexible laryngoscopy
- Alternative management
- Advantages of endoscopic evaluation

CLINICAL FEATURES RELATED TO TIME AFTER EXTUBATION

ACUTE INJURIES DURING PROLONGED INTUBATION
- Early non-specific changes
- Oedema
- Granulation tissue
- Ulceration
- Miscellaneous injuries

CHRONIC CHANGES AFTER EXTUBATION
- Consequences of granulation tissue
  - Post-intubation granuloma
  - Healed fibrous nodule
  - Interarytenoid adhesion
- Consequences of ulceration
  - Healed furrow
  - Posterior glottic stenosis
  - Subglottic stenosis
  - Complete stenosis
- Other changes
  - Ductal retention cysts
  - Vocal cord paralysis
  - Dislocation of arytenoid
  - Fixation of cricoarytenoid joint

GENERAL SUMMARY

BIBLIOGRAPHY

Some degree of injury to the laryngeal mucosa, underlying soft tissue, perichondrium or cartilage due to the presence of an endotracheal tube is more common than is generally realized. Surface injury occurs even during brief intubation for surgical procedures. Most changes are superficial irritation or minor ulceration and heal quickly when the tube is removed. Other more severe, acute injuries, which are related principally to the diameter of the endotracheal tube or the duration of intubation, result in oedema, granulation tissue or ulceration. The changes during or immediately after intubation can be identified by their symptomatology and their appearance at indirect and direct laryngoscopy. Chronic sequelae, seen after prolonged intubation, are caused by persistent granulation tissue and/or scar tissue. The otolaryngologist needs to understand the mechanism of injury and the morbidity which can be caused by prolonged intubation.

Acute injuries

Oedema
Granulation tissue
Ulceration

In most cases intubation for up to 7 days, or occasionally longer, produces no permanent sequelae; the injuries are reversible and readily resolve with normal healing. On the other hand, a few patients, some intubated for just a few days, incur advanced injuries to laryngeal structures caused by prolonged pressure from the indwelling endotracheal tube.

Macewan first reported 'Clinical observations on the introduction of tracheal tubes by the mouth instead of performing tracheotomy or laryngotomy' in 1880. Shortly after, in 1887, O'Dwyer described short metal tubes introduced into the larynx for several days to overcome the airway obstruction in 'croup' or diphtheria. By the early 1900s endotracheal tubes became used routinely in anaesthesia for thoracic surgery, and the acceptance of intubation for all forms of anaesthesia eventually followed. By the 1950s prolonged intubation was applied in unconscious patients for respiratory assistance and support, and thereafter intubation became an acceptable alternative to tracheotomy in neonates and children for a variety of diseases, especially for ventilation of the preterm infant with hyaline membrane disease where long periods of intubation are common.

INTUBATION AND TRACHEOTOMY

Tracheotomy has been almost entirely replaced by endotracheal intubation as the primary airway control for ventilation in patients of all ages. While injuries to the tracheal wall caused by pressure from the cuff of the tube, which were common years ago, are now seldom seen because of high-volume, low-pressure cuffs, there has been no corresponding decrease in the incidence of damage to the larynx.

In 1969 Lindholm first reported injuries to the larynx and trachea as a result of intubation for anaesthesia; his comprehensive study demonstrated that the size and unfavourable shape of the tube and excessive laryngeal activity contributed to the complications of prolonged intubation.

Recognition of the incidence and the long-term morbidity of these injuries has led to replacement of the endotracheal tube by surgical or percutaneous tracheotomy, although the time after which tracheotomy is necessary remains a matter of controversy. As the magnitude of the problem has become recognized and preventative methods have been applied, the rate of complications has decreased to some degree. However, the intensivist, anaesthesiologist or physician may remain unaware of the occurrence and incidence of late complications because the patient usually presents to the laryngologist.

CAUSES

Many factors have been recognized as contributing to laryngeal intubation trauma and, although in an individual patient one or more may have greater or less significance, the role of each is difficult to determine. As Tan et al (1996) have pointed out, there are endotracheal tube factors and patient factors.

Endotracheal tube factors

Size, composition, shape and texture

Size (external diameter), composition, shape, firmness and texture of the tube are of vital importance. There is greater continuous pressure on the surrounding mucosa and cartilage from a tube of excessive diameter than from a smaller tube which allows equally satisfactory ventilation. It seems reasonable

Endotracheal tube factors

Size, shape, composition and texture
Movement
Duration of intubation
Physical intubation trauma

Ideal endotracheal tube

Synthetic composition
Smooth non-irritant surface
Non-toxic
Low porosity
Thermoplastic at body temperature
Low-pressure, high-volume cuff
Inexpensive

that the upper limit should be 8 mm inside diameter in males and 7 mm in females, but in practice the tube size should be chosen for each patient. Infants and children up to approximately 8 years old should have an uncuffed tube whose diameter allows an air leak in the subglottic space with approximately 20 cm of water ventilation pressure.

Contencin and Narcy (1993) have documented the low incidence of neonatal acquired subglottic stenosis in France and relate this to the size of the endotracheal tube. There is a similar low incidence of subglottic stenosis in Australia.

Specially shaped tubes have been recommended to minimize the undue pressure which is exerted by the curvature of conventional tubes in the posterior and lateral larynx, but in practice there is little enthusiasm for using them.

Synthetic tubes made of siliconized rubber or polyvinyl chloride are smooth-walled and less irritating and are considered safest for long-term intubation. On the other hand, the soft and thin-walled siliconized rubber tubes for paediatric use are easily compressed; integration of a thin wire spiral within the wall improves the ability to withstand pressure but makes manufacture more expensive.

The 'ideal' endotracheal tube for prolonged intubation would be made of synthetic material, have a smooth, non-irritating surface, have no toxic components, be of low porosity, be thermoplastic at body temperature to mould itself to body contours and be inexpensive. It would have a low-pressure, high-volume, compliant cuff.

Movement

Tube movement from the piston action transmitted by ventilator activity increases abrasive motion of the tube. Movement during suctioning, coughing or swallowing, during transportation, during light anaesthesia or by an active patient 'bucking' on an endotracheal tube are further aggravating factors.

Duration of intubation

There is no universal agreement about the 'safe' or desirable duration of intubation. Although it is an unresolved question, in most adults up to 7 days can be considered a reasonable time before deciding whether to continue intubation or change to a tracheotomy. This decision depends, to some extent, on the patient's general condition and on whether removal of the tube might soon become possible. Direct endoscopic assessment with telescopes after temporary removal of the tube under general anaesthesia in an operating theatre will reveal the nature and degree of intubation trauma and therefore greatly assist this decision.

In infants the time for prolonged intubation before there is risk of irreversible damage is longer than in adults, and with skilled care in neonatal intensive care units there is almost no limit to the time of intubation. This can be of many weeks duration and still be associated with a low incidence of laryngeal problems. It seems that the hypercellular laryngeal cartilages with a gel-like matrix in infants yield and mould to pressure more than in older individuals.

Patient factors

Abnormality of the larynx
Impaired mucociliary mechanism
Bacterial infection
Gastro-oesophageal reflux
Impaired wound healing
Acute or chronic systemic disease

Physical trauma

Injuries to the larynx may occur during difficult intubation, because of unusual anatomy, in association with the use of a stylet introducer, because of unskilled intubation or after repeated intubations.

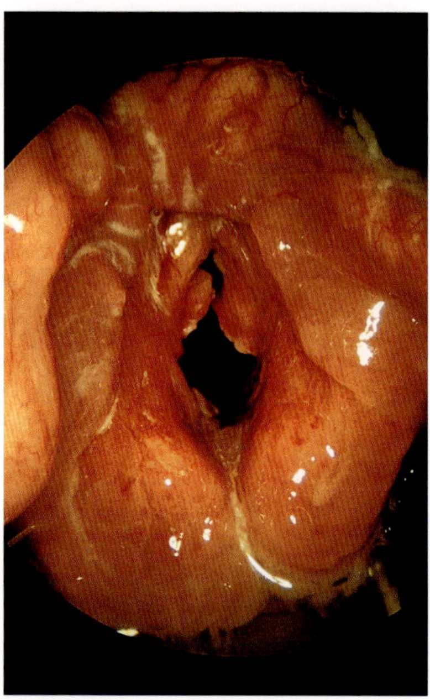

Figure **12.1**
Supraglottic oedema and tongues of granulation. The oedematous supraglottic tissues are bathed in acid gastro-oesophageal reflux fluid. Tongues of granulation tissue arising from each vocal cord are clearly visible.

Patient factors

Abnormal larynx

An abnormal larynx is more prone to damage than a normal larynx, e.g. a larynx crushed by external trauma, a burnt larynx, a congenitally small larynx with subglottic stenosis due to an abnormal cricoid (such as occurs in Down's syndrome) or the small larynx in a preterm, low birthweight infant. It has been found that 12% of paediatric patients intubated for airway obstruction caused by acute laryngotracheitis and subglottic oedema, cannot be successfully extubated after 7 days (McEniery et al 1991). After endoscopic assessment one in three of these were soon extubated, but the remaining two required a tracheotomy which was usually able to be removed within a few weeks.

Impaired mucociliary mechanism

This can be due to excessive secretions, stasis of secretions or bacterial contamination, all aggravated by the presence of the tube itself, trauma to the tracheobronchial mucosa from suctioning and possibly the effect of drugs given systemically.

Bacterial infection

Bacterial infection and sepsis occur quickly, within 24 hours, in tracheotomy wounds, especially in patients in poor general health or those who are immunodeficient. Performance of a tracheotomy below a larynx which is already the site of intubation trauma promotes subsequent contamination of the tracheotomy stoma, prolongs laryngeal healing and influences scar formation as shown by Sasaki et al (1979) who concluded that steps should be taken to minimize infection in these circumstances.

Gastro-oesophageal reflux

Gastro-oesophageal reflux with aspiration of acid into the larynx and subglottic region potentiates the local injury, complicates the healing process, predisposes to infection and ulceration and specifically encourages the development of granulation tissue (Figure 12.1). Patients in an intensive care unit have a high incidence of reflux, made more likely by the presence of a nasogastric tube which not only irritates the lower oesophagus but can also cause pressure necrosis and ulceration in the postcricoid region.

Impaired wound healing

Impaired wound healing may be an important factor for various reasons, e.g. in a diabetic or in a patient who is prone to keloid formation.

Acute or chronic disease states

Acute or chronic disease states with poor tissue perfusion, hypotensive episodes, altered levels of consciousness, hypoxia, anaemia, toxaemia and heart, kidney or liver failure are associated with severe laryngeal damage.

Identification of the above predisposing factors may indicate the likelihood of significant intubation injury in an individual patient and, together with the findings at endoscopic examination, are important in the overall assessment of laryngeal trauma in each patient.

PATHOGENESIS

It is not possible to leave a tube in the larynx without injury due to pressure from the unyielding tube. The important consideration is capillary perfusion. When pressure from the firm wall of the endotracheal tube exceeds mucosal capillary pressure, ischaemia occurs first, with hyperaemic congestion, oedema and eventually ulceration.

Pressure necrosis

Ischaemic necrosis in the posterior and subglottic larynx is a crucial consideration in mucosal injury and results in rapid epithelial erosion, granulation tissue formation (Fig. 12.2) and ulceration, the fundamental lesions from which complications occur. Confluent ulceration progresses to deep stromal necrosis and perichondritis after 90–100 hours and involvement of the nutrition of the perichondrium then produces chondritis with subsequent cartilage necrosis.

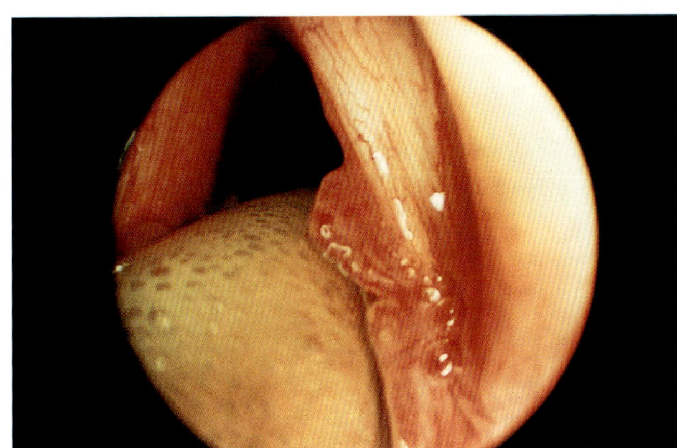

Figure **12.2**
Granulation tissue. The initial reaction occurs at the vocal process of the arytenoid in response to irritation from the endotracheal tube.

Histopathologic evaluation of the posterior glottis shows active inflammatory injury of the arytenoid and cricoid cartilages with lymphocytic infiltration, damage to the cricoarytenoid joints and sometimes frank necrosis of the cricoid. Rarely, in advanced cases (see Figs 12.20, 12.21), a fistula occurs in an area of cartilage necrosis or abscess formation. Ulceration at the site of pressure necrosis from an endotracheal tube can reasonably be likened to a ‘laryngeal bedsore’.

Healing

Granulation tissue proliferates at the margin of the injured area and may even persist after removal of the tube as ulcerative lesions begin to heal by secondary intention. Gould and Young (1992) have shown that in neonates the process of acute injury occurs rapidly in the first few days, but does not necessarily progressively involve more of the subglottic circumference. Ulcer healing may start at the end of the first week, even with the continued presence of the tube, and in many cases healing will be advanced at about 20–30 days despite the nearby presence of deep lesions with cartilage involvement.

If the endotracheal tube is removed at the stage of minor or moderate epithelial erosion, healing by mucosal regeneration and primary re-epithelialization will usually occur. However, if healing is incomplete, microscopic studies show squamous metaplasia replacing normal epithelium at the involved site. More extensive ulcerative lesions heal by secondary intention with granulation tissue and, when this is exuberant, a localized granuloma may proliferate. With extensive or deep change there is production of new collagen which eventually matures to fibrous tissue with contraction of scar tissue, a sequence of events which is fundamental to the development of both subglottic stenosis and posterior glottic stenosis.

Sites of injuries

The endotracheal tube, whether oral or nasal, always lies in, and exerts pressure on, the posterior larynx where there are three major sites of possible damage:

1 the medial surface of the arytenoid cartilage, vocal process and particularly the medial aspect of the cricoarytenoid joint;
2 the posterior glottis and interarytenoid region;
3 the subglottic region, especially the anterior surface of the posterior lamina of the cricoid cartilage on each side, or the damage may be annular affecting the internal circumference within the cricoid; this area is especially vulnerable in infants and small children because of its relatively small diameter.

Sites of laryngeal injury

Medial aspect cricoarytenoid joints
Posterior glottis
Subglottis

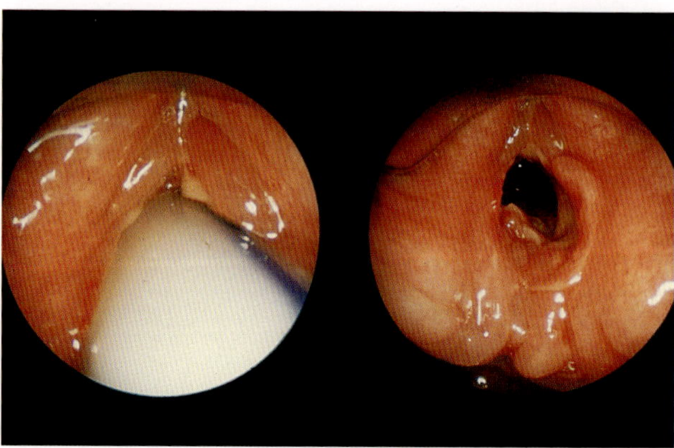

Figure **12.3**
Acute intubation injury seen with and without the endotracheal tube. The vocal cords, the subglottis and the posterior glottis cannot be seen with the tube in place, but oedematous protrusion of the mucosa of the laryngeal ventricles is obvious (left). Removal of the tube reveals the true extent of the laryngeal damage (right).

Intubation injuries can occur in one or more of these glottic and subglottic sites. Damage in the supraglottic larynx is very uncommon.

ENDOSCOPIC ASSESSMENT

Laryngeal injury begins during the first few hours of intubation and, even in an intensive care unit with the best facilities and personnel and with endotracheal tubes of relatively small diameter, the damage worsens each day. This poses the question of what can be done to minimize the injuries and their chronic sequelae.

Experience with patients of all ages has shown that the nature and degree of trauma occurring during prolonged intubation can be precisely assessed only by direct laryngoscopy using rigid telescopes for image magnification. With the patient under general anaesthesia, the endotracheal tube can be temporarily removed to allow complete examination of the upper airway (Fig. 12.3).

Endoscopic assessment performed during intubation to evaluate the severity of damage allows an informed, rational decision on whether to attempt extubation, continue intubation for a further period or perform a tracheotomy.

Continue intubation

Intubation can be safely continued, possibly with an endotracheal tube of smaller diameter, when the observed changes include minor oedema in the membranous vocal folds, oedematous protrusion of the mucosa of the laryngeal ventricles, surface mucosal ulceration, generalized inflammation and congestion, minor granulation tissue at the vocal process and the absence of severe oedema, grossly proliferative granulation tissue and deep ulceration. Removal of the endotracheal tube at this stage allows the damage to resolve.

Continue intubation

Oedema
Surface ulceration
Minor granulation
Absence of deep ulceration

Consider tracheotomy

Changes that indicate severe injury and the need for tracheotomy include deep ulceration through the mucoperichondrium into the cartilage of the arytenoid, the cricoid or the cricoarytenoid joint and/or widespread ulceration in the subglottic region, especially if the ulceration affects the whole circumference of the cricoid. In other cases, when attempted removal of the tube is followed by obstruction caused by large masses of granulation tissue or severe oedema, re-intubation becomes an urgent necessity, to allow an orderly tracheotomy.

Consider tracheotomy

Deep ulceration
Concentric subglottic ulceration
Obstructing tongues of granulation

Duration of intubation

There are diverse opinions regarding the duration of intubation before tracheotomy becomes necessary to minimize laryngeal trauma. In general, experience indicates a need for endoscopic assessment in adults after approximately 5–7 days, in children after 1–2 weeks and in infants only when attempted extubation has been unsuccessful. Unfortunately it is neither possible nor advisable to formulate 'rules' for the duration of intubation because of the variability and the severity of the changes.

Guidelines for endoscopic evaluation

Adults	after 5–7 days
Children	after 1–2 weeks
Infants	after failed extubation

Flexible laryngoscopy

Use of a flexible fibreoptic laryngoscope in the intensive care unit without general anaesthesia, with the endotracheal tube in situ cannot be recommended as it provides inadequate information. The presence of a tube obscures the vital posterior glottic and subglottic areas. They must be carefully inspected after temporary removal of the tube under general anaesthesia using the clarity provided by rigid telescopes.

Alternative management

When continued ventilation is required, another approach to management is to perform a tracheotomy in an adult after an arbitrary period of approximately 7 days and many intensivists now perform percutaneous tracheotomy in the intensive care unit. Endoscopic evaluation is required in those few cases where the tracheotomy cannot be removed later.

This approach ignores the possibility of safe continuation of intubation if endoscopy shows only mild intubation injuries, thus avoiding a tracheotomy. Some patients intubated for 7 days will have minor lesions while others will have more severe injuries – the reasons for this difference in susceptibility to injury are not known.

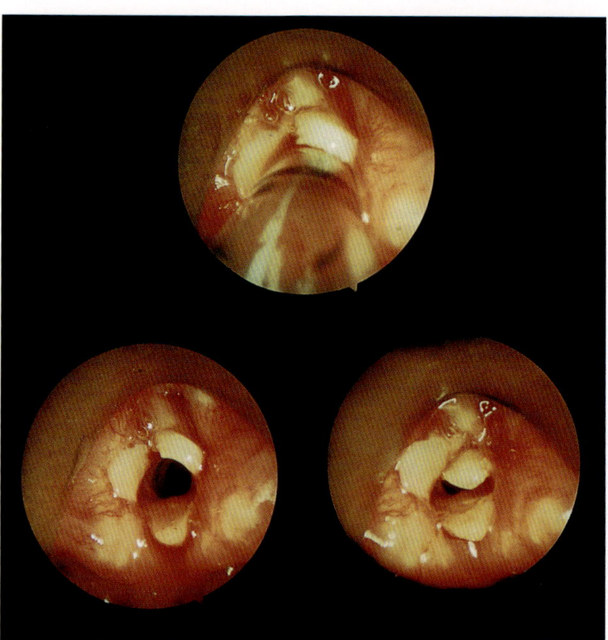

Figure **12.4**
Extensive granulations. Even with the tube in situ, extensive pale granulations can be seen. After extubation, inspiratory stridor is caused by the flap-like reactive granulation tissue.

Advantages of endoscopic evaluation

Thorough endoscopy gives information which will assist in an informed and rational decision on whether to attempt extubation, continue intubation for a further period, possibly with a tube of smaller size, or perform tracheotomy. Endoscopy allows removal of obstructing granulation tissue in some cases to improve the airway prior to attempted extubation. The removed tissue should be submitted for microbiological assessment.

CLINICAL FEATURES RELATED TO TIME AFTER EXTUBATION

Successful removal of the endotracheal tube after prolonged intubation in the intensive care unit often leaves the patient with a husky voice and sometimes with minor stridor, but in most cases these features resolve over hours or days, by which time the patient will usually have been discharged from the hospital. However, some patients may develop symptoms of airway obstruction immediately after extubation, others shortly after discharge or others sometimes weeks, months or years later (Table 12.1). The clinical features and their relationship to time after removal of the tube are as follows:

- in the first seconds or minutes, severe obstruction caused by oedematous flap-like tongues of granulation tissue at the glottic level (Fig. 12.4);
- in the first hours progressive obstruction caused by increasing oedema in the larynx, usually in the subglottic region;
- in the first days, partial obstruction and a husky, weak voice caused by persistent oedema and proliferative granulation tissue;
- weeks later, husky voice caused by a chronic intubation granuloma or sometimes by persistent oedema in the vocal folds;

Table 12.1 Acute injuries during prolonged intubation

Injury	*Endoscopic appearance*	*Outcome*
Early nonspecific	Hyperaemia	
	Oedema	Resolution
	Patchy surface ulceration	
Oedema	Protrusion of ventricular mucosa	Resolution
	Oedema of vocal folds	Chronic Reinke's oedema
	Subglottic oedema	Subglottic obstruction
Granulation tissue[1]	'Tongues' from vocal processes	Resolution
		Intubation granuloma
		Healed fibrous nodule
		Interarytenoid adhesion
Ulceration[1]	Superficial	Resolution
	Ulcerated troughs	Healed furrows
	Annular in posterior glottis	Posterior glottic stenosis
	Subglottic, within cricoid	Subglottic stenosis
Miscellaneous	Laceration	Local scarring
	Bleeding	Haematoma
	Arytenoid dislocation	Fixed cricoarytenoid joint
	Perforation	Neck infection or abscess
	Cricoid ulceration	Chronic sinus or fistula

[1]Note that granulations and ulceration often occur together.

- many months later, increasing obstruction with dyspnoea on exertion as posterior glottic or subglottic stenosis contracts to narrow the airway.

In the patient who has left hospital and complains of husky voice or airway problems indirect examination permits easy recognition of oedema, intubation granuloma, healed fibrous nodule and vocal cord paralysis. Posterior glottic stenosis, healed furrows, interarytenoid adhesion and subglottic stenosis may be difficult to recognize because accurate visualization of the interarytenoid, posterior glottic and subglottic region is seldom possible with indirect laryngoscopy. Vocal cord movement is, without question, best assessed at indirect laryngoscopy. Further, it is difficult, usually impossible, to differentiate a paralysed vocal cord from a fixed cricoarytenoid joint until arytenoid movement is tested at direct laryngoscopy.

Comprehensive, precise evaluation and documentation is obtained only when the larynx is examined using telescopes under general anaesthesia. Attention must be directed to the posterior glottis, the subglottis, mobility of the cricoarytenoid joints and the medial surfaces and vocal processes of the arytenoids. In this way posterior glottic stenosis, subglottic stenosis and limitation of movement or fixation of the cricoarytenoid joints will not be overlooked. The airway diameter should be measured using endotracheal tubes or telescopes of known external diameter or, more accurately, by passing serially larger probes of known diameter. We use the

Benjamin–Jackson oesophageal bougies to calibrate the subglottic airway in millimetres. Less obvious chronic sequelae of prolonged intubation, such as a healed fibrous nodule or scar tissue or linear healed furrows on the medial surface of the cricoarytenoid joints, will be recognized at direct laryngoscopy.

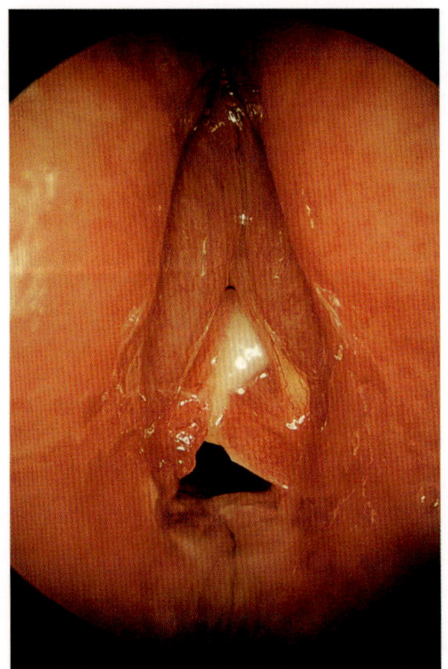

Figure **12.5**
Oedematous protrusion of the mucosa of the laryngeal ventricles and bilateral tongues of granulation. The tube has just been removed but the subglottic region has not yet been evaluated.

ACUTE INJURIES DURING PROLONGED INTUBATION

Changes in the intubated larynx depend on tube pressure causing oedema, infection, ulceration and necrosis, first of the underlying mucous membrane, then of the perichondrium and lastly the cartilage. The degree of damage varies from patient to patient; some incur minimal injury whereas others, intubated for the same time, manifest severe and dramatic changes (see Table 12.1).

Observation of the changes, whether in infants, children or adults, has allowed separation into five categories: early non-specific changes, oedema, granulation tissue, ulceration and miscellaneous injuries.

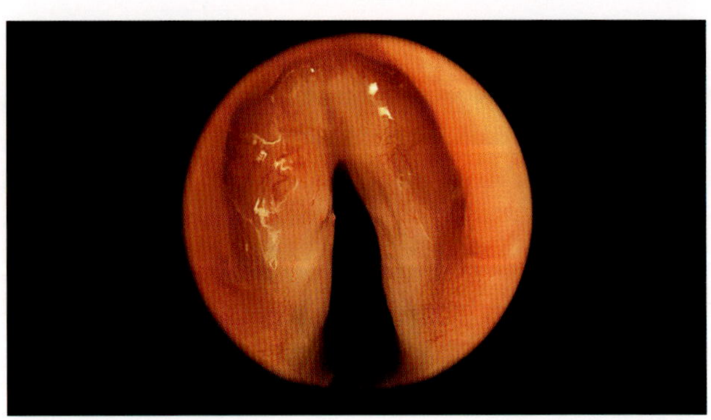

Figure **12.6**
Chronic oedema in the vocal folds of an infant who was intubated for 4 weeks as a premature baby. After extubation he had a persistent weak, husky cry.

Early non-specific changes

Whether oedema or superficial exfoliation of the cells is the first change is unknown; they probably occur more or less at the same time. Endoscopic examination of larynges with minimal change shows only irritation of the mucosa, oedema and hyperaemia.

Oedema

Oedema occurs readily in the loose submucosal tissue of the laryngeal ventricle. Obvious diffusely swollen mucosa has been called 'prolapse of the ventricle' but a better descriptive term is 'protrusion of oedematous ventricular mucosa' (Fig. 12.5).

Oedema in the vocal folds themselves occurs, especially in infants, and sometimes persists after extubation as chronic oedema in Reinke's space (Fig. 12.6) where it causes voice dysfunction.

Oedematous swelling of the supraglottic tissues (Fig. 12.1) is occasionally seen affecting the epiglottis, aryepiglottic folds and arytenoids. Oedematous swelling in the subglottic region, in the mucosal lining of the cricoid cartilage is common, sometimes

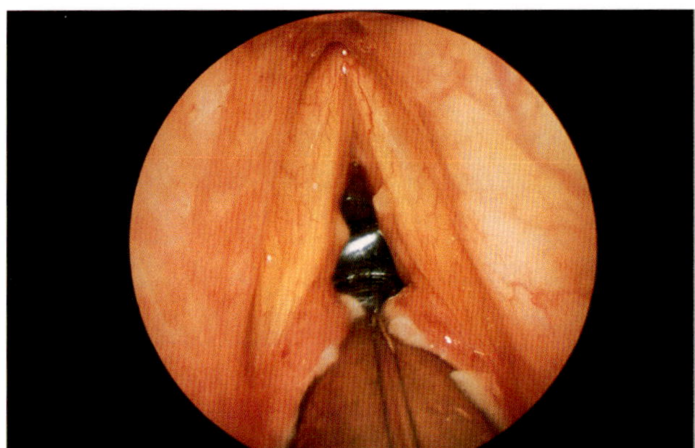

Figure **12.7**
Tongues of granulation tissue with superficial ulceration on their edges. Illustrating extension around the anterior surface of the endotracheal tube.

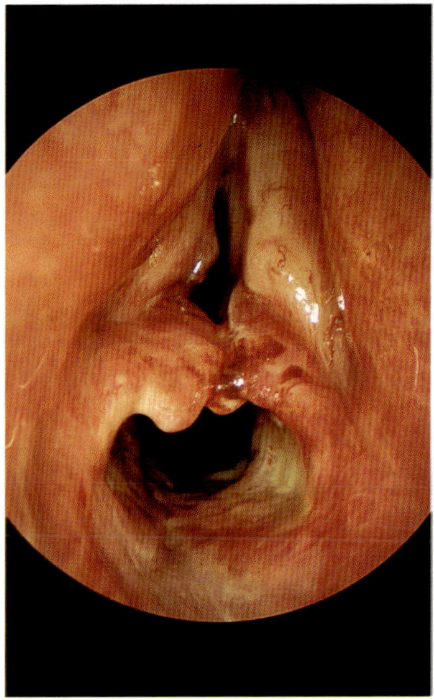

Figure **12.8**
Bilateral tongues of granulation tissue and ulcerated troughs. The posterior glottic mucosa appears to have a non-ulcerated intact strip of mucosa in the midline.

progressing slowly and causing airway obstruction minutes or hours after removal of the endotracheal tube. Its presence will be manifest by inspiratory stridor commencing some minutes after extubation.

Granulation tissue

Granulations form at the sites of ulceration of mucous membrane, perichondrium and cartilage and are often detectable within 48 hours, arising first from the region of the vocal process of the arytenoid (Fig. 12.2). Continued proliferation on each side around the anterior surface of the endotracheal tube (Fig. 12.7) represents tongues of granulation tissue (Fig. 12.8) which are to be found in many larynges during prolonged intubation. Sometimes large, flap-like tongues (Fig. 12.9) cause obstruction after attempted removal of an endotracheal tube making immediate re-intubation necessary.

Surgical removal of these persistent, obstructive granulations is usually unnecessary, although in selected cases removal of the flaps of granulation tissue (which should be submitted to microbiology for culture) may assist extubation.

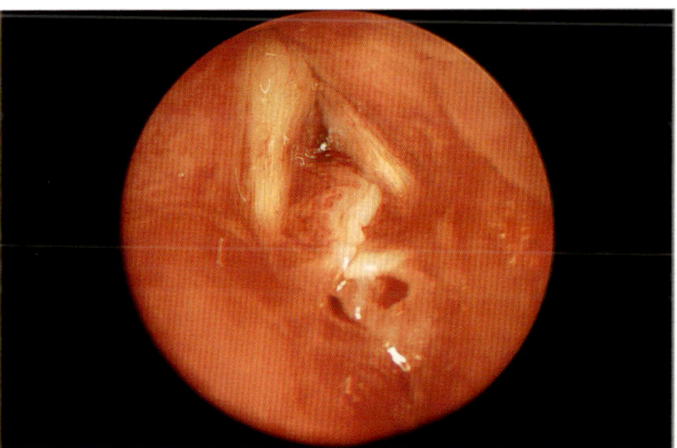

Figure **12.9**
Multiple exuberant flap-like granulations causing total obstruction after removal of the endotracheal tube.

Extubation removes the foreign body irritation of the endotracheal tube and resolution of non-obstructing granulations is usually rapid and complete.

Incomplete resolution of glottic granulations produces several distinct, recognizable chronic problems

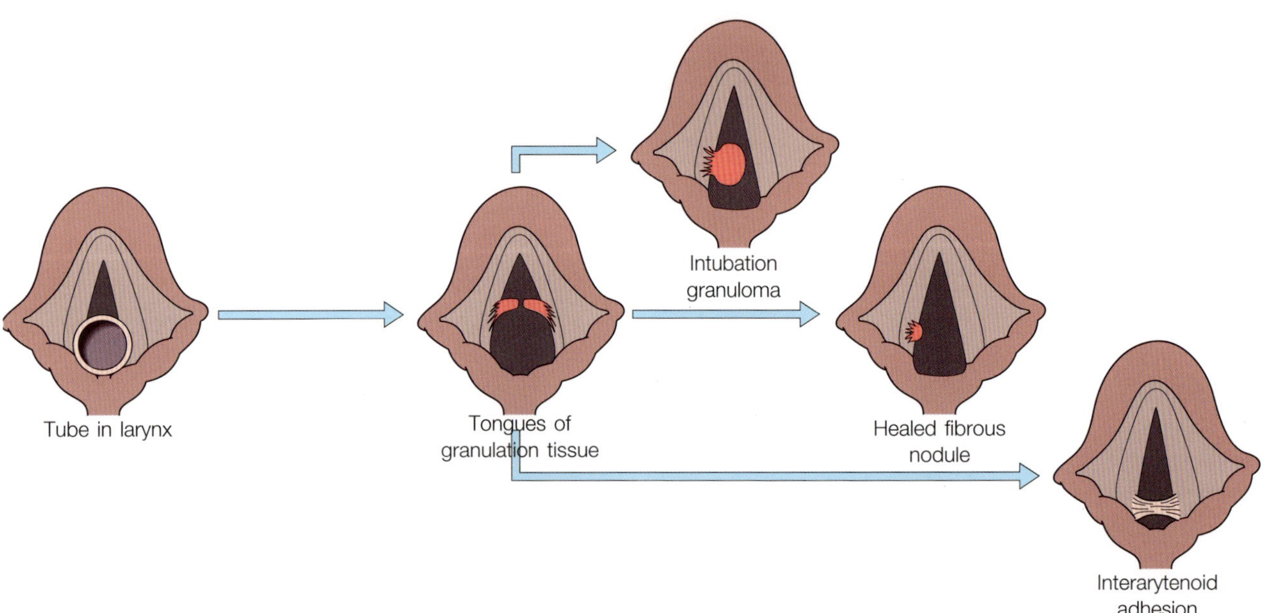

Figure **12.10**
Flow chart showing the chronic end-results of granulation tissue. The final result can be complete resolution, post-intubation granuloma, healed fibrous nodule or interarytenoid adhesion.

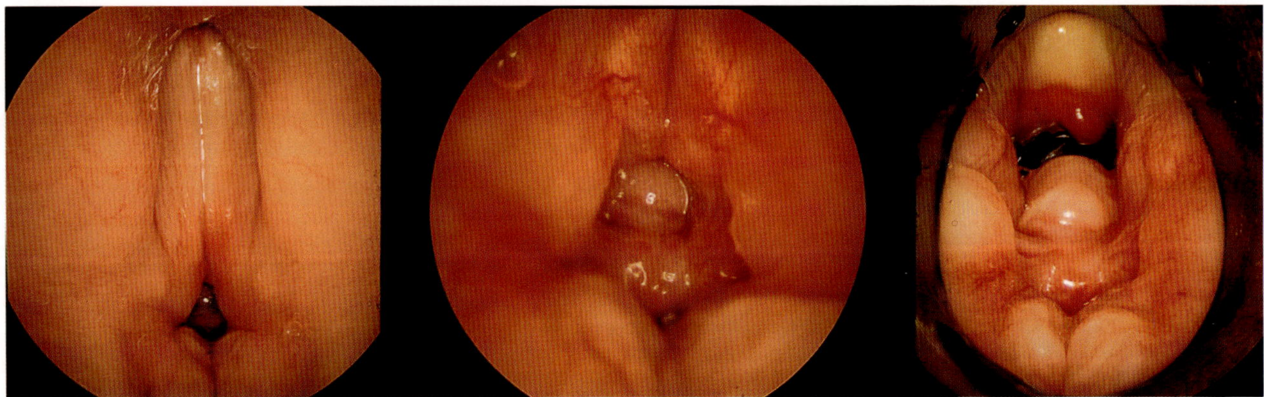

Figure **12.11**
Granulation tissue and ulceration. Initial laryngoscopic view (left) does not reveal pathology. As the laryngoscope is advanced, multiple granulations are seen (centre) in the posterior glottis, and when the cords are separated (right) ulceration is visible in the anterior subglottic region.

(Fig. 12.10). Sometimes the granulation tissue persists to form a rounded, mature intubation granuloma on one or occasionally both sides. Occasionally there is partial but incomplete healing on one side, leaving a small, firm, permanent, healed fibrous nodule of scar tissue near the vocal process. Rarely the granulations become adherent across the midline between the vocal processes at the glottic or subglottic level and this forms an interarytenoid adhesion which ultimately matures to a firm fibrous band.

When the granulation tissue is associated with ulceration (Fig. 12.11) secondary healing takes place

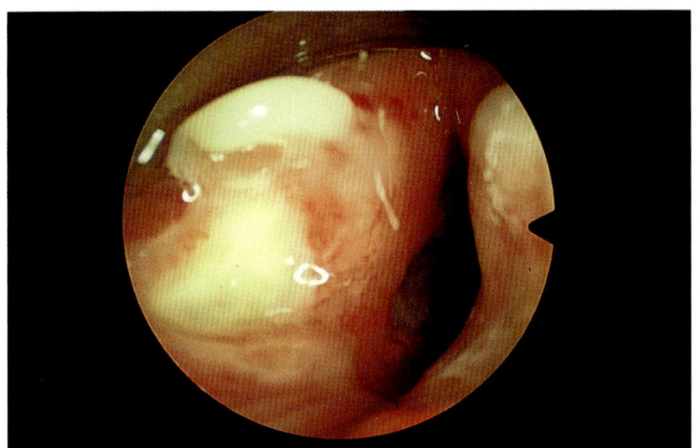

Figure **12.12**
Ulcerated trough. A deep ulcer is clearly seen on the left side with peripheral granulation tissue. The line of the cricoarytenoid joint lies within the ulcer.

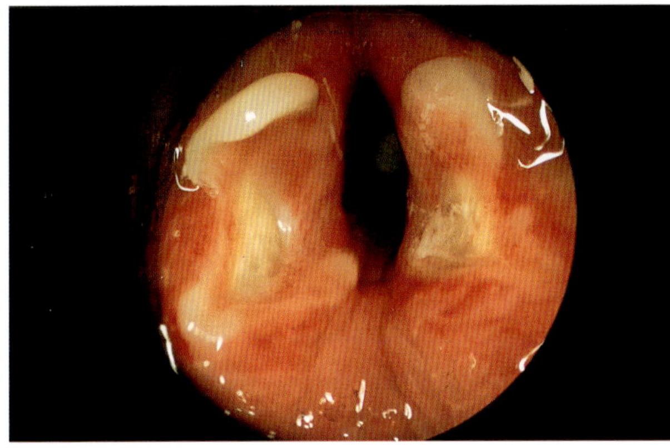

Figure **12.13**
Bilateral ulcerated troughs surrounded by granulations. Note the intact median strip implying that later development of posterior glottic stenosis is unlikely.

in the underlying connective tissue with fibrous tissue formation in the posterior glottic and subglottic area. In the latter case, stenotic scarring is found either on the anterior surface of the posterior cricoid lamina or circumferentially within the cricoid cartilage forming subglottic stenosis. As the collagen contracts and forms scar tissue, upper airway obstruction becomes progressively more pronounced.

Ulceration

Ischaemia induces necrosis and ulceration which penetrates the perichondrium and cartilage causing perichondritis and chondritis. Endoscopic examination at this stage clearly reveals exposed, white, shining cartilage on each side, an appearance referred to as an ulcerated trough (Fig. 12.12). The ulcers involve the medial surface of the arytenoid, the joint itself and the upper surface of the cricoid with the line of the cricoarytenoid joint sometimes visible. Ulceration also occurs on the anterior surface of the cricoid lamina or circumferentially within the cricoid cartilage. Deep ulceration into perichondrium and cartilage heals by scar tissue formation and may later cause stenosis.

An ulcerated trough (Fig. 12.12) is an obvious, wide, deep area of erosion and rounded ulceration usually surrounded by a rim of granulation tissue which proliferates at the vocal process of the arytenoid. Ulcerated troughs can be seen only after the endotracheal tube has been removed. They are usually similar on each side (Fig. 12.13).

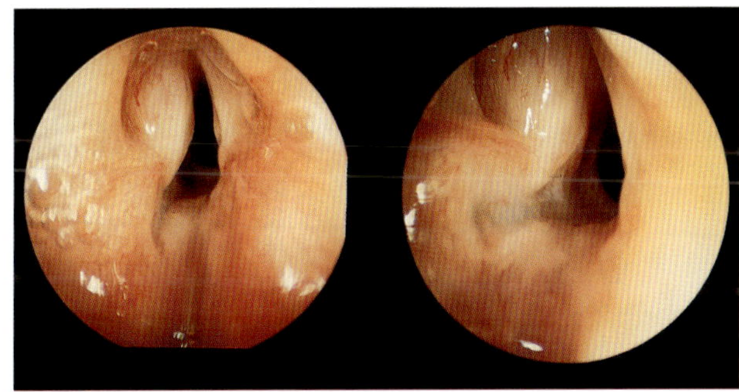

Figure **12.14**
Healed furrow. Here displayed only on the left but almost certainly bilateral. With a 0° telescope (left) the extent of the furrow is not as well seen as with a 30° telescope (right).

The presence, during or immediately after extubation, of a posterior central strip of intact mucosa with ulceration and granulation on each side is a favourable sign that posterior glottic stenosis is less

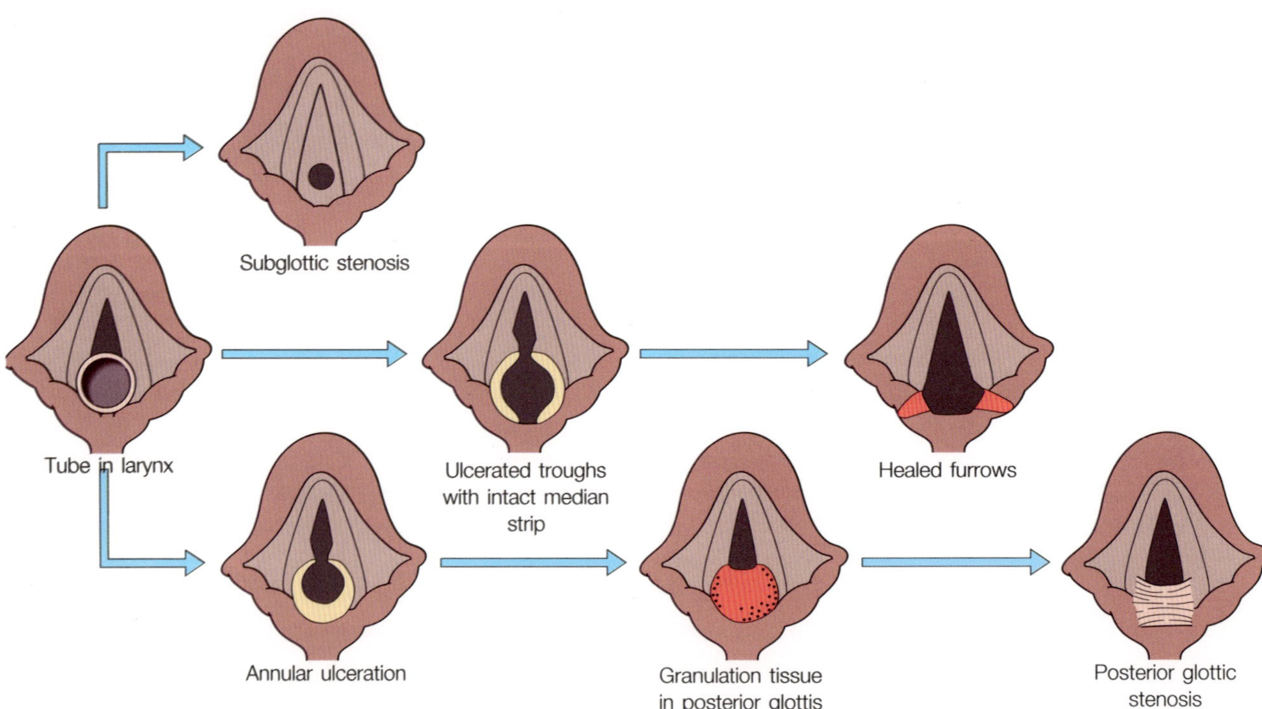

Figure **12.15**
Flow chart showing the results of ulceration during prolonged intubation. The chronic end result might be resolution, subglottic stenosis, healed furrows or posterior glottic stenosis.

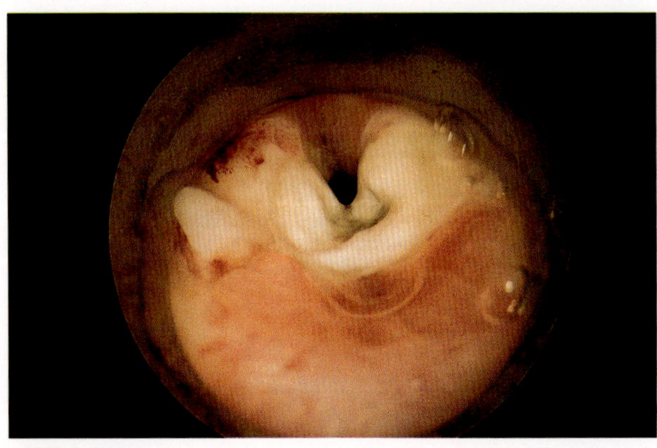

Figure **12.16**
Extensive, deep ulceration in the posterior glottis. This will cause a posterior glottic stenosis with or without fixed cricoarytenoid joints.

likely to occur later, but partial or complete cricoarytenoid joint fixation may still occur.

In the weeks following extubation, as healing and fibrosis occur, the area of the acute ulcerated trough can be recognized as a chronic healed furrow (Fig. 12.14). Detection of an acute ulcerated trough during or immediately after intubation, or of a chronic healed furrow later on, implies dysfunction of the cricoarytenoid joint which may cause dysphonia.

Thus, healing of ulceration produces distinct pathological entities in the larynx (Fig. 12.15): namely, subglottic stenosis, healed furrows and posterior glottic stenosis.

Deep ulceration in the posterior glottis without an intact strip of mucosa in the midline (Fig. 12.16) is likely to form scar tissue and posterior glottic fibrosis.

Miscellaneous injuries

Injuries occur either during the initial intubation or during later intubations. They are more likely when laryngoscopy is difficult because of anatomic problems, after 'blind' intubation or when an intro-

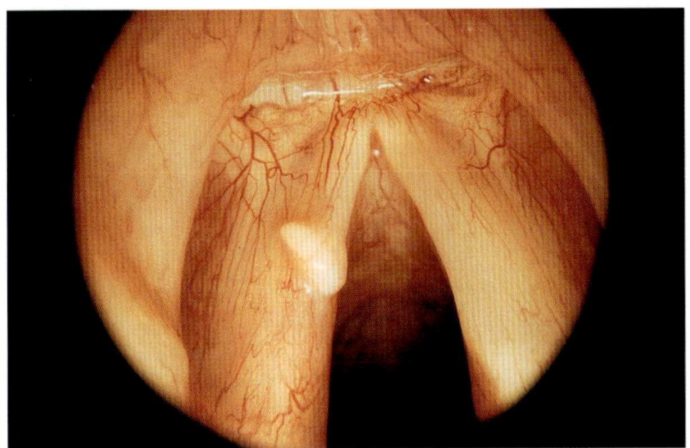

Figure **12.17**
Post-intubation vocal cord scarring. The irregular tag caused a persistent husky voice following intubation for 1 hour. The original laceration may have been due to the tip of the endotracheal tube or the tip of an introducer.

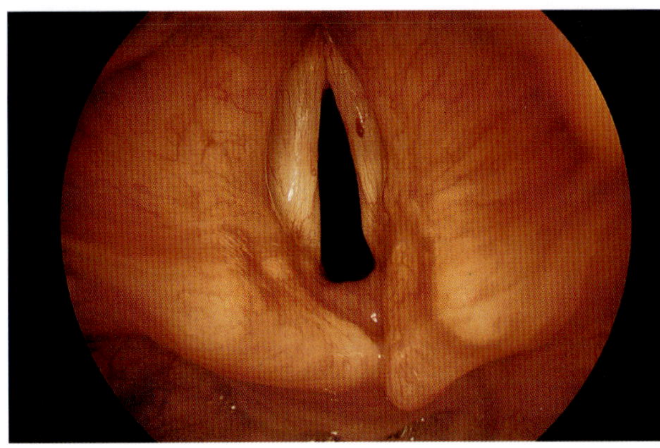

Figure **12.18**
Dislocation of the right arytenoid. There was no movement in the right vocal cord and the cricoarytenoid joint was fixed. After endoscopic removal of the arytenoid, right vocal cord movement could again be seen.

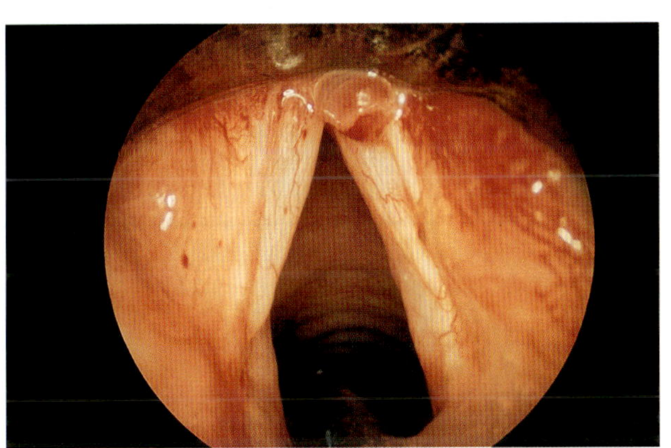

Figure **12.19**
Post-intubation granuloma. An atypical site at the anterior end of the right vocal fold.

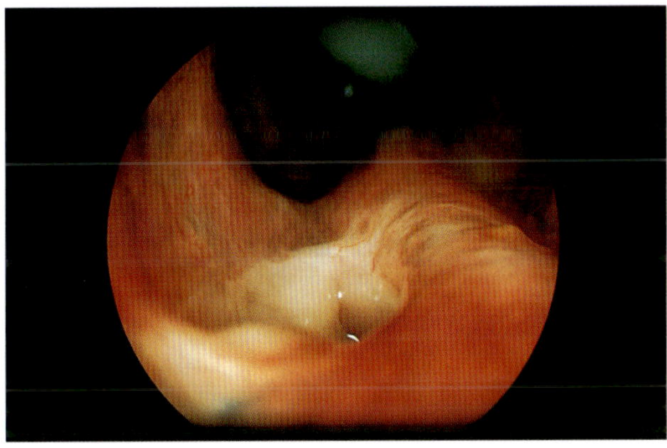

Figure **12.20**
Fistula of the posterior surface of the cricoid cartilage.

ducer is used in the endotracheal tube. Miscellaneous injuries to the larynx inflicted during intubation but not necessarily related to prolonged intubation include:

- laceration, haematoma or bleeding in a vocal cord (Fig. 12.17);
- dislocation or subluxation of an arytenoid cartilage (Fig. 12.18);
- perforation of the airway with spreading surgical emphysema and soft tissue infection;
- a granuloma in an atypical site (Fig. 12.19);
- very rarely an acute pressure injury forms an infected sinus (Fig. 12.20) into the posterior cricoid cartilage in the subglottis;
- if an indwelling nasogastric tube ulcerates the posterior surface of the cricoid at the same site, a fistula will form (Fig. 12.21);
- other unusual injuries will occasionally be seen (Fig. 12.22).

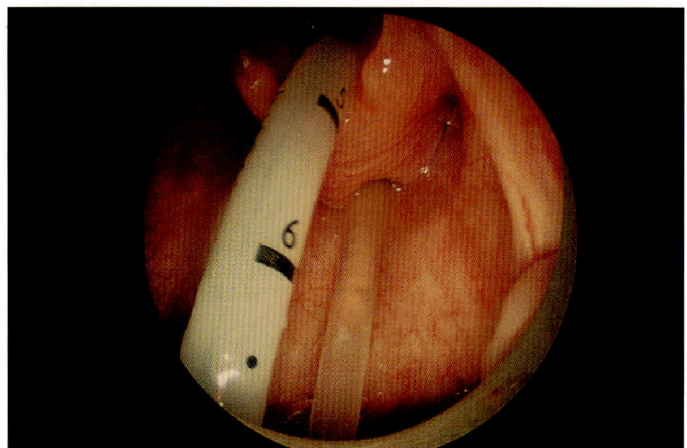

Figure **12.21**
Endotracheal tube and nasogastric tube in situ. Either tube can cause ulceration of the posterior lamina of the cricoid cartilage and rarely can lead to a persistent fistula. Potential trauma from a nasogastric tube must not be forgotten.

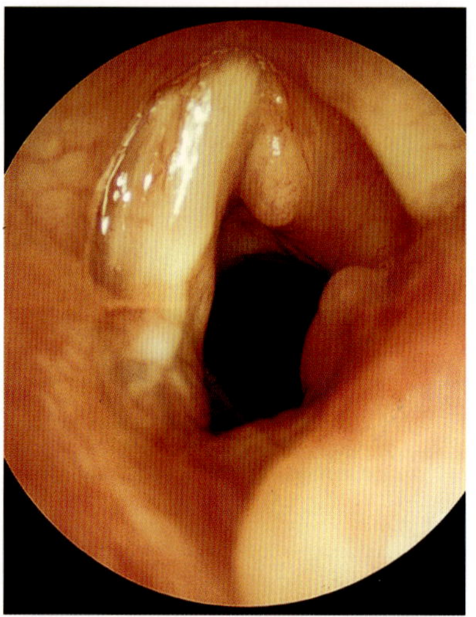

Figure **12.22**
Avulsion in the right vocal cord. A difficult, traumatic intubation as a neonate left this child with a very poor, breathy voice.

CHRONIC CHANGES AFTER EXTUBATION

The need for endoscopic assessment under general anaesthesia will be indicated by a history of stridor, progressive shortness of breath, a husky voice and the findings at indirect laryngoscopy. After extubation the outcome is a spectrum from rapid resolution with regeneration of mucosa and return to a normal state to progressive stenosis. There may be life-threatening airway obstruction or chronic interference with voice production. A number of specific pathological entities may be found either as a consequence of granulation tissue or of ulceration.

Consequences of granulation tissue

Post-intubation granuloma

Post-intubation granuloma is a well-known complication. It appears to be more common in adults although it can occur at any age. The incidence is unknown. If healing of the mucosa is incomplete and perichondritis persists, granulation tissue remains as a chronic, localized intubation granuloma (Fig. 12.23) which is commonly a globular, yellow–red, pedunculated mass arising from the vocal process and medial surface of the arytenoid where the mucoperichondrium is thin. Granulomas may also be found at atypical sites in the subglottis or the anterior larynx (Fig. 12.19) where the initial traumatic laceration was probably caused by the tip of an endotracheal tube or by an introducer projecting from the distal tip of the tube.

Consequences of granulation tissue

Post-intubation granuloma
Healed fibrous nodule
Interarytenoid adhesion

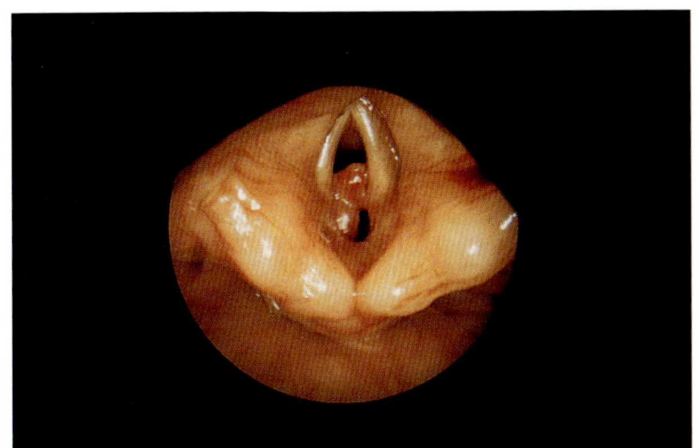

Figure **12.23**
Bilateral intubation granulomata. These granulomas formed after brief intubation, for about 72 hours, in a child who had inhaled the products of combustion in a fire.

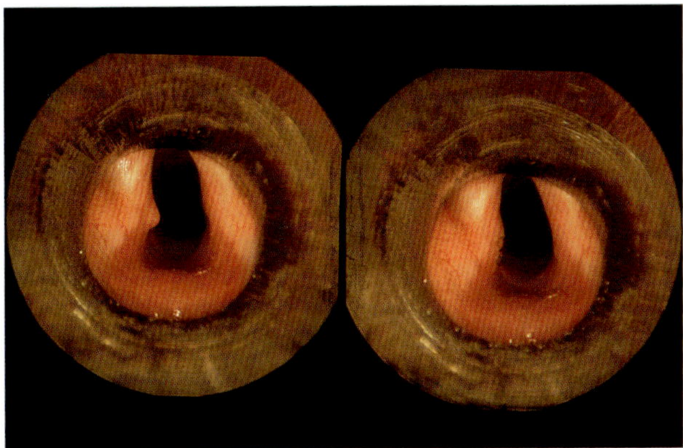

Figure **12.24**
Healed fibrous nodule. The firm, smooth, rounded nodule on the left has been vaporized with the carbon dioxide laser but there was no improvement in the voice.

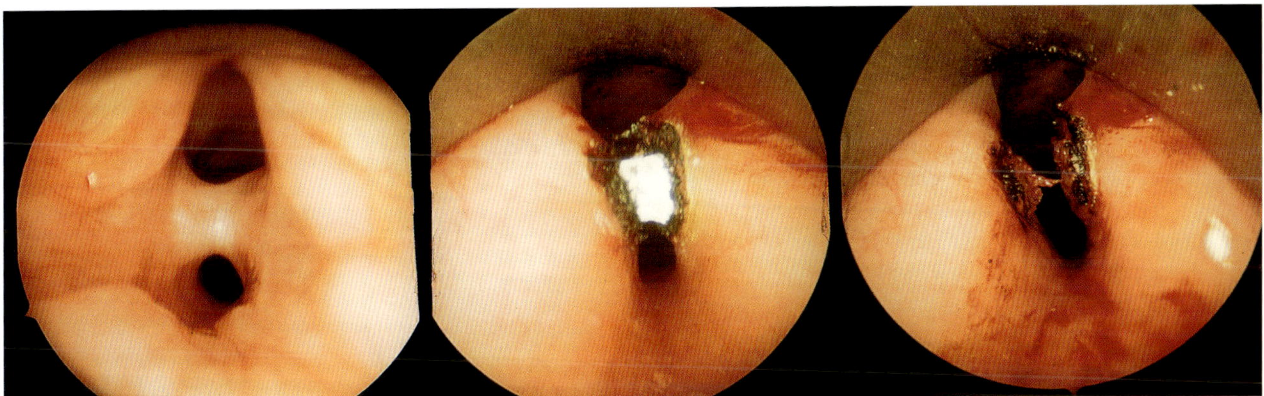

Figure **12.25**
Interarytenoid adhesion and calcification. A patient with severe shortness of breath, wrongly diagnosed as bilateral vocal cord paralysis. During laser division of the adhesion, a bar of bone was found (centre); following treatment symptoms were totally relieved.

The patient complains of 'something' in the throat or dysphonia and presents weeks or even months after the episode of intubation. If the granuloma is large enough or there are bilateral granulomas there may be partial airway obstruction.

Granulomas can be removed using the carbon dioxide laser or by microlaryngeal surgery using forceps and scissors. The latter technique causes troublesome bleeding sometimes making it difficult to identify the attachment of the mass. Accurate removal is important as inadequate removal allows the remainder to proliferate into a recurrent granuloma. Removal too deep into the cartilage and perichondrium of the vocal process again predisposes to recurrence. At histologic examination a vocal granuloma is similar to a pyogenic granuloma.

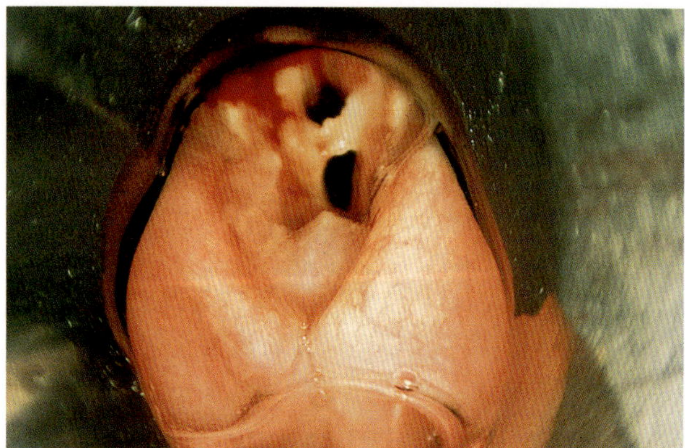

Figure **12.26**
Recently formed interarytenoid adhesion. The child, extubated 6 days previously, had persistent stridor. At endoscopy this developing adhesion was divided. Subsequent endoscopy 2 weeks later showed no recurrence.

Healed fibrous nodule

This small, persistent, rounded area of scar tissue on the medial edge of the vocal cord has seldom been described and may go unrecognized. Most of the reactionary granulation tissue resolves leaving only a small, inconspicuous, rounded, fibrotic nodule or nodules covered by mucous membrane (Fig. 12.24). Removal seldom improves the voice.

Interarytenoid adhesion

Tongues of granulation on the right and left vocal processes may adhere to one another and heal, thus occasionally forming a transverse interarytenoid adhesion (Fig. 12.25) at the level of the vocal folds or below. Interarytenoid adhesion is more likely to occur in patients with vocal cord paralysis or with diminished cord movement because of a depressed level of consciousness. If the adhesion is discovered early, in the first week or two (Fig. 12.26), it can be broken down and will usually not recur, but if it is undetected it will mature to an interarytenoid fibrous band which occasionally undergoes dystrophic calcification. There is an anterior triangular opening in front of the band with a circular or oval opening behind.

As the posterior glottis is difficult to see at indirect laryngoscopy, the anterior opening is often mistaken for the glottis. Bilateral vocal cord paralysis is diagnosed because the vocal cords are tethered to one another preventing abduction and causing partial airway obstruction. A mature adhesion can simply be divided with the laser (Fig. 12.27) or microsurgical scissors (Fig. 12.28); the result with either method is excellent.

Interarytenoid adhesion must be differentiated from posterior glottic stenosis which has thick, firm, scar tissue filling the posterior glottis and sometimes extending into the subglottis.

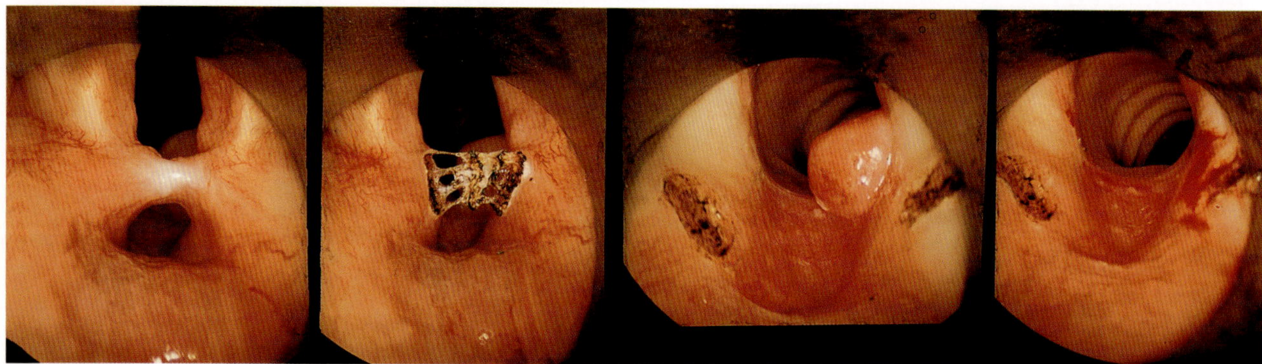

Figure **12.27**
Interarytenoid adhesion and post-intubation granuloma. Thick bridge of scar tissue (left); during laser division (centre left); after complete removal to expose subglottic post-intubation granuloma (centre right); and after laser removal of granuloma (right).

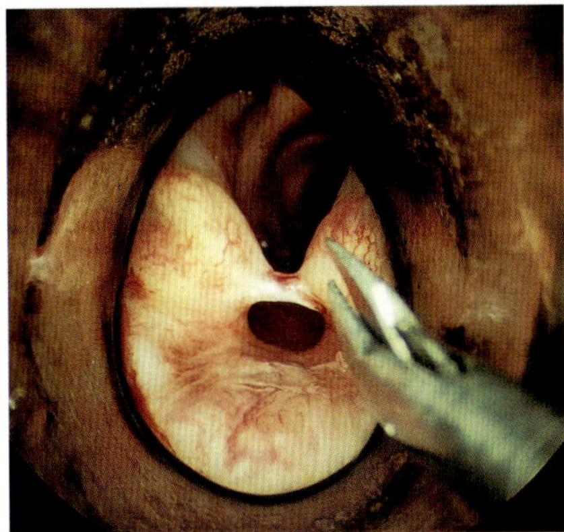

Figure **12.28**
Division of thin interarytenoid web. A subglottiscope has been used to apply pressure to the arytenoid cartilages and put the web on stretch before division with scissors.

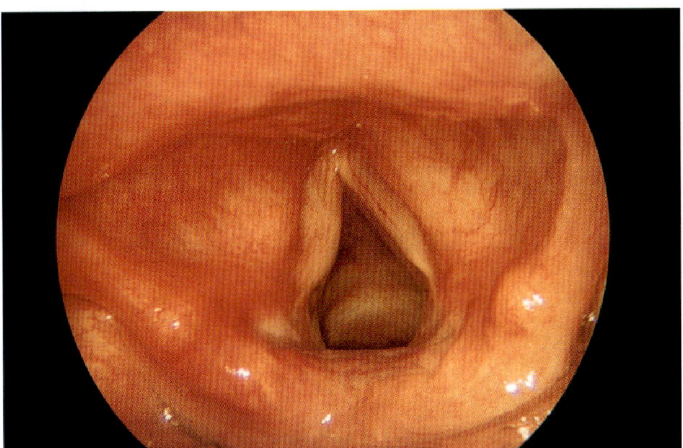

Figure **12.29**
Healed furrow and oedema of vocal fold. Indirect laryngoscopy clearly shows the healed furrow with associated oedema in the left vocal fold.

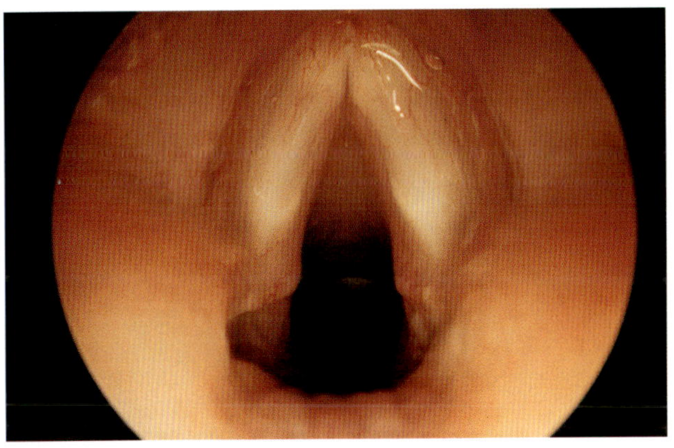

Figure **12.30**
Bilateral healed furrows, worse on the left. The appearance, with a telescope or the microscope, shows relatively normal vocal cords, but a 'divot' appears to have been removed from the posterior aspect over the medial surface of the arytenoid.

Consequences of ulceration

Healed furrows
Posterior glottic stenosis
Subglottic stenosis
Complete stenosis

Consequences of ulceration

Healed furrows

Healed furrows are a not uncommon finding after prolonged intubation. There are narrow, linear, pale scars representing healing of ulcerated troughs which form as an acute injury during intubation as described earlier. They are usually difficult to identify at indirect laryngoscopy (Fig. 12.29). The appearance at direct laryngoscopy with a 0° telescope or the operating microscope (Fig. 12.30) suggests a posterior defect of the vocal cord. The true nature of depressed scars running craniocaudally across the cricoarytenoid joint on the adjacent medial surfaces of the arytenoid and cricoid can be identified at laryngoscopy with a 30° angled telescope (Fig. 12.30). Healed furrows are often associated with some degree of chronic oedema in Reinke's space, and sometimes there is diminished cricoarytenoid joint mobility. Patients with these findings have minor but annoying dysphonia. There is no known effective treatment.

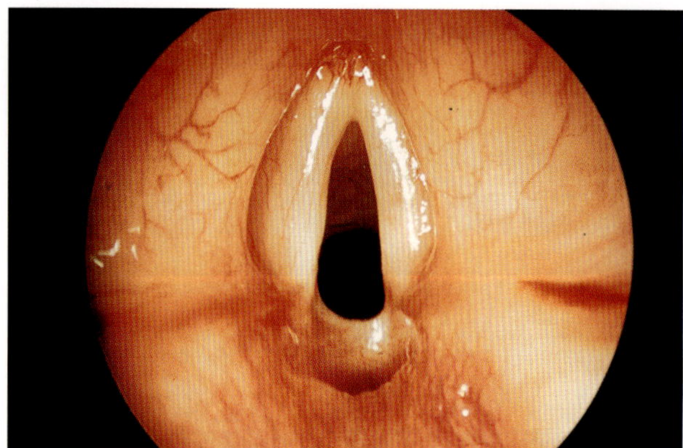

Figure **12.31**
Posterior glottic stenosis. Typical appearance of a stenotic web with a sharp, rounded anterior edge and a concavity behind it.

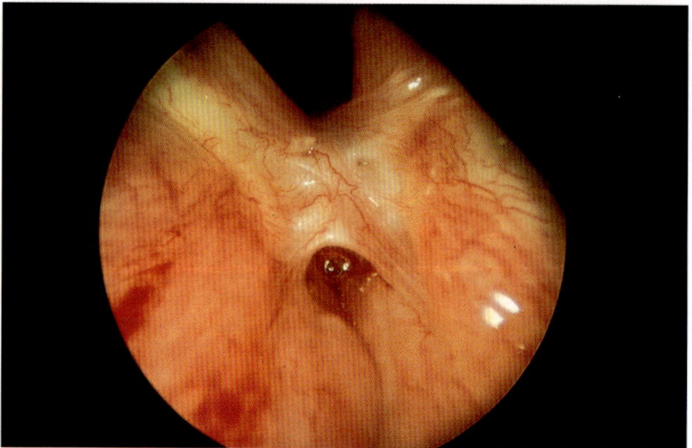

Figure **12.32**
Close-up of posterior glottic stenosis. The arytenoids have been displaced laterally by the laryngoscope stretching the scar tissue. The posterior depression was a blind fistula and did not connect to the subglottic lumen.

Posterior glottic stenosis

The posterior glottic space is sometimes the site of thick scar tissue following prolonged intubation in both adults and children.

It causes major morbidity as the patient usually has inspiratory stridor on exertion or in severe cases at rest, but the reason may not be immediately apparent at indirect laryngoscopy. The arytenoids are tethered together, cannot abduct on inspiration and a misdiagnosis of bilateral vocal cord paralysis may be made. There may be some dysphonia but in many cases the voice is near normal.

The primary pathology is acute ischaemic pressure necrosis and ulceration in the posterior glottic space followed by proliferation of granulations after extubation. Collagen then matures to scar tissue which fills the posterior glottis, holds the posterior borders of the vocal cords together, replaces the interarytenoid muscle by fibrous tissue and thereby produces partial or total fixation of one or both cricoarytenoid joints (Fig. 12.31). The resultant posterior glottic stenosis is often unrecognized or poorly assessed. There may be little functional deficit at first but, as scar tissue matures and contracts during the weeks or months after prolonged intubation, the patient experiences breathing problems which range from dyspnoea on exertion to severe obstruction which can produce alarming manifestations. A larynx with posterior glottic stenosis is sometimes erroneously described as having non-specific 'laryngeal stenosis', an indefinite and imprecise term that neglects assessment of the nature, site and degree of the problem.

At direct laryngoscopy the condition is best seen with a 30° telescope; there is firm fibrous tissue in the interarytenoid region (Fig. 12.32), often with downward extension into the posterior subglottic region with deeper scarring, which cannot be seen but causes fibrous ankylosis affecting mobility of the cricoarytenoid joints.

The stenosis has a transverse anterior edge that may be sharp or rounded and blunt. The web may extend upwards but always includes the glottic level and cricoarytenoid joints and usually extends downwards to the subglottic region. In some cases there is also a separate subglottic stenosis, treatment of which will be ineffective if posterior glottic stenosis remains unidentified and untreated.

An experienced laryngologist, aware of the importance and incidence of posterior glottic stenosis, will suspect the condition clinically when indirect laryngoscopy shows a 'tear drop'-shaped glottic opening and lack of abduction.

Treatment is not always successful. Severe posterior glottic stenosis with fixation of the joints remains

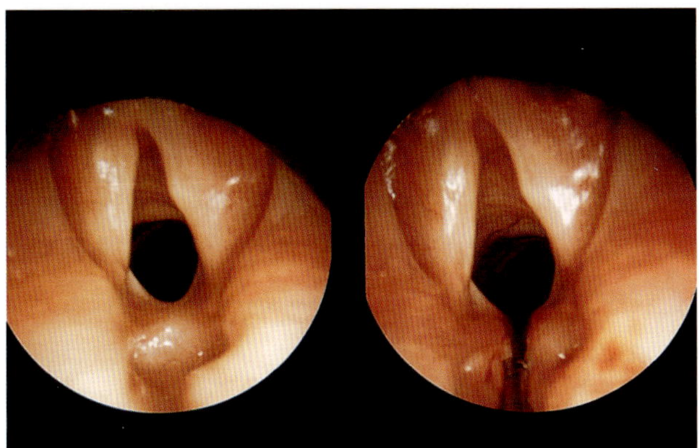

Figure **12.33**
Surgical division of posterior glottic stenosis. Division using a scalpel blade on a long handle leaves a deep V-shaped defect and the stenosis has been temporarily 'released' (right). Re-stenosis is likely.

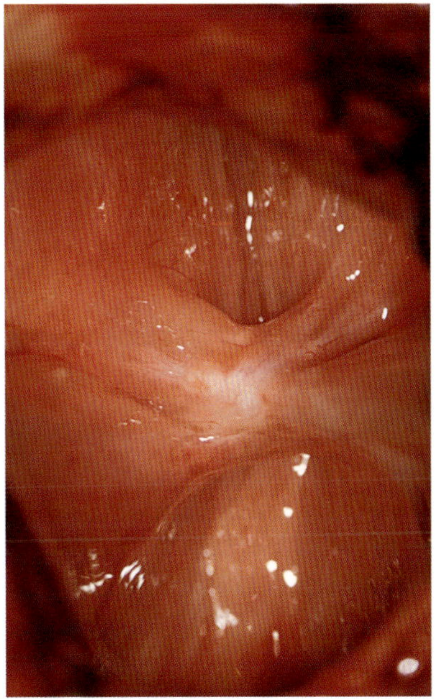

Figure **12.34**
Posterior glottic stenosis seen at laryngofissure. The mature tight scar tissue in the posterior glottis is clearly visible prior to its removal and placement of a mucosal flap. Some cases also require arytenoidectomy.

one of the most difficult laryngeal problems. Endoscopic treatment may be simple vertical division of the scar tissue either with the carbon dioxide laser or, more effectively, with a curved no. 11 scalpel blade on a long handle (Fig. 12.33). The scar is boldly divided in the midline from the subglottic region below to the interarytenoid region above, deep enough to feel the tip of the scalpel blade on the cricoid lamina. If the tissues spring apart leaving a deep V-shaped gap the stenosis is temporarily 'released', the patient gains partial but dramatic relief of airway obstruction, but subsequent re-stenosis may require repeated division or, more likely, open surgery.

Laryngofissure provides good exposure (Fig. 12.34) and allows excision of the web of scar tissue and the fibrosed non-functioning interarytenoid muscle. The denuded area is covered by a free buccal or nasal mucosal graft or a flap of mucous membrane developed from the interarytenoid area above and behind the stenosis and sutured in place. Arytenoidectomy and a cartilage graft to widen the posterior cricoid lamina may be required. A laryngeal stent should be left in place for 2–3 weeks.

Subglottic stenosis

Subglottic stenosis occurs when there is narrowing of the subglottic space above the level of the inferior margin of the cricoid cartilage. The normal diameter in a healthy newborn should be greater than 4 mm. There are many causes of subglottic stenosis including various congenital forms and specific diseases in older patients which are addressed in Chapter 14. Here attention will be turned to acquired subglottic stenosis following prolonged intubation which occurs mostly in children.

A 'soft' stenosis and critical airway obstruction in the post-extubation period is caused by oedematous swelling in the loose submucosal connective tissue comprised of granulation tissue, glandular hyperplasia and ductal retention cysts. Treatment by anterior cricoid split with or without placement of a cartilage graft to widen the cricoid is designed to relieve soft tissue compression and restore circulation. If therapeutic re-intubation, which is considered the alternative treatment of choice by some authorities (see page 194), should fail, tracheotomy may be necessary.

A 'hard' subglottic stenosis can be caused by post-intubation damage alone but is more likely in a

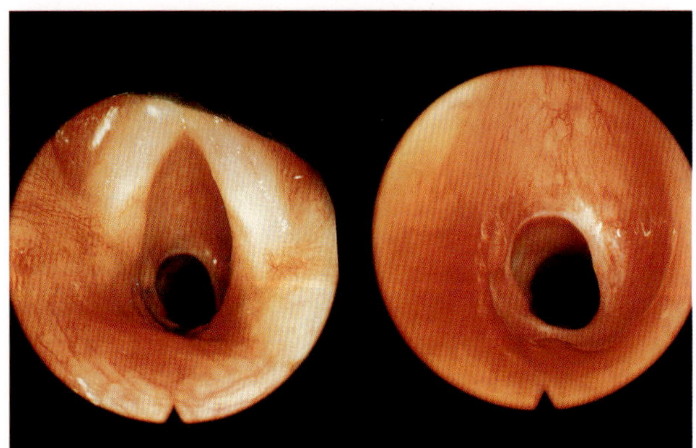

Figure **12.35**
Moderate subglottic stenosis post-intubation. The concentric stenosis is relatively thin and responded to serial laser vaporization with 4 weeks between treatments.

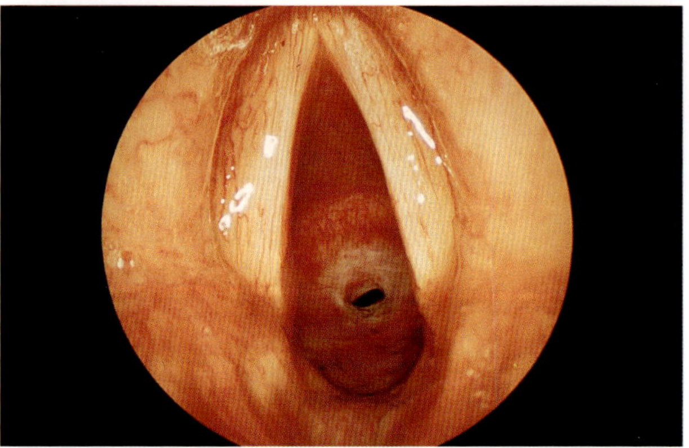

Figure **12.36**
Severe subglottic stenosis. A thick stenosis which required augmentation laryngotracheoplasty using rib graft.

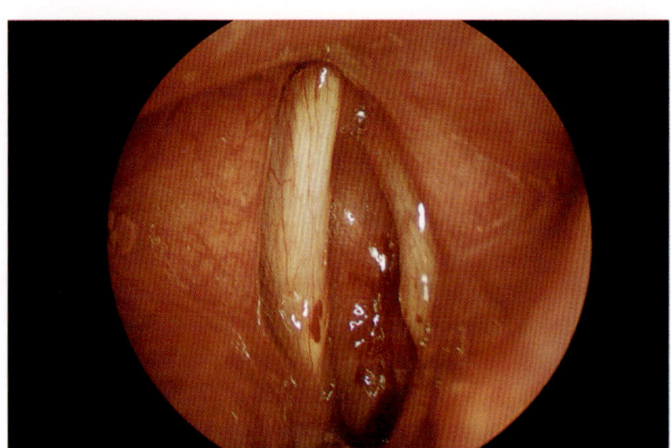

Figure **12.37**
Complete subglottic stenosis. Although the left vocal fold is relatively normal, the right is involved in the scar tissue which completely closed the subglottic lumen. The chance of successful laryngotracheoplasty is small.

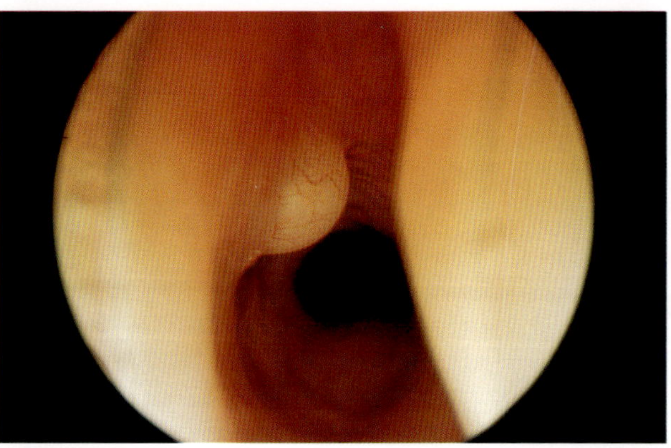

Figure **12.38**
Subglottic ductal retention cyst. An infant intubated and ventilated for hyaline membrane disease was found to have a single, small subglottic cyst which was ablated with laser.

congenitally small larynx which has been intubated. Infants with congenital cartilagenous subglottic stenosis develop oedema, granulation tissue and scarring more quickly and more easily following intubation than infants with a normal larynx.

Each case of subglottic stenosis has a different appearance; there is a spectrum of abnormalities (Figs 12.35, 12.36). There can be a thin membranous diaphragm-like web, a firm fibrotic circumferential scar or irregular eccentric scarring. Although subglottic stenosis is confirmed and evaluated best at endoscopy, a lateral airways X-ray film is very helpful in assessing the length and thickness of the stenosis. This may be the most important prognostic factor.

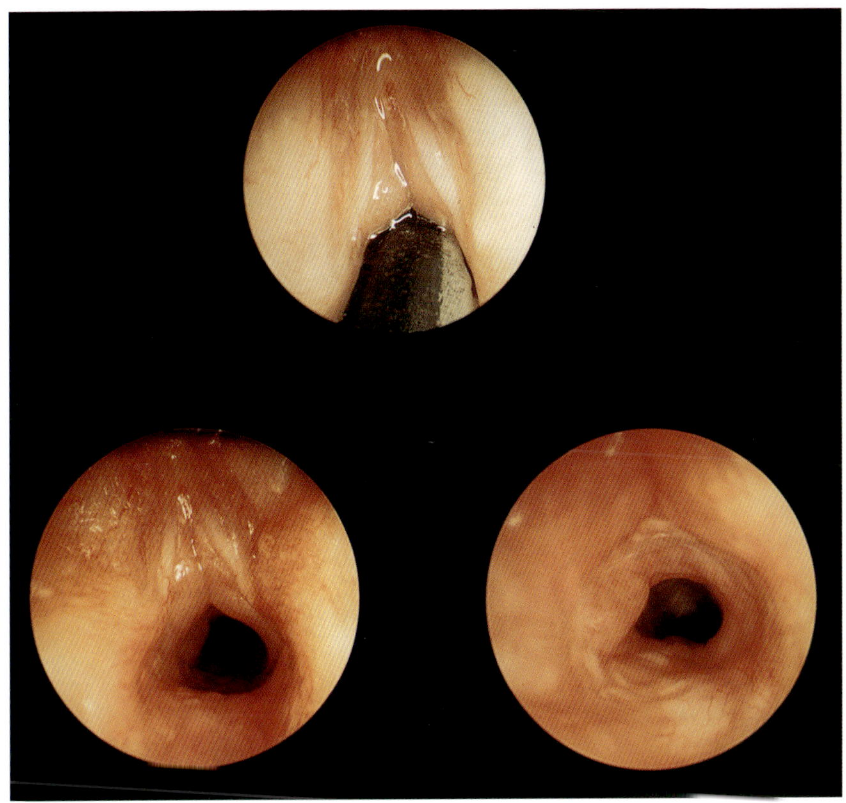

Figure **12.39**
'Soft' subglottic stenosis. The anterior subglottic oedema on each side can be seen both before and after the endotracheal tube is removed. Close-up in the subglottic region shows a flattish ductal retention cyst on the left side. Oedema and glandular hyperplasia account for most of the subglottic swelling.

Laser excision is useful for thin web-like stenoses but inadequate for thick extensive scar tissue. In severe cases rib-cartilage augmentation laryngotracheoplasty with anterior and sometimes posterior grafts in the cricoid is necessary to achieve decannulation. In some cases resection of the stenotic segment and end-to-end anastomosis may be the treatment of choice. The reader is referred to the section on subglottic stenosis in chapter 14 for details of operative techniques.

Complete stenosis

Total obliteration of the lumen sometimes occurs at the glottic and/or subglottic levels (Fig. 12.37). Iatrogenic trauma from ill-judged repeated attempts at dilatation or from excessive laser surgery may worsen the damage initially caused by prolonged intubation. Treatment is difficult, prolonged and often disappointing.

Other changes

Ductal retention cysts

Submucosal ductal retention cysts in the preterm infant may be large or small and usually develop in the subglottic region (Fig. 12.38) in infants who have undergone prolonged intubation. Large cysts can be obstructive and cause stridor some months after extubation. Ductal cysts commonly occur in association with other manifestations of laryngeal intubation trauma (Fig. 12.39) and, although they may resolve without therapy, careful follow-up and treatment of potentially obstructive cysts is recommended. The diagnosis may be suggested by asymmetric, subglottic, smooth lateral or posterior masses on lateral soft tissue X-rays and it is confirmed at direct laryngoscopy. Small cysts of different sizes are sometimes found incidentally as single or multiple, flat or rounded swellings a few millimetres in diameter. Laser is the treatment of choice.

Other miscellaneous injuries

Ductal retention cysts
Vocal cord paralysis
Arytenoid dislocation
Cricoarytenoid joint fixation

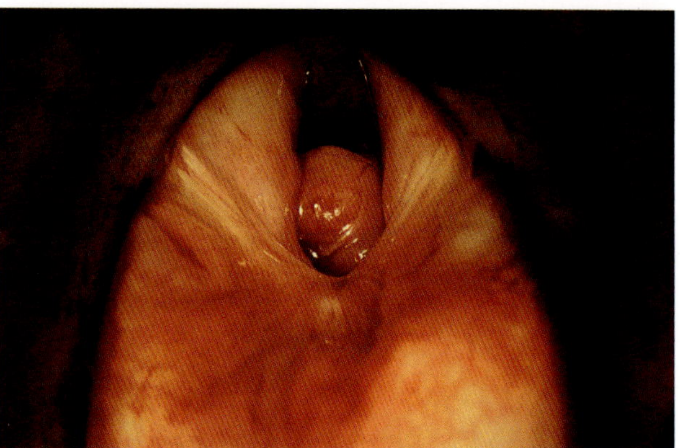

Figure **12.40**
Posterior glottic stenosis and associated granuloma. This atypical post-intubation granuloma can easily be removed, but the posterior glottic stenosis is more difficult to treat.

Vocal cord paralysis

Unilateral and rarely bilateral vocal cord paralysis may be a complication of either short-term or prolonged intubation. Damage to the recurrent laryngeal nerve is thought to be a compression injury of the anterior ramus of the nerve as it passes between the arytenoid and the thyroid cartilage. Spontaneous recovery usually occurs within 6 months; laryngeal electromyography may be helpful in predicting recovery of function.

Dislocation of the arytenoid

The term dislocation should be used strictly when there is complete separation of the opposing articular surfaces of the cricoarytenoid joint, whereas subluxation refers to persistence of contact between the joint surfaces with the cartilage in an abnormal position. The patient may complain of hoarseness, dysphagia, odynophagia, cough or sore throat. Post-intubation malposition of the arytenoid is usually due to trauma following blind intubation or use of an introducer which may have protruded from the endotracheal tube. Dislocation more commonly affects the left arytenoid since intubation is through the right side of the mouth with the tube tending to go to the left side of the larynx. Laryngoscopy shows a displaced arytenoid (Fig. 12.18) with limitation of movement of the arytenoid and the vocal cord. Attempts to manipulate the cartilage into position in the acute stage are seldom successful and most cases present later with limited movement or fixation of the joint. Endoscopic arytenoidectomy may be beneficial in some cases, vocal cord medialization procedures in others.

Fixation of the cricoarytenoid joint

An immobile vocal cord detected at indirect laryngoscopy is usually caused by paralysis, sometimes by cricoarytenoid joint fixation and occasionally by both paralysis and fixation. Passive mobility of the arytenoid on the articular facet of the cricoid cartilage can be assessed only during direct laryngoscopy with the patient under general anaesthesia. A blunt instrument or suction tip is used to test both lateral and medial displacement of the arytenoid on the cricoid articular surface. A fixed or partly fixed arytenoid, usually bilateral, is commonly associated with posterior glottic stenosis (Figs 12.31, 12.32), healed furrows or granuloma (Fig. 12.40). Minor joint abnormalities may be difficult to demonstrate with certainty but can be suspected from surrounding associated changes such as posterior glottic stenosis, healed furrow or healed fibrous nodule.

GENERAL SUMMARY

Prolonged laryngeal intubation causes similar pathologic changes in patients of all ages, but infants tolerate intubation for a longer period than adults. Nevertheless, subglottic stenosis is commoner in

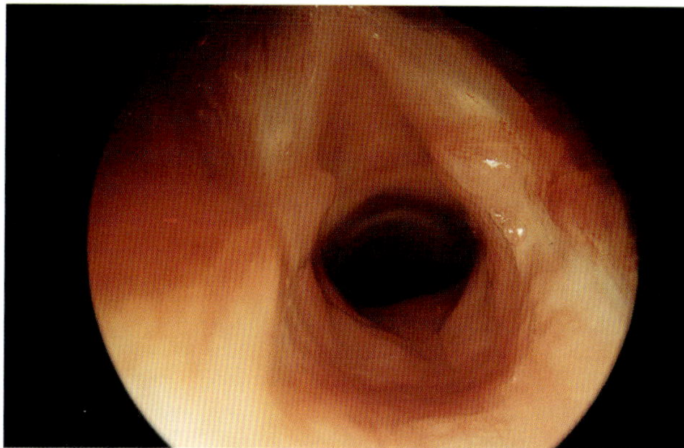

Figure **12.41**
Mild acute intubation injury. The granulation tissue at each vocal process and the minimal subglottic oedema will resolve quickly when the endotracheal tube is removed.

Cases suffering the worst damage

Unconscious patients with a severe head injury
Children in an adult hospital
Children with a large cuffed tube
Those where intubation is followed by tracheotomy
Patients with multiple systemic problems
Patients intubated after smoke inhalation
Infants with congenital subglottic stenosis
Infants where a 'shouldered' tube is used
Very small preterm infants

infants and children than in adults. Subglottic stenosis and posterior glottic stenosis, with or without fixation of the cricoarytenoid joints, are the most serious airway injuries and often require reconstructive surgery or repeated operations over a long period.

There are many post-intubation changes which may cause change in the voice. The patient may complain of hoarseness, tiring of the voice, inability to sing high registers and lesser changes that are most worrying to professional voice users. Minor physical changes in the larynx are detectable only by careful examination at indirect and, if necessary, direct laryngoscopy. Pathology such as post-intubation granuloma, interarytenoid adhesion and dislocation of the arytenoid can be treated, but there is no effective treatment for some patients with dysphonia.

Some of the worst laryngeal damage occurs in certain clinical situations.

Endoscopy under general anaesthesia provides the only accurate assessment of the site, nature and degree of acute laryngeal injuries from intubation. The information obtained allows a rational decision to be made as to whether to continue intubation or to perform a tracheotomy. In the days, weeks or months following extubation, the patient may develop persistent or progressive upper airway obstruction or voice change. Again, evaluation by direct laryngoscopy under general anaesthesia allows the laryngologist to identify important pathology. These changes should be acknowledged by medical specialists in anaesthesia and intensive care. Undoubtedly, future methods for control of the airway and supportive ventilation will be developed to minimize or even prevent laryngeal intubation trauma.

Lastly, it is important to emphasize that most intubation injuries will heal after removal of the endotracheal tube leaving a larynx which is normal in appearance and function.

BIBLIOGRAPHY

Bauman N, Benjamin B (1995) Subglottic ductal cysts in the pre-term infant: association with laryngeal intubation trauma. *Ann Otol Rhinol Laryngol* **104**: 963–8.

Benjamin B (1993) Prolonged intubation injuries of the larynx: endoscopic diagnosis, classification, and treatment. *Ann Otol Rhinol Laryngol* **102** (Suppl 160): 1–15.

Chen J-C, Holinger L (1995) Acquired laryngeal lesions. Pathologic study using serial macrosections. *Arch Otolaryngol Head Neck Surg* **121**: 537–43.

Contencin P, Narcy P (1993) Size of endotracheal tube and neonatal acquired subglottic stenosis. *Arch Otolaryngol Head Neck Surg* **119**: 815–9.

Gould S, Young M (1992) Subglottic ulceration and healing following endotracheal intubation in the neonate: a morphometric study. *Ann Otol Rhinol Laryngol* **101**: 815–20.

Hoeve L, Eskici Verwoerd C (1995) Therapeutic re-intubation for post-intubation laryngotracheal injury in pre-term infants. *Int J Pediatr Otorhinolaryngol* **31**: 7–13.

Lindholm C-E (1969) Prolonged endotracheal intubation (a clinical investigation with specific reference to its consequences for the larynx and the trachea and to its place as an alternative to tracheostomy). *Acta Anesthesiol Scand* (Suppl 33): 1–131.

McEniery J, Gillis J, Kilham H, Benjamin B (1991) Review of intubation in severe laryngotracheobronchitis. *Pediatrics* **87**: 847–53.

Montgomery W (1973) Posterior and complete laryngeal stenosis. *Arch Otolaryngol* **98**: 170–5.

Richardson M, Inglis A (1991) A comparison of anterior cricoid split with and without costal cartilage graft for acquired subglottic stenosis. *Int J Pediatr Otorhinolaryngol* **22**: 187–93.

Sasaki C, Horiuchi M, Ross N (1979) Tracheotomy related subglottic stenosis: bacteriologic pathogenesis. *Laryngoscope* **6**: 857–65.

Tan HKK, Holinger LD, Chen J-C, Gonzales-Crussi F (1996) Fragmented, distorted cricoid cartilage: an acquired abnormality. *Ann Otol Rhinol Laryngol* **105**: 348–55.

Weymuller E (1988) Laryngeal injury from prolonged endotracheal intubation. *Laryngoscope* **98** (Suppl 45): 1–15.

Zalzal G, Cotton R (1993) Glottic and subglottic stenosis. In: Cummings C, Fredrickson J, Harker L, Krouse C, Schuller D, eds, *Otolaryngology – head and neck surgery*, Vol. 3, 2nd edn (St Louis: CV Mosby); 981–2000.

13 Laryngeal trauma

The laryngeal structures can be traumatized by internal or external trauma or injured by inhalation (Fig. 13.1) and by ingestion (Fig. 13.2) of caustics, fire, smoke, etc. This section deals only with external trauma, a relatively uncommon event, which can be either penetrating or blunt. The incidence of blunt laryngeal trauma, usually the result of motor vehicle accidents, is decreasing, probably due to the use of seat belts and air bags and better driver education. The incidence of penetrating trauma due to gunshot or knife wounds is on the increase due to an overall increase in the level of crime and personal assault.

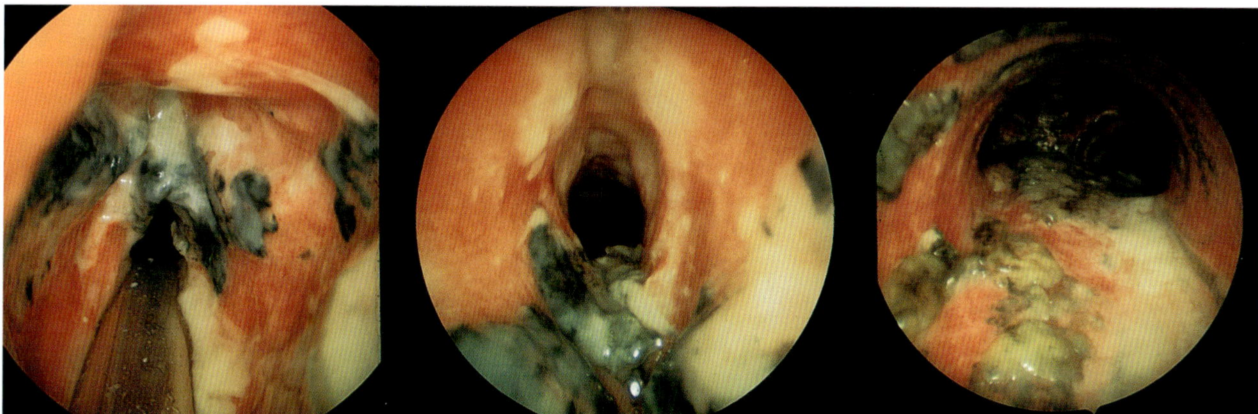

Figure **13.1**
Laryngeal burn. Two days after patient trapped in a burning room. The tracheal mucosa was similarly affected by inhalation of the products of combustion.

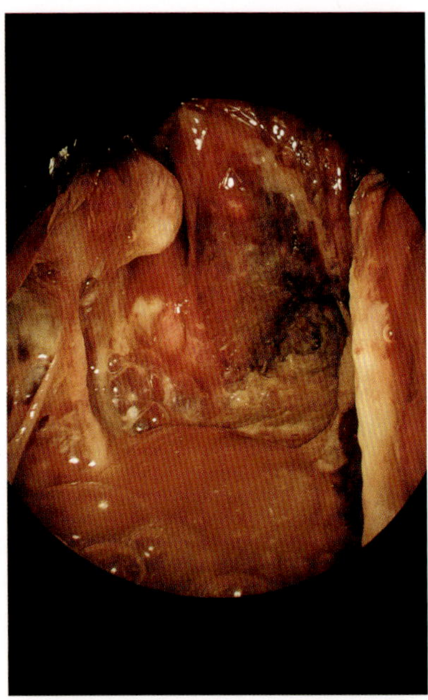

Figure **13.2**
Caustic burns of laryngopharynx. Three days after swallowing liquid caustic. Gross trauma with disruption and distortion of normal anatomical details.

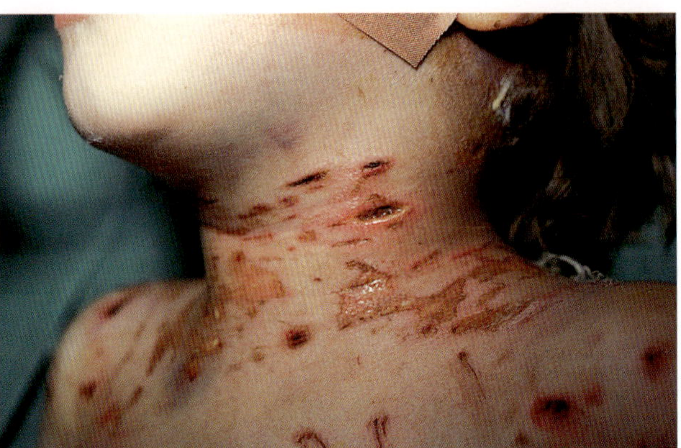

Figure **13.3**
Multiple dog bites on neck and upper chest. Penetrating injuries resulted in surgical emphysema.

Laryngeal trauma

Iatrogenic post-surgical
Post-intubation
Inhalation or ingestion
External, blunt or sharp

MECHANISMS OF INJURY

The larynx is partly shielded by surrounding anatomical structures; the mandible superiorly, the sternum inferiorly and the cervical spine posteriorly, and there is a protective tendency to flex the neck when threatened. Blunt trauma involves sudden force applied to the anterior aspect of the larynx, crushing it against the rigid cervical spine, an injury classically represented in a motor vehicle accident by rapid deceleration which extends the neck to expose the larynx, which is crushed between the dashboard or steering wheel and the bony cervical spine.

The 'clothes line' injury occurs when the unprotected larynx strikes a fixed horizontal object such as a stretched wire or rope so that a large amount of energy is sharply impacted across a small area, resulting in laceration and extensive open trauma. The larynx can also be traumatized in a variety of sports or in an assault. Irrespective of the cause of blunt laryngeal trauma, the mechanism of injury is similar, the nature of the injury depending on the amount of energy and the anatomical area involved. The nature of injury in penetrating trauma (Fig. 13.3) depends upon the weapon and, in the case of gunshot injuries, the distance from the gun to the patient. Knife injuries represent the lowest velocity injuries, usually with little trauma other than the obvious wound. At the other end of the spectrum, high-velocity weapons cause an unpredictable amount of trauma distant to the path of the bullet. Sometimes there is delayed necrosis of damaged but what initially appeared to be viable tissue.

Laryngeal trauma is less common in children because they are less likely than adults to be in risk situations and because they have a higher larynx which is better protected by the mandible. The better flexibility and mobility of the cartilaginous laryngeal framework makes fractures less likely, but the loose attachment of mucosa, lack of fibrous support and relatively small cross-sectional area of the airway compared with the adult places the paediatric airway at greater risk. Laryngeal trauma to children and adults will be discussed together.

TYPES OF INJURY

The nature of the injury depends on the cause and the anatomical location affected. The severity varies from mild oedema, contusion and haematoma to severe crush injury with irreparable destruction of the laryngeal framework and mucosa. Certain injuries which are well recognized and occur alone or in combination are discussed in the following sections.

Surgical emphysema

Rupture of the airway at or below the larynx, or oesophageal perforation initially causes air to escape into the tissues of the neck. The air may track to the face, chest and abdomen causing pneumomediastinum or pneumothorax and will show clearly on X-ray or CT. Continuing or uncontrolled air leak is an indication for surgical exploration to repair the site of rupture.

Fractured hyoid bone

The hyoid is the only bone of the supportive structures of the larynx, and when fractured it usually heals without any sequelae, although occasionally the fractured ends form a bursa which tends to allow movement and may require excision.

Fractured thyroid cartilage

An uncalcified thyroid cartilage compressed against the cervical spine is less likely to fracture than a calcified cartilage (Fig. 13.4). The uncalcified cartilage tends to fracture in the midline with little bleeding and mucosal trauma, whereas the calcified cartilage is likely to sustain a comminuted fracture with more extensive mucosal trauma and bleeding into the paraglottic space which may narrow the supraglottis and compromise the airway. In rare instances, if the clot is allowed to organize it may heal by fibrosis and cause supraglottic stenosis.

Injury sites

- Fractured hyoid bone
- Fractured thyroid
- Fractured cricoid
- Dislocated arytenoid
- Cricotracheal separation
- Disruption of anterior commissure
- Soft tissue injuries

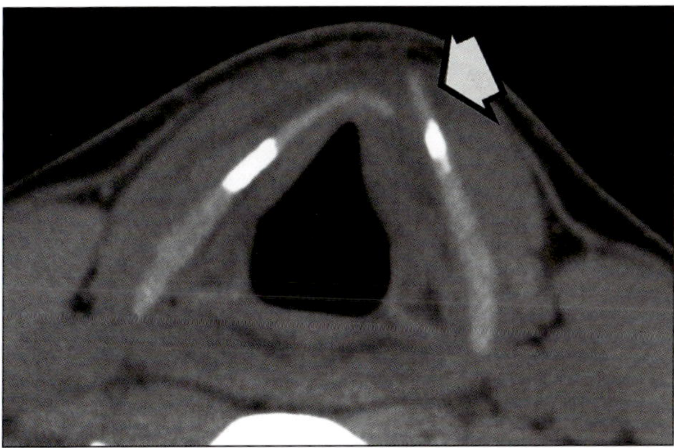

Figure **13.4**
CT of a fractured thyroid cartilage. Direct injury from a plank of wood. Vertical fracture through left thyroid lamina, some widening of the soft tissues in the left paraglottic area. Repaired with sutures and miniplate.

Fractured cricoid cartilage

The fracture lines are usually vertical. Bleeding into the subglottis can heal by fibrosis and eventually cause subglottic stenosis. In injuries to the cricoid cartilage the recurrent laryngeal nerves are at risk.

Dislocation of the arytenoid

Compression of the arytenoid cartilages against the cervical spine can cause subluxation or dislocation of one or both arytenoids (Fig. 13.5) and if untreated can result in fixation of the cricoarytenoid joint and an immobile, fixed vocal cord. Haematoma in the interarytenoid tissues can produce interarytenoid fibrosis.

Cricotracheal separation

This rare and life-threatening injury may result in rapid death at the accident site. The airway is always severely threatened and is difficult to secure, especially if the distal tracheal segment retracts into the mediastinum. Transection or avulsion of both recurrent laryngeal nerves is a possible complication of tracheal separation and bilateral vocal paralysis may be a long-term disability.

Disruption of the anterior commissure

In this classical injury caused by anterior blunt trauma, Broyle's ligaments and the thyro-epiglottic ligament are separated from the thyroid cartilage causing posterior displacement of the epiglottis and allowing the vocal cords to be displaced posteriorly.

Disruption of the anterior mucosa can allow herniation of the fat of the pre-epiglottic space into the airway and associated disruption of the thyro-epiglottic ligament results in backward displacement of the petiole and lower part of the epiglottis – the long-term result may be laryngeal inlet stenosis.

Soft tissue injuries

Laryngeal trauma is accompanied by variable degrees of soft tissue injuries including oedema, contusion, haematoma (Fig. 13.6), laceration and loss of mucosa. Oedema usually resolves spontaneously, although in Reinke's space it may persist and may cause voice change. Haematoma has already been mentioned and large collections may require removal. If left in contact with cartilage, blood is absorbed into the cartilage, altering its shape and strength. Lacerated mucosa may result in granulation tissue formation.

Although discussed separately, these injuries rarely occur in isolation, and due regard must be given to other injuries such as fractured skull, brain damage, facial injuries, chest, abdominal or other injuries.

DIAGNOSIS

Diagnosis depends upon maintenance of a high index of suspicion in accident victims, especially those in

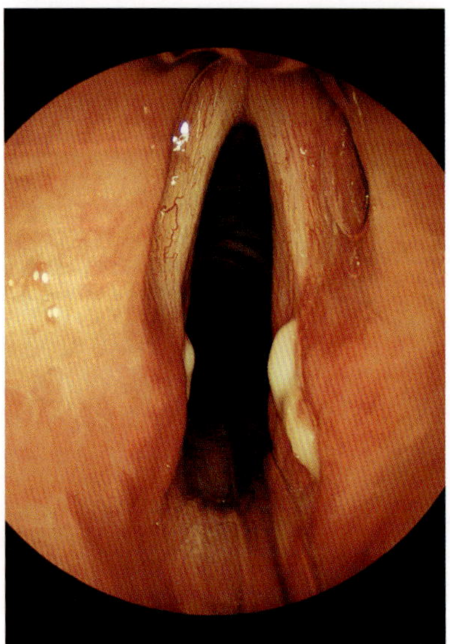

Figure **13.5**
Arytenoid injury. Struck on the neck by a heavy piece of wood. Pale granulations on each side indicate laryngeal compression injury and mucosal disruption at vocal processes.

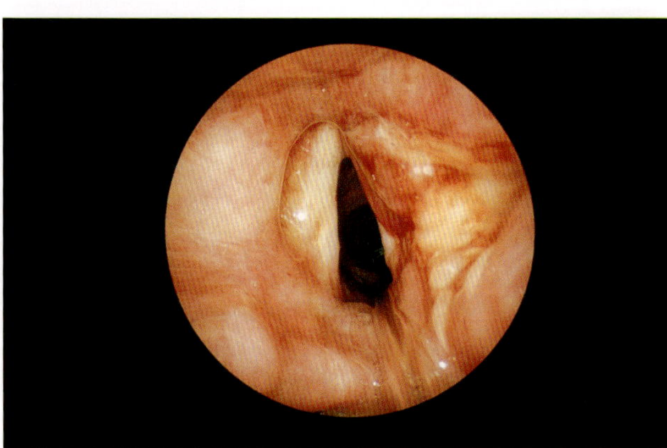

Figure **13.6**
Organizing haematoma. One week after suffering a blow to the neck at football. Bleeding into the right hemilarynx caused severe dysphonia but no airway problem.

Table 13.1 Blunt laryngeal injuries (proposed by Schaefer et al, 1989, modified by Fuhrman et al, 1990); the classification indicates the severity of the injuries

Classification of injuries
1 No detectable fractures, no significant airway problem
2 Minor mucosal lacerations, no exposed cartilage; airway problems from oedema or haematoma; undisplaced fractures
3 Mucosal lacerations, exposed cartilages, massive oedema, airway obstruction; unilateral or bilateral immobile vocal cords
4 More than one fracture line; massive derangement of the endolarynx
5 Cricotracheal separation

Diagnosis

High index of suspicion
May go undetected initially
Mechanism of injury
Effect on laryngeal functions
Skin and soft tissue trauma
Surgical emphysema
Indirect laryngoscopy is vital
CT scan is often vital

the front seat involved in a motor vehicle accident who have sustained trauma to the upper body. At one end of the spectrum is the patient who sustains a seemingly insignificant blow to the anterior neck and complains of hoarseness, while at the other end is the patient with a threatened airway from complete cricotracheal separation (Table 13.1). The diagnosis of subtle laryngeal injury may initially go undetected in the patient where other major injuries dominate the clinical picture. The long-term sequelae of laryngeal injury may well be of greater significance than the other injuries; prompt treatment may avoid or minimize these complications.

History and examination

On history one needs, where possible, to establish the timing, mechanism and forces involved in the acute injury and to correlate this information with the clinical picture. In penetrating trauma, information concerning the ballistics of the weapon and the distances involved must be obtained.

The cardinal signs and symptoms relate to the effect on laryngeal functions, i.e. patency of the airway, prevention of aspiration, and production of voice. The airway may be unaffected, severely threatened or, on rare occasions, temporarily maintained by a laryngocutaneous fistula. There may be a spectrum from mild dysphonia to complete aphonia. The effectiveness of cough must be assessed.

The skin and soft tissues of the neck need to be examined for the degree of damaged skin which may belie the extent of the underlying laryngeal injury. The laryngeal cartilages are palpated and normal laryngeal crepitus on the cervical spine is tested. Surgical emphysema implies disruption of the airway, and blood in the upper airway may be of significance. In penetrating injuries, entrance and exit wounds should be identified but not probed.

Indirect laryngoscopy

Patients suspected of laryngeal trauma demand meticulous indirect laryngoscopy by one or other technique, often using a flexible laryngoscope, looking for mucosal oedema or disruption, exposed cartilage,

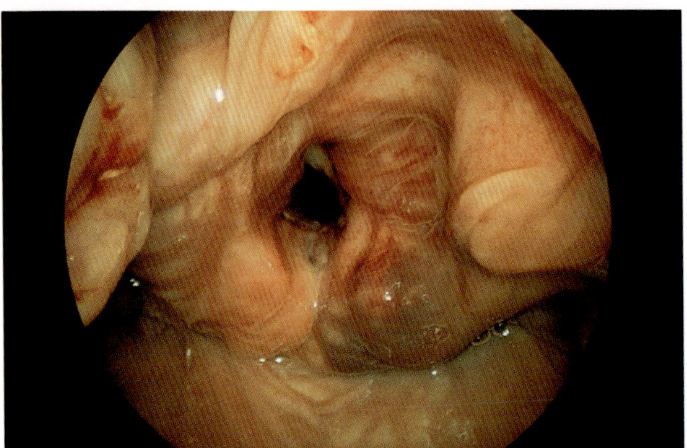

Figure **13.7**
Severe oedema and haematoma. Young male struck on the neck by a baseball. Severe swelling, partial airway obstruction, almost complete aphonia.

blood, vocal cord mobility, and patency of the airway (Fig. 13.7). The otolaryngologist is usually consulted in the emergency room and must be aware of other injuries, particularly to the cervical spine, before undertaking any operative procedure.

Radiological investigation

Computed tomography has rendered most other forms of radiological investigation obsolete, with the exception of contrast swallow in suspected oesophageal trauma and angiography in expanding haematoma. There is no doubt of the ability of CT to demonstrate laryngeal injury, but there is some debate about the indication for and the timing of the scan, and this may be influenced by factors other than injury. Where the CT scanner is readily available, it could be argued that ideally all patients with suspected laryngeal trauma should undergo a CT scan, that the scan is necessary for complete evaluation and for medico-legal documentation. Even a patient with minor trauma evidenced by minor oedema and normal cord movement may show an unsuspected laryngeal fracture on CT. Cases with minimal midline displacement and/or lateral thyroid fractures which are left unrepaired may result in permanent dysphonia: the disruption should be corrected surgically.

CT findings in laryngeal trauma

- Fractures of laryngeal framework
- Large haematoma
- Surgical emphysema
- Arytenoid dislocation
- Degree of airway obstruction
- Cricotracheal separation

If the larynx cannot be examined adequately by clinical means or if the airway is threatened, a prompt CT scan is certainly necessary. In cases with life-threatening obstruction, no investigations are undertaken until an airway is restored. (See also page 36.)

MANAGEMENT

Airway

Initial management of the airway is of crucial importance, but there is some disagreement whether obstruction should be controlled by endotracheal intubation or by tracheotomy. Gussak et al (1986) proposed that patients could be safely managed by orotracheal intubation using a small-diameter endotracheal tube, but trauma may be inflicted during attempted intubation and cause bleeding, further mucosal injury, create a false passage or precipitate complete obstruction of an already compromised airway. Tracheotomy under local anaesthesia may be the safest way to secure the airway, and sometimes an urgent 'crash' tracheotomy may be required in critical circumstances. The airway might occasionally be temporarily secured by intubation of a large laryngocutaneous fistula.

Laryngeal injury

Conservative management

Patients with minor endolaryngeal injuries, no skeletal fractures or non-displaced fractures and no airway

Exploration not indicated

No airway obstruction
Minor oedema ± haematoma
Undisplaced fractures
Normal vocal cord movement
No arytenoid dislocation
No injury to anterior commissure
Satisfactory CT findings

compromise can be managed conservatively by bed rest and observation. There must be an awareness of the possibility of progressive airway compromise, and patients with threatened airway obstruction should be observed in intensive care.

Surgical management

Injuries which disrupt the anterior commissure, expose cartilage, have multiple or displaced skeletal fractures, an uncontrolled air leak, serious airway obstruction, an immobile cord, a dislocated arytenoid or are associated with serious soft tissue neck injury are likely to require open exploration. Direct laryngoscopy, tracheobronchoscopy and oesophagoscopy are undertaken prior to open repair. Particular attention is paid to the mobility and location of the arytenoids with care not to worsen the laryngeal problems or any other injuries. Endoscopic treatment may be satisfactory for subluxation of an arytenoid or evacuation of a limited blood clot.

However, attempts to reduce a dislocated or subluxated arytenoid are often unsuccessful.

The decision to proceed to open exploration is based on the indications mentioned earlier, after correlating the information gained from indirect laryngoscopy, CT scan and direct laryngoscopy. In general, laryngeal repair should be undertaken as soon as possible, preferably within the first 24–48 hours.

Operative technique Using a horizontal or U-shaped skin incision, subplatysmal flaps are elevated above to the hyoid and below to the inferior extent of the injury; separation of the strap muscles provides exposure of the framework of the larynx and upper trachea.

Suspected internal laryngeal injury requires laryngofissure. Displaced or comminuted thyroid fractures are managed by open reduction, mobilization of the fragments and stabilization of the skeletal fragments as described below.

Mucosal injury Mucosal injuries are, where possible, repaired by primary closure with fine, absorbable submucosal sutures. Local mucosal flaps are used to cover exposed cartilage. Loose cartilage fragments are removed. Haematomas are evacuated and potential spaces obliterated with a quilting suture if there is concern that bleeding may continue. Extensive debridement of mucosa is necessary only in high velocity gunshot wounds.

Skeletal injuries Skeletal injuries are addressed after mucosa has been reapproximated. Cartilage is minimally debrided, reduced and fixed using either wire, an internal stent, sutures or external miniplates. Muscle flaps may be used to replace lost cricoid cartilage.

Stenting Although stenting is avoided when possible, a stent may be required to support a severely damaged laryngeal skeleton, maintain the lumen of the larynx and diminish the likelihood of adhesions. Stents should be considered when the laryngeal skeleton is unstable, badly displaced, comminuted or when extensive mucosal damage might predispose to formation of adhesions and subsequent stenosis.

The stent should be soft, made in an anatomically appropriate shape, e.g. the Montgomery silicone rubber solid stent (Fig. 13.8) and, if possible, secured in such a way that allows endoscopic removal (Fig. 13.9). The stent is usually left in situ for 10–14 days, but a severely damaged larynx may need stenting for several months.

The anterior end of the vocal cord may need to be repositioned by suturing it to the external perichondrium of the thyroid cartilage prior to closure of the laryngofissure. The wound is drained, and a nasogastric tube inserted under direct vision.

An irreparably damaged larynx, as might be sustained from a high-velocity gunshot wound, may require total laryngectomy.

Postoperative care Antibiotics are given for at least

Indications for open exploration

Disruption by crush injury
Displaced or multiple fractures of framework
Cricotracheal separation
Airway obstruction – intubation
– tracheotomy
Uncontrolled air leak
Massive haematoma
Widely exposed cartilage
Disruption of anterior commissure
Vocal cord instability – paralysis
– joint dislocation

More than one indication may be present

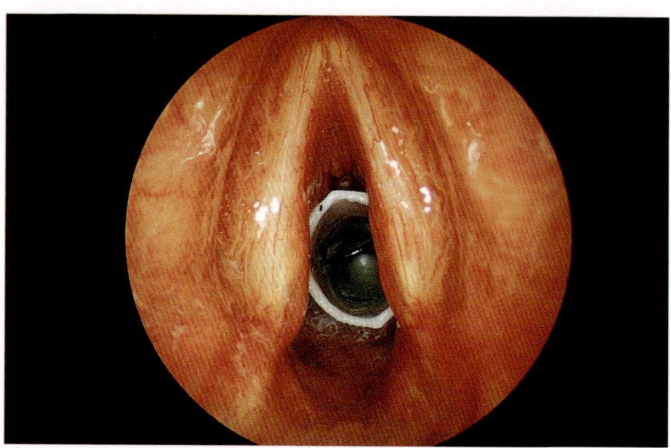

Figure **13.8**
Stent. Aboulker stent sewn into subglottic region, suture placed for endoscopic removal. The upper end can be closed with a round 'cap' if desired.

10 days. Decannulation should be attempted only after endoscopic removal of granulations and confirmation that the repaired tissues have healed leaving an adequate airway. Follow-up of at least 12 months will detect recurrent granulations or fibrous stenosis.

RESULTS

Results are measured by successful restoration of laryngeal functions within the parameters set by the nature of the injury. Most patients will have a good airway and a satisfactory voice, depending on the severity of the initial injuries.

COMPLICATIONS

Granulation tissue at the site of repair or in relation to the stent may be a recurring problem and requires endoscopic removal as often as there is significant recurrence. Aspiration is a rare complication.

Several external and endoscopic techniques have been described for dealing with a larynx which has a fixed, immobile arytenoid. Vocal cord medialization may be necessary eventually for patients with permanent damage to the recurrent laryngeal nerve.

Chronic laryngeal stenosis is the commonest long-term problem. Prompt and appropriate management of laryngeal injury will diminish the incidence of this complication whose management is described in chapter 14.

BIBLIOGRAPHY

Fuhrman GM, Steig FH, Buerk CA (1990) Blunt laryngeal trauma: classification and management protocol. *J Trauma* **30**: 87–93.

Gluckman JL, Mongal AK (1991) Laryngeal trauma. In: Paparella MM, Shumrick DA, Gluckman JL, Meyerhoff WL, eds (1991) *Otolaryngology* (Philadelphia: WB Saunders, 3rd edn) **3**: 2231–44.

Gussak GS, Jurkovitch GJ, Luterman A (1986) Laryngotracheal trauma: a protocol approach to a rare injury. *Laryngoscope* **96**: 660–5.

Schaefer SD, Close LG (1989) Acute management of laryngeal trauma. *Ann Otol Rhinol Laryngol* **98**: 98–104.

14 Laryngeal stenosis

INTRODUCTION

Narrowing or constriction of the larynx can occur in the supraglottic, glottic or subglottic region.

In infants and children the commonest problem is subglottic stenosis which can be congenital but is more often acquired, commonly as a complication of prolonged endotracheal intubation. The incidence of acquired subglottic stenosis in paediatric patients has increased as more low birthweight preterm infants survive after prolonged intubation and ventilation in a neonatal intensive care unit (NICU). Up to 8% of these patients have been reported to have clinically significant subglottic stenosis.

In adults both posterior glottic stenosis and subglottic stenosis occur most commonly as complications of prolonged endotracheal intubation. They sometimes follow severe external laryngeal trauma, iatrogenic trauma following ill-judged or over-enthusiastic laser, microcautery, cryosurgery or electrosurgical treatment of diseases such as papillomas and attempts to treat posterior glottic or subglottic stenosis which worsen the existing problem.

SUPRAGLOTTIC STENOSIS

Supraglottic stenosis (Fig. 14.1) is the least common form of laryngeal narrowing. It usually results from external blunt trauma which damages the hyoid bone, thyrohyoid membrane and sometimes causes a

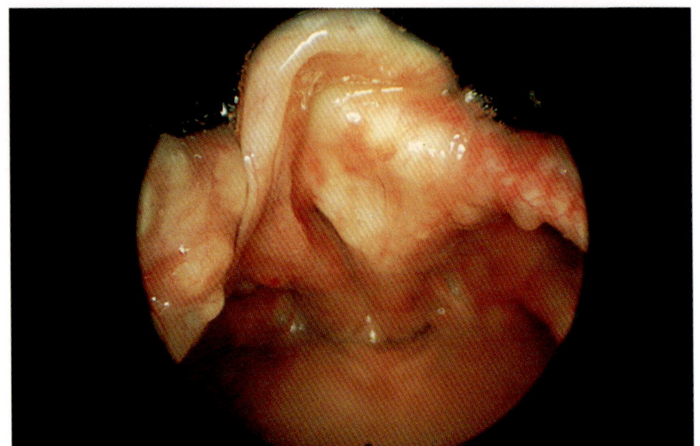

Figure **14.1**
Severe supraglottic stenosis. Distortion, fibrosis and severe obstruction in a child who had been inappropriately managed by repeated laser treatments.

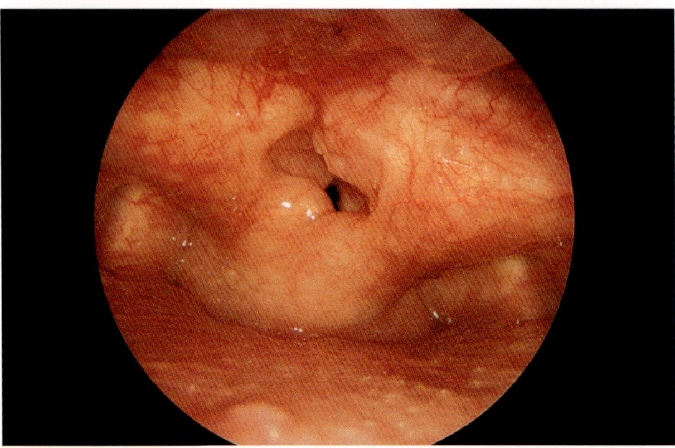

Figure **14.2**
Post-radiation laryngeal stenosis. Radiation therapy 4 years previously caused perichondritis resulting in supraglottic and glottic stenosis.

fracture of the thyroid cartilage. The thyro-epiglottic ligament may be torn causing the epiglottis to be either displaced posteriorly or become adherent to the lateral or posterior pharyngeal walls, and this, in combination with a fractured hyoid bone, can cause a serious laryngeal inlet stenosis. Other causes include post-radiation stenosis (Fig. 14.2), pemphigoid (Fig. 14.3) and sarcoid.

The patient presents with increasing dyspnoea on exertion; severe cases have respiratory distress at rest with a harsh inspiratory stridor. Indirect laryngoscopy shows a displaced, distorted epiglottis obstructing the supraglottic laryngeal airway usually preventing visualization of the vocal cords, but flexible laryngoscopy should allow assessment of cord movement.

Imaging using CT is essential to assess fractures or displacement of the hyoid bone or the thyroid cartilage. In addition, arytenoid dislocation with or without shortening of one or both vocal cords can be detected.

Direct laryngoscopy under general anaesthesia will confirm the supraglottic stenosis, detect arytenoid dislocation or fixation, shortening or laxity of the vocal fold and any other associated pathology.

Endoscopic laser removal of a redundant aryepiglottic fold or a floppy segment of epiglottis will sometimes be adequate treatment, but the most comprehensive, effective surgical approach is through a horizontal skin incision as for a suprahyoid pharyngotomy. If the hyoid bone is fractured or displaced it should be either re-positioned and wired or the body of the hyoid removed. The supraglottic laryngeal space is entered. Adhesions of the epiglottis to the pharyngeal walls are divided with excision of the scar in the submucosal plane and primary closure.

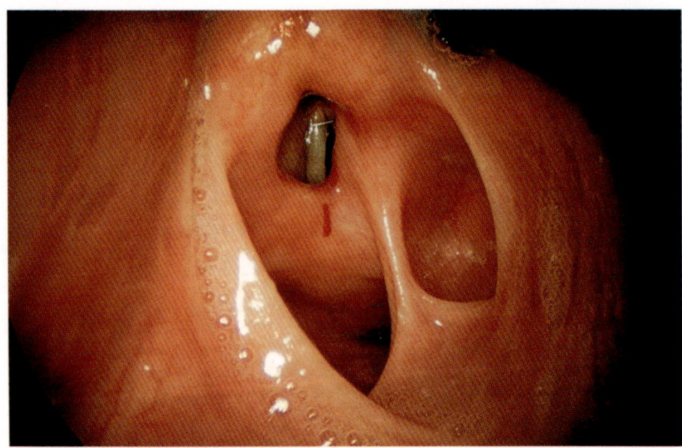

Figure **14.3**
Supraglottic stenosis. The result of pemphigoid, inactive at the time of the photograph. Multiple fibrous bands in the laryngopharynx and supraglottis treated with the laser.

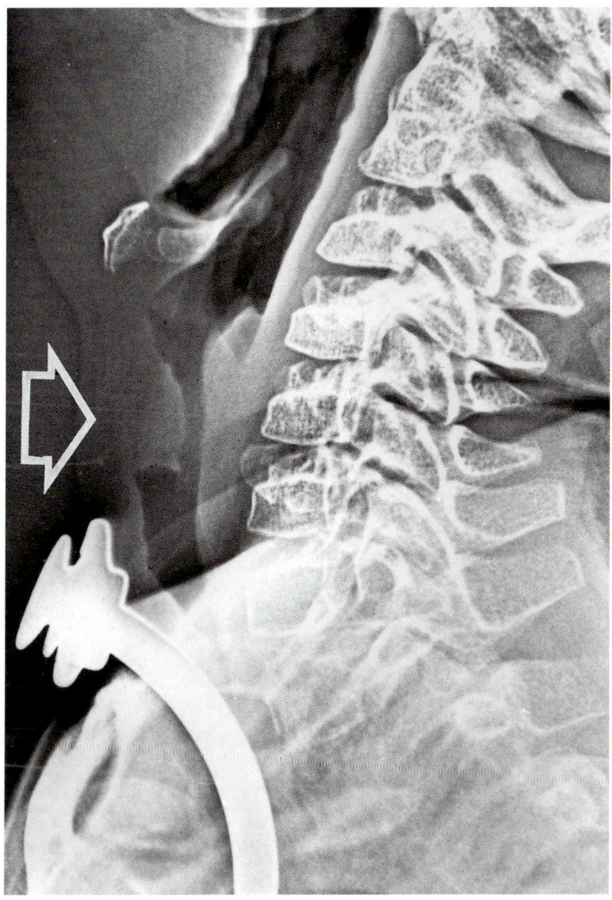

(a)

(b)

Figure **14.4**
Severe congenital glottic web and subglottic stenosis. Lateral xerogram (a) demonstrates the thickness and length (arrow) of the subglottic stenosis. The small posterior airway represents the laryngotracheal groove. (b) Endoscopy shows the outlines of the vocal ligaments through the membranous web. The laryngeal ventricles are prominent.

Montgomery (1973) has described the cause of and treatment by laryngofissure of laryngeal inlet stenosis due to direct trauma causing posterior displacement of the epiglottis, often with an associated fracture of the thyroid cartilage at the level of the notch. Division of the thyrohyoid membrane and a midline thyrototomy gives access to the laryngeal lumen and base of the epiglottis. An incision is made through the fascia and the perichondrium anterior to the base of the epiglottis, and a plane is established anterior to the cartilage. Another plane posterior to the epiglottic cartilage is dissected to allow an inverted V-shaped segment of cartilage and perichondrium to be excised between the submucosal planes. A vertical midline incision through the posterior mucoperichondrium enables the flaps on each side to be turned outwards and sewn to the free edge of the perichondrium; no stent is required.

GLOTTIC STENOSIS

Anterior glottic stenosis

Anterior glottic stenosis in paediatric patients is caused by a congenital glottic web; the largest webs (Fig. 14.4) are often associated with a congenital subglottic stenosis. Small webs (Fig. 14.5) cause a

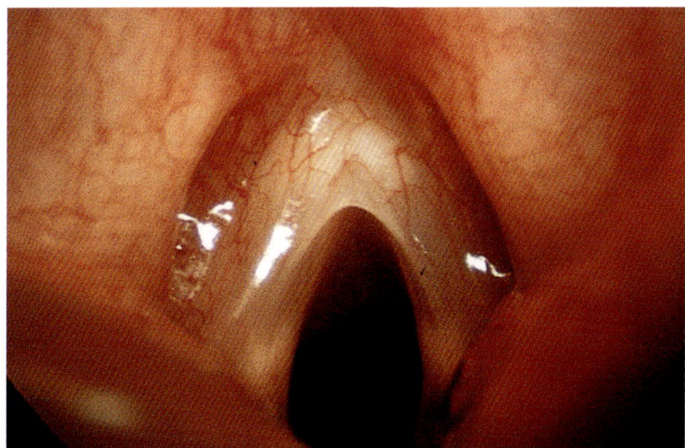

Figure **14.5**
Small congenital glottic web. This baby had a weak cry. After division of the web with microlaryngoscopy scissors, the cry became almost normal.

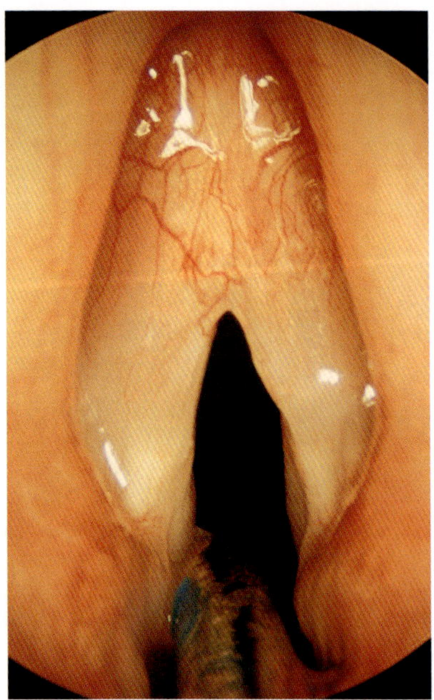

Figure **14.6**
Vocal fold adhesion. Simultaneous removal of vocal nodules caused synechiae of moderate thickness. The voice was worse than before treatment.

weak or husky cry and larger webs cause airway obstruction and stridor. For further information the reader is referred to the section on congenital laryngeal webs in chapter 25.

External laryngeal trauma with fracture of the thyroid cartilage and laceration or disruption of the mucosa can cause anterior glottic stenosis. In other patients, usually adults, anterior glottic stenosis can be due to iatrogenically induced internal laryngeal trauma following removal of mucosal lesions from the anterior surfaces of both vocal folds, e.g. Reinke's oedema, papillomas, vocal nodules (Fig. 14.6) or 'stripping' or removal of dysplastic epithelium. The two opposing raw mucosal edges heal together creating an adhesion which becomes an acquired anterior glottic web. The patient has a husky voice and may develop airway obstruction if severe narrowing of the glottic opening occurs.

Indirect laryngoscopy provides a two-dimensional evaluation of the web, and vocal cord mobility can be assessed. The thickness of the web is all-important

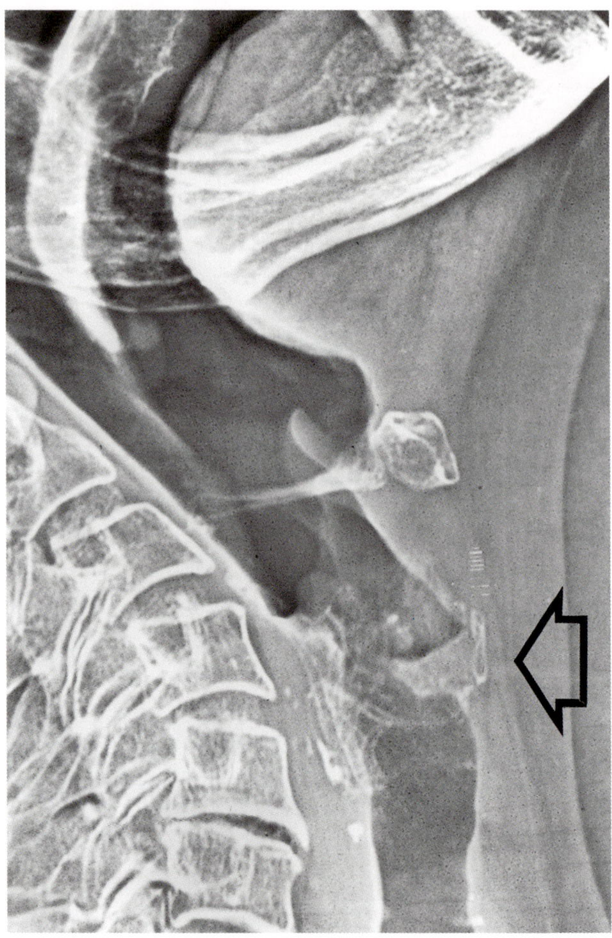

Figure **14.7**
Iatrogenic web. Thick anterior acquired glottic web (arrow) following bilateral 'stripping' for Reinke's oedema.

Causes of anterior glottic stenosis

Congenital glottic web
Blunt or open external trauma
Adhesion after endoscopic surgery

Treatment of anterior glottic webs

No treatment for minor asymptomatic webs
'Rupture' of fine, thin web
Endoscopic division ± keel for moderate webs
Laryngofissure ± keel for severe webs

and can be best judged by a combination of lateral airway X-ray (Fig. 14.7) and direct laryngoscopy using 30° or 70° angled telescopes. The posterior edge of the web is crescentic and thin, but anteriorly it becomes thicker. This assessment is critical as the results of surgical treatment are determined by the overall size of the web and by the anterior thickness. For moderate and severe webs, treatment results for voice improvement are often disappointing.

Minor anterior glottic webs which cause no voice disability require no treatment. When huskiness or weakness of the voice is significant, the web can be divided under suspension microlaryngoscopy using either microscissors or the CO_2 laser.

A very thin, diaphanous, membranous web in infants can be ruptured by anterior pressure with a bronchoscope, endotracheal tube or telescope, and the web seems to 'disappear'.

Small- and medium-sized webs which are less than 2- or 3-mm thick anteriorly can be treated by endoscopic division and placement of a keel. We prefer Lindholm's technique of placing a thin silastic 'flag' between the cut edges of the web, the keel being held in place for 7–10 days by non-absorbable sutures (see section on congenital glottic webs in chapter 25).

Thick, large glottic webs, congenital webs with an associated subglottic stenosis and isolated anterior subglottic stenosis require laryngofissure. The web and the underlying thyroid cartilage should be accurately divided along the line of one vocal fold at endoscopy prior to laryngofissure. Following skin incision the thyroid cartilage is divided exactly in the midline with a scalpel, scissors or saw to meet the endoscopic incision. The larynx is opened and the remains of the web on the anterior edge of the contralateral vocal fold can be carefully trimmed, attempting to preserve as much mucous membrane as possible. Fine suture repair of the cut edges of the web may be possible before placement of a keel and closure of the thyrotomy. In some cases, with good mucosal repair, no keel or stent is required. We prefer the Montgomery T-shaped 'umbrella' silicone keel (Fig. 14.8) which is removed after 10–14 days. Granulation tissue may require removal at one or two further endoscopic procedures in an attempt to prevent partial re-formation of the original web.

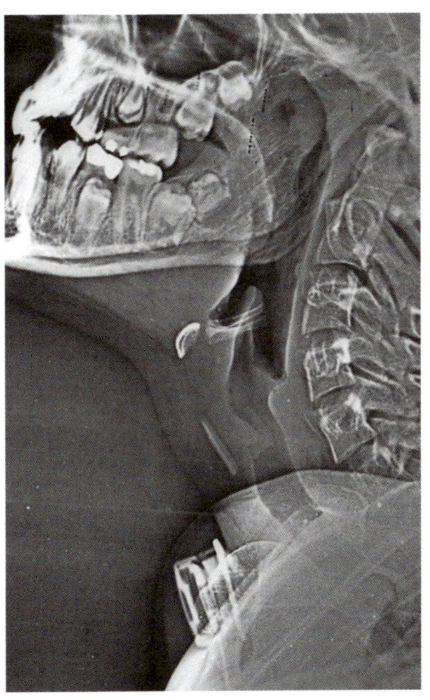

Figure **14.8**
Montgomery umbrella keel. Lateral xerogram showing the keel positioned between the cut edges of an anterior glottic web.

Posterior glottic stenosis

This has been covered in chapter 12, emphasizing that prolonged intubation is usually the cause. Other

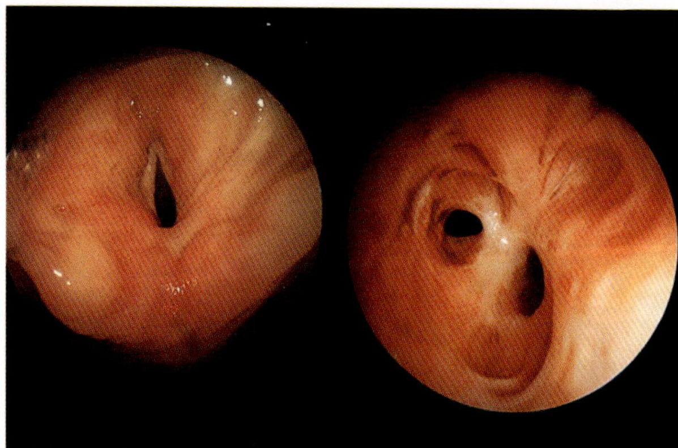

Figure **14.9**
Laryngeal and upper tracheal stenosis from burns. The child was locked in a motor vehicle which caught fire. There is a severe posterior glottic stenosis and several severe tracheal stenoses, one of which is shown.

causes of posterior glottic stenosis include caustic burns and flame burns (Fig. 14.9), prolonged stenting following laryngotracheoplasty and traumatic endoscopic surgery in the posterior larynx, e.g. repeated removal of posterior glottic papillomas or simultaneous bilateral aryepiglottoplasty as a treatment of severe laryngomalacia.

Causes of posterior glottic stenosis

Prolonged endotracheal intubation
Burns ± short or long intubation
Prolonged stenting through the glottis
Traumatic endoscopic surgery in posterior glottis, e.g.:
- Repeated removal of posterior papillomas
- Bilateral, simultaneous aryepiglottoplasty

Treatment of posterior glottic stenosis will be covered with treatment of subglottic stenosis later in this chapter.

SUBGLOTTIC STENOSIS

Classification

The reported incidence of subglottic stenosis has increased partly because of improved survival of premature babies and partly because of more accurate diagnosis. As Tan et al (1996) have stated, subglottic stenosis can be classified in three different ways:

1 by aetiology: congenital or acquired;
2 by clinical anatomy: hard or soft;
3 by histopathology: based on analysis of macrosections (see Table 14.1).

Table 14.1 Histopathologic classification of subglottic stenosis (Chen and Holinger 1995)

Cartilaginous stenosis, which is usually congenital
- Cricoid cartilage deformity
  - Small cricoid
  - Elliptical cricoid
  - Flattened cricoid
  - Thickened cricoid
  - Ossified cricoid
  - Fragmented, distorted cricoid
  - Abnormally shaped cricoid associated with laryngeal cleft
- Trapped first tracheal arch

Soft tissue stenosis which is usually acquired
- Submucosal hyperplasia of mucous glands
- Ductal retention cysts
- Submucosal fibrous connective tissue
- Granulation tissue

'Definition' of subglottic stenosis

Less than 4 mm in full-term infant
Less than 3 mm in a preterm infant
Without clinical features there is no significant stenosis

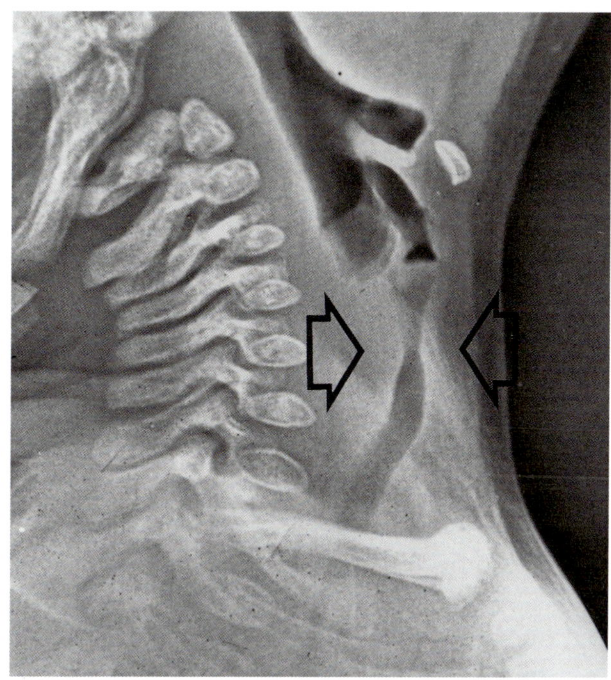

Figure **14.10**
Congenital subglottic stenosis. The narrow area (arrow) in the subglottic region represents a congenital cricoid cartilage abnormality.

Definition

Because the size of the subglottis in an infant increases rapidly with normal growth it is difficult to define subglottic stenosis, but an acceptable definition would be a subglottic airway less than 4 mm in a full-term infant or less than 3 mm in a premature infant. These diameters are likely to be associated with clinical symptoms.

Aetiology

Pre-existent congenital subglottic stenosis may be the basis for acquisition of superadded subglottic stenosis after laryngeal intubation so that a diagnosis of congenital subglottic stenosis (Fig. 14.10) requires that there is no history of previous intubation. For example, a patient with a small cricoid or an elliptical cricoid (where the transverse diameter is smaller than the antero-posterior diameter) may (Fig. 14.11) develop acquired subglottic stenosis after intubation, but it will then be difficult to know if there was a prior congenital abnormality. How many preterm infants who undergo prolonged intubation and fail extubation have an underlying congenital subglottic stenosis is unknown, but there is no doubt that acquired subglottic stenosis from intubation is more common than congenital stenosis.

In adults subglottic and upper tracheal stenosis are sometimes the result of a motor vehicle accident

Causes of subglottic stenosis

Infants
- Congenital ± prolonged intubation
- Acquired after prolonged intubation
- Congenital subglottic haemangioma

Adults
- Prolonged intubation
- Crush injury of larynx
- Cricotracheal separation
- Mucosal burn ± intubation
- Iatrogenic surgical trauma
- Neoplasm, benign or malignant
- Rhinoscleroma
- Wegener's granulomatosis (Fig. 14.12)
- Idiopathic subglottic stenosis (Fig. 14.13)
- Amyloid

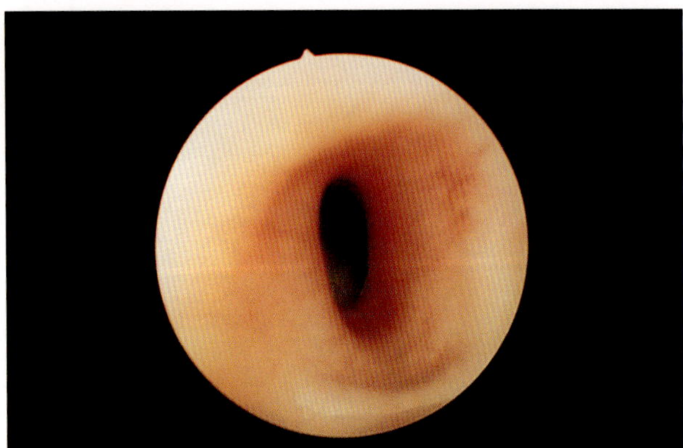

Figure **14.11**
Congenital elliptical cricoid. In the immediate subglottic region, the lumen is narrowed in the shape of an ellipse.

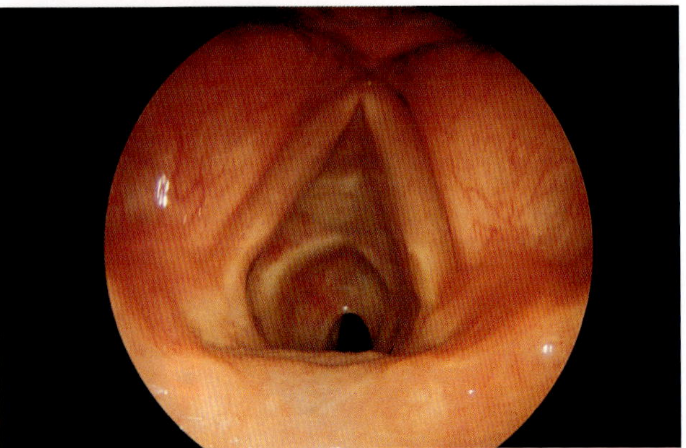

Figure **14.12**
Subglottic stenosis from Wegener's granulomatosis. Indirect laryngoscopy photograph showing mature scar narrowing the subglottic region. Laser treatment on three occasions over 6 years maintained a satisfactory lumen.

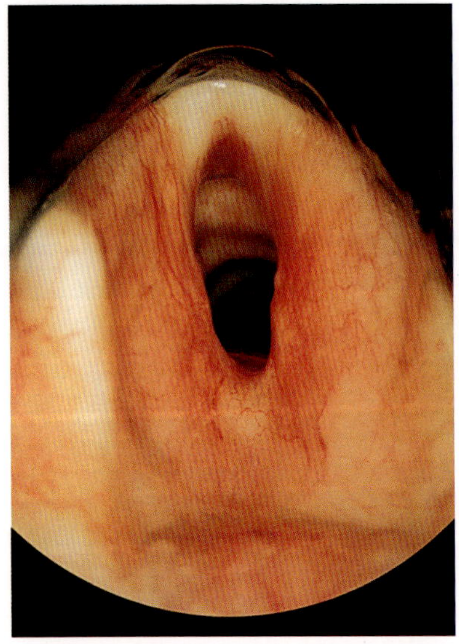

Figure **14.13**
Idiopathic subglottic stenosis. Characteristic pink, moderately vascular tissue narrows the subglottis.

where the larynx and trachea strike the dashboard or the steering wheel causing a fracture of the laryngeal framework. Where indicated, primary repair should be undertaken as soon as possible, as healing by secondary intention and subsequent scarring (Fig. 14.14) may produce an acquired subglottic stenosis. Avulsion of the first tracheal ring from the cricoid requires end-to-end repair, preferably without tracheotomy. A 'clothes line injury' where the neck of a bicycle rider strikes a clothes line or stretched wire, rope or branch of a tree and sustains laryngeal fracture or cricotracheal separation is another cause of acquired subglottic stenosis in adolescents and adults.

Clinical features

The clinical features include inspiratory or biphasic stridor, respiratory distress and sometimes voice changes. Mild to moderate subglottic stenosis usually remains asymptomatic until an aggravating factor, such as an upper respiratory infection or a period of intubation for general anaesthesia, causes oedema and further narrowing of the subglottic airway. The result is inspiratory stridor and respiratory distress – features which simulate croup in younger children. Moderate to severe cases manifest biphasic stridor and persistent respiratory distress, sometimes with a change in the cry or voice.

The most common presentation of acquired subglottic stenosis is that of a preterm, low birthweight infant, intubated and ventilated for treatment of hyaline

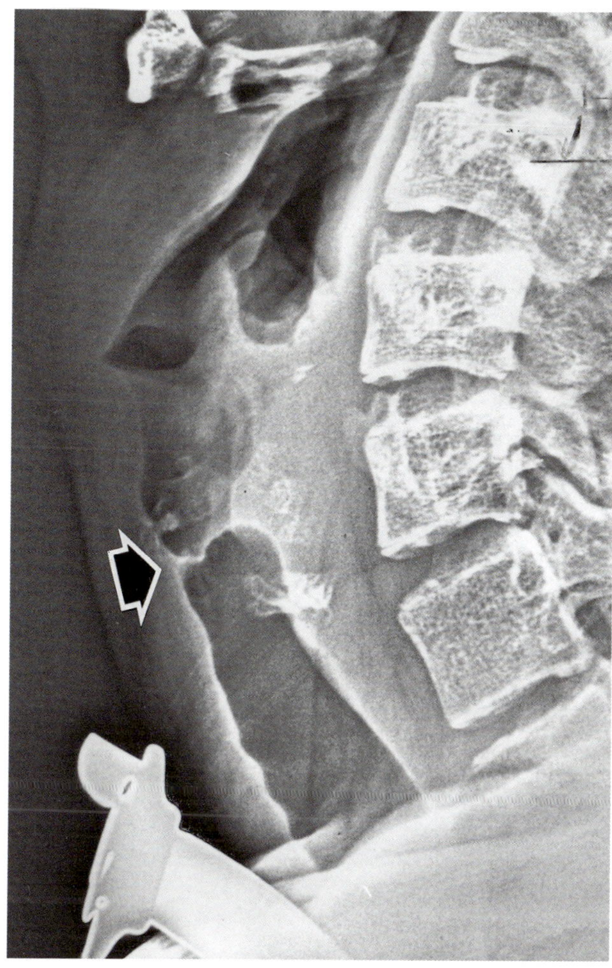

Figure **14.14**
Total subglottic obstruction. Immediate repair of cricotracheal separation after the patient's neck struck a wire strung between two trees. Subsequent scarring caused total stenosis by a thin web (arrow) which was treated by laser. There was permanent bilateral vocal cord paralysis.

membrane disease, who has failed multiple attempts at extubation. It may be possible to remove the tube for several hours but stridor increases, respiratory distress worsens, the infant tires, hypoxia and hypercarbia progress and re-intubation becomes necessary. In other patients, presentation may sometimes be with atypical repeated 'croup' or with stridor after intubation during anaesthesia for some unrelated surgical procedure. Older patients and adults usually develop slowly progressive inspiratory stridor.

Presentation of subglottic stenosis

Failed extubation after prolonged intubation
Repeated atypical croup
Post-anaesthetic stridor after brief intubation
Slowly progressive inspiratory stridor

In some infants general examination may detect other abnormalities, such as a syndromal pattern or congenital abnormalities of the heart, great vessels or respiratory system which must be considered when deciding management.

Pernasal, flexible fibreoptic indirect examination of the larynx may show supraglottic intubation effects such as oedema and allows assessment of vocal cord mobility but in most cases the supraglottis and pharynx will be normal.

Radiologic examination

Radiologic evaluation gives little information in the presence of an endotracheal tube or a tracheotomy tube. In the absence of a tube radiography may assist identification of the site and length of a chronic stenosis or of an airway which is completely obliterated. Computed tomography and magnetic resonance imaging (Fig. 14.15) seldom provide useful information and are not worthwhile in infants and small children.

Direct endoscopic examination

Direct laryngoscopy and bronchoscopy using spontaneous respiration general anaesthesia and employing open-tube laryngoscopes and rigid telescopes

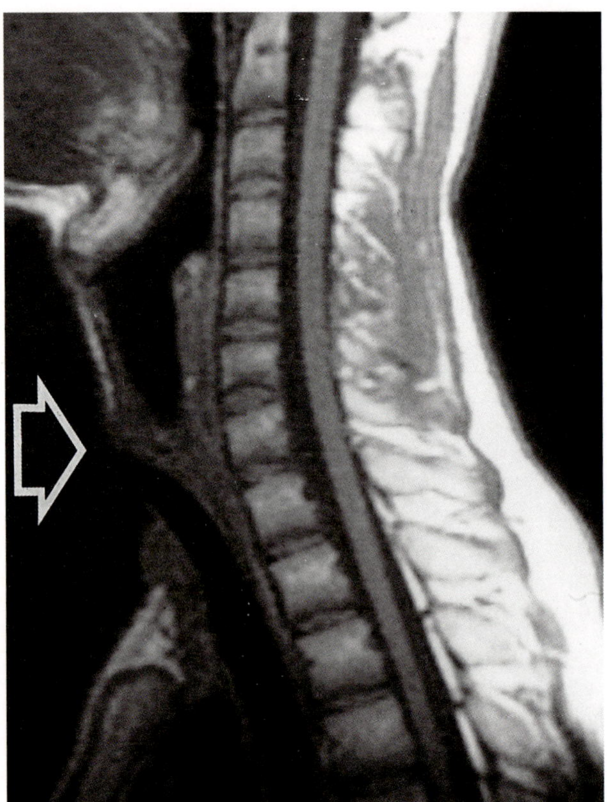

Figure **14.15**
Total obstruction above a tracheotomy. MRI shows soft tissue obstruction (arrow), the site of a percutaneous tracheotomy which was through the cricoid cartilage and caused subsequent perichondritis and scarring.

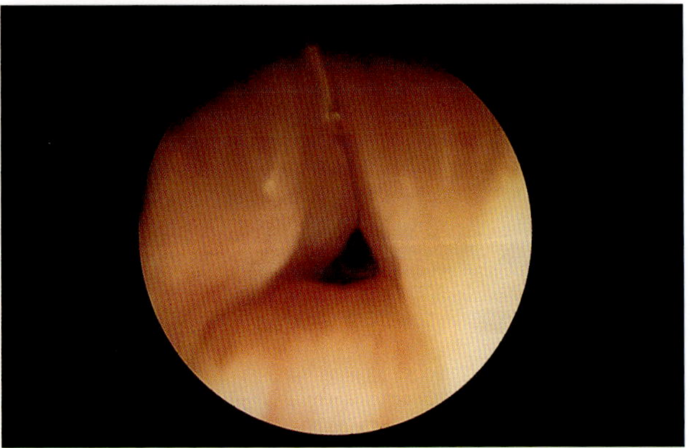

Figure **14.16**
Soft subglottic stenosis. One week after tracheotomy in a neonate who could not be extubated. A moderately large, left subglottic ductal retention cyst and generalized oedema.

'Soft' subglottic stenosis

Oedema
Granulation tissue
Glandular hyperplasia
Ductal retention cysts

provide the most accurate assessment of subglottic stenosis and other associated pathologic changes. There is usually no necessity to pass a bronchoscope; a slim telescope causes no trauma to the airway and provides a comprehensive view of the entire airway.

Endoscopy during intubation or shortly after extubation will document acute changes in the larynx caused by the presence of the endotracheal tube. Acute injuries in the subglottic region include oedema, granulation tissue and ulceration, especially posteriorly, involving the perichondrium and the cricoid cartilage. Oedema and tongues of granulation tissue in the posterior glottis and subglottis are the most likely cause of failed attempts at extubation.

On the other hand, if the patient has been extubated for days or weeks, chronic changes caused initially by granulation tissue and/or ulceration may be observed. In the subglottic region these chronic changes may be those of so-called 'soft stenosis' or of so-called 'hard stenosis'.

Soft stenosis (Fig. 14.16) can cause critical obstruction in the post-extubation period because of swelling within the cricoid cartilage due to oedema, granulation tissue, glandular hyperplasia and formation of ductal retention cysts. The latter may be seen endoscopically as flattish or rounded protrusions, especially in the posterior aspect of the subglottis.

Hard subglottic stenosis (Fig. 14.17) is caused by cartilage and/or acquired scar tissue and is more

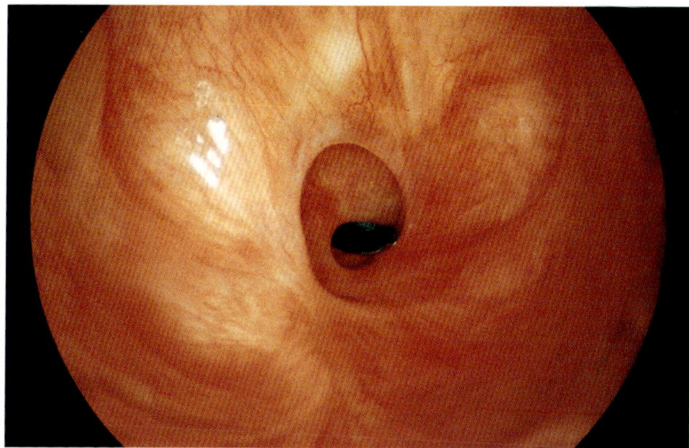

Figure **14.17**
Hard subglottic stenosis. Close-up of firm mature Grade III subglottic stenosis which require laryngotracheoplasty.

Table 14.2 Subjective grading of subglottic stenosis (Cotton and Seid 1989)

Grade	*Estimated percentage of obstruction of subglottic lumen*
I	Less than 70%
II	Between 70 and 90%
III	Greater than 90%: some small lumen identifiable
IV	Complete obstruction; no lumen.

'Hard' subglottic stenosis

Cartilage
Mature scar tissue

'Calibration' of subglottic stenosis

Benjamin–Jackson paediatric bougies
Endotracheal tubes
Bronchoscopes
Telescopes

The measurement is recorded in millimetres

likely to occur in a congenitally abnormal cricoid which will develop intubation changes more readily.

Grading systems

The degree of airway narrowing and the percentage of obstruction (Table 14.2) can be judged approximately by naked-eye examination, but is better measured objectively even if the subglottic lumen is eccentric or spiral rather than circular. Use of the Benjamin–Jackson graduated paediatric oesophageal and laryngeal bougies (Karl Storz) whose smallest diameter is 6 Fr. (2 mm) and whose largest is 30 Fr. (10 mm) is recommended. A lubricated bougie, endotracheal tube, bronchoscope or telescope which gently slips into the lumen, more or less passing under its own weight, effectively calibrates the diameter in millimetres.

Although several grading systems have been proposed, none are universally accepted. The subjective grading scale devised by Cotton and Seid (1989) is most commonly used (Table 14.2).

This system of subjective measurement gives some idea of the prognosis for decannulation which, to a great extent, is dependent upon the severity of the obstruction. For instance, there is little chance of successful re-establishment of the airway and removal of the tracheotomy tube in a Grade IV stenosis. This

Cotton classification considers lumen size only; other important factors are length, site and consistency of the stenosis, and the presence of other pathology such as vocal cord paralysis, posterior glottic stenosis, suprastomal collapse or tracheomalacia.

Other studies

Pulmonary function tests are not possible in infants and small children, but they may be useful in older children and adults as an objective measurement of airway obstruction to be compared with post-treatment results.

The effect of subglottic stenosis and its on-going treatment on speech and language development has seldom been studied, but psycho-acoustic evaluation and acoustic analysis of the voice before and after surgery have recently been reported.

Aims of treatment of subglottic stenosis

Restore an adequate airway
Permanent removal of tracheotomy
Maintain the voice
Restore speech and language
Normal swallowing function

TREATMENT OF SUBGLOTTIC STENOSIS

General considerations

For the acute airway problem in ICU, where extubation has failed, re-intubation will be necessary. When a patient presents with increasing, life-threatening airway obstruction, immediate relief must be provided by intubation or tracheotomy.

The ultimate long-term goal in the treatment of established acquired subglottic stenosis in tracheotomy-dependent patients is to restore an airway which is not only adequate for everyday activities including exercise and exertion, but is also sufficient to withstand the added respiratory demands which occur during an upper or lower respiratory tract infection. Voice quality must be maintained; surgery should not worsen the voice. A further consideration is the possible delay in the development of speech and language in a small child who has a long-term tracheotomy; intensive therapy may be necessary to improve and restore these communication abnormalities.

Treatment must be individualized and appropriate for each case; there is no 'standard' operative procedure. The patient must have adequate pulmonary function for anaesthesia, the surgical procedure and for the postoperative period which may be complicated by pulmonary infections and often includes repeated endoscopic examinations. The effect of prematurity, associated congenital heart defects or other major congenital anomalies must be considered. The laryngologist should work in close co-operation with the anaesthesiologist, neonatologist and paediatric physician.

Attention is concentrated on correcting the subglottic stenosis, but other contributing causes of airway obstruction must be searched for, evaluated and treated for a successful final result; for instance other chronic sequelae of prolonged intubation may occur with subglottic stenosis. They include posterior glottic stenosis with varying degrees of loss of mobility or complete fixation of the cricoarytenoid joints, interarytenoid adhesion, post-intubation granuloma and ductal retention cysts. In addition allowance must be made for vocal cord paralysis, tracheomalacia and congenital abnormalities of the tracheobronchial tree. One or more of these problems may affect the timing of surgery (e.g. delay until tracheomalacia is of less significance) or modify the operation (e.g. addition of posterior cricoid graft for posterior glottic stenosis).

Usually the most important consideration in deciding the timing of surgery is adequacy of pulmonary function particularly in preterm, very low birthweight babies with bronchopulmonary dysplasia. It has been recommended by Willging and Cotton (1995) that, as an arbitrary guide, definitive surgery might be delayed until the patient's weight is 10 kg or greater. The optimum time for surgery is therefore difficult to define. In a patient with moderate to severe obstruction which shows no sign of improving, who has adequate pulmonary status, no aspiration, and where the stenosis is 'mature' with no granulation tissue or infection, surgery should be considered.

The approach to laryngotracheoplasty is often different in adults who more often have posterior glottic stenosis with cricoarytenoid joint fixation, compared to children who tend to have subglottic stenosis. Both can occur together in adult or paediatric patients.

Methods of treatment

Many methods of treatment have been used, depending on the severity of the stenosis, the patient's age, weight and general progress, pulmonary function, presence of gastro-oesophageal reflux and the wishes of parents or of an adult patient. Reconstructive surgery is not always successful in providing a good result with satisfactory expansion of the airway. The first operation gives the best chance of success. There is usually no urgency for surgery.

Methods of treatment of subglottic stenosis

- Conservative - expectant observation
- Dilatation (doubtful value)
- Endoscopic laser
- Anterior cricoid split ± cartilage graft
- Therapeutic reintubation
- Tracheotomy
- Laryngotracheoplasty repair

Observation

For patients with a mild to moderate degree of congenital subglottic stenosis, it is reasonable to adopt a conservative 'wait and see' philosophy, in the expectation that the subglottic airway will improve as growth proceeds. In congenital subglottic stenosis, and in some cases of acquired subglottic stenosis, normal growth and development for 6–12 months with a long-term tracheotomy in place may allow a 'natural' improvement of the subglottic airway as growth proceeds. Operative treatment is indicated if there is no improvement.

Severe congenital stenosis, e.g. associated with a large glottic web, will ultimately require surgical correction. In the meantime, the patient requires a tracheotomy and regular endoscopic assessment, e.g. every 3 or 6 months for evaluation and calibration of the subglottic stenosis, treatment of granulations at the tracheostome and inspection for ulceration or granulation at the distal tip of the tracheotomy tube.

Endoscopic techniques

Several endoscopic treatments have been used including dilatation, laser (usually CO_2 but also argon or KTP), and the micro-flap technique. Microcauterization and cryosurgery have been advocated but have little support. Currently CO_2 laser is accepted as being beneficial in a stenosis which is neither thick nor long (Fig. 14.18), but excessive laser treatment can promote more scar tissue and worsen the stenosis.

There are different opinions about the usefulness of dilatation. It can be argued that serial dilatations for 'soft' stenosis might be useful over a long time, although the apparent beneficial effect may actually be due to steady growth and expansion of the cricoid cartilage. It can also be argued that repeated, forcible dilatation is traumatic, breaks down tissue, causes bleeding in the soft tissues and causes formation of more scar tissue. Further, the cricoid cartilage itself cannot have its diameter increased by dilatation. Attempted dilatation of a congenital carti-

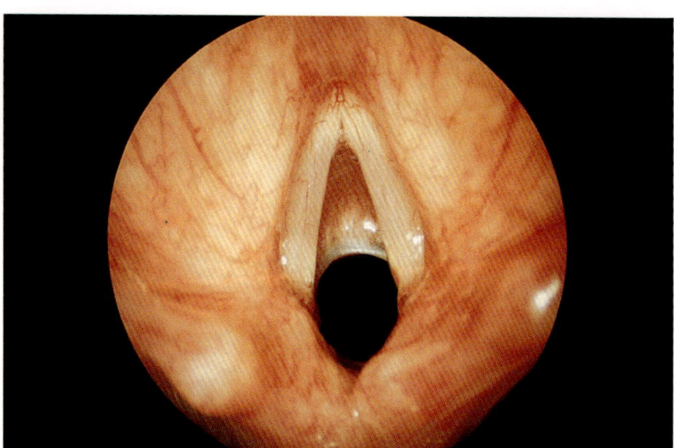

Figure **14.18**
Thin subglottic web. Caused by intubation, this thin web resulted in stridor and some hoarseness. Treated by laser.

laginous stenosis is of no benefit. It has been advocated that so-called 'dilatation treatment' should be supplemented by administration of systemic steroids or injection of local steroids into the scar tissue (which is technically difficult), but this is controversial as there is no proof that steroid administration decreases scar formation.

We use the Benjamin–Jackson paediatric oesophageal bougies to calibrate the diameter of the subglottic stenosis, recording the size as the largest lubricated dilator which 'slips' through. In the rare case where there is a thin membranous web, passage of a dilator, a bronchoscope or an endotracheal tube may disrupt it with beneficial results. Laser vaporization of the thin tissue using a subglottiscope gives a more precise and predictable result.

Certain factors indicate that endoscopic treatment is unlikely to be successful: scar tissue thicker than 8 mm, circumferential scarring, continued activity indicated by granulation tissue or infection, loss or fragmentation of cartilage, and exposure of cartilage during laser treatment.

Cricoid splits

Anterior midline cricoid split is a common procedure, but the cricoid cartilage may also be divided posteriorly, and it is occasionally divided on each lateral aspect to gain further expansion with a severe stenosis.

The anterior cricoid split operation was introduced by Cotton and Seid in 1980 as an alternative to tracheotomy for a neonate who had had several unsuccessful attempts at extubation. In 1991, Richardson and Inglis reported that a modification of cricoid split using an interposition cartilage graft (costal cartilage or auricular cartilage) to achieve and maintain distraction of the cricoid for enlargement of the lumen was more often successful.

The technique of anterior cricoid split according to Willging and Cotton (1995) will be briefly described. Adequate pulmonary function must be present.

A small horizontal skin incision exposes the anterior cricoid lamina which is divided vertically in the midline, together with the inferior third of the thyroid lamina and the upper two tracheal rings, to ensure adequate distraction to enlarge the lumen. The indwelling endotracheal tube is removed and is replaced by one of appropriate size not only to maintain the airway but also to stent the cartilaginous framework. The skin is loosely closed over a small drain.

Ventilatory support, sedation and muscle paralysis in the NICU may be required during the postoperative period. Extubation is attempted in 7–14 days and after the administration of steroids. In the few days after extubation chest physical therapy, humidification and nebulized racemic epinephrine treatment may be needed. Failure of extubation indicates the need for tracheotomy.

Patient selection is critical in the success or failure of a split as only those with adequate lung function can be decannulated.

Therapeutic reintubation

In 1995 Hoeve et al advocated what they termed 'therapeutic reintubation' as the treatment of choice in preterm infants with subglottic obstruction due to oedema, superficial lesions or ulceration. They indicated that this procedure was less successful in patients with granulations and they would then consider the anterior cricoid split operation. Our own experience confirms this line of treatment. We place a smaller endotracheal tube (2.5 mm, even 2 mm in a very small baby) for 24–48 hours, administer steroids and provide support for independent respiration after

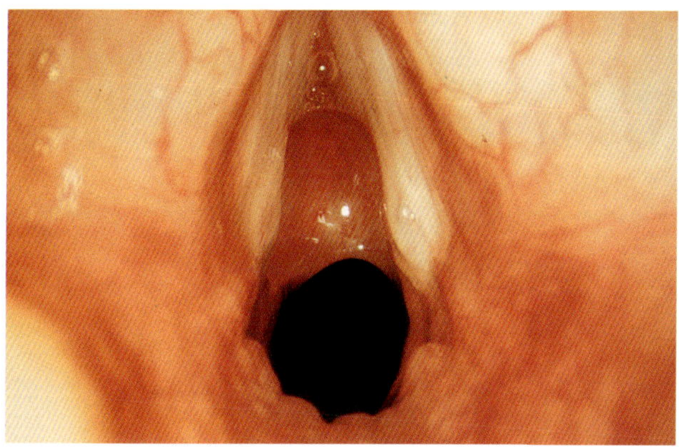

Figure **14.19**
Moderately severe acquired subglottic anterior stenosis. The stenosis was too thick for laser treatment. An anterior rib graft tracheoplasty was required.

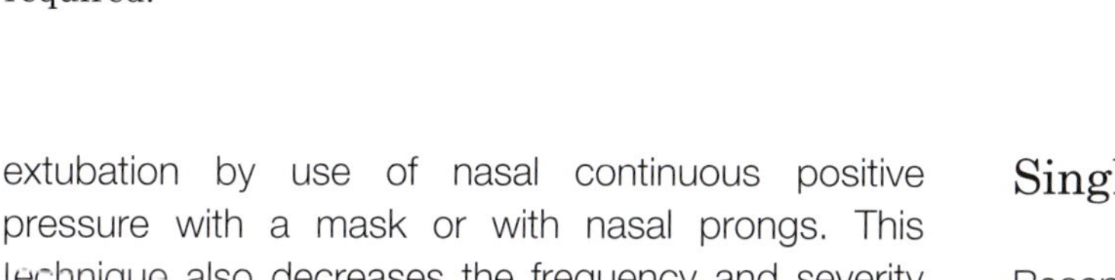

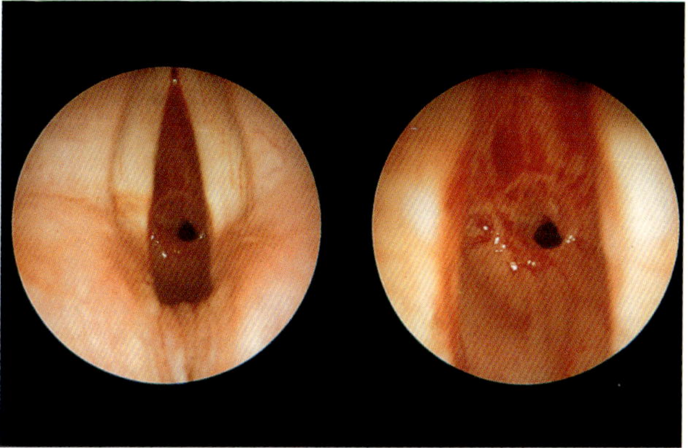

Figure **14.20**
Severe circumferential subglottic stenosis. There is still some oedema. The stenosis will require anterior and posterior rib grafts.

extubation by use of nasal continuous positive pressure with a mask or with nasal prongs. This technique also decreases the frequency and severity of apnoea and bradycardia which often contribute to respiratory failure.

Repeated failure using any of these techniques indicates the need for tracheotomy.

LARYNGOTRACHEOPLASTY

Laryngotracheal reconstruction surgery has the primary goal of enlarging the lumen of a narrowed subglottis to permit removal of a tracheostomy. Other secondary goals are to maintain or improve the voice, aid in the development of speech and maintain normal swallowing function.

The commonest reconstructive procedure involves harvesting rib cartilage which is sculptured and used as an autogenous graft to widen the anterior subglottic lumen. A horizontal skin incision gives exposure and access to the subglottic airway for midline division of the cricothyroid membrane, the cricoid itself and one or two of the upper tracheal rings. This use of an anterior cartilage graft has a high success rate in the treatment of mild or moderate anterior subglottic stenosis (Fig. 14.19).

Single stage and two stage

Recently, 'single-stage' laryngotracheoplasty has been introduced. Correction of the stenosis and removal of the tracheotomy tube are achieved with a single surgical procedure and the airway is maintained by an endotracheal tube which remains in place for 10–15 days. There are potential complications, similar to those reported after anterior cricoid split.

The patients require prolonged intubation, often with assisted ventilation and meticulous skilled care in a paediatric intensive care unit. Sedation and paralysis with muscle relaxants are usually employed to eliminate excessive motion of the operated area, to allow healing of the graft and to minimize the chance of self-extubation. The time of extubation is usually decided on the basis of an air leak with 20 cm or less water pressure. Removal of the tube is undertaken, usually in the operating theatre, within 24 hours of starting steroids. The patient is re-intubated if extubation fails, and if further attempts also fail, a tracheotomy is again necessary.

A 'staged' or 'two-stage' laryngotracheoplasty is performed when a graft with or without an airway stent is placed at operation but the tracheotomy remains in situ awaiting decannulation at a later date.

The indications for both anterior and posterior grafts at the same operation are severe circumferential (Fig. 14.20) or total subglottic obstruction,

Indications for simultaneous anterior and posterior grafts

Total obstruction
Severe circumferential stenosis
Subglottic and posterior glottic stenosis
Subglottic + tracheal stenosis, loss of supporting cartilage

Technique of laryngotracheoplasty

Cricoid cartilage incisions
? Removal of scar tissue
? Mucosal graft
Expansion graft, usually cartilage
Stenting
Stabilization
Postoperative care
Complications

combined subglottic and posterior glottic stenosis and moderate to severe subglottic and upper tracheal stenosis with contraction or loss of support of the cartilaginous framework.

Surgical techniques

There are many techniques of laryngotracheal reconstruction and new methods are constantly evolving. The methods will be covered under the following headings: cricoid incisions; dealing with scar tissue; lining mucosal graft; interposition expansion graft; stenting and stabilization.

Cricoid incisions

After skin incision and elevation of subplatysmal skin flaps, an anterior vertical midline incision is made above, through and below the cricoid. The incision is extended superiorly to a laryngofissure when exposure of the posterior larynx is inadequate. A posterior midline incision through scar tissue, through the posterior cricoid lamina and below it may be necessary to allow simple expansion when placing an anterior graft. For interposition of a posterior graft it is always necessary. Lateral vertical releasing incisions at 3 o'clock and 9 o'clock may occasionally be necessary but may destabilize the cricoid. Grafts are not used in these incisions.

Dealing with scar tissue

Current concepts do not usually advocate removal of scar tissue unless the underlying denuded area is to be covered by a skin or mucosal graft. Scar tissue is usually disturbed as little as possible although it is always divided by the anterior incision. A posterior incision is made when attempting to expand a severe subglottic stenosis or separate and widen a posterior glottic stenosis.

Lining mucosal graft

Skin, nasal mucosa, buccal mucosa or local mucosal grafts have been used as replacement over denuded areas. The graft is sewn directly into place or is fixed around an indwelling stent which then holds the graft in the desired site. Because surrounding respiratory mucosa grows quickly to cover the internal surface of the grafted area, current techniques seldom call for the use of a mucosal graft except for some techniques used in the repair of posterior subglottic stenosis.

Interposition expansion graft

Grafts can be placed in the midline anteriorly and/or posteriorly or a supplementary transverse graft can be used inferiorly for suprastomal collapse or to close the

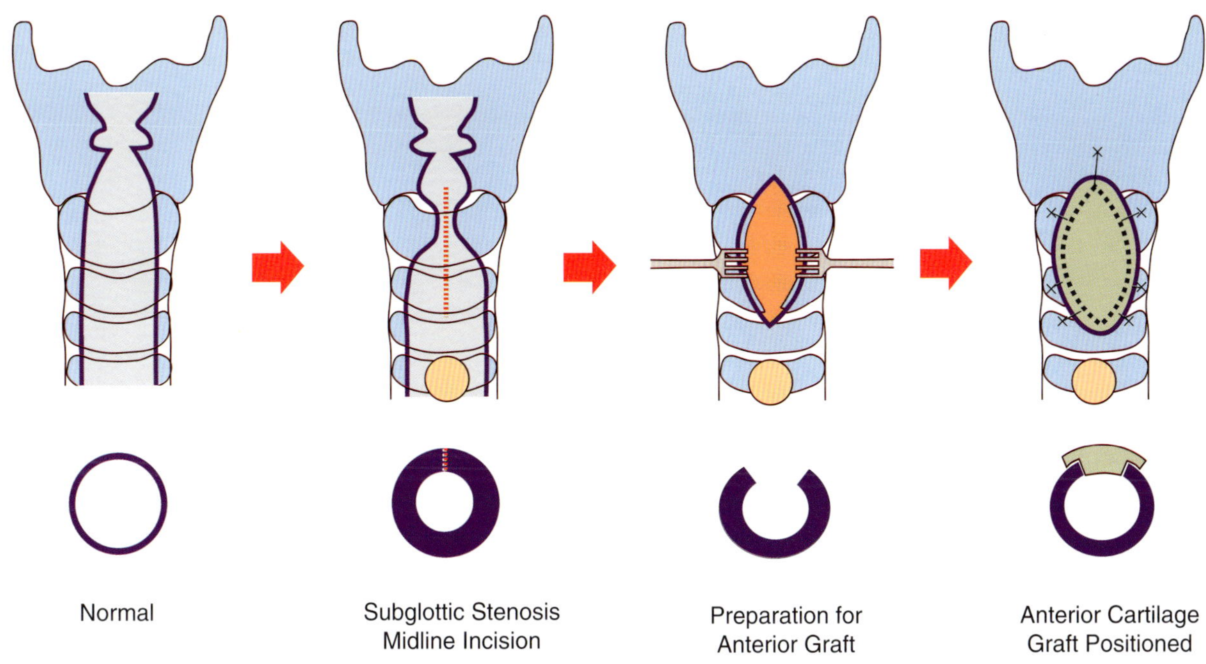

Figure **14.21**
Operative steps in augmentation laryngotracheoplasty for moderate subglottic stenosis, using rib cartilage. Anterior graft for subglottic stenosis alone.

defect of a tracheostomy. Various grafting materials have been used including costal, auricular, thyroid or nasal cartilage, hyoid bone (free or pedicled) and sternocleidomastoid myoperiosteal clavicular flap.

A thyroid cartilage–sternohyoid muscle pedicled composite graft can be harvested using the perichondrium as an internal lining for the repair of a limited subglottic stenosis.

Hyoid bone grafts have lost favour because of the limited length of graft available, the tendency to have too much curvature, the difficulty shaping the bone compared to cartilage and because small drill holes are usually necessary to pass sutures through the graft.

Some techniques do not use an interposition graft of any kind, relying on the development of dystrophic calcification in the perichondrium and strap muscles which have been sutured across the anterior defect. The lumen must be supported by a long-term indwelling stent. This technique has been used successfully in adolescents and young adults.

The most common graft is autogenous rib cartilage harvested from the patient's submammary region, usually from the right side at the costochondral junction without consideration to which particular rib is being used.

The costal cartilage graft is carved with a scalpel and tailored to fit the defect formed in the subglottic region. The anterior graft is shaped into a boat-shaped ellipse with bevelled sides and overhanging edges. When sutured into position (Fig. 14.21) these outer flanges prevent prolapse into the lumen. The graft should not protrude into the lumen and its inner surface should be flush with the cut edges of the inner mucoperichondrium of the cricoid. A layer of perichondrium may be left on the graft facing the lumen as it may encourage epithelialization.

A posterior cartilage graft for posterior glottic stenosis and/or a severe subglottic stenosis (Fig. 14.22) is shaped differently. The stenotic scar tissue is divided but not resected. The cricoid cartilage is divided (in adults an oscillating saw is usually necessary) from upper to lower edge exactly in the midline to expose the inner mucoperichondrium of the

Anterior cartilage graft	Posterior cartilage graft
Thicker and firm	Thinner, less robust
Boat-shaped	Shield-shaped
Bevelled sides	Straight edges
Sewn into position	Difficult to stabilize
May not need stenting	Requires stenting

postcricoid hypopharyngeal region. The incision is extended superiorly only when fibrotic interarytenoid muscle requires division and inferiorly for about 5–10 mm into the membranous tracheal wall exercising care not to enter the oesophagus. The two halves of the cricoid are retracted laterally with hooks and the shaped cartilage graft is interposed, sometimes with difficulty, between the medial edges of the incised cricoid (Fig. 14.23). The graft may be held in place with absorbable sutures, by a transverse pin or by the shape of the graft (refer to the section on stabilization later in this chapter). An Aboulker, a Cotton–Lorenz stent (Fig. 14.24) or a Montgomery T-tube is necessary to maintain a posterior graft. Arytenoidectomy, especially when the arytenoid is fixed, can be a useful additional operation when dealing with posterior glottic stenosis.

Note that anterior grafts are larger and thicker than posterior grafts. The anterior graft is elliptical with wide flanges and the posterior graft is thinner and shield-shaped.

For severe or total obstruction, some scar tissue must be removed, a lining mucosal graft is optional, and combined anterior and posterior grafts are necessary (Fig. 14.25).

If the suprastomal area of the trachea or the tracheostomy requires augmentation, the midline incision is extended to the stoma and a longer graft (Fig. 14.26) or a second horizontal cartilage graft interlocking with the primary anterior vertical graft can be used. The stoma is closed by the graft and a single-stage laryngotracheoplasty is performed.

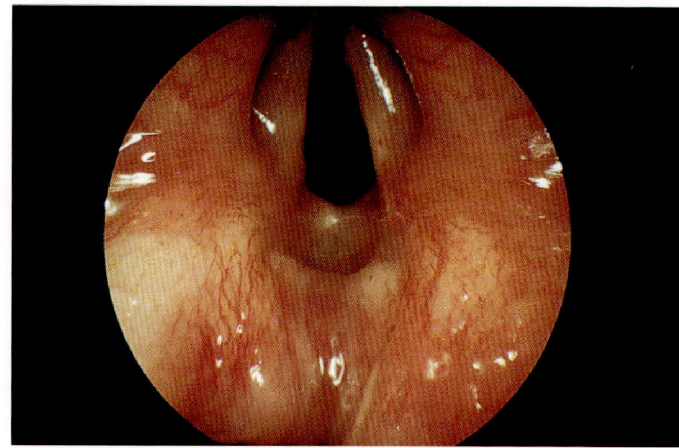

Figure **14.22**
Posterior glottic stenosis. Typical posterior glottic stenosis with fixed cricoarytenoid joints, in this case requiring a posterior cartilage graft.

Stenting

Many kinds of stent have been used including an endotracheal tube, finger cot, Montgomery T-tube, Aboulker or Cotton–Lorenz stent (Fig. 14.27), roll of silastic sheeting ('Swiss roll') and silastic or PVC tubing (Fig. 14.28). Many surgeons prefer to avoid the use of a stent, but when the cricoid cartilage has been divided both anteriorly and posteriorly stenting is required to provide stability. The duration of stenting varies from 1–2 weeks to 6 months. Mucosal grafts require stenting for at least a week.

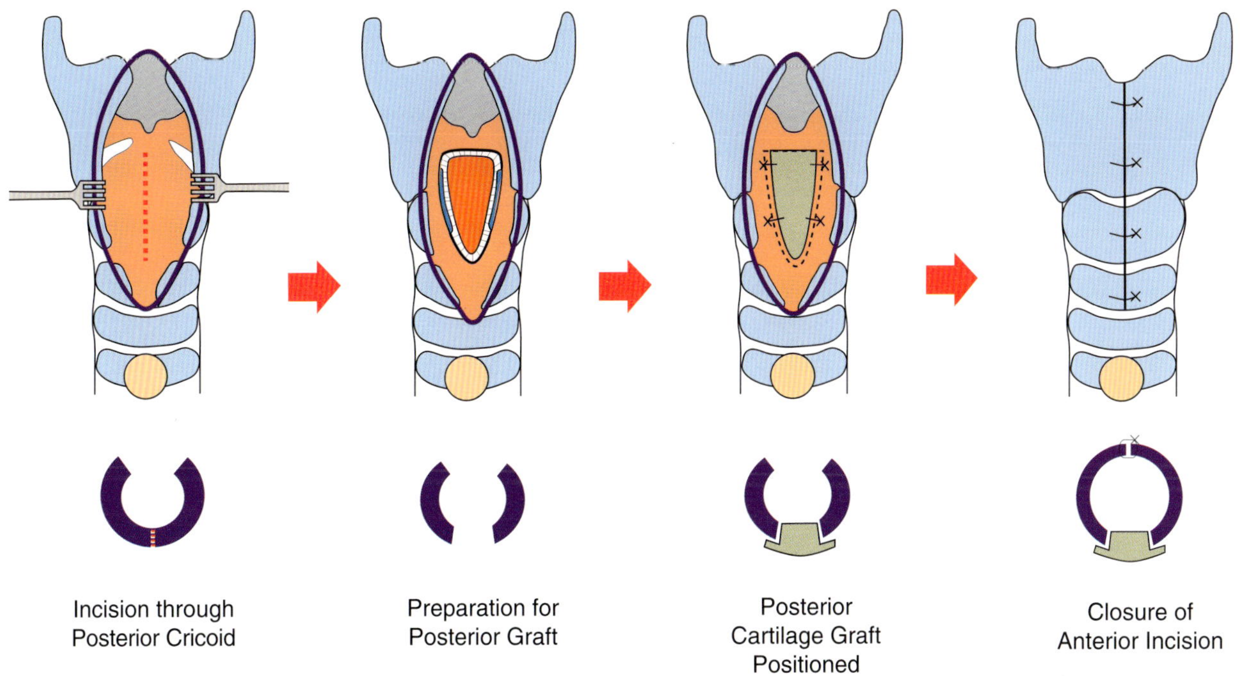

Figure **14.23**
Operative steps, following laryngofissure for posterior glottic stenosis; rib cartilage in the posterior lamina of the cricoid cartilage.

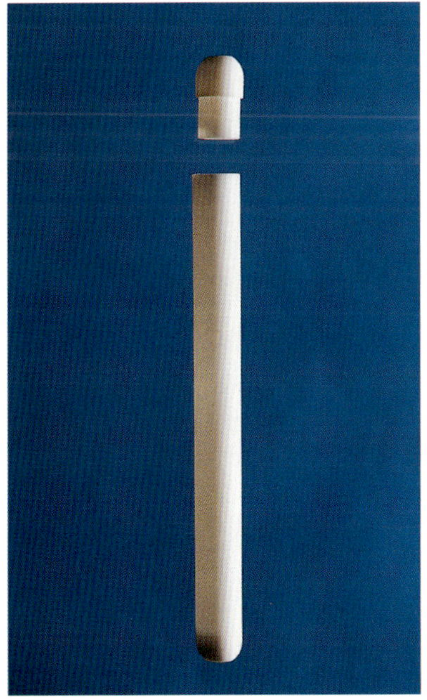

Figure **14.24**
Cotton–Lorenz stent. Upper end has a cap so that both ends are smooth.

Types of stents

Endotracheal tube
'Swiss roll' of silastic sheet
Montgomery T-tube
Aboulker or Cotton–Lorenz
Silastic or PVC tube

Placement is important; a stent with an open end above the vocal cords can predispose to aspiration, ulceration of the posterior surface of the epiglottis and formation of granulation tissue in the vocal cords. A stent whose upper end is below the vocal cords can cause ulceration of the subglottic region.

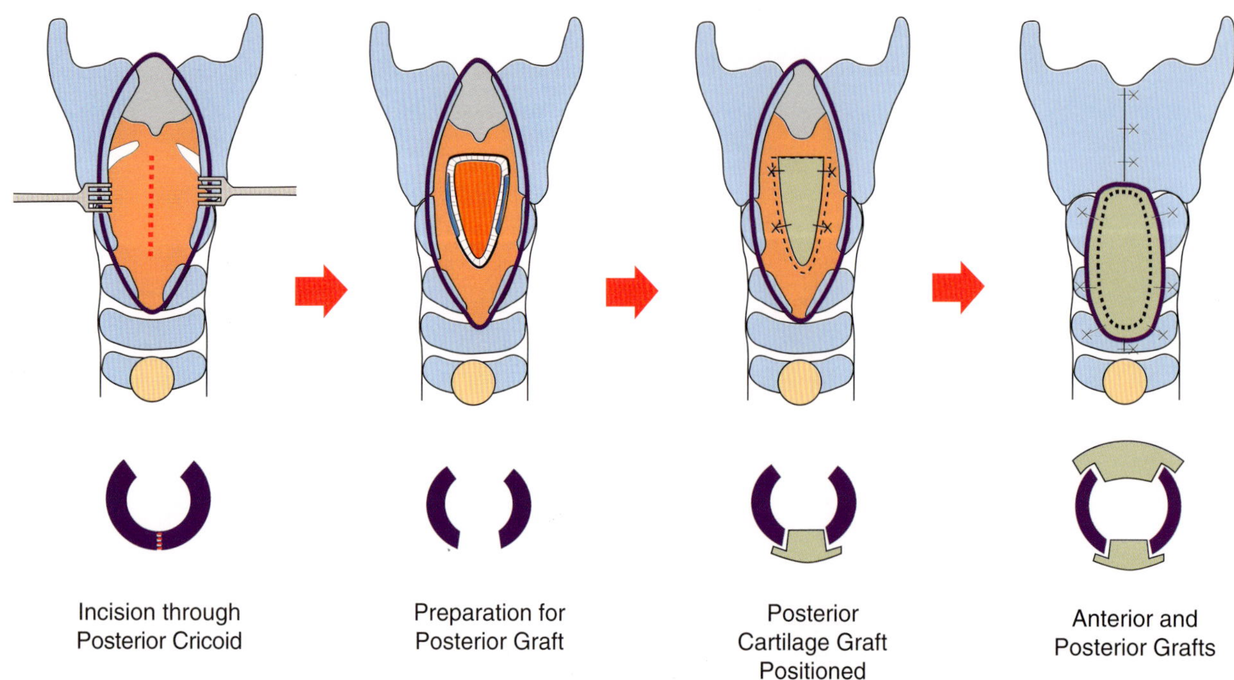

Figure **14.25**
Operative steps in combined anterior and posterior laryngotracheoplasty for severe glottic stenosis.

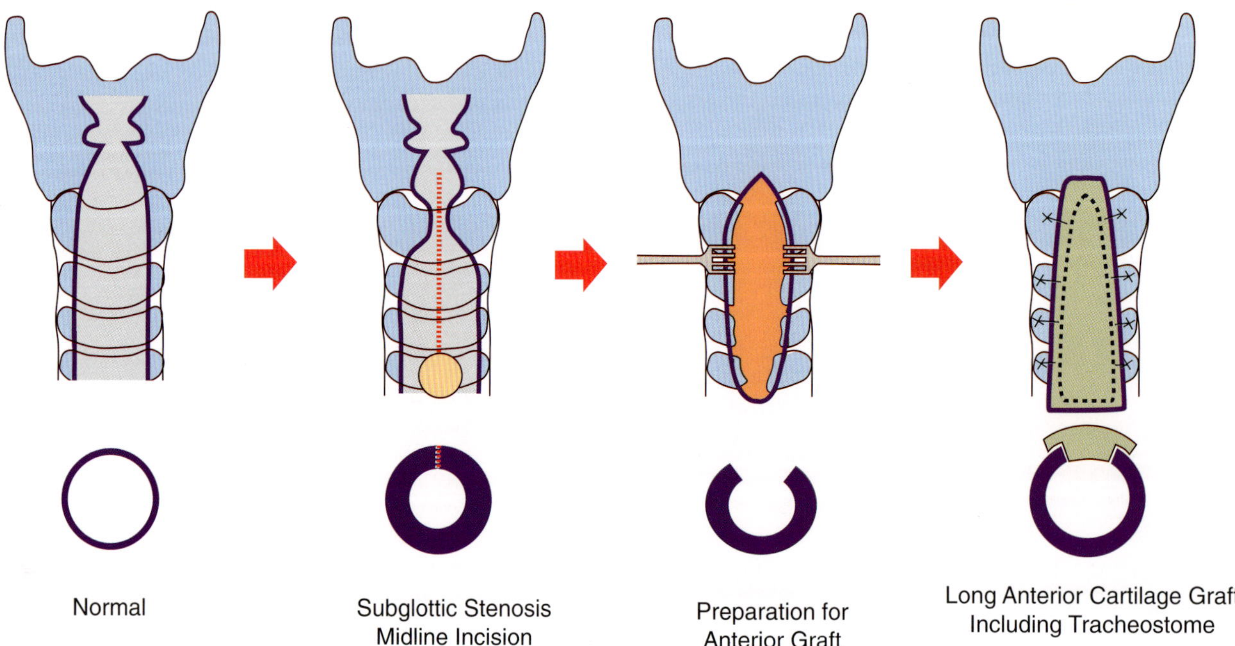

Figure **14.26**
Operative steps using an extended anterior graft to cover the tracheotomy.

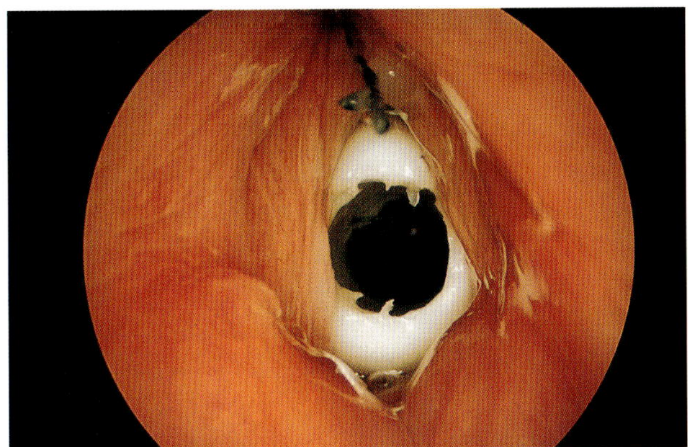

Figure **14.27**
Cotton–Lorenz stent in situ. The upper end of the stent lies just below the vocal cords.

Stabilization of grafts

Sutures
Shaped, fitted graft
Wire pinning
Miniplates
Internal stenting

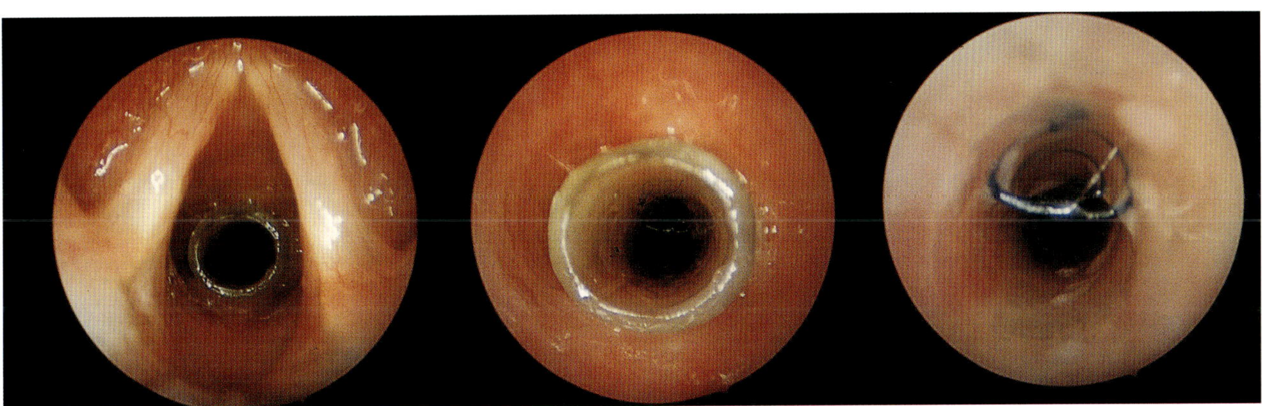

Figure **14.28**
Silastic tube used as a stent. Showing relation below the glottis; close-up of upper end and nylon retaining suture; the suture is within the tube so that the tube can be removed endoscopically.

A short stent is used when the lower end is positioned above an indwelling tracheotomy tube. A long stent is used when the tracheotomy tube is incorporated in a full-length stent; a double-lumen metal Holinger tracheotomy tube is usually wired to the stent.

Prolonged stenting is necessary for the repair of severe, widespread or long stenosis, where the graft in the operative field is unstable, and for all posterior grafts.

Stabilization

The sculptured shape of the anterior graft prevents it from prolapsing into the lumen, and placement of six to eight sutures holds it firmly in position preventing up or down movement.

A posterior graft may be difficult to position and may be held in place by shaping it (Fig. 14.23) or by one or two small-diameter stiff wires passed in a coronal direction through the upper and lower part of the graft, with sharpened projecting ends of

1–1.5 mm length which are pushed into the distracted edges of the cricoid lamina. In other cases two small non-absorbable sutures on each side, with the knots buried, are used to position and stabilize the graft. An indwelling stent is used in all cases of posterior grafting.

Metal alloy miniplates can be shaped and placed anterior to the cartilaginous airway to provide external support for a fascial or cartilaginous graft. One miniplate with four holes can be bent to the appropriate curve to fit over the graft and fixed in place with sutures; sometimes more than one miniplate is required.

Thus, stabilization is achieved by a combination of a shaped, well-fitting graft with side flanges held in position by sutures, stabilized by a suitable internal stent and in some cases with one or more external miniplates.

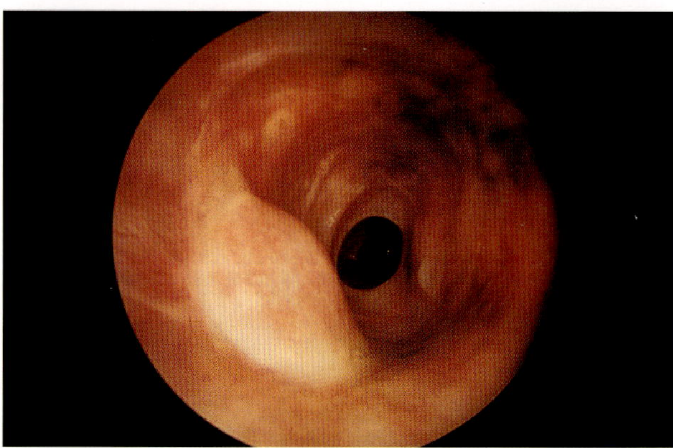

Figure **14.29**
Granulation after stent removal. Small mass of granulations, left postero-lateral aspect of upper trachea, seen after removal of silastic tube which had been in place for 6 months.

Postoperative care

After an anterior cricoid split, with or without cartilage interposition graft, infants are nursed in an intensive care ward with skilled, experienced personnel in attendance. Most surgeons prefer paediatric patients to be sedated, paralysed and ventilated to minimize movement around the graft, giving it an opportunity to heal in position, and to minimize the chance of accidental extubation. If accidental extubation occurs, re-intubation must be carefully performed. Stay sutures placed on each side of the incised cricoid at the time of operation can be used as retractors to assist later re-introduction of the endotracheal tube. Where a cartilage graft has been used in an anterior cricoid split, re-intubation appears to be less prone to complications.

Anti-reflux treatment is used arbitrarily in most cases, particularly in paralysed ventilated patients who are necessarily lying supine. Antibiotics are given during the stenting period.

Endoscopy with a flexible fibreoptic instrument or, more usually, with rigid instruments under general anaesthesia is required for removal of the stent and for removal of any granulation tissue masses which might form, particularly at the bottom end of the stent. Repeated endoscopy may be required to remove granulations. Sometimes a further stenosis occurs because of the persistent granulations and attendant perichondritis.

Complications

The major complication of laryngotracheoplasty is failure of the graft or grafts. Revision surgery will be necessary at a properly selected time.

Other complications (Zeitouni and Manoukian, 1994) include instability of the graft, wound infection or haemorrhage, granulation tissue from the presence of the stent (Fig. 14.29) or from the surgical incision (Fig.

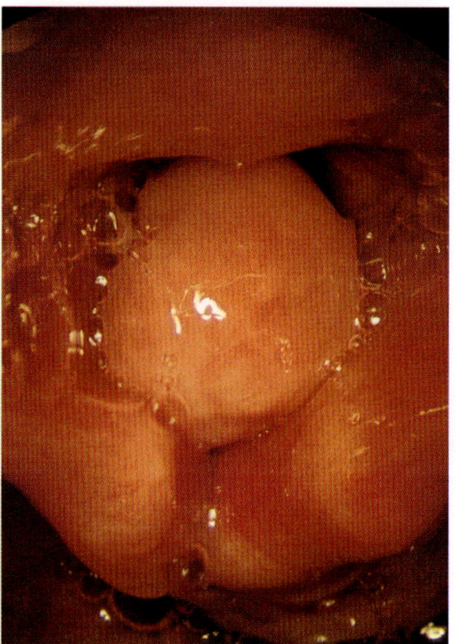

Figure **14.30**
Massive granuloma. Three weeks after laryngofissure. No recurrences after removal.

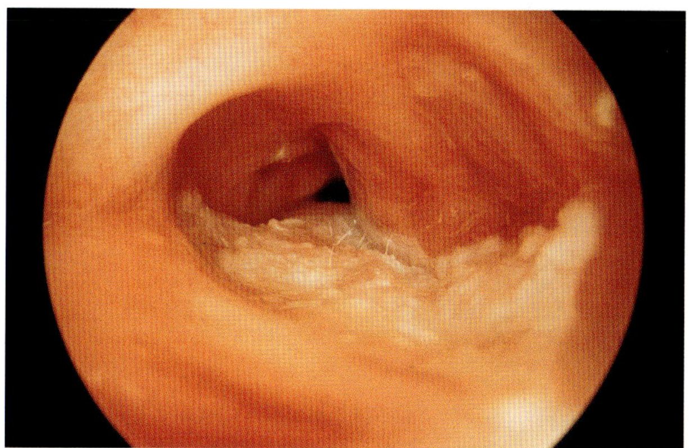

Figure **14.31**
Skin graft with hair. Skin graft performed in another country.

Major complications of laryngotracheoplasty

Graft instability or failure
Migration or breakage of stent
Obstruction of endotracheal tube
Accidental or self-extubation
Pneumonitis, atelectasis or pneumothorax
Wound infection or disruption

14.30), subcutaneous emphysema, movement or migration of the stent, broken stent and cerebral hypoxia which might result in transient blindness or brain damage. Withdrawal of sedation, narcotics or neuromuscular blockers may lead to agitation, tremulousness or transient muscular weakness. Other complications which have been reported include myocardial infarction, wound breakdown, accidental or self-extubation, obstruction of the endotracheal tube, tracheocutaneous fistula and prolapse of soft tissue through a cricoid split. Skin grafting with hair-bearing skin (Fig. 14.31) sometimes creates problems.

The most common complications in patients who have been paralysed and ventilated are pulmonary, such as segmental or subsegmental atelectasis, pneumonia or pneumothorax.

Conclusion

Anterior cricoid split or elective laryngotracheoplasty can be 'routine' operative procedures, usually with good results, but many complications can occur, and these need to be detected and treated promptly. Failure occurs especially in severe, long-segment stenosis, in total obstruction or in cases where the cartilaginous framework has been distorted, fragmented or is badly contracted and surrounded by dense scar tissue.

It is important that consideration be given now and in the future to refinements which will allow maintenance or improvement of the voice, rehabilitation of speech and language and maintenance of a normal swallowing mechanism.

Prognosis and success rate

The reported success rates of laryngotracheoplasty range from 50% to over 90%. Success depends not only on the severity of the stenosis being repaired, but also on the skill and experience of the operator together with the quality of the postoperative care. For example, repair of a Cotton Grade I stenosis has a very good success rate, but attempted repair of a Grade IV obstruction has a poor success rate.

Success should be measured not only by the surgeon's ability to remove the tracheotomy tube but also by the patient's respiratory capability. The effect of upper respiratory tract infections causing soft tissue swelling and further obstruction must be taken into account. Of most importance, and receiving more attention recently, is the effect on the voice and the swallowing mechanism (Smith et al, 1992).

No long-term follow-up studies have been reported and the success rates and prognosis currently quoted assume a favourable outcome will be maintained throughout further growth and development. Further follow-up studies are needed to determine long-term results.

RESECTION

A short segment of the upper cervical trachea can be resected without difficulty and can be repaired by primary end-to-end anastomosis, taking care not to damage the recurrent laryngeal nerves in the tracheo-oesophageal groove. Long-segment stenoses may require laryngeal release when the gap is greater than 2.5–3 cm. This can be achieved by multiple incisions in the annular ligaments of the trachea or by mobilization of the distal trachea from the thorax by transsection of the left main bronchus and by primary anastomosis with the right main stem bronchus, but this is a major procedure with inherent risks.

The release procedure which is usually used is a superior laryngeal release – either infrahyoid or more often suprahyoid. The suprahyoid release requires transsection of the muscles from the superior border of the hyoid, transsection of the stylohyoid insertions and transsection of the body of the hyoid on each side medial to the insertion of the digastric tendon. Thus, the body of the hyoid, the thyroid cartilage and the cricoid cartilage are able to be lowered by several centimetres. It is usual to maintain flexion of the neck in the postoperative period either by a flexion splint behind the neck and the head or by sutures holding the chin towards the sternum.

Partial cricoid resection with anastomosis of the upper trachea to the remaining cricoid and thyroid cartilages is difficult in small children but has a place in a small group of older patients who have an entirely subglottic stenosis. The upper resection line removes the inferior border of the thyroid cartilage and is directed inferiorly and posteriorly to the lower margin of the cricoid lamina, taking care to preserve the recurrent laryngeal nerves. The lower resection line is just below the lower border of the stenosis and the posterior incision is often bevelled superiorly so that a wide tongue of posterior membranous tracheal wall can be brought up into the subglottic and posterior glottic region. This operation is usually combined with one or other laryngeal release procedures.

BIBLIOGRAPHY

Chen JC, Holinger LD (1995) Acquired laryngeal lesions. Pathologic study using serial macrosections. *Otolaryngol Head Neck Surg* **121**: 537–43.

Cotton RT, Seid AB (1980) Management of the extubation problem in the premature child: anterior cricoid split as an alternative to tracheotomy. *Ann Otol Rhinol Laryngol* **89**: 508.

Cotton RT, Gray SD, Miller RP (1989) Update of the Cincinnati experience in pediatric laryngotracheal reconstruction. *Laryngoscope* **99**: 1111–19.

Friedman M, Mayer AD (1991) Laryngotracheal reconstruction in adults with the sterno-cleido-mastoid myoperiosteal flap. *Ann Otol Rhinol Laryngol* **102**: 897–908.

Hoeue LJ, Eskici O, Verwoerd CDA (1995) Therapeutic re--intubation for post-intubation laryngotracheal injury in preterm infants. *Int J Paediatr Otorhinolaryngol* **31**: 7–13.

Liu H, Chen JC, Holinger LD, Gonzalez-Crussi F (1995) Histopathologic fundamentals of acquired laryngeal stenosis. *Pediatr Pathol Lab Med* **15**: 655–77.

Montgomery W (1973) Laryngeal inlet stenosis. In: Montgomery W, ed. *Surgery of the upper respiratory tract*, Vol. 2 (Philadelphia: Lea and Febiger); 557–64.

Richardson MA, Inglis AF (1991) A comparison of anterior cricoid split with and without costal cartilage grafts for acquired subglottic stenosis. *Int Pediatr Otorhinolaryngol* **22**: 187–93.

Smith ME, Cotton R, Mortelliti AJ, Meyer C (1992) Phonation and swallowing considerations in pediatric laryngotracheal reconstruction. *Ann Otol Rhinol Laryngol* **101**: 731–8.

Tan H, Holinger L, Chen J-C, Gonzales-Crussi F (1996) Fragmented, distorted cricoid cartilage: an acquired abnormality. *Ann Otol Rhinol Laryngol* **105**: 348–55.

Weisberger E, Nguyen C (1996) Laryngotracheal reconstruction using a vitallium alloy miniplate. *Ann Otol Rhinol Laryngol* **105**: 363–6.

Willging JP, Cotton RT (1995) Subglottic stenosis in the paediatric patient. In: Myer CM, Cotton RT, Shott S, eds. *The paediatric airway* (Philadelphia: JB Lippincott); 111–32.

Zalzal G (1993) Treatment of laryngotracheal stenosis with anterior and posterior cartilage grafts. *Arch Otolaryngol Head Neck Surg* **119**: 82–6.

Zeitouni AG, Manoukian J (1994) Severe complications of the anterior cricoid split operation and single stage laryngotracheoplasty. *Ann Otol Rhinol Laryngol* **103**: 723–5.

15 Cystic disease

CLASSIFICATION

Cystic disease in the endolarynx can be classified as follows:

- congenital saccular cysts
- laryngocoeles
- ductal retention cysts
- cystic hygroma
- intracordal cysts
- rare developmental cysts.

Within this convenient classification there is a developmental spectrum of congenital saccular cysts and laryngocoeles (whether air- or fluid-filled), all of which arise from the laryngeal saccule.

Ductal retention cysts are due to accumulation of secretions in dilated collecting ducts of mucous glands or minor salivary glands. They therefore include larger ‘vallecular’ and ‘epiglottic’ cysts which are named for their anatomical location.

Cystic hygroma is one of three forms of lymphangioma – a developmental anomaly of lymph vessels. Cystic hygroma has multilocular cystic spaces and usually presents in the face and neck, but can extend as an obstructive mass into the larynx and pharynx.

Intracordal cysts are usually epidermoid and, although they often occur alone, they may be associated with abnormalities known as vocal sulcus and mucosal bridge.

PATHOGENESIS OF SACCULAR DISEASE

The normal saccule of the larynx (Fig. 15.1) is a blind out-pouching of the anterior end of the normal

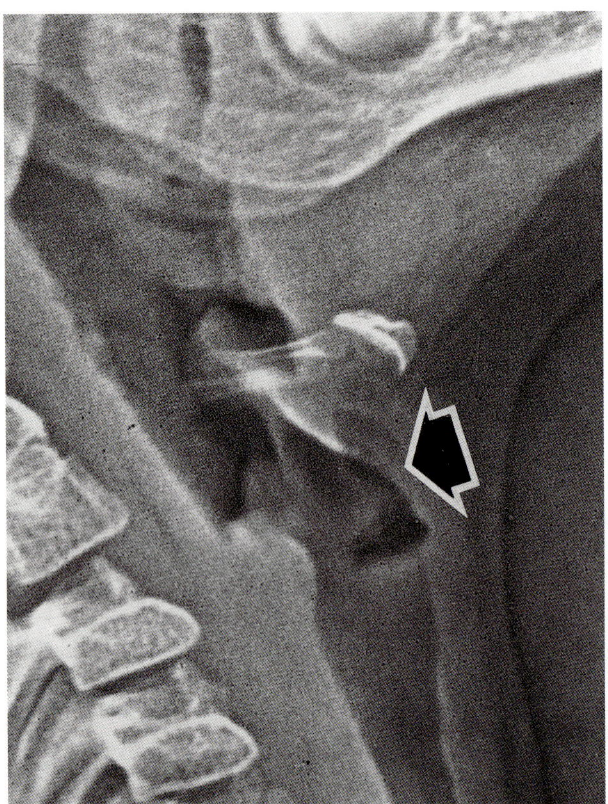

Figure **15.1**
Normal saccule. Xerogram which shows a normal saccule (arrow) in an infant.

Cystic conditions of the saccule

Lateral saccular cyst
Anterior saccular cyst
Laryngocoele (air)
Laryngomucocoele (fluid)
Laryngopyocoele (pus)

ventricle, extending upwards for a variable distance between the false vocal cord and the thyroid cartilage, just postero-lateral to the edge of the epiglottis. The lining contains mucous glands whose secretions assist lubrication as they are expressed by delicate muscles in the wall of the saccule into the anterior ventricle and onto the upper surface of the vocal folds through the orifice of the saccular duct located in the lateral part of the anterior third of the ventricle. Congenital saccular cysts and laryngocoeles are disorders of the saccule which has undergone abnormal dilatation, usually with mucus, sometimes with air, because of obstruction of the saccular duct.

Saccular cysts, whether anterior or lateral, are filled with glandular secretions because the duct is occluded. An air-containing laryngocoele occurs when the saccular duct allows filling – as air pressure in the larynx increases – but does not allow emptying so that the laryngocoele becomes progressively larger.

Saccular disease is congenital when occlusion or partial occlusion of the saccular duct is developmental, but saccular disease is acquired when occlusion is secondary, e.g. to neoplasm, infection or trauma.

CONGENITAL SACCULAR CYSTS

These cysts have also been called 'congenital cysts of the larynx', 'laryngeal mucocoeles' and 'saccular mucocoeles'.

Congenital saccular cysts occur when the duct or orifice of the saccule is obstructed, with consequent dilatation of the saccule by secretions. There are two types and, although both are rare, the more common is the lateral saccular cyst which distends and expands the false vocal cord and aryepiglottic fold in the supraglottic region. A lateral saccular cyst (Fig. 15.2) is the same thing as an internal laryngomucocoele, a diagnostic term usually applied to adult disease. If it continues to enlarge, it may pass through the thyrohyoid membrane and appear in the neck as a swelling – an external laryngocoele.

An anterior saccular cyst is smaller and more anterior than a lateral saccular cyst and may be seen at indirect laryngoscopy in adults and older children. At direct laryngoscopy, an anterior saccular cyst (Fig. 15.3) is seen as a rounded swelling, deep in the

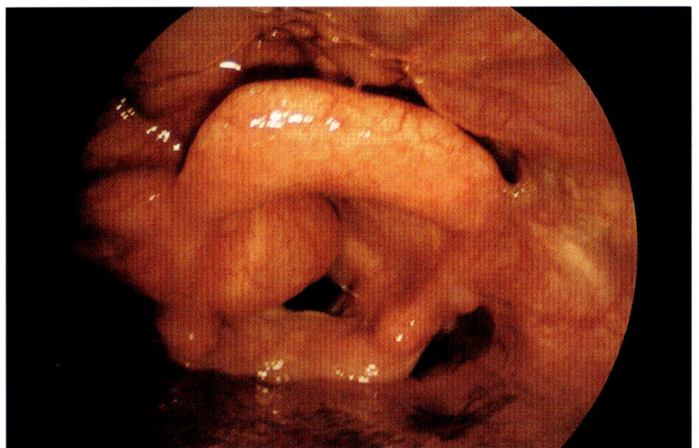

Figure **15.2**
Lateral saccular cyst. Large left lateral saccular cyst at indirect laryngoscopy. The 45-year-old female patient had respiratory obstruction, worse at night. The cyst was removed endoscopically.

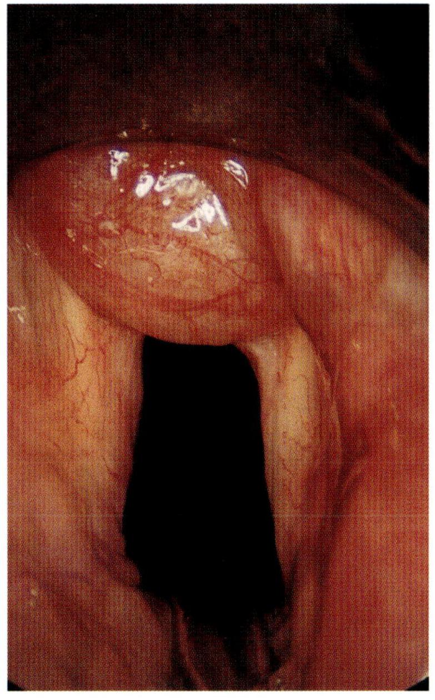

Figure **15.3**
Anterior saccular cyst. Large right anterior saccular cyst at direct laryngoscopy before removal using the laser. Male aged 67 years with husky voice and minor airway symptoms.

anterior part of the hemilarynx, bulging medially to obscure the ipsilateral vocal fold and the anterior part of the contralateral vocal fold.

Thus, congenital saccular cysts are the counterparts of adult laryngocoeles, whether internal, external or both. A cyst is distinguished from an air-filled laryngocoele because the latter may sometimes be filled with air and may sometimes be empty.

Clinical features

Air-containing laryngocoeles are not seen in infants. The distended saccule presents as a mucus-filled cyst, sometimes at birth, more often in older children. A saccular cyst which presents at birth may be large enough to cause severe respiratory distress, inspiratory stridor, episodes of cyanosis, inaudible or muffled cry and difficulty swallowing. Although very rare, an external swelling may exist in the neck and, if so, investigation is required to confirm the presence of both an internal and an external laryngocoele (Fig. 15.4). Lateral soft tissue radiographic studies will show a cyst which is large enough to cause airway obstruction (Fig. 15.5).

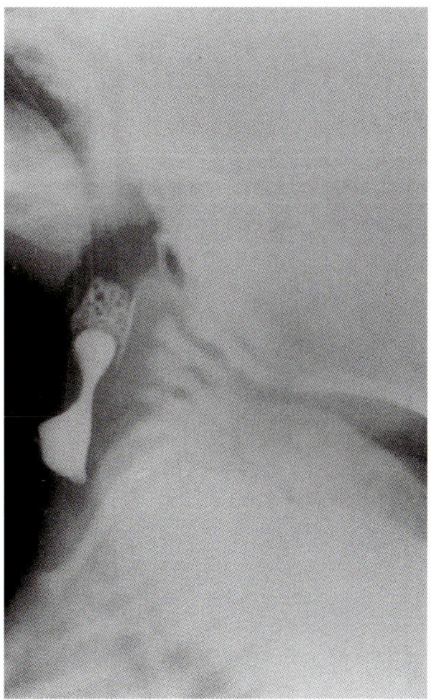

Figure **15.4**
Internal and external laryngocoele in a baby. Radio-opaque dye injected into the internal component revealed the combined nature of the lesion.

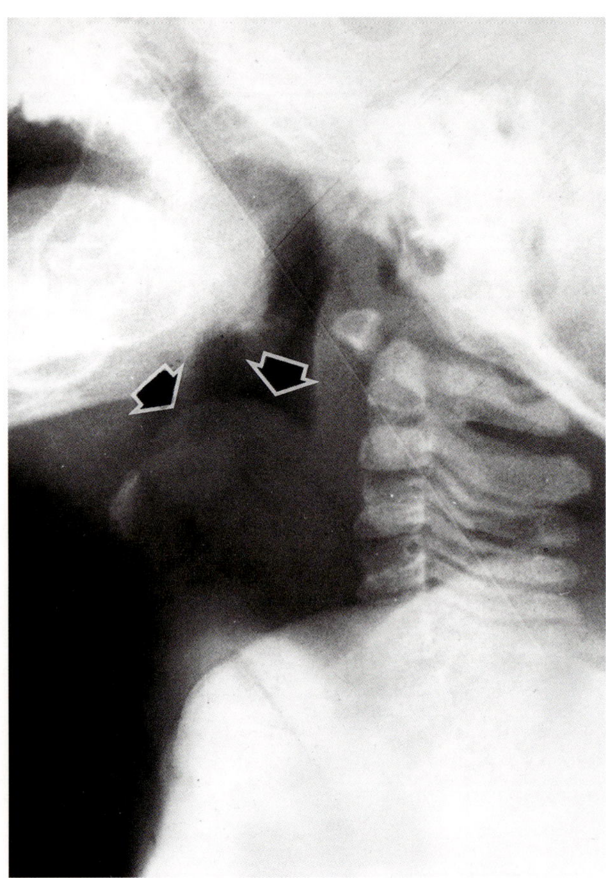

Figure **15.5**
'Congenital laryngeal cyst' X-ray. Very large lateral saccular cyst (arrows) causing severe airway obstruction at birth. Treated endoscopically at 4 hours of age.

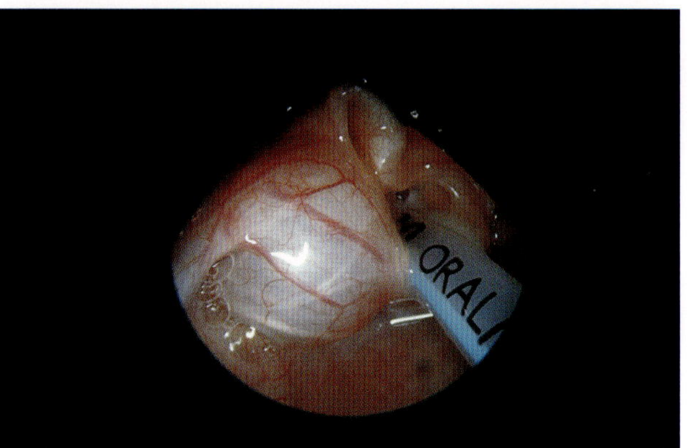

Figure **15.6**
'Congenital laryngeal cyst'. Endoscopic appearance. Large, obstructive, rounded, lateral saccular cyst before operative laser treatment. Intubation is very difficult.

Treatment

Endoscopy reveals a large bluish or pink fluid-filled cyst distending one side of the supraglottic tissues and making intubation very difficult (Fig. 15.6). When X-ray has shown a large cyst, induction of anaesthesia for laryngoscopy can precipitate severe or total airway obstruction. If attempted intubation fails, the surgeon must be prepared to restore the airway by decompressing the cyst either by sucking out its content through a large bore needle or by incising it with a scalpel. Immediate removal of the dome of the cyst, although more difficult, will also achieve drainage of the thick fluid and restoration of the airway.

Wide removal of the roof of the cyst and marsupialization using the carbon dioxide laser is the recommended treatment, but may have to be repeated if the cyst reforms. Tracheotomy should seldom be required even in a patient who requires surgery through an external incision for a cyst which persistently recurs.

The less common anterior saccular cyst is also filled with mucus, does not reach such a large size and causes only partial airway obstruction. Because of its position in the ventricle between the false cord and the vocal fold, in infants the cry is absent or muffled and in adults the voice is altered. Laser removal of most of the cyst wall is the treatment of choice.

LARYNGOCOELES

It is emphasized that a lateral saccular cyst is the same as an internal laryngomucocoele and that:

- a laryngocoele is distended with air (Fig. 15.7);
- a laryngomucocoele is distended with mucus;
- a laryngopyocoele is an infected laryngomucocoele and is distended with pus.

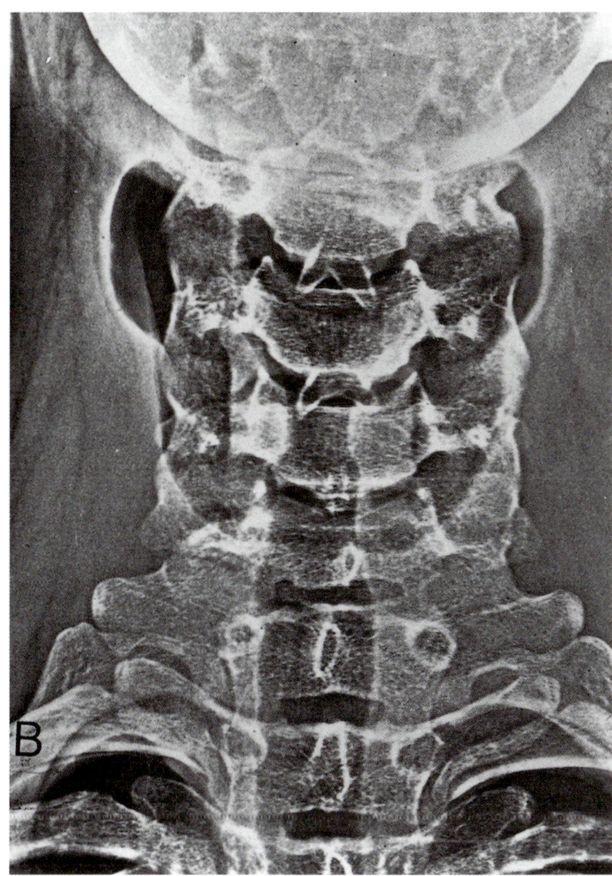

Figure **15.7**
Laryngocoeles. Bilateral air-containing laryngocoeles distended with air.

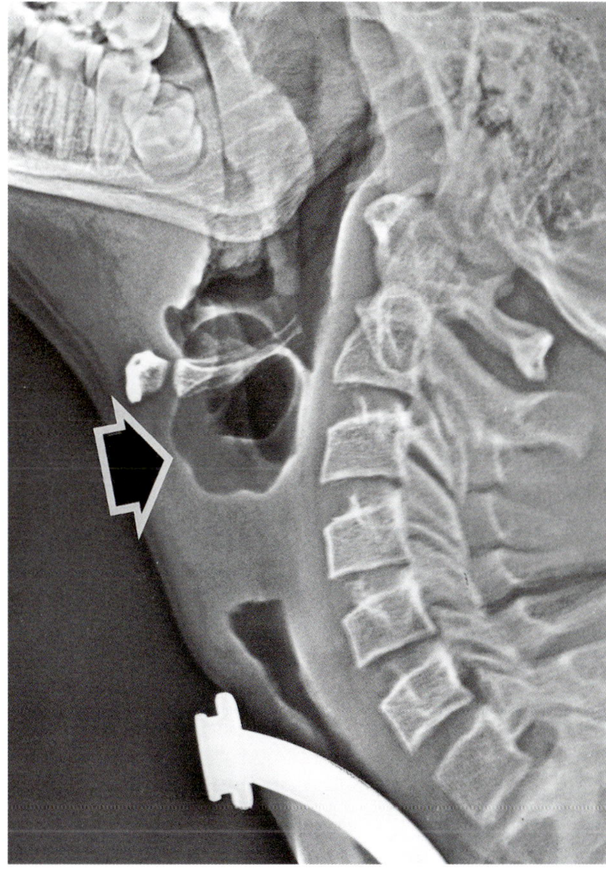

Figure **15.8**
Secondary laryngocoele. Air-containing laryngocoele (arrow) which occurred after a 15-year-old boy with a mass of papillomas in his larynx had been shouting.

Pathogenesis

Laryngocoeles occur internally, externally or as a combination of both. Although the cause of laryngocoeles is said to be increased glottic air pressure, such as occurs in glass blowers or wind instrument players, this is not so in all patients. In some cases, primary pathology, e.g. a laryngeal neoplasm such as squamous cell carcinoma or papilloma or trauma in the ventricle, results in obstruction of the saccular duct with formation of a secondary laryngocoele (Fig. 15.8). The lateral and anterior ventricle must be carefully inspected with a 30° or a 70° telescope after retraction of the false cord, to exclude primary pathology in this region before surgical treatment of a laryngocoele.

Laryngocoeles are usually unilateral but can be bilateral; in fact, an air-filled laryngocoele can occur on one side with a mucus-filled laryngocoele on the

Laryngocoeles

Internal
External
Combined

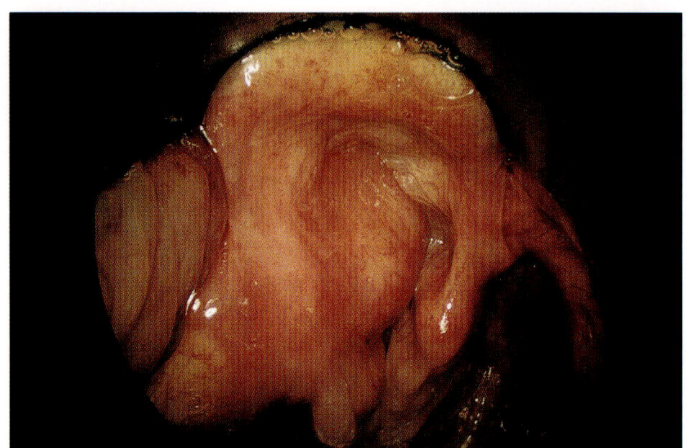

Figure **15.9**
Internal laryngocoele. Indirect laryngoscopy. Photograph at indirect laryngoscopy reveals a swelling distending the supraglottis.

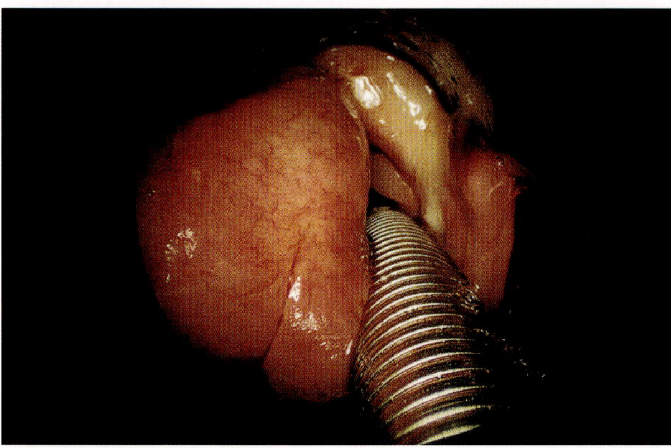

Figure **15.10**
Internal laryngocoele. Direct laryngoscopy. Satisfactory visualization for endoscopic laser treatment.

other side. They are more common in men than women, and can be found in adults from approximately 15 years of age.

Clinical features

The mode of presentation depends on the size of the laryngocoele and on whether it is internal, external or combined. Symptoms from an internal laryngocoele include hoarseness, a feeling of 'something' in the throat, sore throat and difficulty swallowing. Stridor can occur with a large obstructive swelling. The external component presents in the lateral neck as a rounded swelling which has passed through the thyrohyoid membrane where the superior neurovascular bundle pierces it.

At indirect laryngoscopy (Fig. 15.9), an internal laryngocoele is seen as a unilateral, supraglottic, rounded swelling deep in the aryepiglottic fold and false cord, projecting medially into the supraglottis to obscure the vocal cords and laterally to partly fill the piriform fossa.

A combined internal and external laryngocoele creates the same swelling as seen in an internal laryngocoele due to the internal component in the supraglottic larynx. The external component is detected as a palpable rounded mass in the neck at a level between the hyoid bone and the thyroid cartilage. The extent of the swelling depends on the size of the external component. An external laryngocoele must have an internal component whether or not there is an easily detectable intralaryngeal mass.

Radiographic imaging

Although a laryngocoele may be diagnosed on plain films, CT or MRI are preferred and show a supraglottic mass which passes through the paraglottic area to the level of the ventricle, with deformity of the supraglottic soft tissues. An air-filled laryngocoele is seen as a large, rounded, air-filled sac which may be made more prominent by the Valsalva manoeuvre.

Treatment

A laryngocoele which intermittently fills with air but which promptly empties, does not usually require treatment. However, a mucus-filled laryngomucocoele producing persistent, troublesome symptoms will require surgical treatment, either by endoscopic

Methods of surgical treatment of laryngomucocoele

Immediate decompression for severe obstruction
Endoscopic dissection and marsupialization
External operation for persistent recurrence or if combined internal and external
Antibiotics, drainage of laryngopyocoele

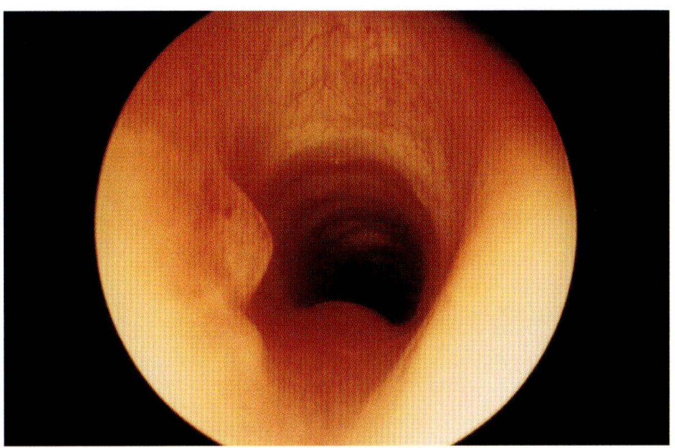

Figure **15.11**
Subglottic ductal cyst. Moderate-sized ductal retention cyst in left subglottis in an infant following prolonged intubation.

marsupialization or by removal via an external approach.

A large internal laryngocoele causing airway obstruction requires a careful technique for induction of anaesthesia and intubation. The ventricle is always examined endoscopically to rule out any possible hidden primary pathology. An internal laryngocoele can usually be treated endoscopically if wide visualization of the supraglottic larynx can be obtained through a large-diameter laryngoscope (Fig. 15.10). Mucosa covering the prominence of the cyst is incised and reflected. Combined laser and cold instrument dissection is painstakingly carried out until either a large part of the cyst is exposed or the cyst wall is breached. As much of the wall as possible is removed to marsupialize the cyst, which is left open to heal. Persistent recurrences may need external operation.

An external operation at the level of the thyrohyoid membrane allows an external laryngocoele to be dissected out and followed through the thyrohyoid membrane, taking care to preserve the superior laryngeal nerve. If necessary, part of the upper portion of one side of the thyroid cartilage is removed to reach the internal component which is freed from the deep substance of the aryepiglottic fold and false cord. Thus, combined external and internal laryngocoeles require external surgical removal via a lateral thyrotomy approach.

Histologically, the wall of the cyst is lined with ciliated or columnar epithelium with a fibrous wall. Squamous metaplasia may be seen in places or may even completely replace the respiratory epithelium in an infected cyst.

Laryngopyocoele is treated initially by incision, drainage, and intravenous antibiotic therapy. After infection is totally controlled, surgical excision is undertaken.

DUCTAL RETENTION CYSTS

The non-specific terms ‘retention cyst’ or ‘inclusion cyst’ are in common use. However, ‘ductal cyst’ seems to be a more appropriate term because the lining is usually ductal epithelium. Other cysts originate from minor salivary glands. Ductal cysts can occur anywhere submucosal mucus-producing glands are found, thus being common in the valleculae, the lateral surface of the epiglottis and the supraglottic larynx, but they are rare in the vocal folds which normally have no mucous glands. The cysts contain mucus in dilated collecting ducts and whether large or small the cystic swellings are usually superficial, often projecting into the lumen.

In infants, especially preterm babies who have been intubated for a long time, ductal retention cysts occur

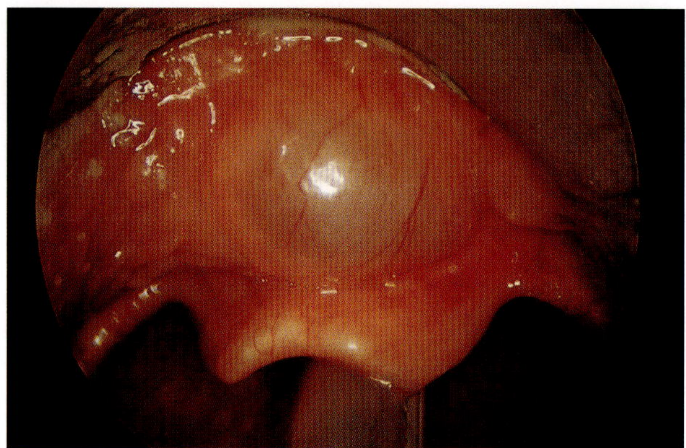

Figure **15.12**
'Vallecular cyst'. Distended, large, rounded, thin-walled retention cyst.

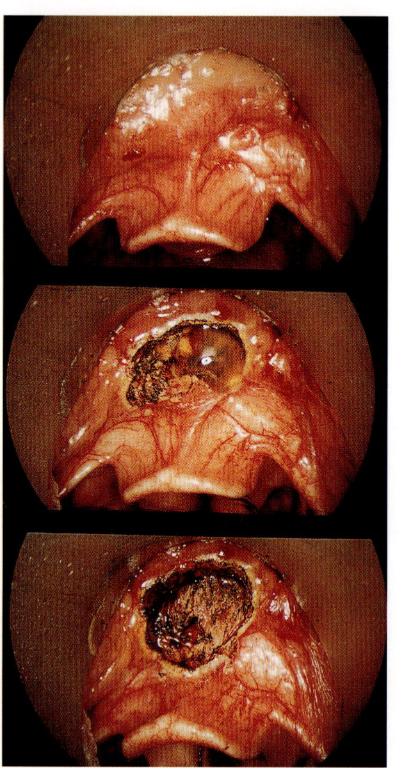

Figure **15.13**
Laser treatment. Vallecular cyst 'removed' five times at another hospital. Wide removal into muscle, using the laser, with no further recurrences.

mostly in the subglottic region (Fig. 15.11) and sometimes in the upper trachea or supraglottic tissues. They are directly related to mucosal trauma during prolonged intubation (see chapter 12 for intubation injuries of the larynx).

'Vallecular cysts' occur on one side or sometimes near the midline at the base of the tongue anterior to the epiglottis (Fig. 15.12), and as most cysts are large with a broad base they can easily be seen at indirect laryngoscopy; occasionally they are discovered by an anaesthetist performing translaryngeal intubation.

A mucus-containing cyst on or in the vocal fold can usually be differentiated from an intracordal epidermoid cyst as a unilateral, translucent, greyish, superficial, rounded swelling. The contents are a clear or greyish colour.

Cysts in the pharynx, supraglottic larynx, subglottis, or upper trachea are treated by removal or by marsupialization using forceps and scissors or the carbon dioxide laser (Fig. 15.13). The site should be re-examined later for possible recurrence.

CYSTIC HYGROMA

Pathogenesis

Lymphangioma is an uncommon endodermal anomaly of lymphatic vessels generally considered to be a congenital disorder. Lymphangiomas have been classified by Batsakis (1979) into three morphologic groups:

- lymphangioma simplex, consisting of capillary-sized lymphatic vessels
- cavernous lymphangioma, composed of dilated lymphatic spaces
- cystic lymphangioma or cystic hygroma containing cystic spaces from a few millimetres to several centimetres in size.

Sometimes combinations of patterns coexist. In the loose, clearly definable fascial planes of the neck the endothelial-lined spaces of cystic hygroma expand freely and insinuate themselves among muscles, vessels and nerve trunks in an invasive pattern that makes complete excision impossible. There is no malignant potential.

Classification of lymphangiomas

Lymphangioma simplex
Cavernous lymphangioma
Cystic lymphangioma (hygroma)

When abnormal blood vessels occur with the lymphatic vessels the anomaly is known as lymphangiohaemangioma.

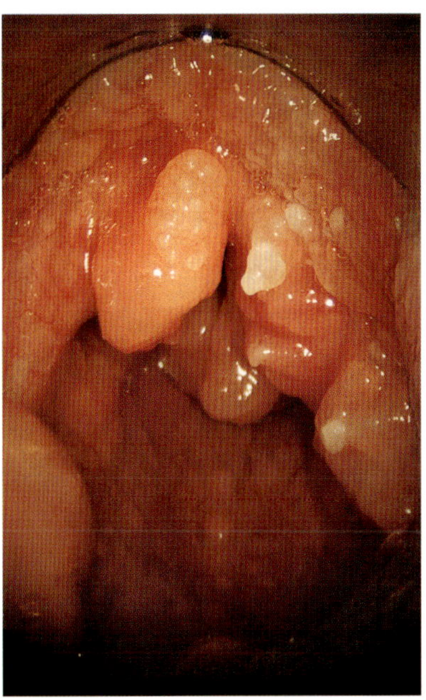

Figure **15.14**
Cystic hygroma in the larynx. Primary supraglottic, irregular mass, causing partial obstruction. No lesion in face or neck.

Clinical features

Large cystic hygromas are obvious at birth, while others become prominent in the first year or two as the cystic spaces fill with fluid, or increase rapidly in size because of spontaneous bleeding. Most occur in the soft tissues of the neck and face as a diffuse, compressible, smooth, non-tender mass that transilluminates. Involvement of the larynx is usually secondary to the external mass. Primary cases confined to the larynx (Fig. 15.14) are very rare.

Clinical features include cosmetic distortion of the neck and/or face, speech problems, difficulty swallowing, regurgitation and choking, cyanosis or respiratory distress and stridor. Small cystic hygromas may be asymptomatic but large masses cause deformity as they stretch or compress tissues of the neck, pharynx and larynx (Fig. 15.15) or, by virtue of their size and position, produce airway obstruction. They have a tendency to become larger as lymph accumulates following upper respiratory tract infection or bleeding and, if the laryngopharyngeal internal segment becomes distended, airway obstruction can occur. Cystic hygromas usually have no natural tendency to involution and are not self-limiting. They may become progressively larger, regress or even apparently spontaneously disappear in exceptional cases.

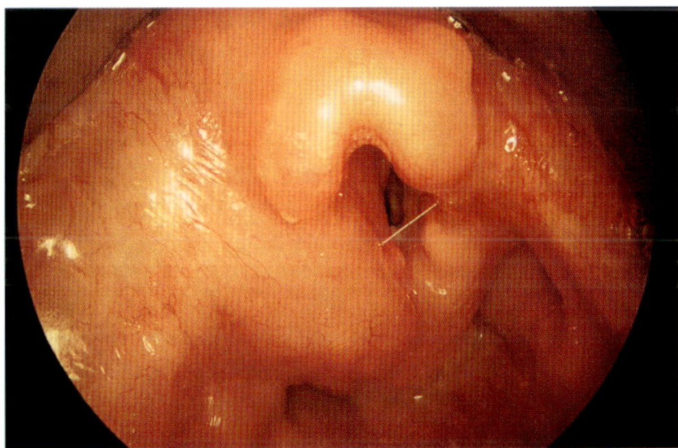

Figure **15.15**
Obstructive cystic hygroma. Large lesion, part of larger face and neck cystic hygroma.

Treatment

Treatment is often frustrating. Surgical removal is necessary for larger cosmetically deforming lesions or for those causing alimentary and respiratory obstruction.

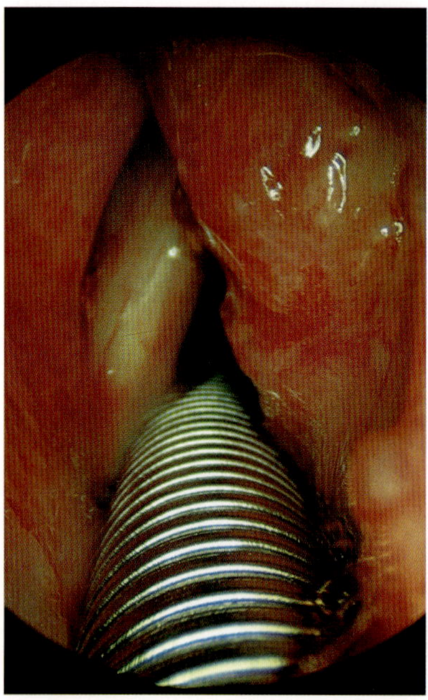

Figure **15.16**
Laser treatment. Cystic hygroma about to be treated with carbon dioxide laser. Note the laser-proof anaesthetic tube.

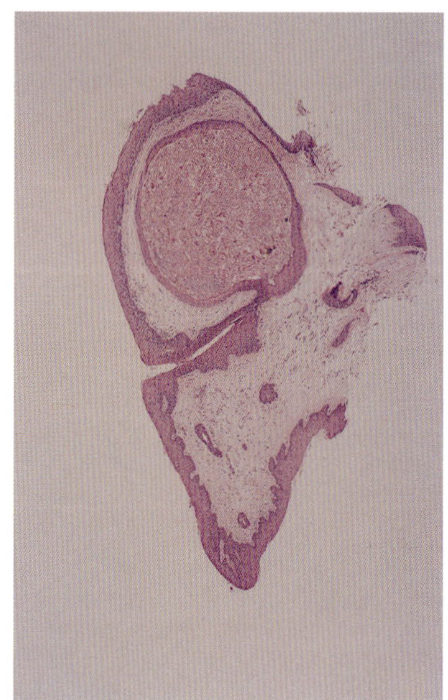

Figure **15.17**
Epidermoid cyst and vocal sulcus. Coronal cross-section of operative specimen showing association of round epidermoid cyst and vocal sulcus.

Tracheotomy may be necessary either for airway obstruction or to allow one or more staged operations to remove not only the major primary mass in the neck but also the lymphangiomatous tissue in the laryngopharynx. When considering the diagnosis, note that cystic hygroma occurs as a supraglottic mass whereas congenital haemangioma causing airway obstruction in infants is almost always subglottic.

Treatment of cystic hygromas

- Sometimes no treatment necessary
- Surgery is often frustrating
- Staged removal of large neck and face lesions
- Laser reduction of internal obstructive lesions

Sometimes serial laser excision of supraglottic cystic hygroma tissue (Fig. 15.16) will be necessary to relieve airway obstruction; the laser is the ideal instrument to remove the tissue by vaporization as there is usually no appreciable bleeding. More than one removal is usually necessary. The aims of surgery are both relief of obstruction and a satisfactory cosmetic appearance.

Transcutaneous needle aspiration of tense, distended cystic spaces may be helpful when a sudden increase in cyst size threatens airway compromise. Radiation therapy is contraindicated, and the use of various sclerosing agents has had little success.

INTRACORDAL CYST, GLOTTIC SULCUS AND MUCOSAL BRIDGE OF THE VOCAL FOLD

These benign disorders are discussed together because they are on or in the edge of the vocal fold

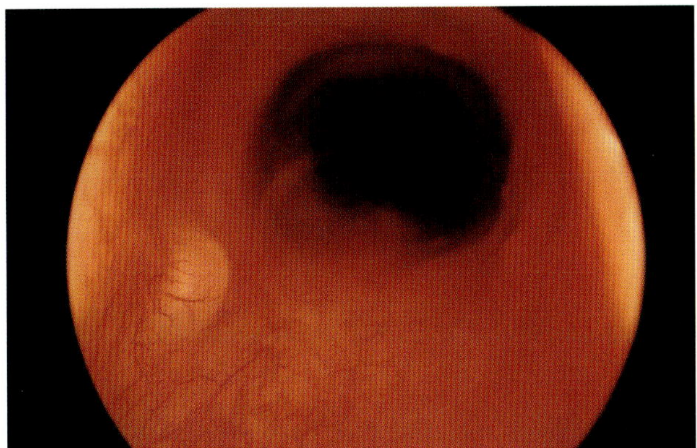

Figure **15.18**
Subglottic ductal retention cyst. Single, small, superficial subglottic cyst caused by prolonged intubation in an infant.

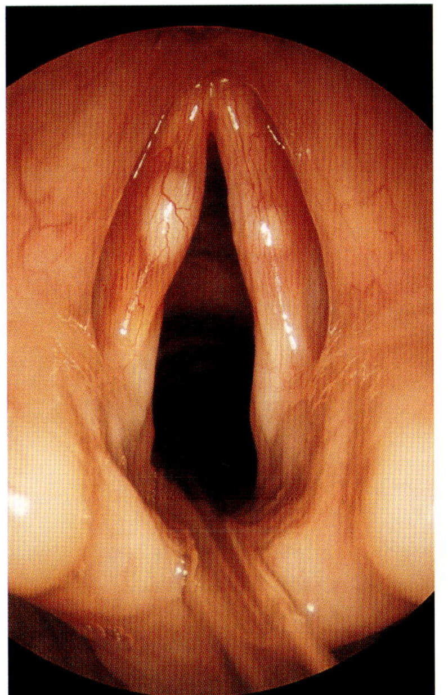

Figure **15.19**
Bilateral intracordal cysts. The appearance should not be confused with vocal nodules.

and sometimes occur together, e.g. an epidermoid cyst can occur with glottic sulcus (Fig. 15.17) or mucosal bridge with glottic sulcus.

Intracordal cyst

A cyst in the vocal fold can be either an epidermoid cyst or a mucous retention cyst.

An intracordal epidermoid cyst is lined by several layers of epithelium. Desquamated keratin and glittering, milky, turbid contents with cholesterol crystals accumulate in the cavity. The cyst is in a submucosal plane in the vocal fold, superficial or deep, depending on its size and site. Sometimes there is surrounding chronic inflammatory reaction with adhesions to the overlying epithelium or to the vocal ligament.

A mucous retention (or ductal) cyst arises when the duct of a mucous gland becomes obstructed and secretions accumulate, but such a cyst is uncommon as the vocal fold has few mucous glands. Ductal cysts are much more likely to occur in the subglottic region in preterm infants after prolonged intubation (Fig. 15.18) or in older patients in the supraglottis or pharynx.

Pathogenesis

There are two theories of the origin of epidermoid cysts. The congenital theory supposes they arise from buried epithelial cell rests which slowly become larger and clinically important in later years. The second theory suggests that they are acquired during healing of injured mucosa, supposing that buried epithelial cells form an epidermoid cyst. It has been suggested that rupture of a cyst forms a vocal sulcus.

Clinical features

The presenting symptom is chronic, slowly progressive hoarseness, often accompanied by vocal hyperfunction, occasionally presenting in childhood, sometimes in teenage, but usually presenting in adults. Some patients have been diagnosed as, or even operated on, for what was described as a 'polyp' or a 'nodule', the true nature of the pathology having been unrecognized. Bilateral cysts (Fig. 15.19) are easily confused with vocal nodules.

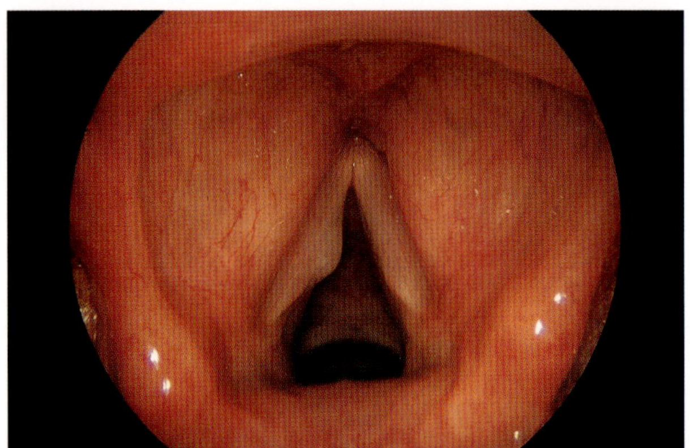

Figure **15.20**
Epidermoid cyst. Indirect laryngoscopy. Superficial epidermoid cyst which can be easily recognized in the central part of the left vocal fold.

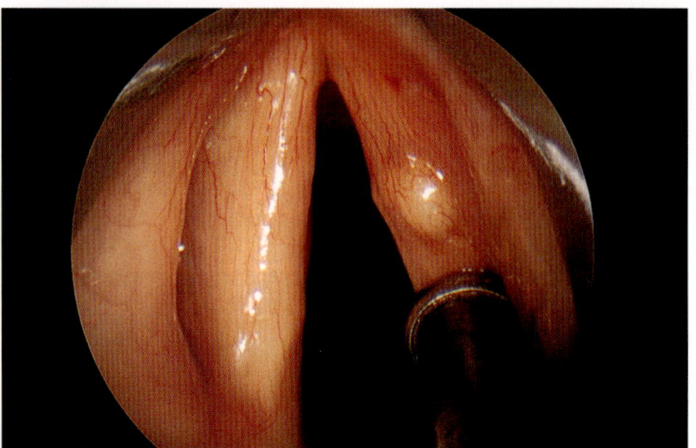

Figure **15.21**
Epidermoid cyst. Direct laryngoscopy. Right cyst bulging the upper surface of the centre of the vocal fold, made more prominent by depressing the vocal fold with the sucker.

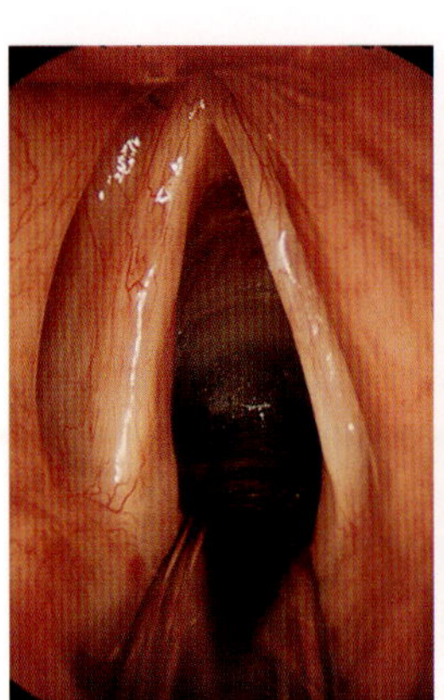

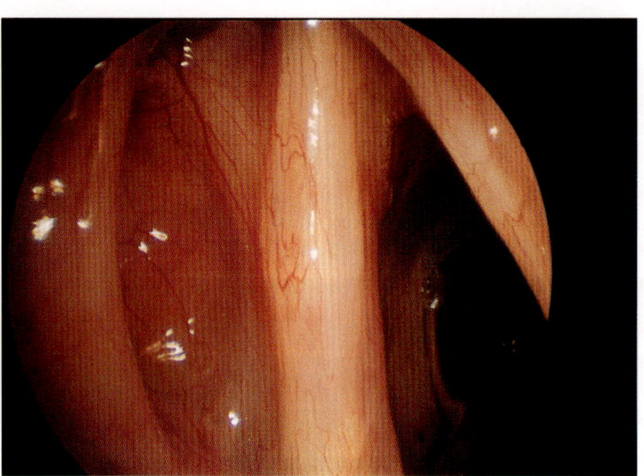

Figure **15.22**
Epidermoid cyst. Under general anaesthesia a fusiform swelling in the left vocal fold indicates a submucosal cyst (left) more easily recognized with a 30° telescope (right).

Indirect laryngoscopy

Indirect laryngoscopy usually confirms the diagnosis of intracordal cyst with reasonable confidence (Fig. 15.20) but a small cyst or a cyst deep in the vocal fold may be seen only as an ill-defined fusiform swelling on one side, with an adynamic mucosal segment on stroboscopic examination. There may be minor reactionary vascularity and oedema on the opposite vocal fold. The diagnosis is obvious when a superficial or large whitish-yellow epidermoid cyst bulges the upper surface or edge of the vocal fold in its middle third (Fig. 15.21). In cases where doubt exists, diagnosis can be confirmed only by close inspection at direct laryngoscopy, and even then an incision in the upper surface of the vocal fold with dissection to expose the wall of the cyst may be necessary for final diagnosis (Fig. 15.22).

Epidermoid cysts are usually large, ovoid, yellow, sometimes bilateral and affect the voice more than mucous retention cysts which are small, grey and unilateral.

Small mucous cysts distend the vocal fold, may be sausage-shaped, and lie longitudinally in the subepithelial space superficial to the vocal ligament. They usually contain opaque or thick fluid in contrast to the yellowish, milky or glistening (cholesterol crystals) fluid in an epidermoid cyst.

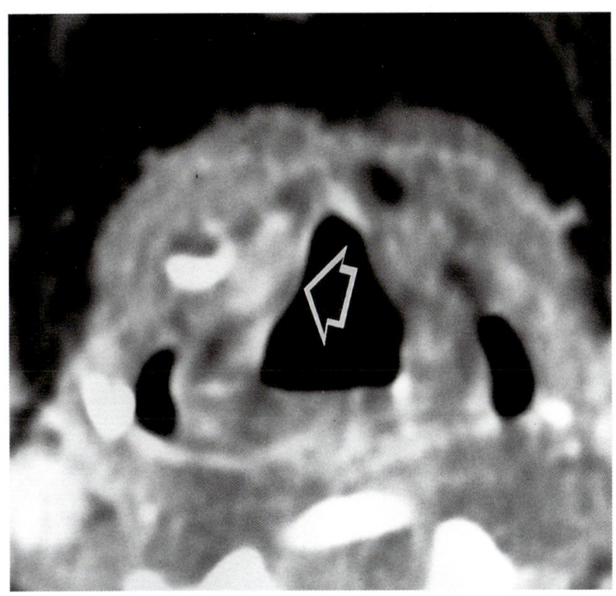

Figure **15.23**
Right intracordal cyst. CT scan performed by referring specialist shows mass (arrow) deep in the right vocal fold.

CT scan (Fig. 15.23) will show a large lesion but is not a necessary investigation.

Treatment

Voice therapy cannot correct the problem but may be useful in the postoperative period. Surgical excision is necessary.

Operative removal requires good exposure, preferably using a laryngoscope whose beak will push the false cord to one side to expose the upper surface of the vocal fold (Fig. 15.24).

Adrenaline 1 : 200 000 can be injected in the vocal fold around the cyst using a 28 gauge laryngeal infusion needle. A short, shallow, linear incision is made on the upper surface of the fold just lateral to the cyst using a knife or a laser with a small-diameter cutting spot (Fig. 15.24). Careful dissection is carried down to the wall of the cyst to confirm its nature. The mucosal cover is elevated medially from the cyst which is delicately dissected free and almost 'shelled out', keeping the medial mucosal edge of the vocal fold intact. When the cyst is superficial or the mucosa is attached to the cyst, the edge of the vocal fold may inevitably be traumatized. Laterally, the vocal ligament and the vocalis muscle are preserved unless previous inflammation has caused adhesions. The overlying mucosa, undamaged as far as possible, is redraped along the superior surface of the vocal fold; trimming of excess mucosa or suturing is seldom necessary. The opposite cord is examined to exclude the possibility of bilateral cyst formation.

Results of treatment

Larger cysts are sometimes partly adherent to the vocal ligament or even push into the vocalis muscle so that some surgical trauma is inevitable. Postoperatively, the vocal fold may be hyperaemic and slightly oedematous for weeks or months, and vocal

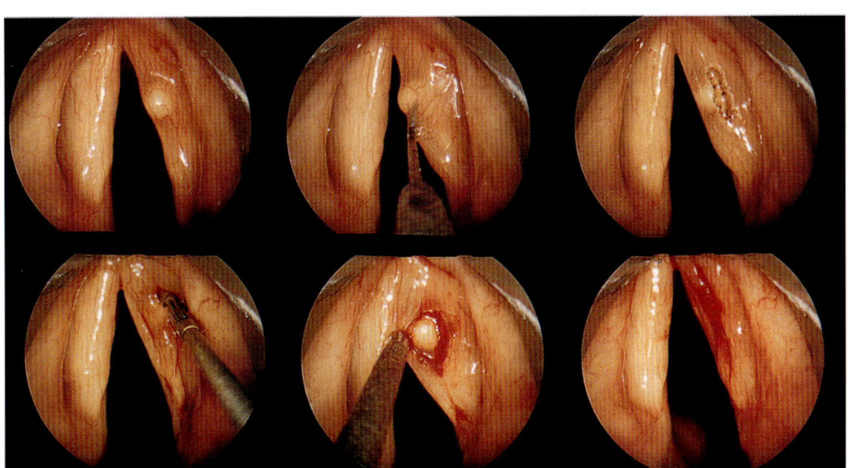

Figure **15.24**
Microdissection of cyst. Steps in removal of the cyst shown in Fig. 15.23. Mucosal incision, dissection and removal, preserving the vocal ligament and membranous edge of the vocal fold.

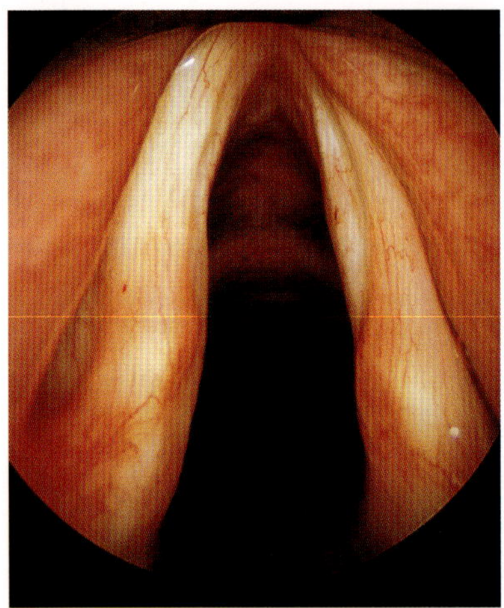

Figure **15.25**
Bilateral vocal sulci. Longitudinal furrow grooving the right and left vocal folds.

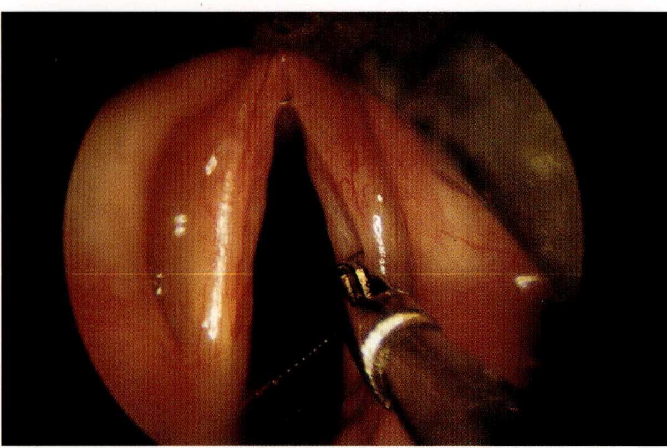

Figure **15.26**
Vocal sulcus. An angled, cupped forceps has been used to probe and palpate the abnormality which was bilateral Type 2 sulcus.

fold stiffness can be recognized on stroboscopic examination.

Some patients regain an excellent voice after cyst removal but others continue to have minor dysphonia and fatiguability of the voice. The mucosal wave may not return fully.

Glottic sulcus

Also known as vocal sulcus, sulcus vocalis and 'reduplication' of the vocal cord. Vocal sulcus is an epithelium-lined linear groove or furrow in the edge of a vocal fold. It is commonly bilateral (Fig. 15.25).

Pathogenesis

There is disagreement on whether vocal sulci are congenital or acquired. The spindle-shaped linear depression along the medial edge of the vocal fold or both vocal folds is occasionally seen in children, but more often in adults and sometimes associated with 'bowed' vocal cords in older patients. Bouchayer et al (1985) point out that sulci may be congenital anomalies derived from the 4th and 6th branchial arch, possibly explaining why cysts, sulci and mucosal bridges can be associated with one another. Support for a congenital origin includes the fact that symptoms may start in childhood, sulci occur in patients with no history of voice abuse or laryngitis and sulci do not recur after adequate treatment. Familial occurrence has been described.

The acquired hypothesis is supported by the fact that glottic sulcus patients often present in adulthood and that oedema and inflammation sometimes surround the lesion.

Clinical features

The patients, whether children, adolescents or adults, complain of chronic hoarseness. They may have seen other consultants without the correct diagnosis being made. Sulci can often be diagnosed at indirect laryngoscopy, taking advantage of the brightly lit, magnified image obtained with a large-diameter telescope. Sometimes there is associated bowing of the vocal folds or oedematous fusiform swelling of the margins.

In some patients sulci are recognized only after careful examination and palpation at microlaryngoscopy (Fig. 15.26). One suspects that some cases of vocal sulcus are labelled 'chronic laryngitis' because the generalized bilateral vocal fold oedema seen at indirect examination does not appear to warrant microlaryngoscopy. In other cases the diagnosis will be suspected at indirect examination

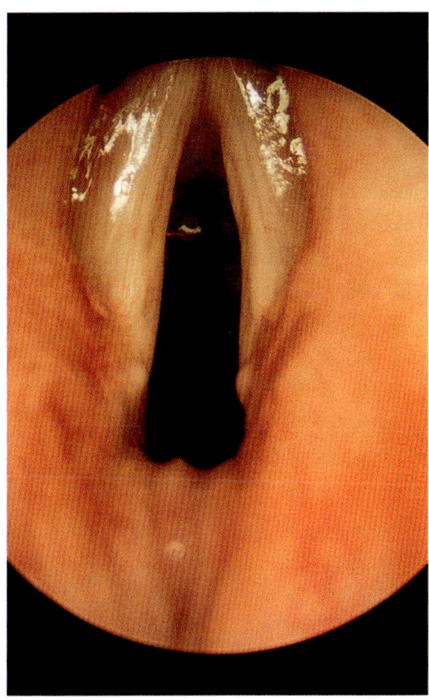

Figure **15.27**
Bilateral vocal sulci at direct laryngoscopy.

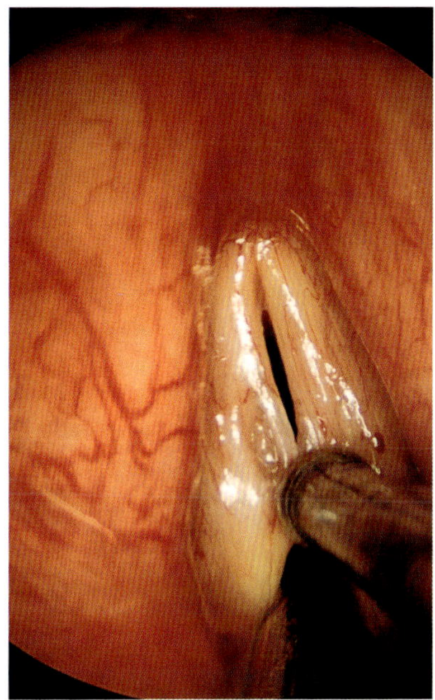

Figure **15.28**
Vocal sulcus. Type 3 deep sulcus causing severe dysphonia.

and vibratory changes will be seen under stroboscopic examination.

Treatment

Vocal therapy alone will not resolve the symptoms.

Microlaryngoscopy allows confirmation of the diagnosis and assessment of its severity. Ford et al (1996) point out that sulcus vocalis is a spectrum of disorders from minor vocal fold indentation to destructive lesions causing severe dysphonia. They propose:

- Type 1, or physiological, sulcus (Fig. 15.27) occurring in individuals who have essentially normal voices; the sulcus is recognized on videostroboscopy during phonation.
- Type 2 sulcus patients (Fig. 15.26) have dysphonia, vocal fold oedema, capillary dilatation, vibratory disturbance and are consistent with Bouchayer et al's (1985) description of 'sulcus vergeture'. Histologically, there is epithelial thinning, loss of lamina propria structure and adherence of the epithelium to the intermediate and deep layers of the lamina propria, i.e. the vocal ligament.
- Type 3 sulcus vocalis patients have severe dysphonia, there are deep sulci (Fig. 15.28) with pathologic alteration of the vocal fold. This is the most specific pathologic sulcus designation. Histologically, Type 3 sulcus may be associated with an epidermoid cyst (Fig. 15.17) or there may be intense inflammation with neovascularization and fibrosis involving the vocal ligament. The loss of separation of the epithelial cover from the vocal ligament causes severe dysphonia because of vocal fold stiffness and incomplete glottic closure.

Pathologic Type 2 and Type 3 sulci can be treated by microsurgery although voice improvement may not be optimal.

Sulci have been treated with collagen injections, medialization thyroplasty and, more recently, by direct surgical intervention to remove diseased tissue and to separate the covering epithelium from the vocal

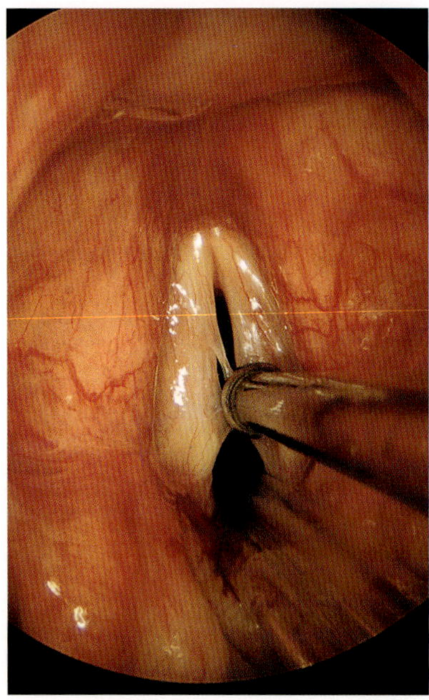

Figure **15.29**
Mucosal bridge. Gentle separation using a sucker for traction.

ligament by freeing mucosal attachments and breaking up linear contractions. After infusion of the cord edge by saline injection or 1 : 200 000 adrenaline to spread the lips of the sulcus, upper and lower antero-posterior incisions are made to circumcise the lips and dissect the adherent mucosa without injury to the vocal ligament, thus peeling away the invaginated pocket of the sulcus through the elongated elliptical incisions (Ford et al, 1996).

More advanced Type 3 sulci are adherent to the vocal ligament and sometimes involve the vocalis muscle. They may require operation as described by Ford et al (1996) by incision, undermining and sectioning (slicing). The sulcus is dissected away from the underlying vocal ligament, breaking down adhesions and four or five vertical incisions are made to produce three or four mucosal segments, each incision a different length to discourage linear contractions. This difficult microsurgery is designed to remove destroyed tissue, release scar contracture and promote mucosal redraping.

Mucosal bridge

In very rare cases a glottic sulcus may be hidden by a mucosal bridge, a strip of epithelialized tissue, entirely separate from the edge of the vocal fold except at the anterior and the posterior ends (Figs 15.29, 15.30) which are attached near the anterior commissure and in front of the vocal process. A blunt instrument or a probe inserted gently under the bridge can display its complete separation from the edge of the vocal fold which is itself intact. Treatment is complete removal by detachment of both the

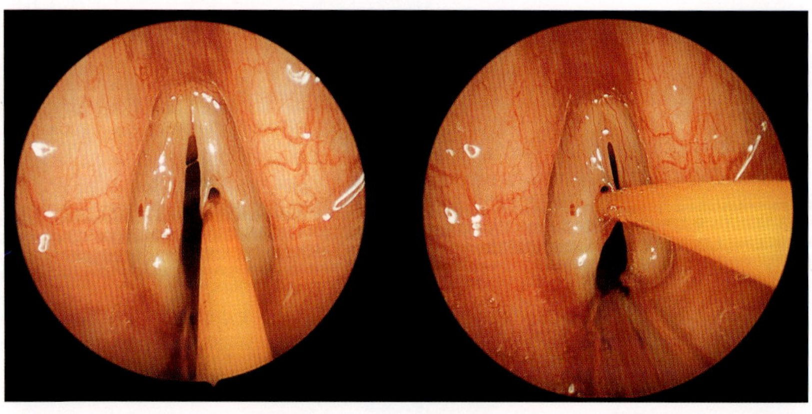

Figure **15.30**
Bilateral mucosal bridges.

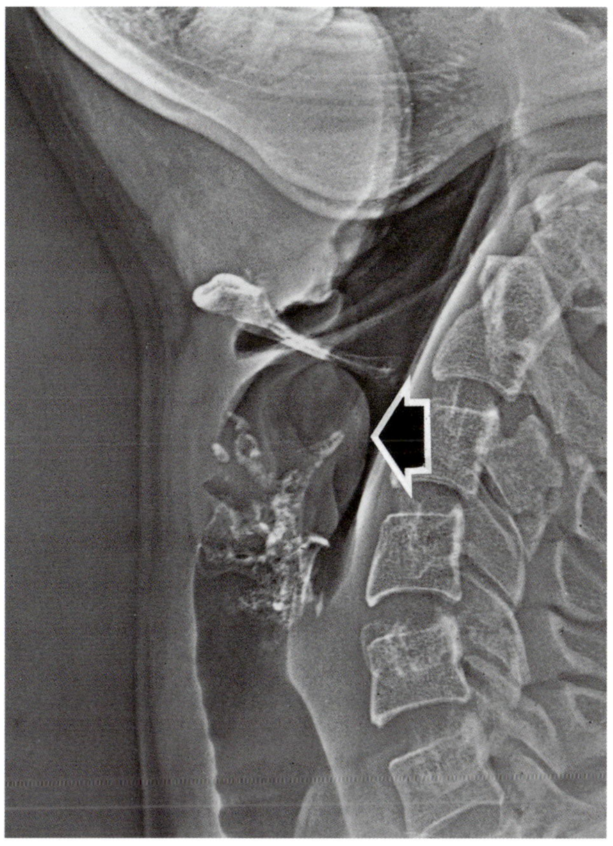

(a)

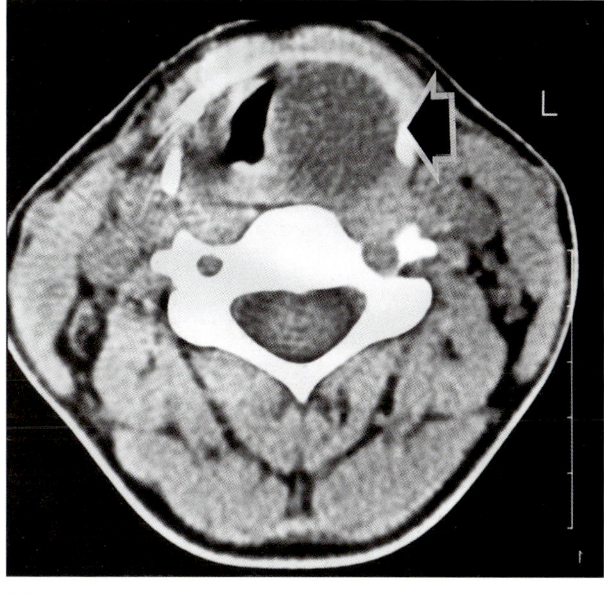

(b)

Figure **15.31**
Very rare developmental cyst. (a) Lateral xerogram and (b) CT of developmental cyst (arrows) of the internal perichondrium of the thyroid cartilage which caused intermittent laryngeal obstruction.

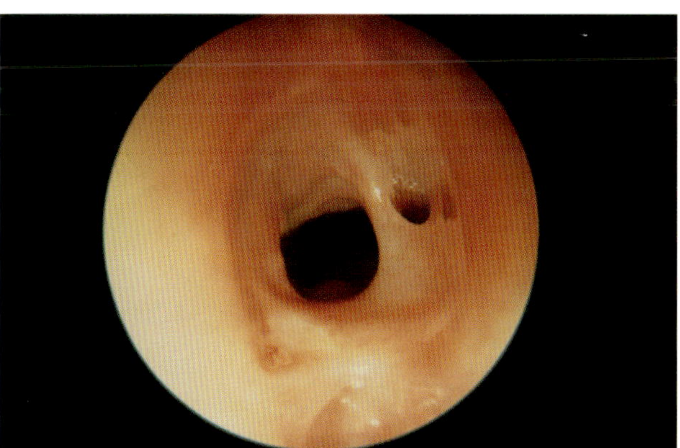

Figure **15.32**
Subglottic duplication cyst. Endoscopic view of slit-like opening on the right, in the subglottic region of an infant with intermittent stridor.

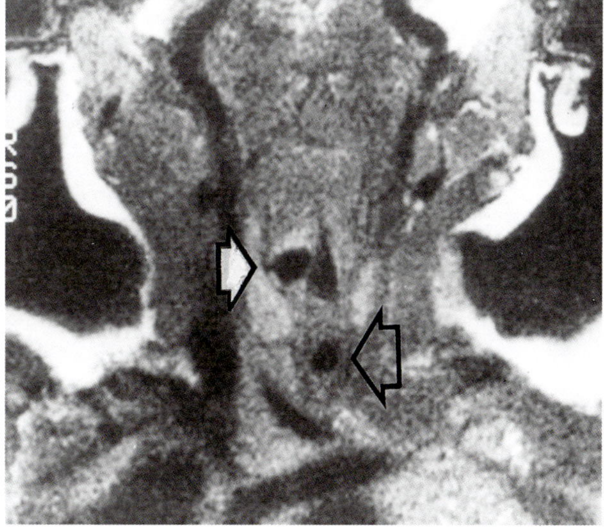

Figure **15.33**
Subglottic duplication cyst. MRI of same patient (Fig. 15.32) showing air-containing cyst (upper arrow) and tracheostome (lower arrow). Removed via external neck incision at 12 months of age.

anterior and the posterior end. Histologically, the bridge has a central core of connective tissue covered by stratified squamous epithelium.

The laryngologist must be careful to identify a sulcus which may be associated with a mucosal bridge.

RARE DEVELOPMENTAL CYSTS

Other cysts are encountered very rarely, e.g. a developmental cyst from the perichondrium lining the thyroid cartilage (Fig. 15.31) or an interesting duplication cyst of the subglottic region (Figs 15.32, 15.33).

BIBLIOGRAPHY

Batsakis JG (1979) *Tumours of the head and neck: clinical and pathological considerations*, 2nd edn (Baltimore: Williams and Wilkins); 221–4.

Bouchayer M, Cornut G, Witzig E, et al (1985) Epidermoid cysts, sulci and mucosal bridges of the true vocal cord: a report of 157 cases. *Laryngoscope* **95**: 1087–94.

Civantos FJ, Holinger LD (1992) Laryngocele and saccular cysts in infants and children. *Arch Otolaryngol Head Neck Surg* **118**: 296–303.

De Santo LW (1974) Laryngocele, laryngeal mucocele, large saccules and large saccular cysts; a developmental spectrum. *Laryngoscope* **84**: 1291–6.

Ford CN, Inagi K, Bless DM, et al (1996) Sulcus vocalis: a rational analytical approach to diagnosis and management. *Ann Otol Rhinol Laryngol* **105**: 189–200.

Holinger LD, Barnes DR, Smid LJ (1978) Laryngocele and saccular cysts. *Ann Otol Rhinol Laryngol* **87**: 675–82.

16 Haemangiomas

CLASSIFICATION

Haemangiomas in the larynx are of two types: adult and paediatric. According to the size of the vascular spaces and the microscopic appearance they can be further classified as capillary or cavernous:

- the adult type is typically glottic or supraglottic and usually cavernous;
- the paediatric congenital type is almost always subglottic and usually capillary.

Congenital haemangiomas often exhibit increased mitotic activity and rapid postnatal growth which are later followed by steady involution after 6–12 months.

Although haemangiomas are benign they can have serious life-threatening complications, such as bleeding in adults or airway obstruction in infants.

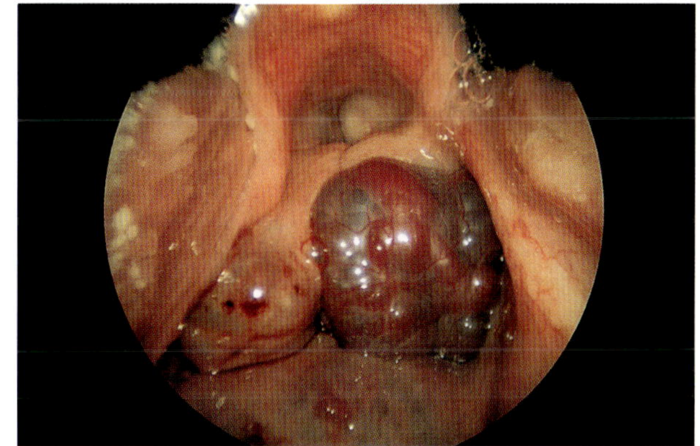

Figure **16.1**
Large cavernous malformation in an adult. Situated in the piriform fossa, postcricoid and right supraglottic region, this malformation had required tracheotomy and had already been unsuccessfully treated by attempted embolization and radiotherapy. Three staged treatments with direct injection of sclerosant gave an excellent response.

ADULT HAEMANGIOMAS

Diagnosis

Diagnosis in adults is more difficult than in infants because the location and size of the tumour are variable and the clinical features are non-specific. The haemangioma occasionally arises on a vocal cord but is usually in the supraglottic tissues or outside the larynx (Fig. 16.1), in the piriform fossa (Fig. 16.2) or postcricoid region. They occur in males much more often than females. Small vascular masses on a vocal fold may interfere with vibration and cause a husky voice – the histopathologist might confuse this lesion

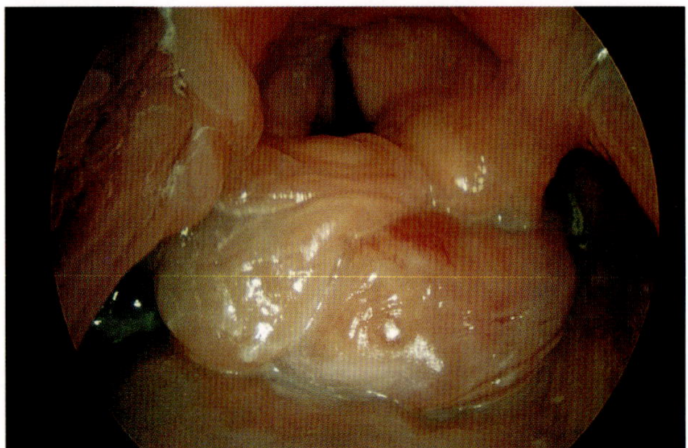

Figure **16.2**
Mixed cavernous and capillary malformation in an adult. Good response to injection of sclerosant as primary treatment.

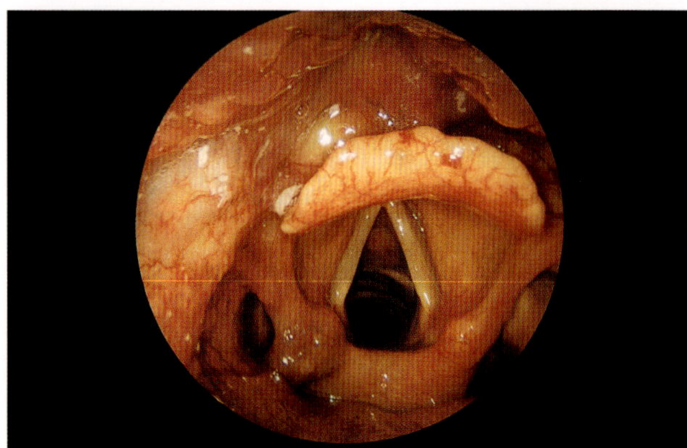

Figure **16.3**
Small lesion of the left arytenoid region. Indirect laryngoscopy. This small vascular malformation found in an elderly woman was asymptomatic. No observed change in 2 years.

with a vocal nodule in a vascular stage, but clinically vocal nodules are bilateral. Larger cavernous haemangiomas or vascular malformations can cause airway obstruction, dysphagia, the sensation of a lump and sometimes bleeding. Usually the diagnosis can be made by the appearance and confirmed by contrast angiography, which may be followed by therapeutic embolization in suitable cases.

In atypical cases biopsy might be necessary, with due respect for the bleeding potential. Localized haemangioma enhances on contrast CT and on MRI it has a fairly high T2W signal intensity.

Management of adult haemangiomas

No treatment for minimal symptoms
Endoscopic removal, laser or cold surgery
Selective arterial embolization
Sclerosant injection
Pharyngotomy, surgical removal

Treatment

Vascular lesions in adults causing no symptoms (Fig. 16.3) or minimal symptoms need no treatment but should be observed. The treatment options for symptomatic lesions depend on the site, size and vascular configuration on angiography:

- endoscopic removal with conventional instrument or the laser, e.g. lesions on the vocal fold;
- selective arterial embolization, e.g. large lesions with one or two feeding vessels;
- direct injection of sclerosant, e.g. large cavernous lesions;
- pharyngotomy, e.g. very large lesions requiring surgical control of the vascular supply.

Other forms of treatment which have been used include radiotherapy, cryosurgery and Nd-YAG laser. A tracheotomy might be required to relieve airway obstruction, allow safe anaesthesia and provide good endoscopic exposure during treatment. Laser treatment of large lesions, whether with the CO_2, argon or Nd-YAG laser, is often complicated by severe bleeding from cavernous spaces.

INFANTILE HAEMANGIOMAS

Haemangiomas are the commonest laryngeal tumours in infants. They are considered congenital abnormalities which represent cellular proliferation from mesodermal nests of vasoformative tissue. In most anatomic sites, such as the soft tissues of the face, neck or trunk, they can be managed conservatively, awaiting slow involution in the first 2–5 years of life, but narrowing of the subglottic and upper tracheal airway threatening serious obstruction requires treatment to avoid asphyxiation.

Pathology

Obstructive haemangiomas in the larynx are consistently subglottic or sometimes upper tracheal. They develop in the submucosa and follow a typical growth pattern with increasing size causing progressive clinical features usually within the first 8–12 weeks of life. Symptoms very seldom start from birth. A review of autopsy cases by Brodsky et al (1983) showed that haemangiomas sometimes extend into the perichondrium and even into the surrounding tissue planes between the tracheal rings or beyond the trachea. This explains the reason for regrowth after treatment directed solely at the subglottic component. A solitary subglottic mass is much more common than multicentric or diffuse lesions. The majority are of the capillary type with vascular spaces surrounded by endothelial cells.

Clinical features

The clinical features include stridor (intermittent at first, then persistent), harsh barking cough and failure to thrive. In about half the patients there is an associated cutaneous haemangioma of the head, face or neck strongly suggesting the diagnosis. An erroneous diagnosis of 'croup' may be made at first. Females are affected twice as often as males. The degree of airway obstruction may increase during periods of agitation, crying and with respiratory tract infections. An haemangioma with a large mediastinal component may cause tracheal compression with retained secretions.

Features of infantile haemangioma

- Subglottic, usually capillary type
- Unilateral, bilateral or circumferential
- Intermittent, then persistent stridor
- 50% have cutaneous haemangioma
- More common in females
- Usually demonstrated on X-ray
- Diagnosed at direct laryngoscopy
- Biopsy seldom necessary

Radiological appearance

Antero-posterior soft tissue studies usually show asymmetric changes consistent with a unilateral soft tissue mass and lateral films often show a sharply defined posterior mass protruding into the subglottic airway (Fig. 16.4). CT with contrast may not only show the subglottic mass but occasionally also soft tissue enhancement in the paraglottic space or in the neck.

Direct laryngoscopy

The appearance of the mass at direct laryngoscopy under general anaesthesia is usually sufficiently characteristic for an experienced observer to make a diagnosis without biopsy, especially when there is an associated cutaneous haemangioma. The subglottic swelling is usually well demarcated, smooth, either pink, red or of slightly bluish appearance, localized in the subglottic region on one side (Fig. 16.5), on both sides (Fig. 16.6) or with a posterior subglottic extension (Fig. 16.7). Sometimes there is a discrete obstructive mass below the subglottis in the upper

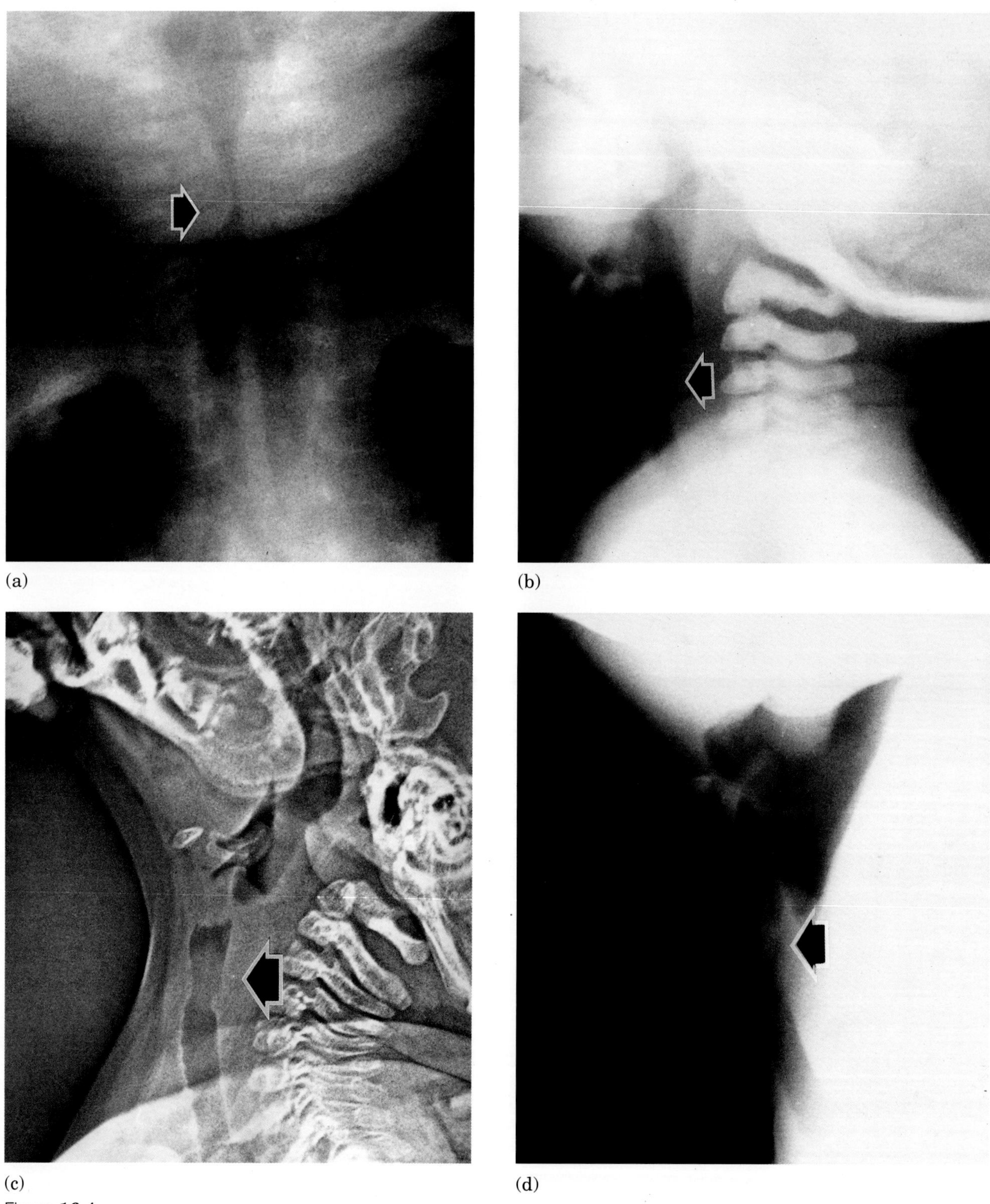

Figure **16.4**

Radiologic appearance of subglottic haemangiomas in infants. a. Antero-posterior X-ray showing rounded, unilateral subglottic swelling (arrow). b. Lateral X-ray with large posterior subglottic soft tissue mass (arrow). c. Lateral xerogram shows upper tracheal lesion (arrow). d. Atypical lobulated, pedunculate mass (arrow) which arose from right supraglottic tissues.

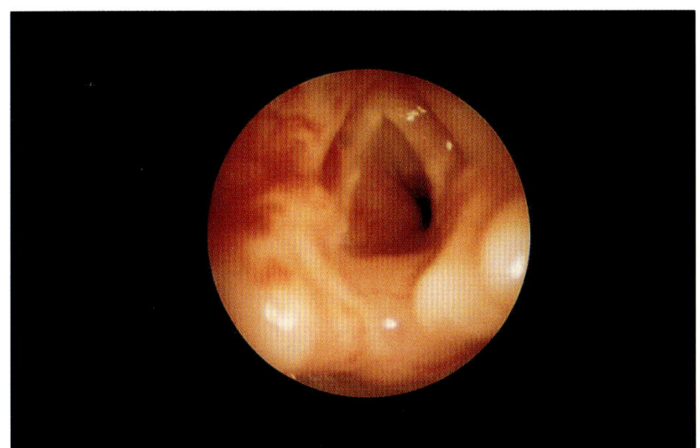

Figure **16.5**
Unilateral subglottic haemangioma. Typical appearance of unilateral subglottic haemangioma which may be amenable to staged laser vaporization.

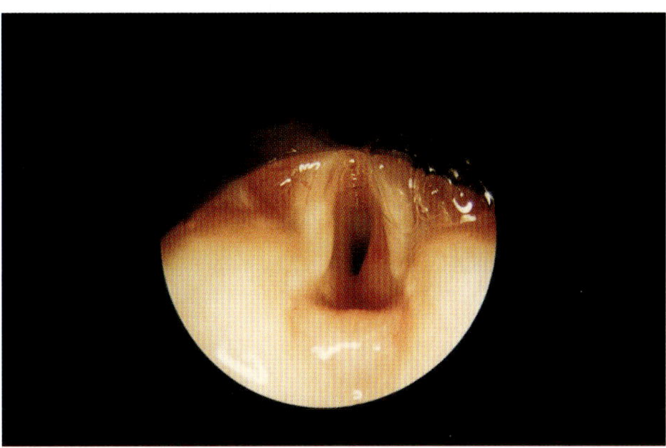

Figure **16.6**
Bilateral subglottic haemangioma. Left and right lesions. Single radioactive platinum-coated gold grain in the left side brought about shrinkage of both sides.

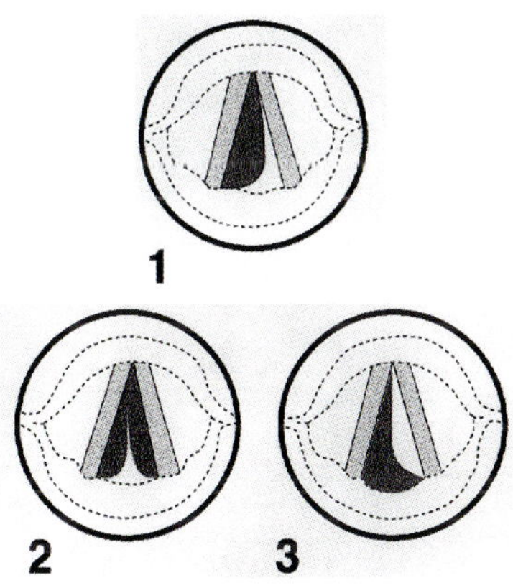

Figure **16.7**
Anatomical classification according to site: 1, unilateral; 2, bilateral; 3, unilateral with posterior extension.

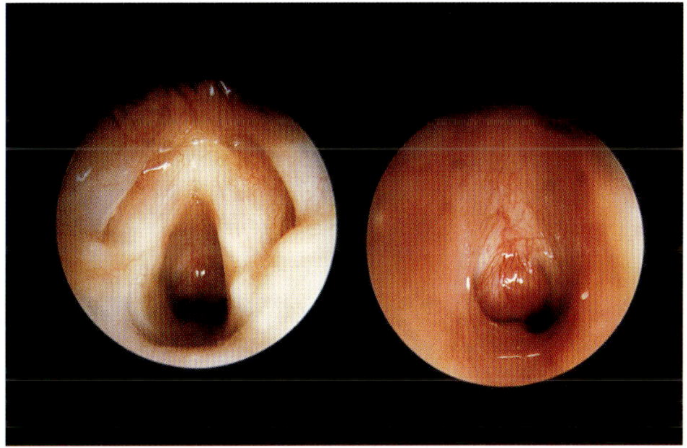

Figure **16.8**
Upper tracheal haemangioma. Situated just below the subglottis (left). An obvious vascular malformation (right). Surgical removal through a neck incision, with postoperative pernasal intubation for 3 days; a tracheotomy was not necessary.

trachea (Fig. 16.8). Biopsy is usually unnecessary but may be performed in atypical cases or if the diagnosis is in doubt. In the unlikely event of excessive bleeding, precautions are taken to maintain the airway.

The degree of airway obstruction and the form of treatment to be used indicates the need for tracheotomy – provision of a safe airway is essential.

Treatment

After an initial period of enlargement for 6–12 months, resolution of cutaneous haemangiomas is to be expected, but the natural history of untreated subglottic haemangiomas is not so predictable. Unrecognized, untreated or poorly treated lesions have a high mortality and active treatment, even though it may be confined to a tracheotomy alone, is justified. Airway compromise is usually severe and progressive during the proliferative phase with some infants presenting with acute, life-threatening obstruction. Many patients therefore require immediate relief of obstruction, either by tracheotomy or by temporary intubation followed by tracheotomy to ensure the patient's safety and to enable treatment to be undertaken.

There is no agreement on treatment and many options have been advocated:

- Tracheotomy, no other treatment, awaiting spontaneous regression; this strategy is reported to be associated with a significant mortality rate from airway obstruction;
- temporary, repeated or prolonged endotracheal intubation with or without systemic or intralesional steroids;
- oral corticosteroids may be useful for 6–8 weeks, or less if there is improvement; the mode of action is poorly understood; large doses often produce unacceptable side-effects; they are seldom effective as the sole treatment;
- interferon α2a for life-threatening haemangiomas unresponsive to laser treatment and/or corticosteroid therapy is advocated (Ohms et al, 1994) for large, platelet-consuming cutaneous haemangiomas; the interferon acts as an antiangiogenic substance;
- injection of sclerosant and direct injection of steroids are difficult to control (neither is currently recommended);
- cryosurgery or electrocautery; precise control of tissue destruction is difficult;
- surgical excision of subglottic haemangioma which might result in subglottic stenosis, or postoperative voice problems; surgical excision is best reserved for discrete upper tracheal lesions;
- laser vaporization for selected cases;
- radiation therapy, either with external beam irradiation or a radioactive gold grain;
- regular observation may be appropriate for small lesions with minimal symptoms, e.g. children with no stridor.

The advocates of each form of therapy have reported successful results and it may be that various treatment methods can achieve similar results. The success of any treatment depends on careful assessment of the size and site of the haemangioma and the avoidance of possible complications, especially subglottic stenosis. The array of options indicates that there is no universally accepted treatment but the most commonly employed therapies are expectant treatment, CO_2 laser using serial staged vaporization, or localized radiation therapy using a gold grain.

External beam irradiation was an acknowledged and reliable therapy for many years, but it is no longer favoured because of the possibility of radiation-induced malignancy of the thyroid gland. In Sydney we have used a radioactive gold grain placed in the haemangioma for maximum tumour dose and minimum radiation of surrounding tissues in over 40 cases in 30 years, achieving very satisfactory results (Fig. 16.9) with no subglottic stenosis.

However, sequential CO_2 laser over several months now appears to be a safe and effective treatment for localized, unilateral lesions, using pulsed mode at 3–5 watts in several stages, usually two to three, with intubation and administration of steroids in the postoperative period if necessary. The risk of post-laser subglottic stenosis is increased if laser treatment

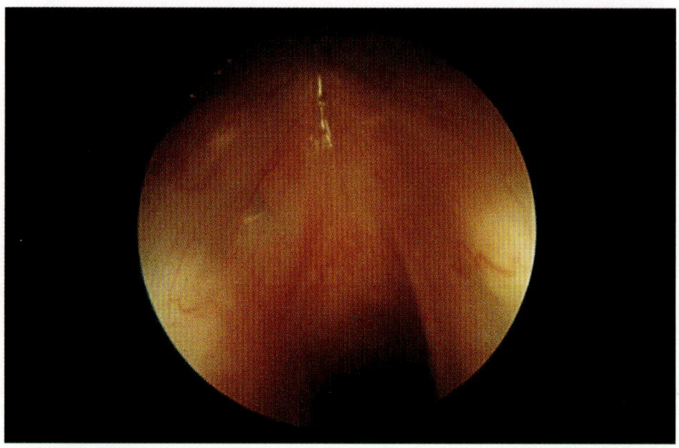

Figure **16.9**
Radioactive gold grain. Four years after treatment of a left, subglottic haemangioma using a radioactive insert which lies inertly in the submucosa. The grain measures 2.5-mm long × 0.8-mm diameter.

Treatment of subglottic haemangioma

Very rarely no treatment necessary
Tracheotomy and await involution
Staged laser for localized, unilateral lesions
Localized radiation using gold grain
Surgical excision for discrete upper tracheal lesions

There is no generally accepted 'ideal' treatment; the risk of subglottic stenosis must be minimized

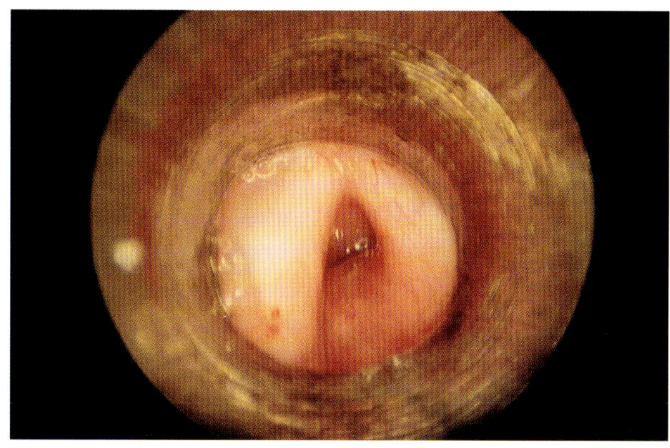

Figure **16.10**
Exposure using subglottiscope. Right subglottic haemangioma exposed using 4.7-mm internal diameter, purpose-designed subglottiscope.

is used for lesions which are bilateral, have posterior extension or a circumferential pattern. Sie et al (1994) report 20% subglottic stenosis when all haemangiomas, both localized and extensive, were treated by CO_2 laser.

The choice of treatment in an individual patient may depend on the age of the patient, the facilities available and the degree of endoscopic surgical exposure of the subglottic region. The purpose-designed Benjamin infant subglottiscopes (Karl Storz), either 3.5-mm or 4.7-mm internal distal diameter, allow binocular microscopic diagnostic inspection and facilitate laser treatment in the subglottis (Fig. 16.10) or upper trachea.

BIBLIOGRAPHY

Benjamin B, Carter P (1983) Congenital laryngeal haemangioma. *Ann Otol Rhinol Laryngol* **92**: 448–54.

Brodsky L, Yoshpen N, Reuben RJ (1983) Clinical pathological correlates of congenital subglottic haemangiomas. *Ann Otol Rhinol Laryngol* **105** (Suppl): 4–18.

Ohms LA, Jones DT, McGill T, Healy GB (1994) Interferon alpha 2a therapy for airway haemangioma. *Ann Otol Rhinol Laryngol* **103**: 1–8.

Sie KCY, McGill T, Healy GB (1994) Subglottic haemangioma: ten years experience with the carbon dioxide laser. *Ann Otol Rhinol Laryngol* **103**: 167–72.

IV ADULT DISEASES

17 Reinke's oedema

Reinke's oedema is also known as polypoidal corditis, polypoidal degeneration and bilateral diffuse polyposis.

ANATOMY

Reinke was an anatomist who described the fine structure of the vocal cords including the space – which corresponds to the superficial layer of the lamina propria – which bears his name. This potential space is normally closed by loose adherence of the covering squamous epithelial layer to the underlying vocal ligament, which consists of the admixture of elastic and collagen fibres of the intermediate and deep layers of the lamina propria. The boundaries of Reinke's space are the anterior commissure, the vocal process of the arytenoid cartilage, the covering epithelium medially, the vocal ligament laterally and, above and below, the superior and inferior arcuate lines, which themselves are the lines of transition from squamous to pseudostratified columnar epithelium.

Layers of membranous vocal cord

- Cover
  - Squamous epithelium
  - Superficial layer of lamina propria
- Transition zone
  - Vocal ligament, composed of elastic and collagen fibres of the intermediate and deep layers of lamina propria
- Body
  - Thyroarytenoid (vocalis) muscle

EPIDEMIOLOGY

Men and women are about equally affected. Symptoms usually start after 40–50 years of age, but occasionally children are seen with Reinke's oedema (Fig. 17.1); they are usually already heavy smokers.

The causative factors include excessive talking, voice abuse (e.g. auctioneers), cigarette smoking and airborne irritants from industrial or environmental fumes. Irritation from chronic sinusitis and postnasal discharge has also been implicated.

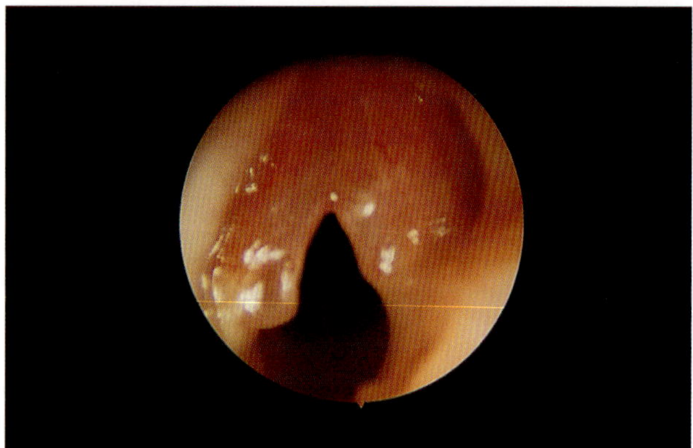

Figure **17.1**
Reinke's oedema in an 11-year-old boy. Photograph taken at direct laryngoscopy of an 11-year-old who had been a heavy smoker for almost 5 years.

Causative factors for Reinke's oedema

Cigarette smoke
Voice abuse
Atmospheric irritants
Chronic sinusitis

PATHOPHYSIOLOGY

Reinke's space is subject to the collection of fluid because of poor lymphatic drainage, venous stasis and vascular congestion. Diffuse polypoid changes develop in the membranous vocal fold from the vocal process to the anterior commissure, become progressively worse and ultimately become permanent. When fully developed, each vocal cord appears as a smooth-surfaced translucent or opalescent distended 'bag'; there may be capillaries or dilated vessels stretched on the surface imparting an angiomatous appearance. The oedema is usually bilateral and symmetrical but when one side is more enlarged than the other a search for nearby primary pathology should be made. Sometimes there are small areas of leukoplakia on the surface and although biopsy may reveal some degree of dysplasia, Reinke's oedema does not have any direct relationship to development of carcinoma.

Histologically there is hyperplasia of the epithelium, especially of the basal layer, but there is usually no hyperkeratosis or keratin formation. The overall histopathologic appearance is benign.

Ultrastructural examination, as opposed to light microscopy, contributes to the differentiation of Reinke's oedema from vocal cord polyp and vocal cord nodules. The basement membrane is thickened, there are oedematous lakes, signs of recent bleeding, increased vessel wall thickness and some fibrin, but there is less capillary endothelial cell damage than in polyps. The areas of oedema contain variable amounts of mucopolysaccharides.

CLINICAL FEATURES

The typical history is of consistent, slowly progressive hoarseness in a smoker who talks a lot. The

Clinical features in Reinke's oedema

Long history of cigarette smoking
Harsh, low-pitched, progressive hoarseness
'Masculinized' voice in females
Airway obstruction in advanced disease
Be alert for myxoedema

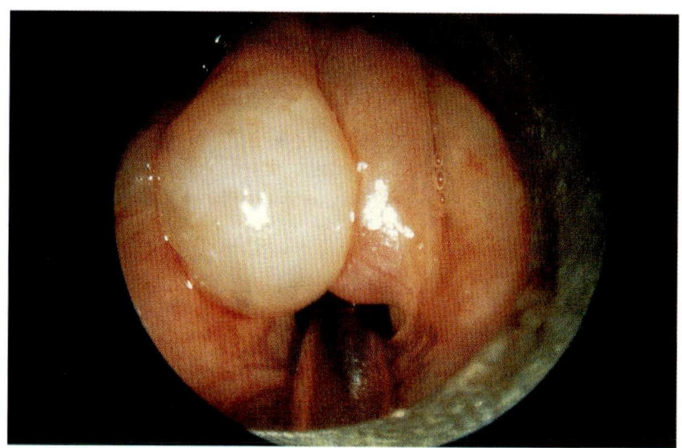

Figure **17.2**
Very severe Reinke's oedema. Extremely large 'polypoidal corditis'. The oedema in Reinke's space is so severe that the vocal folds cannot be identified. Surgical treatment is necessary to overcome airway obstruction.

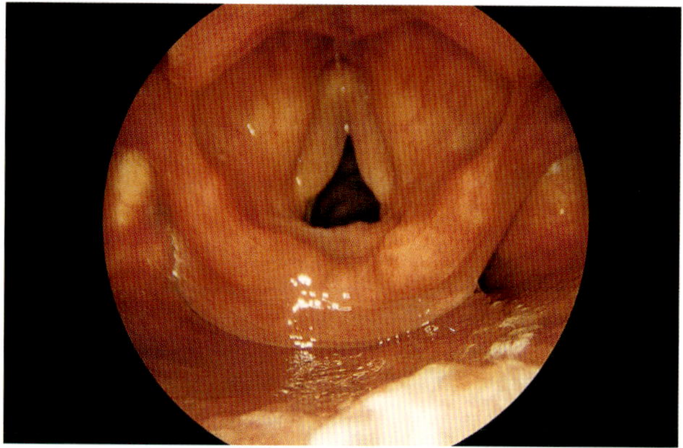

Figure **17.3**
Indirect laryngoscopy. Moderate almost symmetrical swelling of the vocal folds with some dilated vessels on the surface.

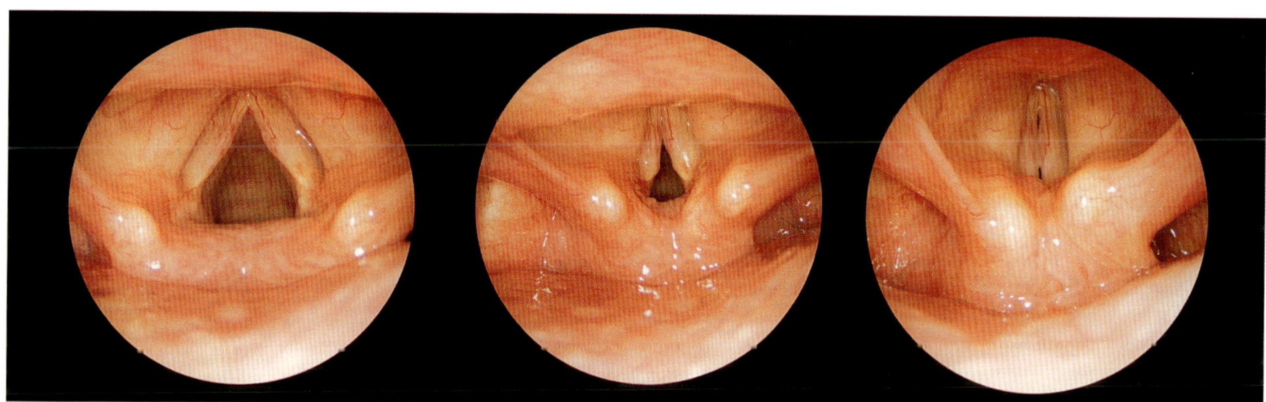

Figure **17.4**
Mild to moderate Reinke's oedema at indirect laryngoscopy. The degree of swelling of the vocal folds is more distinct in the centre photograph. There are some dilated vessels, more marked on the right side.

voice is harsh and low pitched so that the female patient develops a masculinized voice and may find herself taken for a male when speaking on the telephone.

Reinke's oedema is uncommon among classical professional singers but is more frequent in untrained, 'popular' singers, announcers and other professional voice users. Its presence is usually associated with voice abuse and almost always also with smoking.

When Reinke's oedema is severe (Fig. 17.2), the large bags of fluid may 'flap' in and out producing a harsh, snoring, obstructive quality during sleep. The patient may wake, get up, walk about, take a breath of 'fresh air' and go back to bed.

In longstanding Reinke's oedema some patients are unable to phonate with their vocal cords and develop dysphonia plica ventricularis.

The laryngologist should be alert to the clinical features of hypothyroidism which may be present when Reinke's oedema is part of myxoedema.

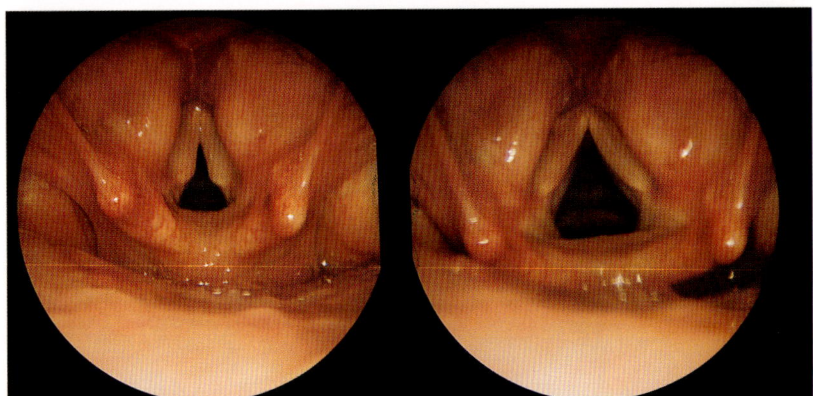

Figure **17.5**
Moderate Reinke's oedema. Indirect laryngoscopy. Even in moderately developed disease the changes are more obvious after phonation as the vocal folds relax.

INDIRECT LARYNGOSCOPY

Diagnosis can be made at indirect laryngoscopy and is immediately obvious in moderate (Fig. 17.3) or advanced cases. In early cases there may be only minimal swelling in the vocal folds (Fig. 17.4) and careful examination, especially with a large-diameter telescope, will assist in confirming suspicion of Reinke's oedema. The diagnosis is made by seeing bilateral, symmetrical, fusiform, thin-walled vocal folds distended by clear or yellow fluid. Phonation on inspiration may make the swellings more obvious. Sometimes the changes are best seen after phonation (Fig. 17.5).

TREATMENT

Non-surgical

Patients who smoke must be strongly advised to stop. An attempt must be made to avoid irritating fumes or dust. Speech therapy may assist in limiting overuse of the voice. The best that can be expected from medical treatment is a slight improvement in voice quality. Regular review and indirect laryngoscopy usually confirms slow progression of the condition.

Where hypothyroidism is suspected, thyroid function should be tested. In myxoedematous patients, firm, non-reddened, symmetrical, bilateral Reinke's oedema results in a hoarse, low-pitched voice. Treatment improves the voice within a few months.

In moderate and severe cases the voice is usually unacceptable, especially in female patients. Surgical treatment should be undertaken only after the patient has been informed that restoration of a 'normal' voice is unlikely.

Microlaryngoscopy and microsurgery

Depending upon the stage of the disease, microlaryngoscopy clearly shows mild (Fig. 17.6), moderate or severe oedematous distention of Reinke's space. In severe cases (Fig. 17.7) the pathology is sharply demarcated at the superior and inferior arcuate lines. The taut, pendulous, bag-like swellings on each side often display dilated capillary vessels in and under the surface epithelium (Fig. 17.8) which is raised off the vocal ligament by the oedema. In early cases the change will be more or less obvious depending upon the tension put on the vocal cords by the particular laryngoscope used and how it is positioned (Fig. 17.9).

Surgical removal is necessary for large or moderate size polyps causing an objectional voice and when large swellings cause airway obstruction (see Fig. 17.2).

The operation of vocal cord 'stripping' has lost favour. Excessive mucosa removal leads to trauma in

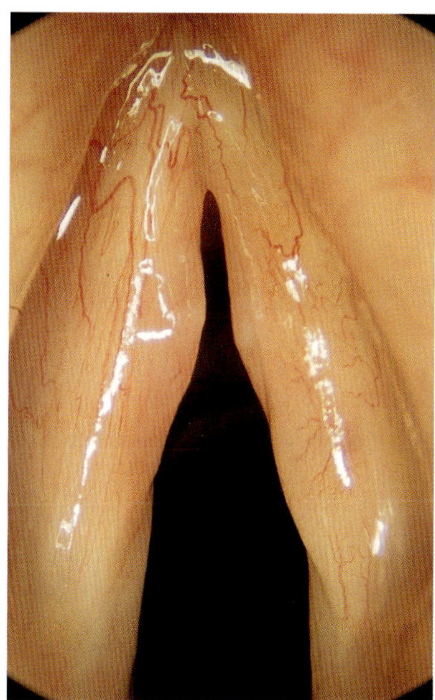

Figure **17.6**
Mild Reinke's oedema at direct laryngoscopy. There is semi-translucent oedema in each vocal fold, with a somewhat irregular edge on the right side; there are several dilated vessels on the surface.

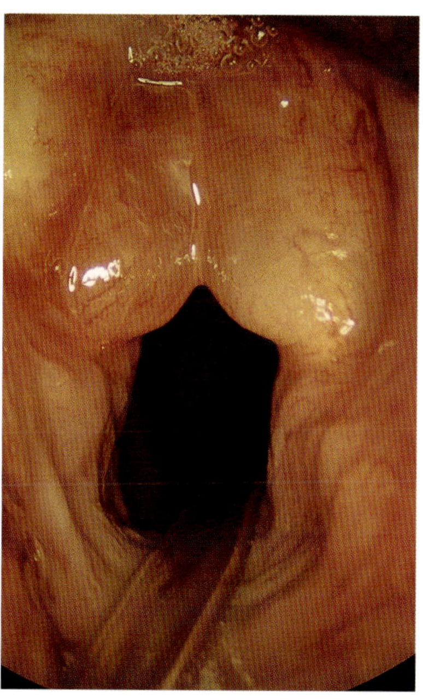

Figure **17.7**
Severe Reinke's oedema at direct laryngoscopy. Severe oedema, limited to Reinke's space, causing partial laryngeal obstruction.

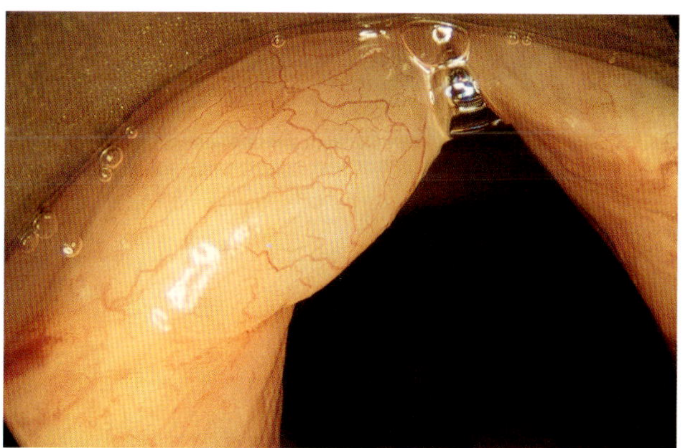

Figure **17.8**
Close-up of left Reinke's oedema. The laryngoscope has been angled to expose the left-sided swelling and the surface vessels can be very clearly seen.

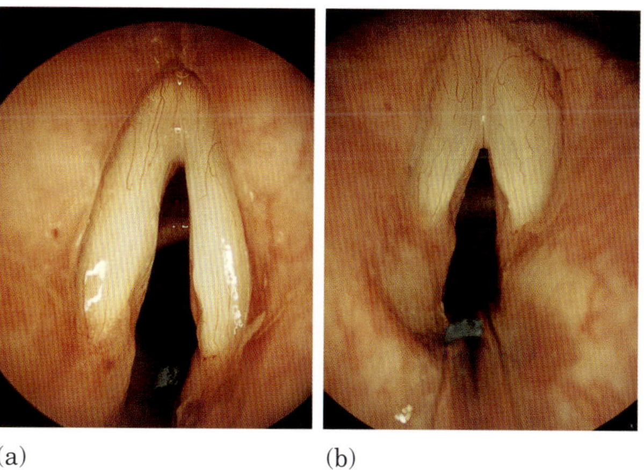

(a) (b)

Figure **17.9**
Reinke's oedema: difference in appearance. Lindholm laryngoscope anterior to the epiglottis (left). Kleinsasser laryngoscope posterior to the epiglottis (right). The difference in appearance relates to the different tension put on the vocal cords by placement of the laryngoscope.

Microsurgical treatment

Extended microflap incision
Suction removal of fluid contents
Trim and redrape mucosal edges

Removal of the superior surface to reduce polyps causing obstruction

Separate, staged procedures in selected cases

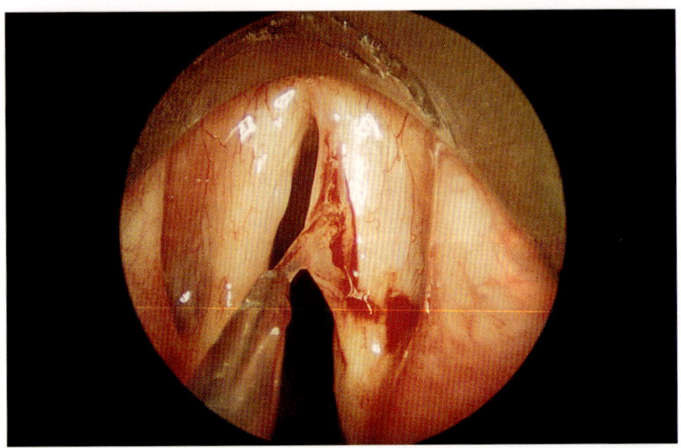

Figure **17.10**
Aspiration of fluid contents. Reinke's space has been opened, dissected and the thick yellow fluid is being suctioned from Reinke's space.

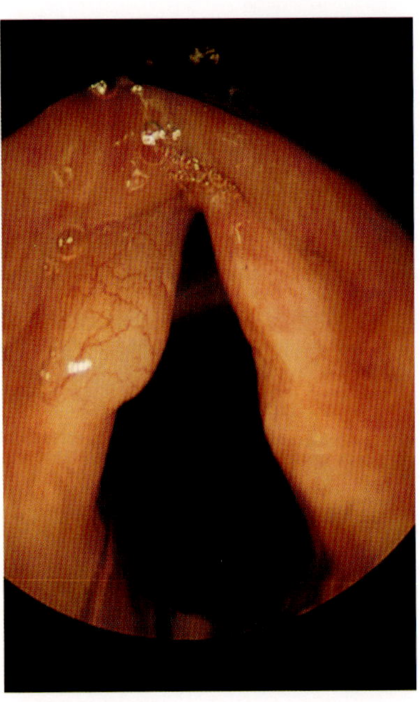

Figure **17.11**
Second stage operation. The right side was operated 4 weeks before this photograph and still has some oedema. Staging will obviate the risk of adhesion.

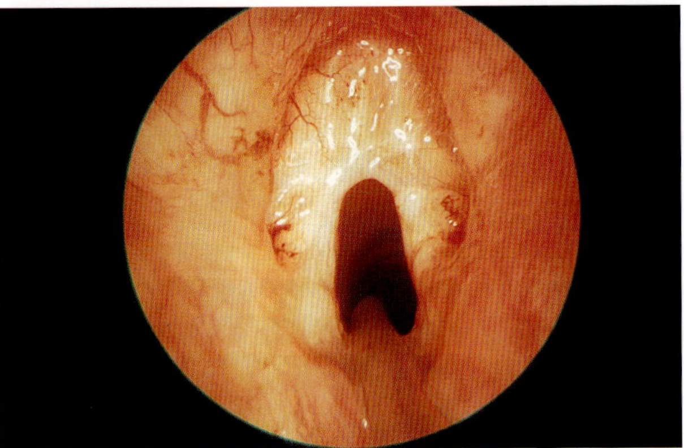

Figure **17.12**
Glottic web after operation. Both vocal cords had been 'stripped' at the same operation some months before this photograph was taken.

Reinke's space and promotes micro-adhesions of the mucosa to the vocal ligament thereby producing a detrimental effect on the vibrating properties of the mucosal cover of the vocal fold. Postoperative dysphonia often persists for weeks and the long-term result may be an unacceptable, high-pitched, poor voice.

A more acceptable, surgically conservative and less traumatic procedure involves excision of a strip of mucosa on the upper surface lateral to the edge of the vocal fold extending from the anterior commissure to the vocal process. This preserves as much mucosa as possible while removing gelatinous fluid. Reinke's space is opened and mobilized by blunt dissection, freeing thick, yellow, gelatinous fluid which

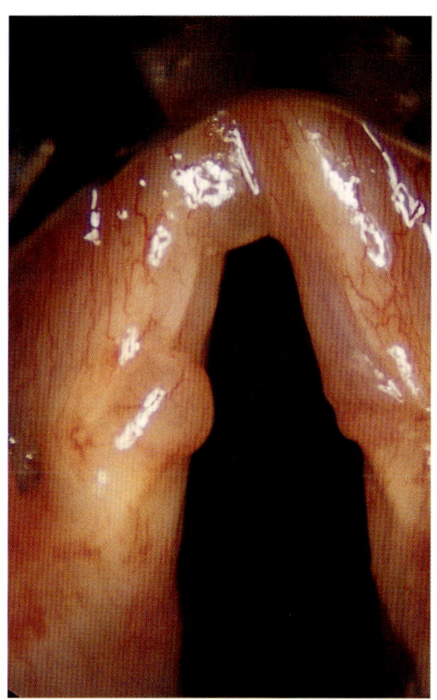

Figure **17.13**
Reinke's oedema and vocal cord polyps. A 59-year-old female patient with chronic laryngitis due both to Reinke's oedema and vocal cord polyps. Staged surgical procedures were necessary.

is suctioned from the mucosal envelope. As the sticky fluid (Fig. 17.10) is lost, the envelope collapses and appears wrinkled. The edges of the mucosal flaps are re-draped and placed together to encourage healing; some surgeons advise use of the laser to assist adherence of the edges. The vocal ligament must, of course, be left untouched. It is wise to stage operations on the two sides (Fig. 17.11) to minimize the chance of adhesion formation if there is a raw surface on one side which would oppose a raw surface on the other. Some of the worst and most disabling glottic adhesions have occurred after ill-judged bilateral vocal cord stripping (Fig. 17.12).

In some cases Reinke's oedema and vocal cord polyps are seen together (Fig. 17.13) making surgical treatment more complicated.

Although considerable improvement is likely the voice seldom returns to 'normal'. The patient should be made aware of the possibility of an indifferent result.

BIBLIOGRAPHY

Dikkers FG, Nikkels PG (1995) Benign lesions of the vocal folds: histopathology and phonotrauma. *Ann Otol Rhinol Laryngol* **104**: 698–703.

Freedom ST, Amadee RG (1990) Reinke's oedema. *J Louis State Med Soc* **142**: 7–9.

Kleinsasser O (1968) Reinke's oedema. In: Kleinsasser O, ed. *Microlaryngoscopy and endolaryngeal microsurgery* (Philadelphia: WB Saunders); 48–54.

18 Vocal cord polyps

Polyps usually occur on the anterior or middle part of the membranous vocal fold and are the commonest laryngeal pathology requiring surgical removal. Polyps are often discussed with Reinke's oedema as both result from increased vessel permeability causing oedema. However, whereas Reinke's oedema affects the whole length of both vocal folds, vocal polyps are more localized and are usually unilateral.

EPIDEMIOLOGY

Polyps are twice as common in men as in women. They are found in adults of all ages with most patients presenting between the ages of 20 and 60 years.

AETIOLOGY

Overuse or abuse of the voice and work in a noisy environment are said to be aggravating factors. In some patients there is a history of increased use of the voice, such as shouting, at a time when the patient felt that the voice 'went'. Some patients have used excessive aspirin or other anticoagulant, increasing the likelihood of haemorrhage into the vocal fold. Tobacco consumption has no association with the development of polyps.

The cause is uncertain and the theories of pathogenesis generally unconvincing. A haemorrhagic unilateral vocal fold polyp (Fig. 18.1) may begin with rupture of a capillary in Reinke's space, with extravasation of blood followed by organization and polyp formation.

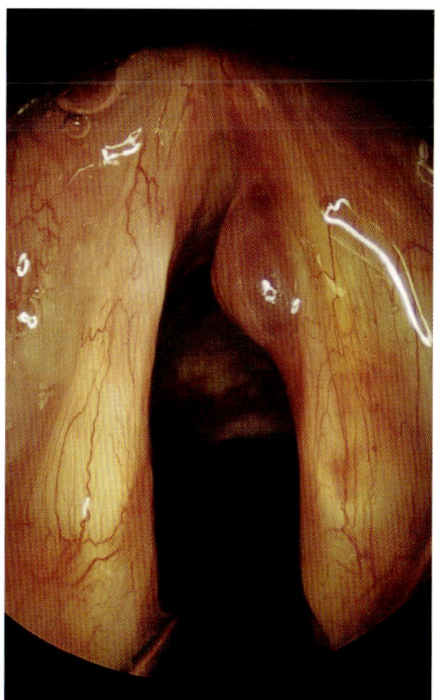

Figure **18.1**
Haemorrhagic polyp. Smooth, blood-filled polyp on the anterior part of the right vocal fold.

Vocal fold polyps

Twice as common in men
Usually 20–60 years of age
May be caused by an intracordal bleed
Usually unilateral
Oedematous, angiomatous or fibrous
Require microsurgical removal
Results are very good

PATHOLOGY

About 80% of vocal cord polyps are unilateral. They occur on the free edge or the undersurface of the vocal fold at the anterior or middle third; 20% are bilateral or multiple.

Polyps may be rounded, elongated, irregular or multilobulated. They are usually pale, translucent and oedematous and there is a red, angiomatous, haemorrhagic type. Therefore, the size, appearance, colour and consistency vary considerably.

Several appearances have been described histologically. The 'oedematous' or 'gelatinous' polyp is pale, translucent, and shows loose, fibre-poor connective tissue. The epithelium is generally normal, sometimes thinned and occasionally ulcerated. Severe oedema accompanied by fibrin is a characteristic finding. Vascular dilatation is sometimes sufficient to simulate an angioma and the lacunae which form may undergo thrombosis. Some polyps have both angiomatous and oedematous components.

The 'angiomatous' or 'telangiectatic' polyp is red and vascular with cavernous blood spaces. The 'fibrous' polyp has a very cellular and fibrous connective tissue which is sometimes vascularized and occasionally accompanied by deposits of amyloid. The covering squamous epithelium is usually normal, sometimes thin, and may undergo hyperplasia with a layer of keratosis on the surface. Histopathologists may then confuse polyps with vocal nodules.

Dysplasia and atypia are very rare – polyps are benign, having no tendency to malignancy.

CLINICAL FEATURES

Abrupt onset of hoarseness while cheering at a sporting event or enjoying a party suggests that a vessel may have ruptured, but this history is certainly not always present. Hoarseness is often insidious, slowly progressive, usually unremitting, and accompanied by a lowered voice intensity and a reduced frequency range. The voice sometimes has a breathy quality. The degree of vocal disability varies with the size, site, nature and pedunculation of the polyp, yet sometimes interference with phonation may be minimal. Occasionally a large polyp causes an irritative cough and very large or multiple polyps may account for partial airway obstruction.

INDIRECT LARYNGOSCOPY

Whether they are loose, gelatinous, shiny masses, firm fibrous polyps or angiomatous lesions, polyps generally arise from the free edge or the undersurface of the anterior one-third of the vocal fold (Table 18.1).

Contact response on the opposite cord may cause a shallow depression. The diagnostic appearance can be easily recognized at indirect laryngoscopy (Fig.

Table 18.1 Differentiation of polyps from nodules, granulomas and papillomas

Disease	*Site on the vocal fold*
Nodules	Central part
Granulomas	Medial aspect behind the vocal process
Polyps	Anterior third usually
Papillomas	Anywhere; predilection for anterior commissure

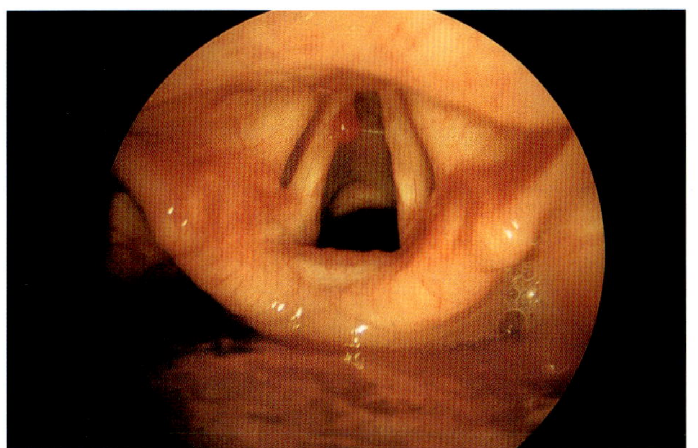

Figure **18.2**
Left vocal cord polyp. Indirect laryngoscopy. Small, pedunculated, red polyp on the left vocal fold.

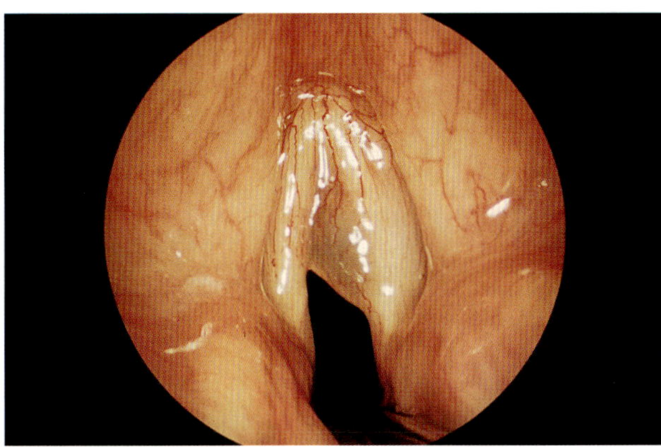

Figure **18.3**
Translucent polyp. Thin-walled, fusiform polyp on the right vocal fold, with small vessels in the epithelium.

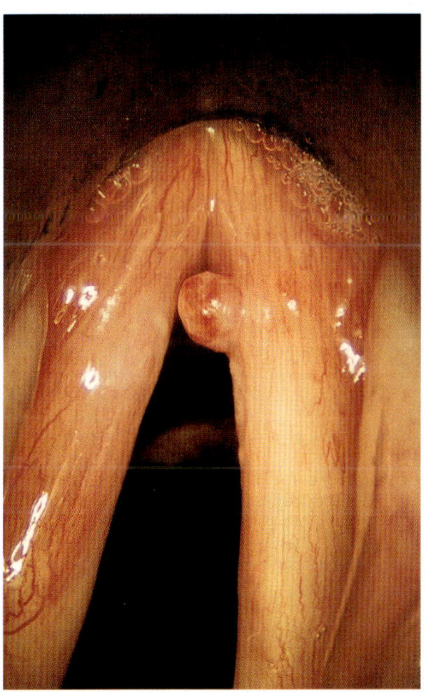

Figure **18.4**
Vascular polyp. History of sudden onset of hoarseness 6 weeks before.

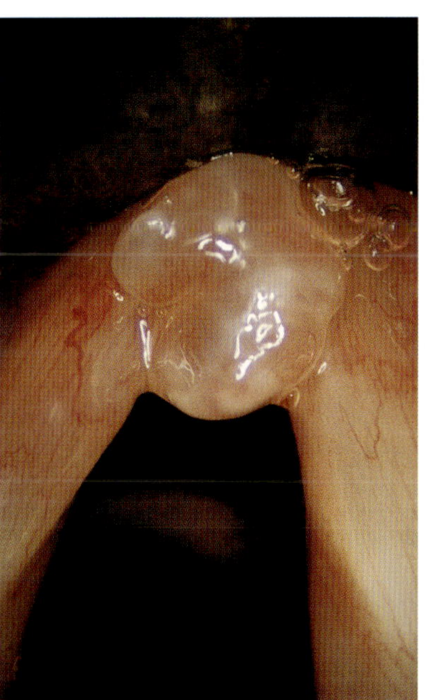

Figure **18.5**
Irregular polyp. Multilobed, gelatinous polyp at the anterior commissure.

18.2) and the polyps, according to their appearance, can be classified as multiple, pedunculated, fusiform or generalized depending on the length of the base attaching to the vocal fold.

The differentiation of polyps from nodules, granulomas and papillomas is usually not difficult (Table 18.1).

MICROLARYNGOSCOPY

The appearance is characteristic but variable. Soft, translucent, broad-based gelatinous polyps have a thin wall and small capillaries in the epithelium (Fig. 18.3).

Vascular polyps (Fig. 18.4) have more blood vessels and have a pink-reddish, oedematous appearance

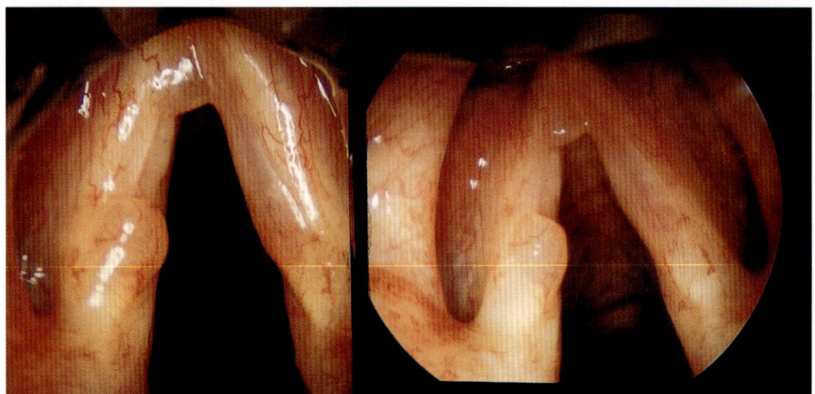

Figure **18.6**
Multiple polyps. Two left-sided gelatinous polyps and Reinke's oedema of the right vocal fold. This is the same patient as shown in Fig. 17.13.

with one or more larger vessels which may appear to run into the base as 'feeders' – these vessels can be vaporized with the carbon dioxide laser on a very low setting.

Other polyps have an uneven surface (Fig. 18.5) and a dark red colour. Multiple polyps (Fig. 18.6) are not unusual.

MICROSURGICAL REMOVAL

Polyps do not improve with medical treatment or speech therapy. Surgical removal is necessary to restore the vocal fold to its normal appearance and vibratory function with a good prognosis for return of normal voice. Precision microsurgery requires that the polyp, whether sessile or pedunculated, is grasped with cupped forceps or Bouchayer forceps so that with gentle traction towards the opposite side it can be neatly excised at the base with scissors, taking care not to damage deeper layers of the vocal fold, especially the vocal ligament (Fig. 18.7).

Voice rest for 7–10 days should be followed by return of a good voice in 1–2 months as the natural elasticity, flexibility and vibration of the vocal fold returns. Recurrences are unusual.

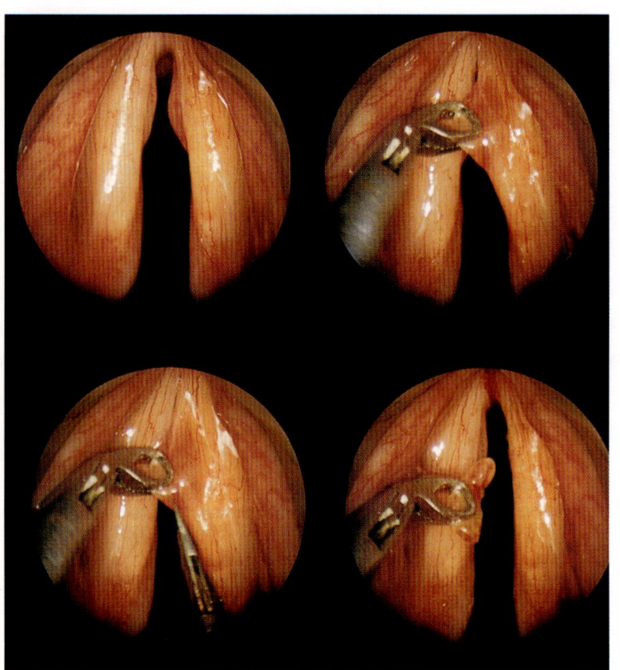

Figure **18.7**
Bilateral polyps. Technique of removal. Steps in the removal of a right polyp using Bouchayer forceps and scissors.

19 Vocal granulomas and contact pachydermia

NOMENCLATURE

There are numerous references in the literature to idiopathic vocal cord granuloma, 'contact ulcer' and even granuloma/ulcer, often in the same context, without discrimination between granuloma and 'ulcer'. But there appears to be no evidence of an interrelationship between the two or of a sequence of events where one lesion leads to the other. Further studies might determine whether they represent different manifestations of a single disease or whether they are separate entities which occur at the same anatomical site (Benjamin and Croxson 1985). Do vocal granulomas commence as an ulcer or even pass through what might be regarded as an ulcer–granuloma stage where, hypothetically, there should be a central crater surrounded by a rim of hypertrophic granulation tissue?

Referring to 'contact ulcer', Kleinsasser (1968) stated that he had not observed the presence of true ulcer with loss of substance in the altered tissue and that he preferred the term 'contact pachydermia' postulating that 'nature is trying to build a protective barrier around the sensitive cartilage tip of the vocal process'.

VOCAL GRANULOMA

Vocal granulomas have been classified according to aetiology as post-intubation, idiopathic, hyperfunctional or hyperacidic. Post-intubation granulomas have been discussed in chapter 12 on intubation injuries.

Idiopathic, hyperfunctional or hyperacidic vocal granulomas (Federer and Michell 1984) are a disease of adult life usually in the fourth or fifth decade and with a strong predominance in males of approximately 10 : 1.

The patient with a hyperfunctional vocal granuloma may be a tense, hard-driving, voice-abusing male; sometimes a salesman who needs to talk over loud noises or to large groups of people. However, this description is not typical of most patients.

Vocal granulomas

- Post-intubation
- Idiopathic
- Hyperfunctional
- Hyperacidic
- Disease specific

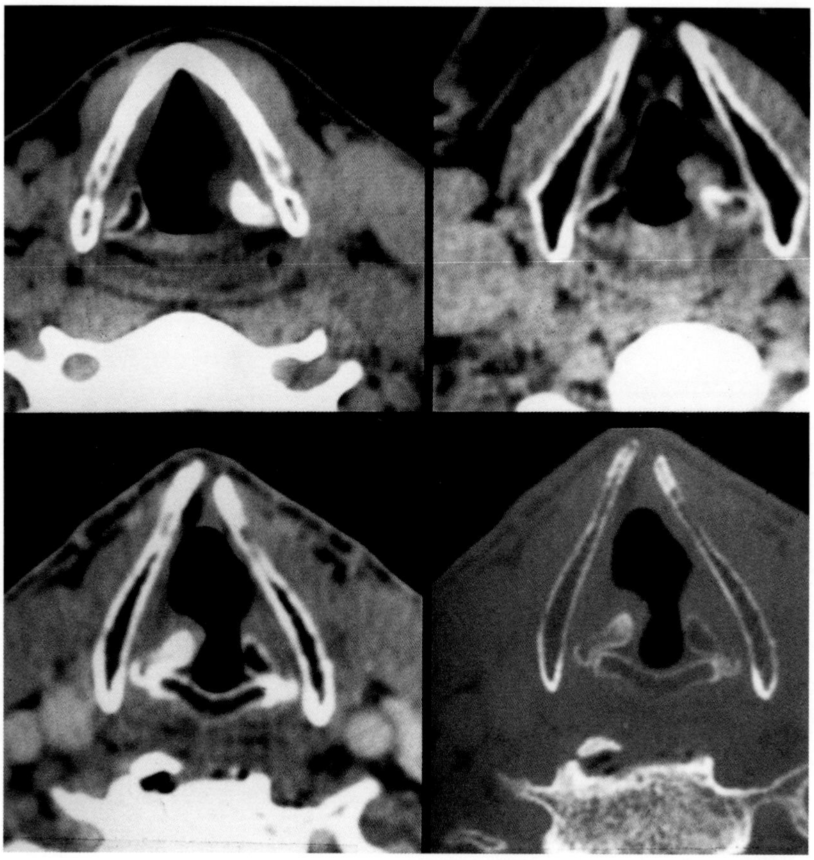

Figure **19.1**
Axial CTs showing sclerosis of arytenoids. In each of the four cases there is partial or complete osteosclerosis of the arytenoid cartilage on the side showing the soft tissue opacity of the granuloma.

A hyperacidic vocal granuloma is said to be related to gastro-oesophageal reflux and caused by gastric contents contaminating the larynx. Some authorities believe this is the cause of most granulomas and advise arbitrary treatment with anti-reflux medication. Other authorities have not found any reflux symptoms nor any radiological, endoscopic or pH evidence of reflux in most patients. Further, the granuloma may not resolve with stringent anti-reflux treatment.

Pathogenesis

The histological features of vocal granulomas include proliferation of non-specific reparative granulation tissue consistent with pyogenic granuloma, chronic inflammatory changes and a covering of squamous epithelium, usually hyperplastic but sometimes showing minor ulceration (not visible to the naked eye) at various sites on the surface. There are no premalignant or malignant features.

Arytenoid osteosclerosis on the side of the granuloma is evident on CT (Fig. 19.1) in all patients and is more often focal than general (Benjamin and Roche 1993). Focal arytenoid sclerosis is nearly always medial. There is no apparent relationship between the duration of symptoms, the size of the granuloma, the number of operations and the degree of arytenoid sclerosis. These radiographic changes in the arytenoid appear to be secondary to the presence of the granuloma and to be a part of the local pathologic process. This osteosclerosis in the arytenoid is likely to be secondary to reactive hyperaemia and to infective changes in the perichondrium around the base of the granuloma and is not present on the other side. This knowledge presents the laryngologist with a wider appreciation of the disease process but does not indicate a change in the current treatment.

It seems likely that the thin mucoperichondrium over the medial side of the vocal process becomes inflamed or acutely ulcerated during a coughing attack, following an irritative upper respiratory tract infection or after voice abuse or shouting. Thereafter, chronic cough or throat clearing, with or without acid reflux, aggravates and potentiates local inflammation and leads to perichondritis and chondritis in the arytenoid cartilage, the visible result being formation of a typical proliferative vocal granuloma on the surface.

In general, the differential diagnosis of disease-specific granulomas occasionally found in the larynx includes conditions such as tuberculosis, histoplasmosis, coccidiomycosis, blastomyocosis, syphilis, leprosy, sarcoidosis, Wegener's granulomatosis, scleroma and Crohn's disease. These granulomas will not be further discussed.

Clinical features

Although some patients have hoarseness the speaking voice may be normal or very near normal. Patients complain of a feeling of irritation, a feeling of 'something', a lump or foreign body in the throat and a constant urge to clear the throat of this sensation or of excessive mucus. There may be pain localized to the side of the throat at the laryngeal level, sometimes radiating to the ear.

The symptoms may be aggravated by excessive voice use, shouting or prolonged talking such as lecturing. Few of our patients have symptoms associated with gastro-oesophageal reflux or oesophagitis such as retrosternal burning pain, regurgitation of acid, waking at night with pain, laryngospasm or excessive coughing. Some patients complain that the extra effort required for phonation causes muscular tiredness and aching in the throat and neck especially after prolonged talking.

Our patients are not hard-driving tense personalities, nor do they seem to abuse their voices or speak excessively as patients with contact pachydermia do. Few have the localized or severe pain radiating to the ear which is such a consistent feature in contact pachydermia, nor is there a granuloma on one side and contact pachydermia on the other side of the larynx.

Features of non-specific vocal cord granulomas

- Almost always in males
- Feeling of something in the throat
- Sometimes slight huskiness
- Constant throat clearing
- Sometimes local pain or otalgia
- Easily visible on indirect laryngoscopy
- CT shows osteosclerosis of cartilage
- Recurrence likely after removal

Indirect laryngoscopy

Vocal granuloma may be suspected from the symptoms and be confirmed by indirect laryngoscopy which reveals a rounded, unilobular or multilobular pedunculated mass arising from the posterior third of the vocal cord, with the base of the granuloma arising near the vocal process, usually just posterior to it on the medial surface of the arytenoid cartilage. A granuloma is better seen during quiet respiration than on phonation (Fig. 19.2). Bilateral idiopathic vocal granulomas are extremely rare but bilateral post-intubation granulomas are sometimes seen.

Our patients do not have surface inflammation and mucosal thickening of the posterior larynx which is said to be due to an irritative effect of chronic gastro-oesophageal reflux.

Treatment

Because causative factors have not been proven, there is no agreement on therapy or prevention of recurrence.

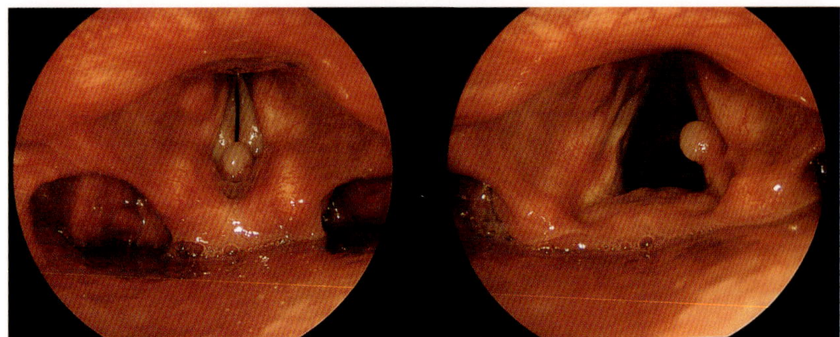

Figure **19.2**
Idiopathic vocal granuloma. Indirect laryngoscopy. Round pale-pink granuloma arising near right vocal process. Seen during both adduction and abduction.

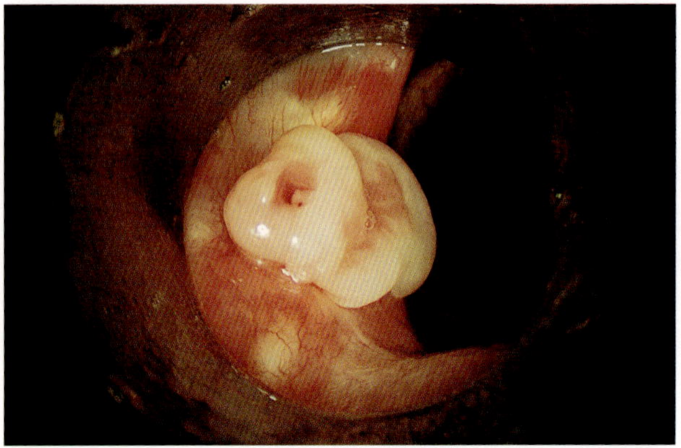

Figure **19.3**
Vocal granuloma. Direct laryngoscopy. Exposure of posterior glottis and left-sided granuloma prior to removal.

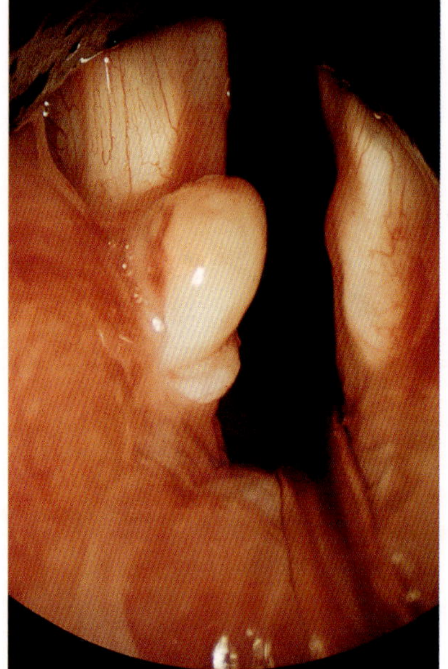

Figure **19.4**
Vocal granuloma. The base arises from the medial surface of the arytenoid in this example.

Many forms of treatment have been advocated including therapy for acid reflux (often on an empiric basis for patients with no symptoms of reflux), prolonged antibiotic therapy, oral steroids, oral zinc sulphate, local injection of steroids and repeated removal using scissors, laser, diathermy or cryotherapy. A voice therapist should advise the patient on voice care.

Medical management should include dietary advice, administration of antacids and histamine antagonists for appropriate patients and consultation with a gastroenterologist for selected patients.

Explanation about the condition and counselling of the patient is important, including reassurance that the granuloma is not malignant and that it will eventually resolve. Idiopathic granuloma is a self-limiting condition; although the natural history has never been established, it seems that when arytenoid sclerosis is complete, and the cartilage becomes calcified, there is no further perichondritis or chondritis and the granuloma resolves.

Surgical granuloma removal can be performed with forceps and scissors but troublesome bleeding often obscures the base of the granuloma and the vocal process. Use of the laser allows more precise granuloma removal with little or no exposure of cartilage and minimal trauma of the mucoperichondrium, because of the absence of bleeding.

A suitable laryngoscope is positioned to expose the posterior larynx (Fig. 19.3). The gross appearance of

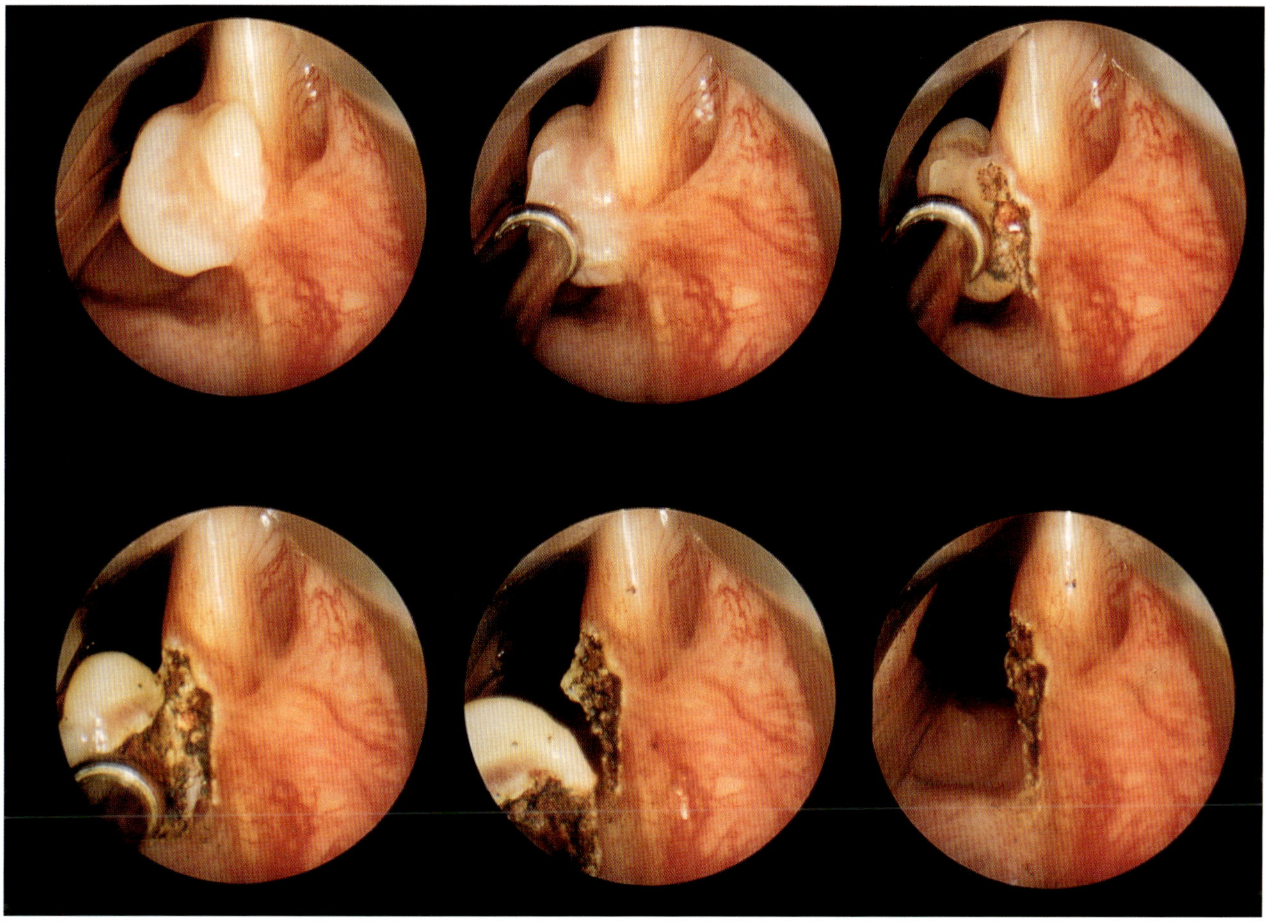

Figure **19.5**
Laser removal of vocal granuloma. Showing steps in operative technique: exposure, traction using suction, line of excision commenced, partially removed, completely amputated, and final result after 'tidying up'.

the granuloma shows a unilobular or multilobular round or oval fleshy mass with a pale irregular surface (Figs 19.4–6), attached by a broad pedicle to the medial aspect of the arytenoid, near the vocal process. The base is exposed using a sucker to exert gentle traction towards the contralateral side (Fig. 19.5); using a small-diameter laser beam on low power, the granuloma is amputated from the base taking care not to expose cartilage.

Vocal granuloma is often a frustrating problem to treat; recurrences are common. Bastian (1993) stated, 'Surgery should be a last resort because operative recurrence of the ulcerative granuloma is very common'. Microlaryngoscopy and biopsy removal of a suspected granuloma when first seen is reasonable to confirm the diagnosis; a malignant

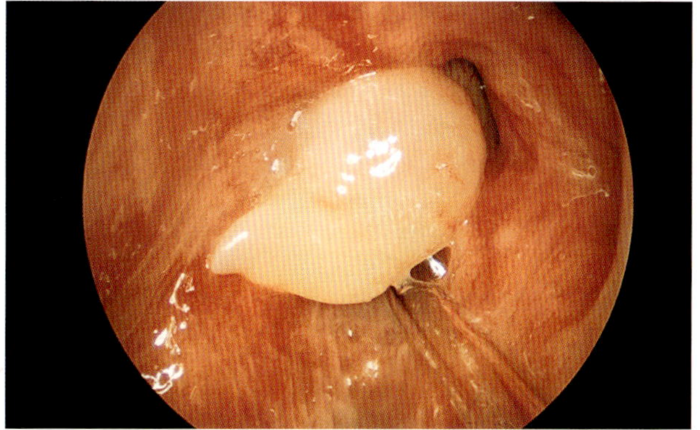

Figure **19.6**
Very large granuloma. Obstructive pale mass almost filling the posterior glottic space. The surgeon and anaesthetist must be aware of possible airway obstruction.

neoplasm in this site, or a specific granuloma (e.g. tuberculosis) can occasionally resemble idiopathic granuloma. Even with careful surgical removal and with strict anti-reflux measures, granulomas can recur or persist for a long time but all eventually resolve and do not recur. The indication for further removal is partial airway obstruction caused by the size of the mass (Fig. 19.6) or interference with phonation. Small granulomas should be regularly observed by indirect laryngoscopy.

CONTACT PACHYDERMIA

Contact 'ulcer' or contact 'pachydermia'?

In 1928, reviewing 127 cases referred to as 'contact ulcer', Jackson made no mention of granuloma when he first presented the clinical and pathological features. Later, in 1935, he reviewed his experience with a further 47 cases and included examples of vocal cord granuloma. He stated, 'necrosis of the epithelium may allow infective agents under the epithelium barrier' and 'in infected areas, trauma to cartilage and perichondrium results in slow healing; reparative processes are retarded by exuberant, flabby granulations that persist so long as they become epithelialised and more or less organised; they constitute granulomas.'

Jackson was the first to use the term 'contact ulcer' in the English language. Previously, Virchow had documented 'pachydermia verrucosa laryngis' to describe the histological appearance seen with epithelial thickening. More recently, Kleinsasser (1968) and others have pointed out that the saucer-shaped appearance with epithelial thickening surrounding a central depression which occurs on the mucosa near the vocal process is not a true ulcer as there is no loss of the surface. Thus the term 'contact pachydermia' is preferred (Fig. 19.7).

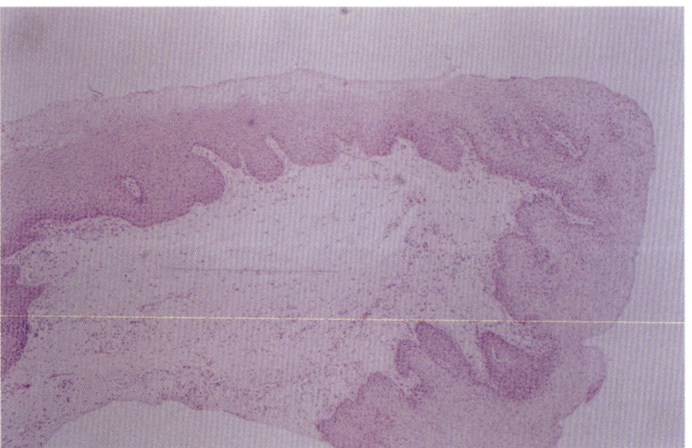

Figure **19.7**
Microscopic examination. Contact pachydermia. Thickened epithelium, some oedema, no ulcer and normal submucosa.

Clinical features

The symptoms of contact pachydermia include feeling 'something' or a foreign body in one side of the throat, localized pain, pain on swallowing or pain radiating to the ear. The primary site of pain is usually so localized that the patient can point confidently with one finger to the side of the neck at about the level of the mid-thyroid cartilage. The patient seldom has hoarseness.

With this symptomatology the diagnosis can usually, but not always, be confirmed at indirect laryngoscopy (Fig. 19.8) if a clear view can be obtained of

Features of contact pachydermia

`Localized pain on one side
Odynophagia
Referred otalgia
'Something' in the throat
Seldom any effect on the voice
Difficult to see on indirect laryngoscopy
May resolve with voice therapy
Chronic cases require surgical removal

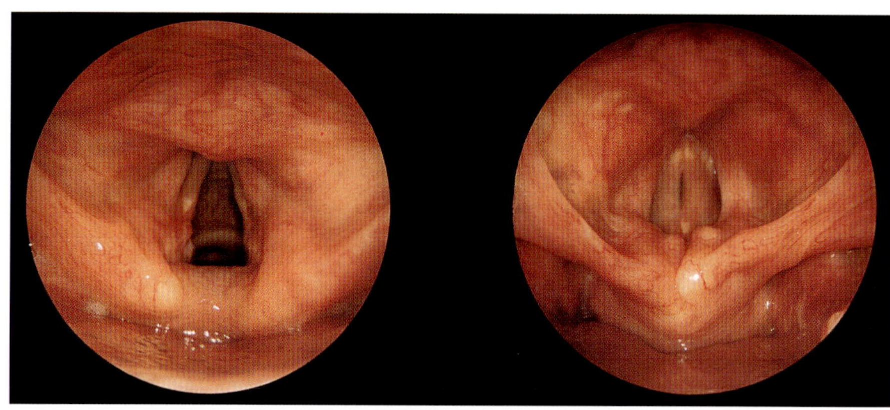

Figure **19.8**
Contact pachydermia. Indirect laryngoscopy. Small lesion near left vocal process can be recognized. Examination should pay particular attention to this area.

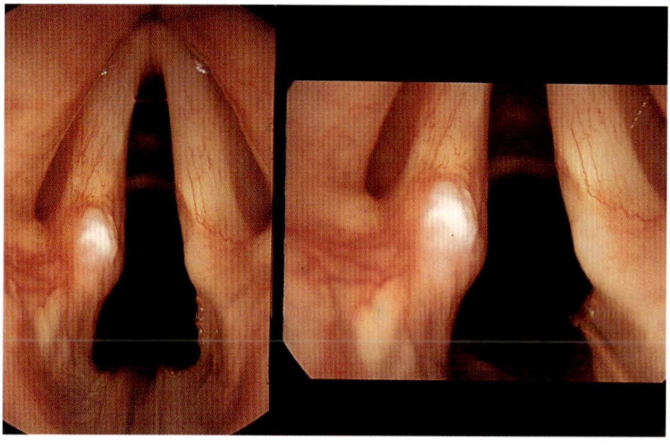

Figure **19.9**
Contact pachydermia. Direct laryngoscopy. Examination with a 0° (left) and a 30° (right) telescope clearly demonstrates the typical white, heaped-up round surface lesion. There is no sign of ulceration.

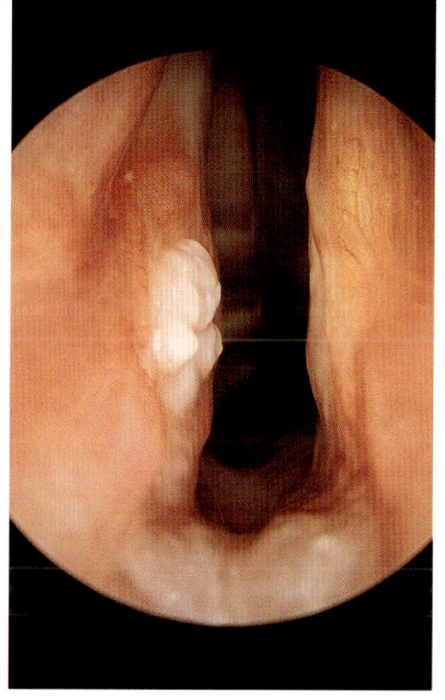

Figure **19.10**
Contact pachydermia prior to removal. Chronic changes include a severely thickened, irregular, heaped-up round lesion with a central depression. Slight depression where it 'fits into' the opposite side.

the posterior larynx. A circumscribed slightly oedematous, circular, raised white swelling over the vocal process on the medial edge of the vocal process will be seen, usually on one side only but sometimes on both.

Treatment

Contact pachydermia with a short history should be treated conservatively by voice rest and voice therapy, and may resolve within 1 or 2 months.

At microlaryngoscopy (Fig. 19.9) to confirm the diagnosis or for biopsy removal, a characteristic saucer-shaped circular lesion with surrounding severely thickened pale epithelium is diagnostic. Sometimes the lesion on one side 'fits into' a second smaller lesion on the opposite side (Fig. 19.10). The vocal folds are usually normal or slightly oedematous. Chronic contact pachydermia with a long history requires careful removal with cup forceps and scissors, although some surgeons prefer the laser. Voice rest and voice therapy post-surgically should allow complete healing.

Malignant degeneration has not been reported from contact pachydermia. It behaves differently to pachydermia in the mucosa of the interarytenoid area in the posterior glottic space.

BIBLIOGRAPHY

Bastian RW (1993) Benign laryngeal tumours. In: Cummings CW, Fredrickson JM, Harker LA, Krause CJ, Schuller DE, eds, *Otolaryngology – head and neck surgery*, 2nd edn, Vol. 3 (St Louis: CV Mosby), 193–5.

Benjamin B, Croxson G (1985) Vocal cord granulomas. *Ann Otol Rhinol Laryngol* **94**: 538–41.

Benjamin B, Roche J (1993) Vocal granuloma, including sclerosis of the arytenoid cartilage; radiographic findings. *Ann Otol Rhinol Laryngol* **102**: 756–60.

Federer RJ, Michell MJ (1984) Hyperfunctional, hyperacidic and intubation granulomas. *Arch Otolaryngol* **110**: 582–4.

Jackson C (1928) Contact ulcer of the larynx. *Ann Otol Rhinol Laryngol* **37**: 227–30.

Jackson C, Jackson CL (1935) Contact ulcer of the larynx. *Arch Otolaryngol* **22**: 1–15.

Kleinsasser O (1968) Contact pachydermia (contact ulcers). In: *Microlaryngoscopy and endolaryngeal microsurgery* (Philadelphia: WB Saunders); 42–5.

20 Laryngeal manifestations of systemic diseases

WEGENER'S GRANULOMATOSIS IN THE LARYNX

Wegener's granulomatosis is considered a generalized autoimmune disease of unknown aetiology characterized by necrotizing granulomatous vasculitis. In the initial acute phase there is preferential involvement of the upper and lower respiratory tracts sometimes resulting in subglottic stenoses as a long-term sequel in the larynx.

Pathology

The vasculitis takes the form of disseminated angiitis involving small vessels: arterioles, capillaries and venules. There is tissue necrosis, sometimes formation of microabscesses, infiltration of inflammatory cells, scattered multinucleated giant cells and histiocytes so that the lesion has a non-specific inflammatory granulomatous appearance. Inflammation of mucous membranes with extensive ulceration and necrosis is often present.

About three-quarters of the cases have respiratory manifestations including nodular masses on chest X-ray, fleeting alveolar infiltrates, atelectasis, pleural effusion, haemoptysis and sometimes cavitation. The kidneys are often involved; proteinuria, red-cell casts and microscopic haematuria are commonly found on urinalysis and renal failure occurs in some cases. Biopsy of the kidney or of extra-renal sites such as the skin is often necessary to confirm the diagnosis.

Clinical features

About 90% of patients have upper respiratory tract features often involving the nose and paranasal sinuses and sometimes involving the ears, orbits, and pharynx. Nasal obstruction and pain over the nasal dorsum or sinuses with abnormalities on sinus X-rays or CTs are characteristic findings together with persistent nasal discharge, bleeding, crusting and perforation of the nasal septum. The initial symptoms are often confused with a prolonged upper respiratory tract infection.

Respiratory distress, cough, shortness of breath, stridor and progressive airway obstruction indicate involvement of the subglottic larynx and tracheobronchial tree, which are affected in the early phase in about 15% of cases. Subglottic or upper tracheal narrowing with inspiratory stridor is a feature of the disease in the acute phase and is caused by reddish friable inflammatory areas which lead to more permanent subglottic or tracheal scarring and stenosis in the chronic phase, after relapse or following treatment.

Hoarseness is sometimes one of the presenting features.

Antineutrophil cytoplasmic antibodies, specifically cANCA (c for cytoplasmic staining as opposed to p for perinuclear staining) titres are high or increase in over 90% of cases and usually correlate with activity of the disease. A positive cANCA test when there are other suggestive clinical features supports the diagnosis.

Wegener's granulomatosis

- Generalized autoimmune disease
- Necrotizing granulomatous vasculitis
- Preferential respiratory tract involvement
- Often renal involvement
- Sometimes acute airway problems
- Often chronic subglottic stenosis
- Laser treatment or laryngotracheoplasty

Laryngoscopy

Indirect laryngoscopy in the acute stage may show red, inflamed or ulcerated areas in the subglottis. In the chronic stage or during remission, mature subglottic stenosis (Fig. 20.1) can be seen.

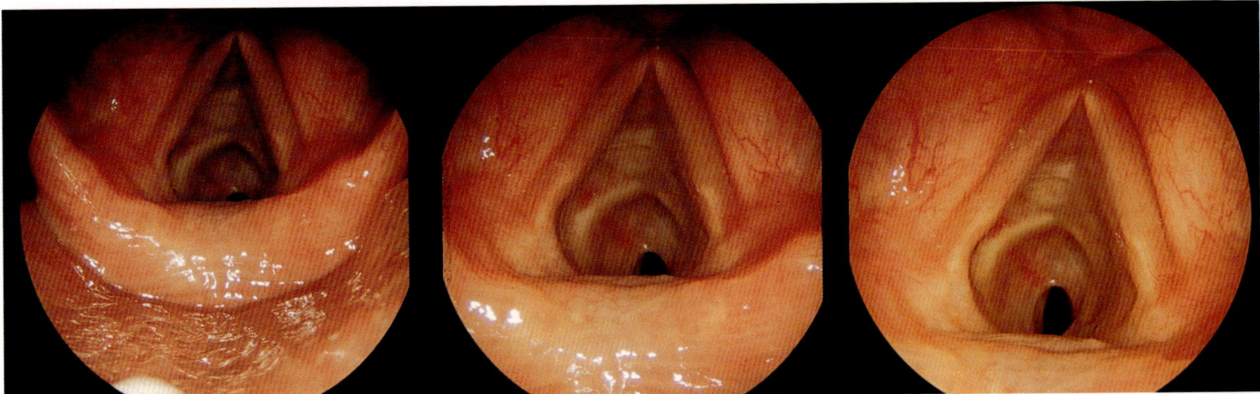

Figure **20.1**
Subglottic stenosis caused by Wegener's granulomatosis. Indirect laryngoscopy. Successive views, as the telescope is re-positioned, finally showing irregular bands of fibrous tissue causing subglottic stenosis, which was treated by staged endoscopic laser vaporization.

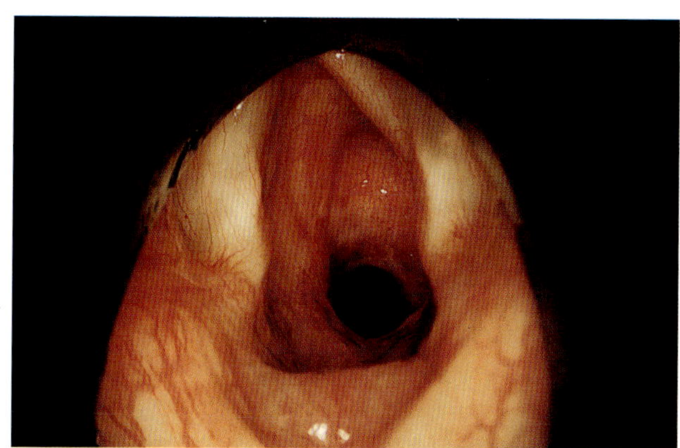

Figure **20.2**
Subglottic stenosis. Wegener's granulomatosis. Direct laryngoscopy. Irregular mature scar prior to laser treatment.

Direct laryngoscopy shows subglottic or upper tracheal stenosis (Fig. 20.2) sometimes with multiple bands of scarring, and if these are severe, relief of airway obstruction can be achieved by either tracheotomy and/or laser treatment. In selected chronic cases, when the disease is under control and no longer active, laryngotracheoplasty may be considered.

Treatment

Medical treatment of systemic disease employs oral cyclophosphamide and methylprednisolone often used in pulsed doses. It appears that limited Wegener's granulomatosis may respond to trimethoprim/sulphamethoxazole. Medical therapy may be beneficial for the laryngeal disease.

Note on nomenclature

The controversial term '**lethal midline granuloma**' should no longer be associated with Wegener's granulomatosis. It described relentless progressive erosion, ulceration and destruction of the soft tissues, cartilage and bones of the central face including the nose, palate and paranasal sinuses. However, many of the patients originally diagnosed with lethal midline granuloma were found to have a different disease during the later course of their illness or at autopsy. Using immunohistochemical and monoclonal antibody techniques a more specific diagnosis can now usually be made, such as malignant lymphoma or specific bacterial, fungal, mycobacterial or protozoan infection.

Lymphomatoid granulomatosis is a rare disease with similarities to malignant lymphoproliferative disorders. There is an intense inflammatory cell infiltrate but, unlike Wegener's granulomatosis, no vasculitis. There is commonly upper and lower respiratory tract involvement but the larynx appears to be spared.

LARYNGEAL AMYLOID

Amyloidosis is a disease of unknown aetiology. There are two types: *primary* (not associated with systemic disease) and *secondary* (associated with systemic disease, e.g. rheumatoid arthritis or tuberculosis). Primary amyloidosis can be *localized* (confined to a single site or organ system), or *generalized* (found in many body tissues). Amyloid of the larynx presents as an obstructive mass or as scattered submucosal deposits.

Pathology

Amyloidosis is characterized by subepithelial and intramuscular extracellular deposits of fibrillar protein–polysaccharide complex. Histological examination shows that under the squamous mucosal layer there is band-like cellular infiltrate, mostly plasma cells, lymphocytes and macrophages, with some giant cells arranged focally around amorphous and sometimes globular homogeneous material.

Primary localized amyloidosis has been found in many sites in the body including the aerodigestive tract, the orbit, nasopharynx, lips, floor of the mouth, tongue, larynx, tracheobronchial tree and oesophagus.

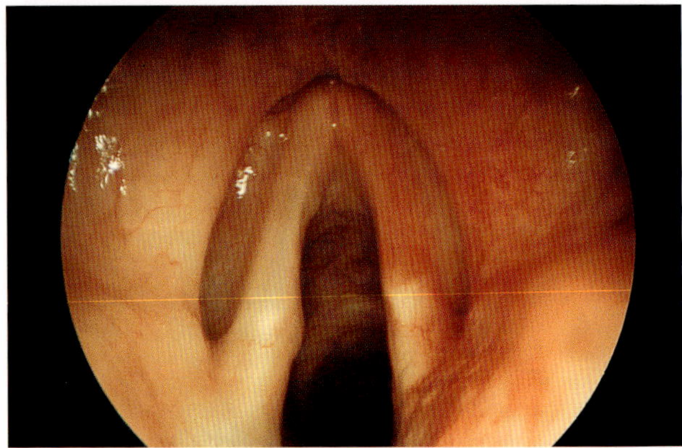

Figure **20.3**
Amyloid right vocal cord. Pink-red, slightly swollen vocal fold in a 26-year-old male with a husky voice. Biopsy proven amyloid; no other organs affected.

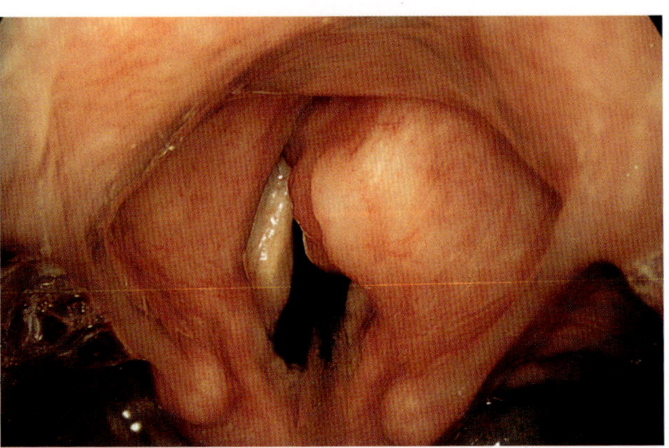

Figure **20.4**
Primary localized laryngeal amyloid. Rounded, solitary mass with surface irregularities in the right anterior supraglottic region in a young woman. Local endoscopic removal.

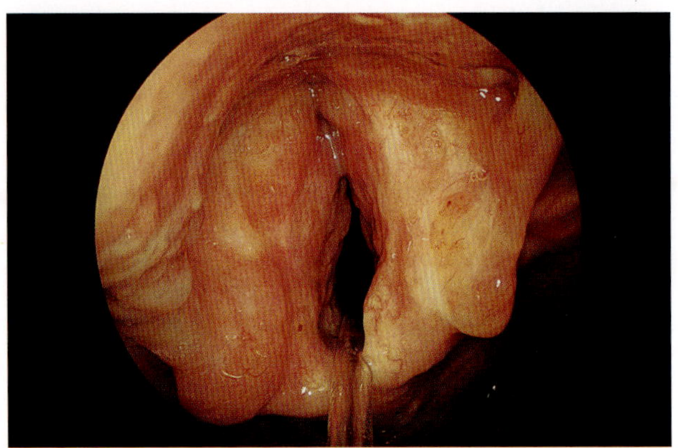

Figure **20.5**
Amyloid of larynx. Diffuse submucosal irregular deposits in the larynx were the only amyloid found in the patient.

Laryngeal amyloid

Primary or secondary
Localized or generalized
Larynx usually primary, localized
Hoarseness, sometimes stridor
Usually laser removal

The larynx is seldom involved with amyloid. Most reported cases have been the localized type, confined to the larynx and not affecting other organs, but some have multiple sites of respiratory involvement indicating that any patient found to have laryngeal amyloid requires complete investigation to rule out disease in other sites.

In the larynx, deposits of amyloid may cause only minimal detectable change (Fig. 20.3), there may be irregular masses (Fig. 20.4) of various sizes or the disease may be more widespread beneath intact epithelium (Fig. 20.5). Under light microscopy, biopsy material appears as amorphous, pink-staining eosinophilic deposits showing green birefrigence under polarization after being stained with Congo red. The diagnosis can be confirmed by electron microscopy, which shows an interlacing mesh of non-branching fibrils. Immunohistochemical features

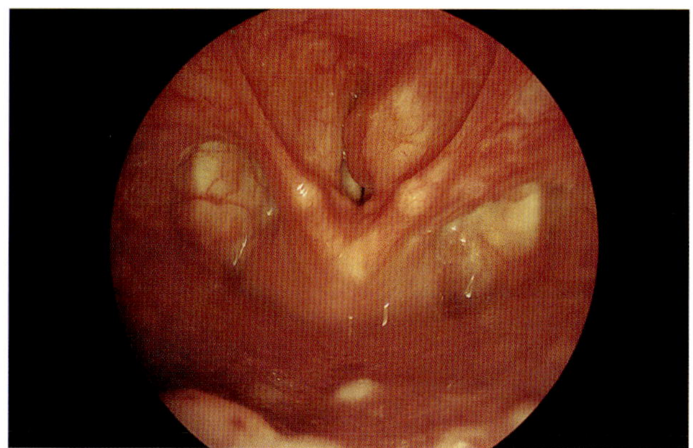

Figure **20.6**
Amyloid mass. Indirect laryngoscopy. Large localized deposit of primary amyloid in the right supraglottic region causing increasing hoarseness by interfering with vocal fold vibration.

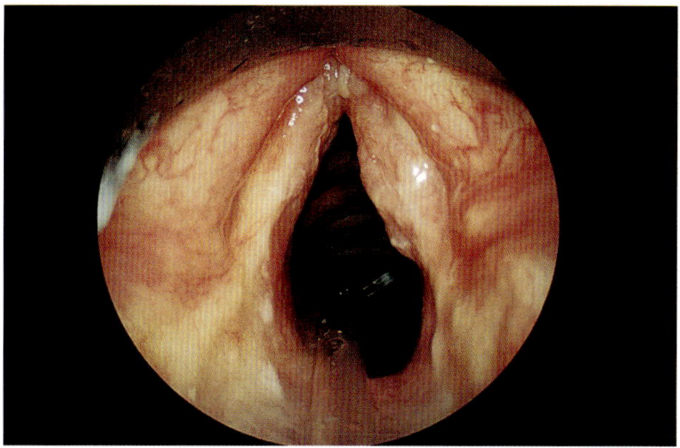

Figure **20.7**
Amyloid in vocal folds. Severe dysphonia caused by primary, localized amyloid infiltration; worse on the right than the left.

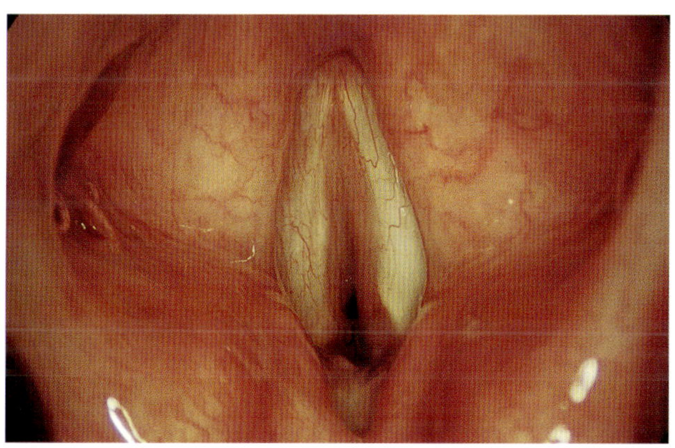

Figure **20.8**
Subglottic amyloid. Bilateral subglottic deposits of primary, localized amyloid causing chronic hoarseness and airway obstruction which required temporary tracheotomy to allow serial endoscopic laser treatment.

provide the possibility of identifying amyloid disease when appropriate antibodies are available.

Localized amyloid of the larynx and trachea has been reported to progress in some cases to tracheobronchopathia osteochondroplastica.

Clinical features and treatment

Patients with laryngeal amyloid most often present with non-specific hoarseness, sometimes stridor and occasionally pain. Large masses (Fig. 20.6) are seen at indirect laryngoscopy. Direct laryngoscopy shows the distribution of the deposits which may be supraglottic (Fig. 20.4), glottic (Fig. 20.7) or subglottic (Fig. 20.8). Biopsy of the deposits is always necessary. Treatment may not be indicated if symptoms are minimal but local removal or removal at intervals using the laser is more rational than radical resection. As recurrences may occur after many years, long-term follow-up is necessary.

LARYNGEAL SARCOID

Sarcoidosis is a poorly understood chronic granulomatous disease of unknown cause which can affect virtually any organ in the body. In the larynx, sarcoid presents as a diffuse, chronic, symmetrical supraglottic swelling.

Pathology

Previously sarcoid was thought to be a variant of tuberculosis because of its histological resemblance,

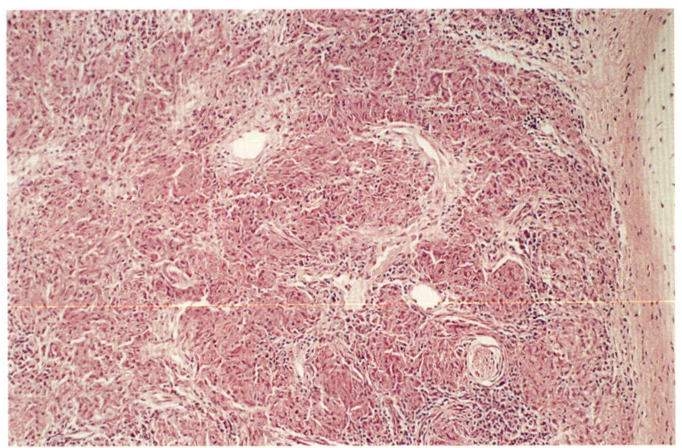

Figure **20.9**
Histologic section of sarcoid. Laryngeal biopsy showing granulomatous change with epithelioid cells, macrophages, and chronic inflammatory cells but no caseation.

but an infective agent has never been identified and sarcoid granulomas have no caseation. Strangely, the incidence of sarcoidosis is greater in developed countries but the reason is not known. It is ten times more common in the black population of the United States than the white, ten times more common in females than males, and, for comparison, the incidence is approximately ten times that of Hodgkin's disease.

The characteristic lesion is a circumscribed granuloma, usually found within the lymphoreticular tissue. The granulomas consist of epithelioid cells, macrophages, a few Langerhans' giant cells, and a variable number of lymphocytes and plasma cells (Fig. 20.9).

Although the lesions resemble tuberculosis, there is neither caseation nor necrosis and there is a conspicuous absence of bacilli. The granulomas may remain for months or years, resolve completely or undergo hyaline fibrosis.

Clinical features

Sarcoidosis is a chronic disease which undergoes exacerbations and remissions and commonly presents in young adults. It is usually found in multiple organs; it often affects the lungs (with an alveolitis consisting mainly of T cells), lymph nodes, spleen, liver, eyes, skin, bone and nervous system. Some cases may be asymptomatic and may be diagnosed only when enlarged hilar lymph nodes, with or without pulmonary infiltrates, are seen on chest X-ray. More often patients present with respiratory complaints such as dyspnoea, cough or non-specific features such as malaise, fever, fatigue and weight loss. They may present with multiple nodules and plaques on the skin, nasal obstruction, cranial nerve palsy, keratoconjunctivitis sicca or arthralgia. Approximately 90% of patients have an abnormal chest X-ray.

Diagnosis

The diagnosis depends on suggestive clinical, radiographic and laboratory findings and is confirmed only when biopsy reveals non-caseating granulomas (which may be difficult to identify and multiple sections may be required). The Kviem test, once considered diagnostic, is now of no practical importance. Hypercalcaemia and increased serum angiotensin-converting enzyme (SACE) are indicators of activity. Investigations to exclude other diseases include cultures for acid-fast bacilli, Ziehl–Neelsen staining, fungal cultures, serologic tests for syphilis and an ANCA titre for Wegener's granulomatosis.

Laryngeal sarcoid

Laryngeal sarcoid is estimated to occur in less than 5% of patients with generalized sarcoidosis. However, laryngeal sarcoid occurs in isolation, with no evidence of systemic disease.

The initial stages of sarcoid may be relatively benign. The symptoms include hoarseness, a feeling of a lump in the throat, dysphagia, cough and, in well-developed cases, dyspnoea secondary to upper airway obstruction. Previously undiagnosed laryngeal sarcoid has been reported to cause severe upper airway obstruction and asphyxiation in advanced cases. The disease characteristically affects the

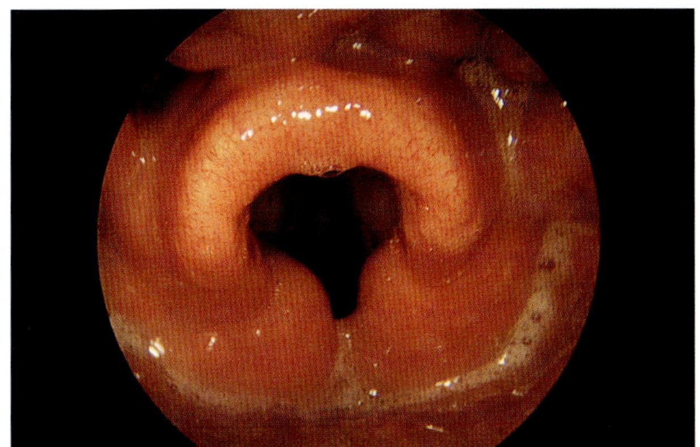

Figure **20.10**
Laryngeal sarcoid. Indirect laryngoscopy. Diffuse, symmetrical supraglottic swelling in a 35-year-old male with a feeling of 'something' in the throat and mild dyspnoea on exertion.

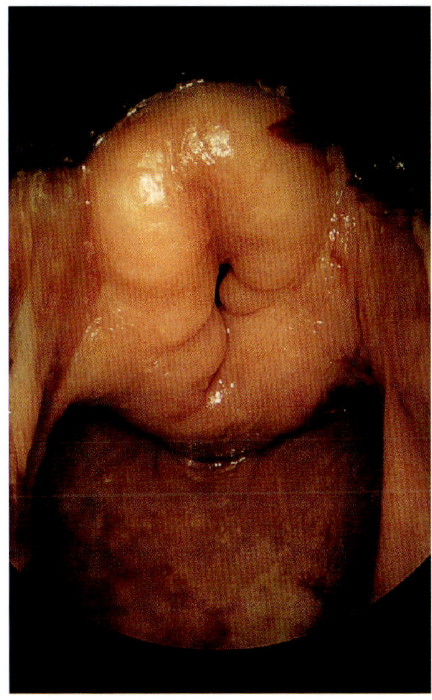

Figure **20.11**
Laryngeal sarcoid. Gross supraglottic swelling. Patient complained of slight voice change and severe shortness of breath.

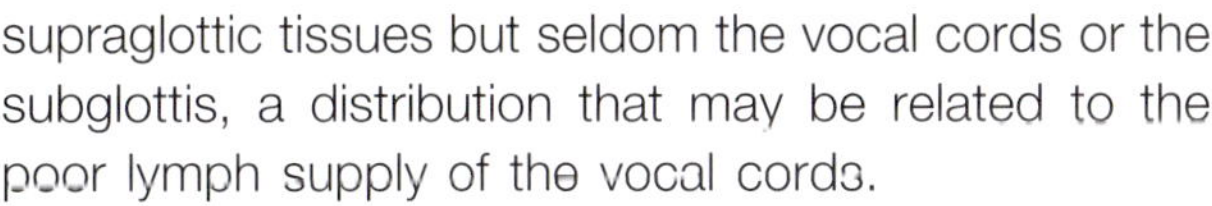

supraglottic tissues but seldom the vocal cords or the subglottis, a distribution that may be related to the poor lymph supply of the vocal cords.

Indirect laryngoscopic appearance

The typical appearance of the supraglottic tissues should be emphasized. There is diffuse, pale pink-red oedematous enlargement of the epiglottis, aryepiglottic folds and arytenoids (Fig. 20.10). The appearance of laryngeal sarcoid at direct laryngoscopy (Fig. 20.11) confirms diffuse generalized, symmetrical non-ulcerated swelling of the supraglottic tissues, usually with normal vocal cords. Vocal cord paralysis can occur by direct involvement of the sarcoid or by indirect involvement of the neural pathways.

The appearance of the supraglottic structures in laryngeal sarcoid is so characteristic that it should alert the laryngologist to the possibility of the disease in a patient with unexplained dysphonia, dysphagia or partial airway obstruction, even before biopsy.

Laryngeal sarcoid

Chronic granulomatous disease
Cause not known
Laryngeal sarcoid often in isolation
Symmetrical supraglottic swelling
May not need treatment

Radiological appearance

Radiography shows smooth swelling of the epiglottis and aryepiglottic folds (Fig. 20.12), an appearance similar to that of acute epiglottitis but the characteristic acute clinical features of localized infection, severe

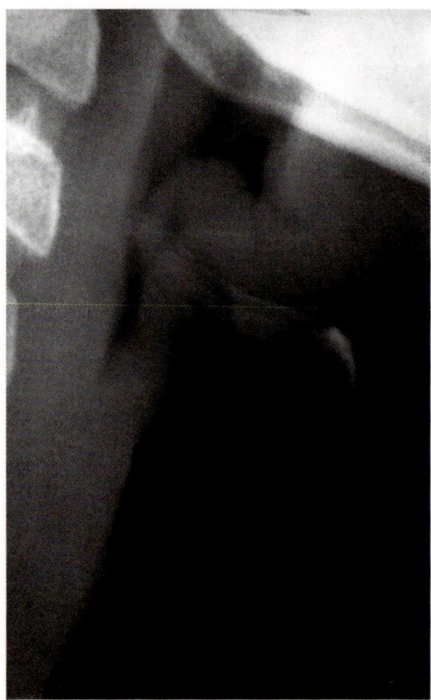

Figure **20.12**
Sarcoid on lateral X-ray. Rounded supraglottic swelling involving epiglottis and aryepiglottic folds.

obstruction and septicaemia are absent. Lateral airways soft tissue radiographs are more valuable than a CT scan. Chest X-ray, and often CT examination, are essential to detect enlarged hilar lymph nodes and disease in the pulmonary parenchyma.

Treatment

The mortality rate is about 5% and usually due to cardiac or pulmonary disease. In most patients the clinical course is prolonged and marked by long periods of remission, often followed by acute exacerbation; this fluctuating course makes the decision to recommend treatment a difficult one. Systemic steroids are usually effective in alleviating symptoms and, although intralesional injections have been advocated for laryngeal disease, in most patients symptoms are relatively minor. For isolated laryngeal sarcoidosis regular observation is all that is required unless there is progressive or significant airway obstruction.

RHEUMATOID ARTHRITIS IN THE LARYNX

Rheumatoid arthritis is a chronic, systemic, inflammatory, autoimmune disease, whose outstanding feature is symmetric, progressive, deforming arthritis with variable extra-articular manifestations. In most patients it affects multiple joints, notably those in the hands and feet, and may be accompanied by rheumatoid skin nodules. Rheumatoid arthritis may be confined to the vertebral column as ankylosing spondylitis. There are many other manifestations, including cardiac, neurologic and pulmonary. When the larynx is affected, swelling and fixation of the cricoarytenoid joints causes slowly progressive airway obstruction.

Pathology

Histologically the disease is characterized by progressive hyperplasia and hypertrophy of synovial lining cells, a proliferation which eventually destroys the articular cartilage probably by the action of collagenase and leads to severe osteoarthritis and joint destruction. Depending on the stage of the disease, the inflammatory process exhibits varying degrees of fibrosis, tissue destruction and pannus.

Clinical features

It is three times more common in women than men and usually begins between the third and seventh decades, although there is a distinct subset of

Rheumatoid in the larynx

Chronic inflammatory autoimmune disease
Multiple manifestations
Swelling and fixation of cricoarytenoid joints
Airway obstruction may need tracheotomy

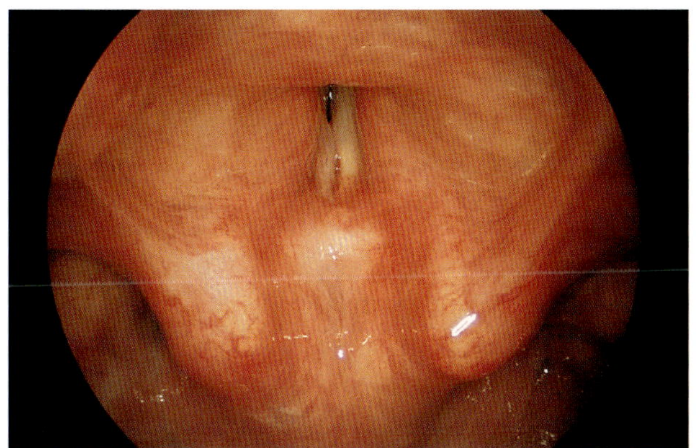

Figure **20.13**
Rheumatoid arthritis of the larynx. Severe chronic, posterior glottic swelling and fixation of both cricoarytenoid joints combining to cause severe obstruction which required long-term tracheotomy. No response to therapy for generalized disease.

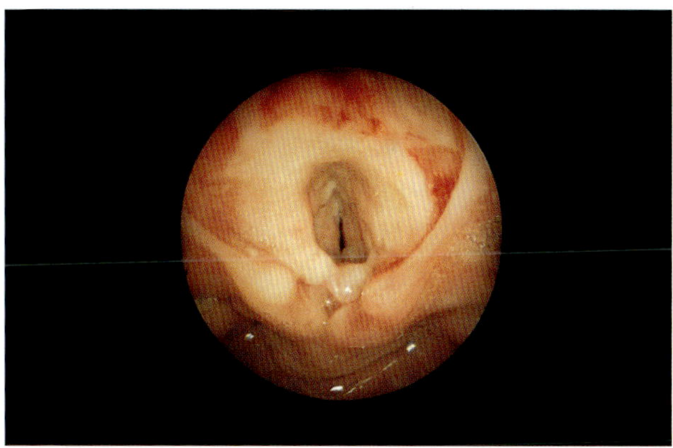

Figure **20.14**
Epidermolysis bullosa dystrophica. Acute on chronic manifestations with partial airway obstruction.

manifestations which constitute juvenile rheumatoid arthritis. The symptoms are very variable in severity and progression, with periods of exacerbation and remission which occur for no obvious reason.

The clinical features range from mild to severe, destructive and mutilating. There is no one specific test result diagnostic of rheumatoid arthritis although there is a high titre of rheumatoid factor or IgM circulating autoantibodies in 80% of patients with the clinical disease.

Involvement of the larynx has been reported in 25–50% of patients with longstanding systemic disease and causes huskiness, stridor, dysphagia and a feeling of fullness. Changes in the larynx include oedematous inflammatory swelling of the posterior larynx (Fig. 20.13), myositis in the intrinsic muscles, rheumatoid nodules in the vocal folds, atrophic changes in the recurrent laryngeal nerves and involvement to a greater or lesser degree of the cricothyroid or cricoarytenoid joints.

Treatment

There are many forms of treatment depending on the extent and severity of the condition. They include nonsteroidal anti-inflammatory drugs; corticosteroids (systemic or by injection) and many other anti-inflammatory, immunopressive and cytotoxic agents whose effect on laryngeal disease is not known.

Inflammatory swelling with obliteration and/or ankylosis of the cricoarytenoid joints causes airway obstruction (Fig. 20.13) which can be severe enough to warrant tracheotomy.

EPIDERMOLYSIS BULLOSA

The term epidermolysis bullosa covers a heterogeneous group of rare hereditary connective tissue disorders in which the basic defect is a flaw in the dermal component of the basement membrane. Loss of adherence between the epidermis and dermis leads to recurring formation of blisters which rupture, ulcerate, and heal with scar formation. The tendency to form blisters at a site of minor trauma varies from a mild nuisance to a life-threatening condition. Epidermolysis bullosa simplex, the milder form, heals without scarring unless there is secondary infection. Epidermolysis bullosa dystrophica, the more serious form, is inherited as a recessive trait and minor trauma often leads to bullae which rupture and heal with scarring in the skin or mucous membranes.

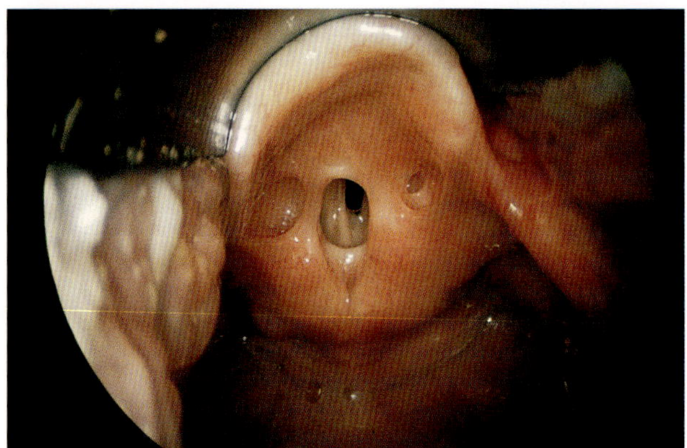

Figure **20.15**
Epidermolysis bullosa dystrophica. Chronic phase with supraglottic and posterior glottic scarring. Same patient as in Fig. 20.14, but 5 years later.

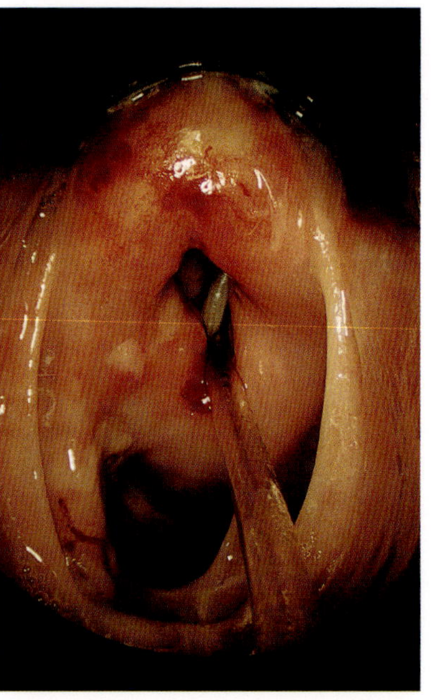

Figure **20.16**
Bullous pemphigoid. During an active stage in a 45-year-old woman. Haemorrhagic surface on an oedematous epiglottis and scarred bands in the pharynx, forming pockets in which food collects.

Involvement of the larynx, e.g. after endotracheal intubation, can lead to haemorrhagic ulceration, denuding of the mucous membranes and severe airway obstruction (Fig. 20.14). Healing eventually forms laryngeal stenotic webs (Fig. 20.15), either supraglottic, posterior glottic or subglottic.

In the severe forms of the disease, intubation for general anaesthesia must be avoided at all costs. In milder or simplex forms careful intubation can usually be safely accomplished with due precautions such as using a small-diameter tube to minimize mucosal trauma.

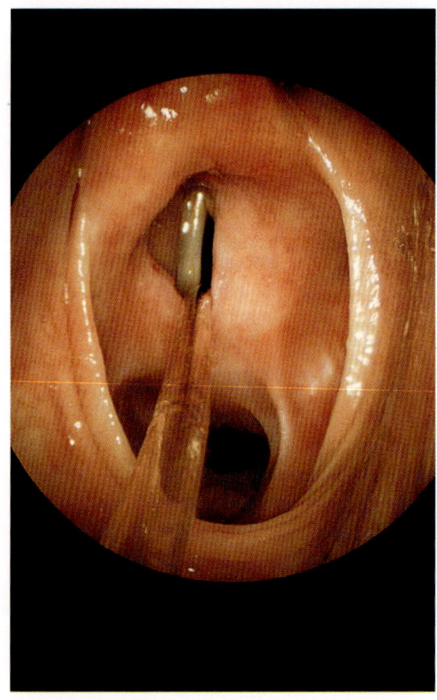

Figure **20.17**
Bullous pemphigoid. The same patient as Fig. 20.16, but the bullous pemphigoid is now inactive; conditions are suitable for laser division and release of the constricting scar tissue causing posterior laryngeal stenosis and narrowing of the airway.

Epidermolysis bullosa

Group of rare connective tissue disorders
Tendency to form blisters and swell after trauma
Intubation may cause airway obstruction
Healing eventually causes laryngeal stenosis

Bullous pemphigoid

Blistering disease
Cause unknown – autoimmune?
Usually elderly women
Supraglottic bands and stenoses

BULLOUS PEMPHIGOID

Pemphigoid or bullous pemphigoid is a blistering disease similar to pemphigus vulgaris. The cause is unknown but it is thought to be an autoimmune disease whose autoantibodies are directed against some components of the basement membrane, whereas in pemphigus they are thought to act against intercellular antigens.

Bullous pemphigoid usually affects elderly women and can cause large, tense blisters with an erythematous base anywhere on the skin but with a predilection for the groin, inner thighs and lower abdomen. The mouth is involved in about one-third of patients and occasionally, following an acute phase (Fig. 20.16), cicatricial stenotic bands and webs (Fig. 20.17) affect the supraglottic region. Laser treatment should be limited to division of scar tissue causing swallowing or airway problems, and if possible should be carried out during an inactive stage of the disease. Systemic or topical steroids may be required; therapy with cyclophosphamide and steroids is used in severe cases.

PACHYONYCHIA CONGENITA

This rare, autosomal dominant disorder with variable penetrance affects membranes and is characterized by nail dystrophy, hyperkeratosis and hyperhydrosis of the palms and soles, leukoplakia of the mucosa of the upper respiratory tract and anus and occasionally laryngeal involvement.

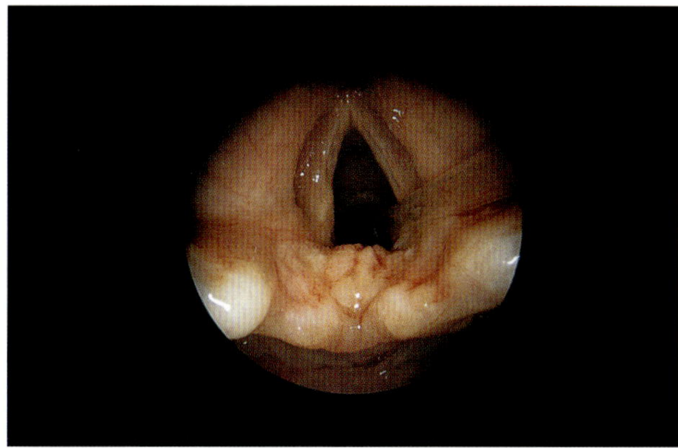

Figure **20.18**
Pachyonychia congenita in the larynx. A multilobed, irregular, pink, exophytic, midline mass in the interarytenoid region prior to subtotal excisional biopsy. Repeated endoscopy and laser vaporization 3 months later.

The laryngeal lesions have all involved the posterior glottis (Fig. 20.18) and appear as white, thickened masses. Histopathological examination reveals thickened epithelium, acanthosis, parakeratosis and extensive vacuolization as seen in white sponge naevus but without evidence of dyskeratosis.

Hoarseness, the symptom of laryngeal involvement, has been reported in less than 10% of patients with the disease. It has been suggested that the larynx has its worst manifestations in childhood and that they may regress in adulthood. Endoscopic surgical debulking using forceps and/or laser seems appropriate as postoperative recurrence appears to be minimal.

Pachyonychia congenita

Autosomal dominant disorder
Lesions in posterior larynx
Laser for debulking

BIBLIOGRAPHY

Benjamin B, Dalton C, Croxson G (1995) Laryngoscopic diagnosis of laryngeal sarcoid. *Ann Otol Rhinol Laryngol* **104**: 529–31.

Roger G, Gallas D, Tashjian G, Baculard A, Tournier G, Garabedian EN (1994) Sarcoidosis of upper respiratory tract in children. *Int J Pediatr Otorhinolaryngol* **30**: 233–40.

Godbersen GS, Leah JF, Hansmann ML, Rudert H, Linke RP (1992) Organ-limited laryngeal amyloid deposits: clinical, morphological, and immunohistochemical result of five cases. *Ann Otol Rhinol Laryngol* **101**: 770–5.

Grum CM, Lynch JP (1992) Tracheobronchial and oesophageal manifestations of systemic disease. In: Cummings CW, Frederickson JM, Harker LA, Krause CJ, Schuller DE, eds., *Otolaryngology – head and neck surgery* (St Louis: CV Mosby); 2304–8.

James DG, Barter S, Jash D, MacKinnon DM, Carstairs LS (1982) Sarcoidosis of the upper respiratory tract (SURT). *J Laryngol Otol* **96**: 711–8.

McIlwain JC, Shepperd HWH (1996) Laser treatment of primary amyloidosis of the larynx. *J Laryngol Otol* **100**: 1079–80.

Neel HB III, MacDonald TJ (1982) Laryngeal sarcoidosis. Report of thirteen patients. *Ann Otol Rhinol Laryngol* **91**: 359–62.

Shumrick KA, Shumrick DA, Vietti MJ (1995) Inflammatory diseases of the larynx. In: Freid MP, ed., *The larynx* (St Louis: CV Mosby); 290–3.

Simpson GT, Strong MS, Skinner M, Cohen AS (1984) Localised amyloidosis of the head and neck and upper aerodigestive and lower respiratory tracts. *Ann Otol Rhinol Laryngol* **93**: 374–9.

Waxman J, Bose WJ (1968) Laryngeal manifestations of Wegener's granulomatosis: case reports and review of the literature. *J Rheumatol* **13**: 308–13.

21 Idiopathic subglottic stenosis

Idiopathic subglottic stenosis is a rare, slowly progressive, inflammatory process of unknown aetiology occurring in the subglottic region and the first tracheal arch and with no systemic manifestation. It appears to occur only in females. There are no indicators of precipitant or concurrent disease either at the time of presentation or subsequently.

CLINICAL FEATURES

The clinical features are progressive stridor, dyspnoea, sometimes minor dysphonia and occasionally progression to life-threatening obstruction if the nature of the problem is not recognized. All reports emphasize the localized subglottic stenosis, the progression of symptoms, the undetermined aetiology and the difficulties with treatment. An association with gastro-oesophageal reflux has been proposed but reflux is not present in all patients. An autoimmune aetiology has been suggested for some cases but remains unproven.

Lateral X-rays or CT of the subglottis (Fig. 21.1) confirm the presence of stenosis but the severity of narrowing is more accurately measured by calibration in millimetres at endoscopy.

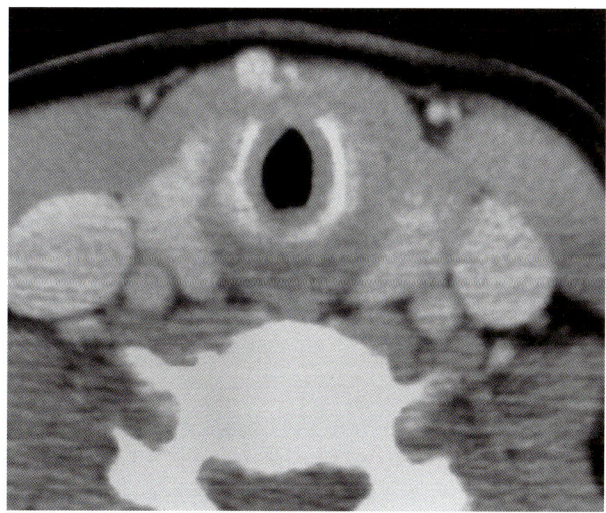

Figure **21.1**
Axial CT through the cricoid. Circumferential, symmetrical soft tissue swelling narrows the airway.

ENDOSCOPY

The appearance of idiopathic subglottic stenosis at direct laryngoscopy (Fig. 21.2) is similar in all cases. Neither vocal cord nor cricoarytenoid joint mobility are impaired. Stenosis commences in the immediate subglottic region and extends to the inferior margin of the cricoid cartilage or to the first tracheal arch. Calibration can be graduated bougies, a series of endotracheal tubes or telescopes of known external diameter. The lesions are circumferential, some are eccentric and some are more prominent in one aspect than another. The mucosa usually has a reddened, finely granular inflammatory appearance, the underlying tissue is soft to firm and the surface bleeds easily on biopsy. The trachea distal to the stenosis is normal.

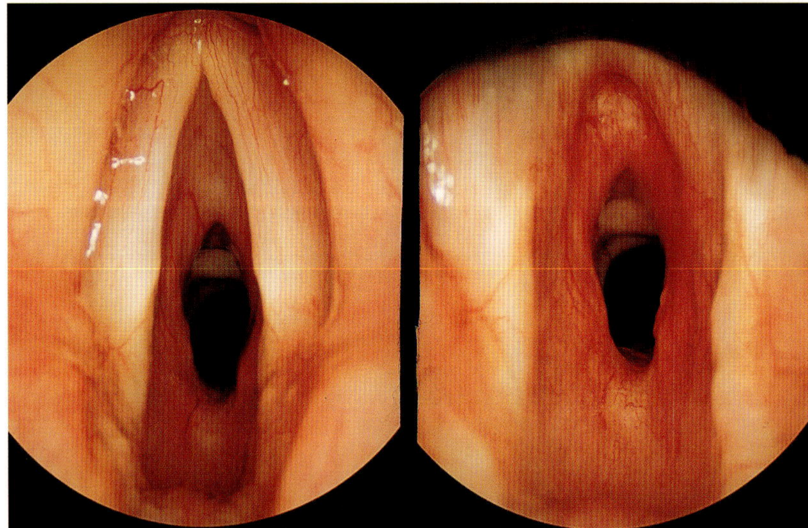

Figure **21.2**
Direct endoscopy. Subglottic site and relation to vocal cords (left) and with subglottiscope positioned for laser surgery (right).

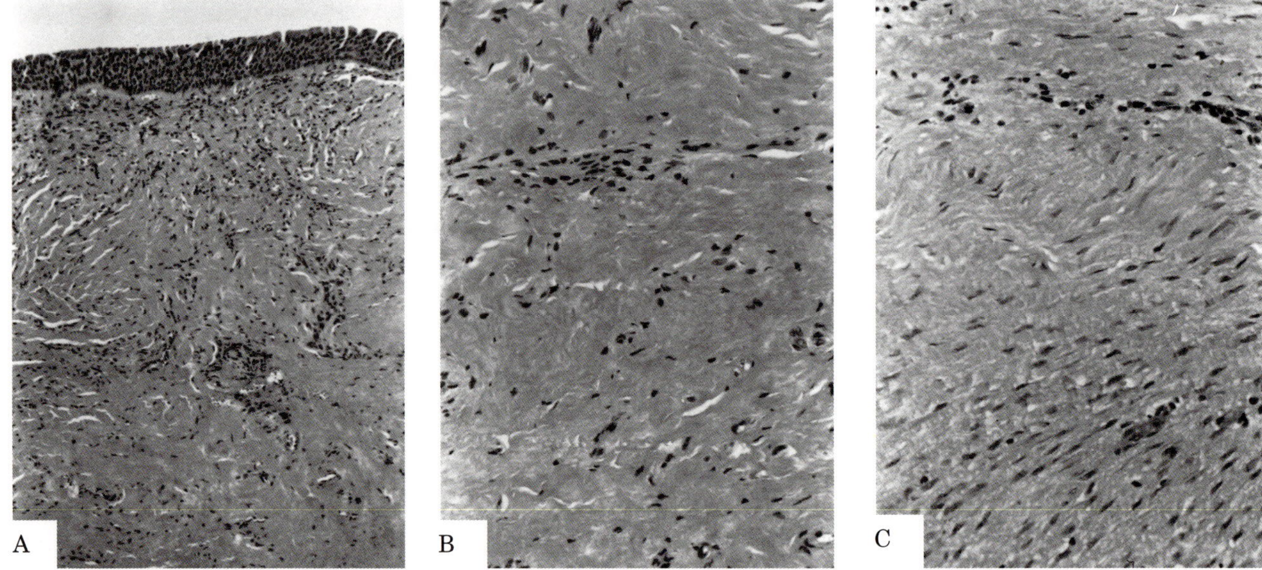

Figure **21.3**
Histopathology of biopsy. A. Transitional surface mucosa and dense fibrous tissue in the lamina propria. Inflammatory cells are sparse. B. Higher magnification of the same biopsy showing hypocellular fibrous tissue. C. Another biopsy showing more cellular fibrous tissue resembling fibromatosis.

HISTOPATHOLOGY

There is a characteristic histopathological appearance (Fig. 21.3). The most striking feature, common to all biopsies, is dense fibrous tissue extending to the epithelial surface. The fibrosis is generally poorly cellular and the collagen is very dense although in some areas cellularity resembles fibromatosis. Blood vessels are scant and tend to be surrounded by a mixed mononuclear inflammatory cell infiltrate. The overlying epithelium may be squamous, respiratory or transitional but shows no dysplastic changes. No

Idiopathic subglottic stenosis

Rare, slowly progressive, cause unknown
Appears to affect females only
Increasing stridor, respiratory distress
Characteristic endoscopic appearance
Non-specific histopathology
Endoscopic laser treatment
May require tracheotomy
Resection for selected cases

vasculitis, granuloma formation or foreign body is seen. There is no amyloid, no sign of acid-fast bacilli or fungi. Cultures of the tissue are negative. Cytoplasmic and perinuclear pattern antineutrophil autoantibodies are absent.

TREATMENT

The clinical course of the disease is unpredictable and it is difficult to treat. Options include observation, tracheotomy, endoscopic laser surgery, or an open surgical procedure including resection as reported by Grillo et al (1993) who described good or excellent results in 32 of 35 selected patients treated by single-stage resection of the stenosis.

For most patients, endoscopic laser therapy with staged vaporization of the subglottic tissue is effective primary therapy to maintain the airway.

BIBLIOGRAPHY

Benjamin B, Jacobsen I, Eckstein R (1997) Idiopathic subglottic stenosis: diagnosis and endoscopic laser treatment. *Ann Otol Rhinol Laryngol* **106**: 770–4.

Grillo HC, Mark EM, Mathison DC, Wain JC (1993) Idiopathic laryngotracheal stenosis and its management. *Ann Thorac Surg* **56**: 80–7.

V LARYNGEAL NEOPLASIA

22 Multiple respiratory papillomas

BACKGROUND

Morrell Mackenzie specified papillomas as the commonest benign tumour of the larynx in children in the late 1800s (Fig. 22.1). The tumours were clearly described by Chevalier Jackson (Fig. 22.2) and the term 'juvenile laryngeal papillomas' was used until the 1960s. At that time it was thought that the papillomas were confined to the laryngeal mucosa and that they were found almost exclusively in children because they had a tendency to regress at puberty. Recent studies make it clear that papillomas in the respiratory tract can occur at any age, with about

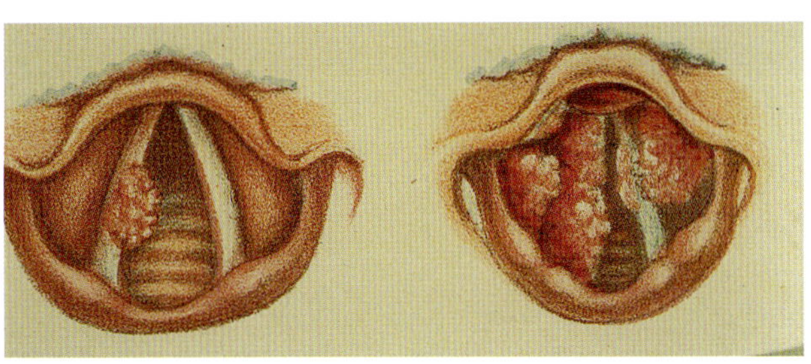

Figure **22.1**
Mackenzie's hand-drawn diagrams of papillomas. Reproduced from Mackenzie (1871).

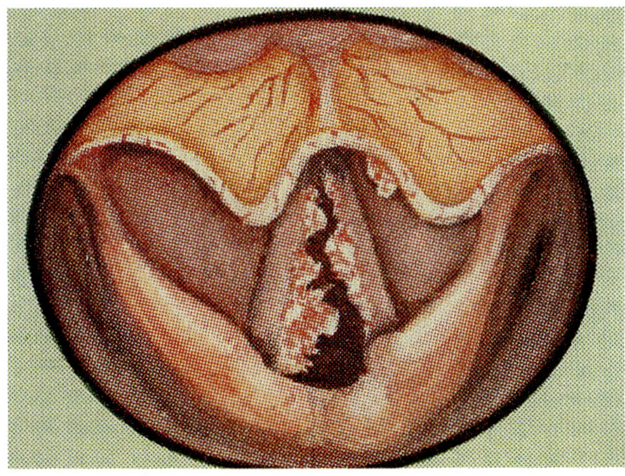

Figure **22.2**
Jackson's hand-drawn diagram of a papilloma. Reproduced with permission from Jackson and Jackson (1942).

Multiple respiratory papillomas

Any age, two-thirds under 15 years, many under 5 years
HPV activated by unknown promoter
Usually in the larynx, may be above or below
Also tracheobronchial tree, lung, pharynx, nose
Onset, control, recurrence not related to puberty
Unpredictable remissions and recurrences

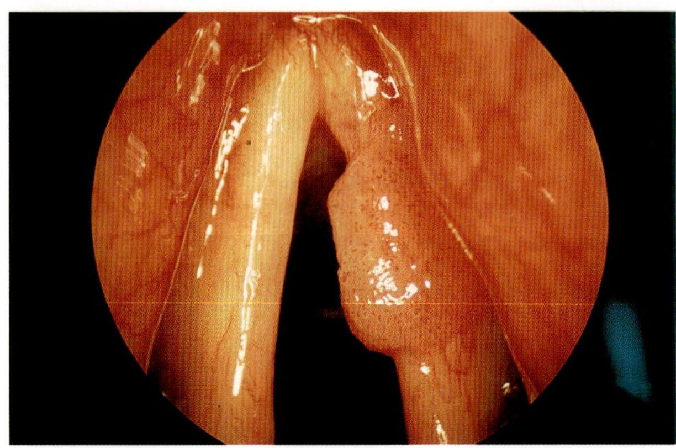

Figure **22.3**
Large solitary papilloma. Large papilloma mass on the right vocal fold of an adult male. A lesion of this kind is less aggressive than multiple lesions in younger patients and less likely to recur after removal.

two-thirds of patients younger than 15 years and one-third older than 15 years, with the highest incidence being before the age of 5 years. Furthermore although papillomas occur most commonly on the mucosa of the larynx, they are found elsewhere in the upper respiratory tract including the anterior nasal cavities, nasopharynx, oropharynx, trachea, bronchi, lung parenchyma and even in the oesophagus. It has been proven conclusively that there is no relationship between puberty and the age of onset, the rate of control or the rate of recurrence, and patients should therefore be treated without regard to age. The preferable and more accurate term for the condition is multiple respiratory papillomatosis (MRP).

Although the disease is almost always benign, many patients require multiple operations for repeated papilloma removal over a long time. When the papillomas grow almost uncontrollably, widespread respiratory papillomatosis becomes a devastating disease which not only disrupts the patient's quality of life but sometimes also becomes life-threatening.

Pathogenesis

Papillomas are relatively common in infants and young children, and in some cases their cause is thought to be related to condylomata acuminata in the mother. But they also occur in older children and less commonly in adults where no such causal relationship has been established. The older the patient the more likely surgical control is to be achieved and, although the disease is notorious for frequent recurrences, unexpected spontaneous improvement does sometimes occur. The natural history of untreated papillomas over a long time is unknown but progressive spread and enlargement is very likely.

In general there is a tendency for recurrence, in some cases despite all forms of treatment. Relentless proliferation of large obstructing masses may threaten life.

Adult onset papillomas are less aggressive in their clinical behaviour than those of juvenile onset. Solitary lesions (Fig. 22.3) which are more often seen in adults are less likely to recur after removal.

There is no significant racial or ethnic difference in incidence but many patients come from socio-economically deprived families.

Human papilloma virus

For many years there has been debate about the aetiology of papillomas but overwhelming evidence has now accumulated to implicate the human papil-

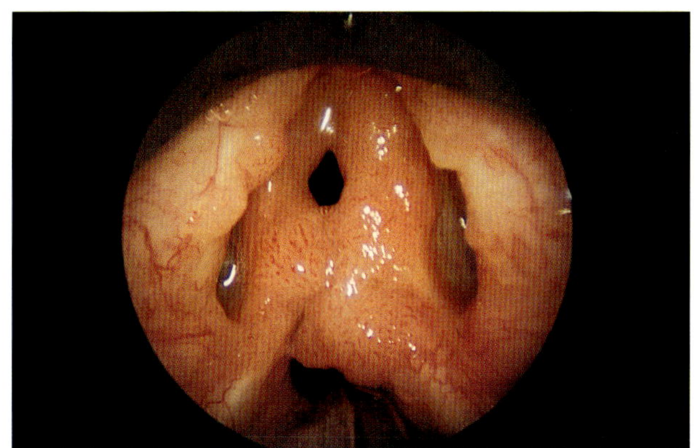

Figure **22.4**
Widespread papilloma seen at direct laryngoscopy. A 63-year-old man with progressive hoarseness for over 12 months. The papillomas are so widespread no normal vocal cord can be seen.

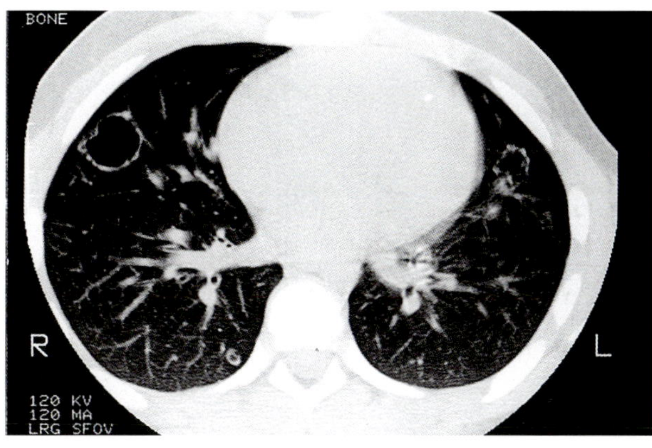

Figure **22.5**
Pulmonary papillomatosis on CT scan. Both solid and cystic spaces can be seen scattered in each lung. This 18-year-old man has had approximately 100 operations, but the papillomas in his larynx, trachea and bronchi are not controlled.

loma virus (HPV) in the genesis of respiratory papillomas. An unspecified 'promoter' is thought to activate HPV in the mucosal cells. It has also been postulated that there is an unidentified immune deficit. Many neoplasms have been shown to contain HPV DNA including warts, papillomas, condylomas, oral precancerous lesions, and verrucous lesions whether in the skin, oral cavity or the genital tract.

Specific types of HPV are associated with particular lesions in different parts of the body. Currently there are approximately 80 subtypes which have been identified. Type 6 and Type 11 are generally associated with laryngeal disease. Recent studies have documented HPV in normal epithelium, the virus apparently residing in the nuclei of cells in the superficial layers of the squamous epithelium. Not only are there viruses in the cell nuclei of the papillomas themselves but there are also latent viruses in the surrounding mucosa, accounting for recurrence at the site of removal and elsewhere. Furthermore, HPV DNA has been found in epithelium that appears to be normal in patients with MRP which is active, as well as in patients in remission, indicating a reservoir for potential re-infection.

It has also been suggested that turbulent airflow may concentrate infectious virus particles at certain sites and that lack of unspecified protective elements in mucous secretions may lower local immunity and sensitize cell receptors.

Laboratory studies of HPV are painstaking and difficult. The Southern blot hybridization has been used to study HPV in various benign and malignant lesions, but it requires tissue for study to be collected and frozen immediately. The polymerase chain reaction can be performed on paraffin sections, has a high sensitivity, requires less tissue and allows for retrospective study, but its sensitivity is so great that contamination can lead to false positive results. HPV can also be identified by in situ hybridization.

There is a strong association between MRP in infants and children and maternal condylomata acuminata or genital warts. Why the lesions sometimes present at or soon after birth and sometimes cause symptoms many months or years later is unresolved. Transmission of HPV during passage through the birth canal is most unlikely as some infants have papillomas already in their larynx at birth; HPV transfer from the mother to the child's laryngeal mucosa is more likely to be due to viraemia.

Growth pattern

Growth may be slow and persistent or irregular and unpredictable with remissions and exacerbations

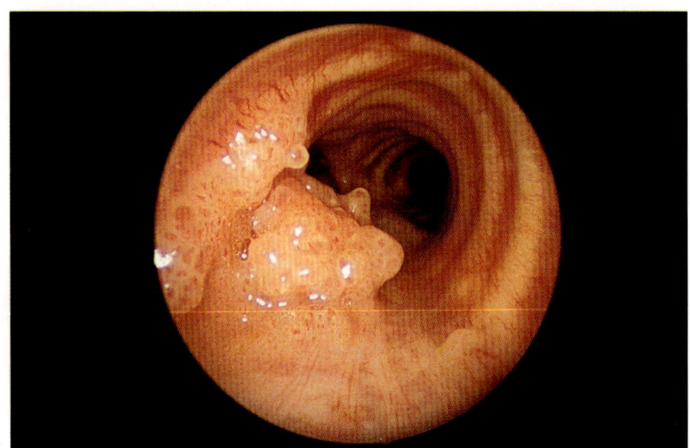

Figure **22.6**
Tracheal papillomas. An adult female who had many operations over 20 years developed papillomas in several sites in the trachea; these were treated with the bronchoscopic laser.

occurring for no apparent reason. Respiratory papillomas in different patients can have an identical histologic appearance but different clinical behaviour.

Papillomas are benign squamous lesions. They tend to occur in clumps or clusters and histologically are composed of a vascular connective tissue core covered by stratified squamous epithelium with little or no tendency to invade submucosal tissues. They are usually multiple, sessile and spread over a wide area (Fig. 22.4) but, in older men, may be small, pedunculated or localized (Fig. 22.3). There are sometimes multiple sites of involvement and this potential for spread in the respiratory tract explains the progression that occasionally occurs into the lung parenchyma where deposits of squamous papilloma appear on a chest X-ray as multiple cystic spaces (Fig. 22.5). Pulmonary parenchymatous seeding is multicentric, progressive and appears to be eventually fatal.

Malignant degeneration is very rare, although it was occasionally seen in the past after radiotherapy was used in a vain attempt to control the disease. Radiotherapy is contraindicated.

Anatomical sites

There is a strong tendency for papillomas to occur in the larynx itself; about half the patients have lesions confined to the larynx. There is good evidence that those with disease confined to the larynx only will continue to have localized and less aggressive disease and that control can be achieved with fewer operations. The other half of the patients have papillomas not only in the larynx but also in other areas above and below and in the trachea (Fig. 22.6), the bronchi, the oropharynx and occasionally the oesophagus.

In the larynx, the anterior glottis, especially the anterior commissure, is the site of predilection for

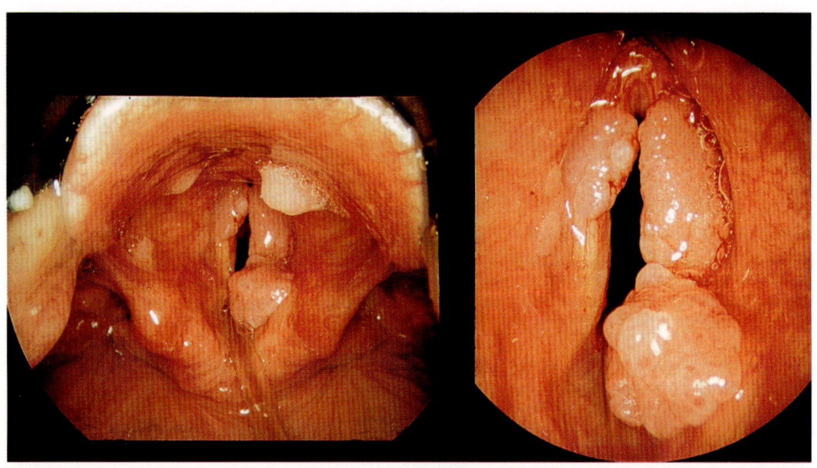

Figure **22.7**
Laryngeal papillomas. Widespread scattered papillomas in the supraglottic and glottic region.

papillomas. Small isolated areas or large clumps of papillomas can be found anywhere in the larynx (Fig. 22.7), often on the posterior surface of the epiglottis, the laryngeal surface of the aryepiglottic folds, within one or both laryngeal ventricles, under the vocal folds and sometimes in the posterior glottic space. However, the commonest site is the vocal folds, which very seldom remain unaffected.

Papillomas are also seen quite commonly isolated from the larynx on the anterior tonsillar pillars, soft palate or uvula; there appears to be no association between these palatal lesions and the presence of papillomas in the larynx.

Macroscopically, and with telescopes, laryngeal papillomas appear as separate sessile masses of different sizes, as a blanket covering the endolarynx or occasionally as a single pedunculated mass. They have an irregular, warty, nodular appearance, and are usually pink or red. They are somewhat friable and bleed when touched.

It has been postulated that papillomas occur at the sites of airway constriction but it seems more likely that the sites of predilection follow a pattern with lesions occurring at anatomic areas where ciliated epithelium changes to squamous epithelium. The laryngeal surface of the epiglottis, the upper and lower margins of the ventricle, the undersurface of the vocal folds and the carina, being sites of squamociliary junction, are often the location of papilloma formation. If, in rare cases, tracheotomy is required, abrasion or injury to the respiratory epithelium apparently leads to metaplastic changes and papillomas occur in the mid-trachea or in the tracheostome.

CLINICAL FEATURES

Presentation

The commonest mode of presentation is a change in the cry or voice. Some patients, mostly children, present with increasing upper respiratory tract obstruction. Thus, paediatric and adult patients present in much the same manner, with stridor a prominent feature in some of the younger patients. These presenting features often lead to a wrong diagnosis such as 'asthma', 'laryngitis', 'bronchitis' or 'croup'. Children are occasionally mistakenly treated for upper airway obstruction by adenotonsillectomy, the papillomas usually being discovered at the time of operation. On average, children with MRP have symptoms for longer than 12 months before the correct diagnosis is made, compared to about 6 months for adults. In our own series (Benjamin and Parsons 1988) of 60 patients treated over 10 years, nine children (15% of all the patients) had symptoms directly attributable to RRP by 60 days of age, a peak of onset of symptoms not previously described. There was a second peak of onset of symptoms between 18 months and 5 years of age, and then a decline to early adolescence. Some of the infants actually had clinical features of papillomas present from birth.

Huskiness in a child, especially if it has been progressive, suggests the possibility of papillomas. Vocal nodules are much commoner and more likely if the hoarseness is variable and worse following overuse of the voice. Some younger children cannot tolerate indirect laryngoscopy and diagnostic laryngoscopy under general anaesthesia may be required where there is doubt about the differentiation between nodules and papillomas.

Effect of puberty and pregnancy

It was traditional in the past to advise that hormonal factors at the time of puberty were likely to lead to regression or remission with resolution of the papillomas. Many recent studies have shown that there is no such tendency for regression during puberty and patients whose disease is controlled before puberty have no tendency to relapse. In fact, some patients continue to have active disease from childhood through pubescence. Patients whose age of disease onset is parapubescent may continue to have active disease as adults. Therefore there is no relationship between puberty, the age of onset and the rate of control or recurrence of the disease.

Patients whose disease appears to come under control during pregnancy sometimes have recurrence, perhaps many years later.

Indirect laryngoscopy

The diagnosis is usually straightforward in adults and older children when indirect examination of the larynx

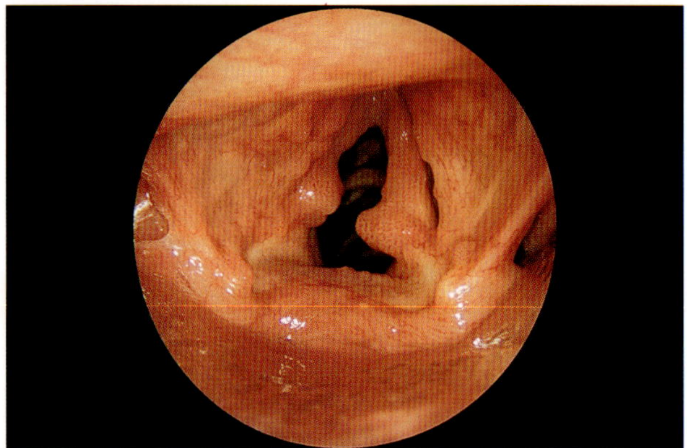

Figure **22.8**
Widespread papillomas at indirect laryngoscopy. This is the same larynx as shown in Figure 22.4 (direct laryngoscopy) showing the appearance before operation.

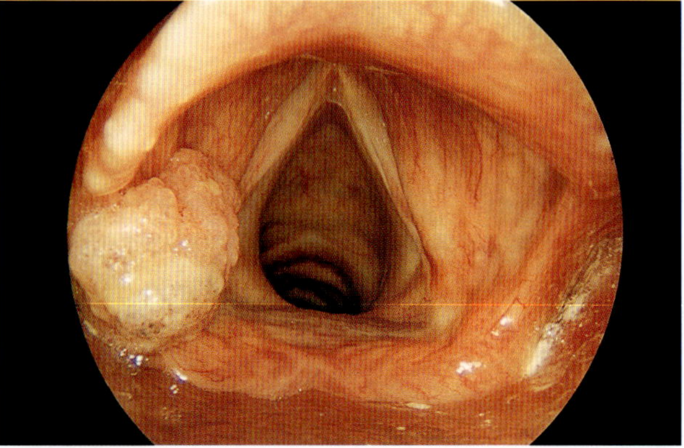

Figure **22.9**
Supraglottic papillomas. Indirect laryngoscopy. The vocal cords are free of disease. There is a single large mass on the left aryepiglottic fold which was removed with the laser and did not recur.

reveals scattered masses of pinkish-red wart-like lesions (Figs 22.8, 22.9). The clearest view is obtained with a 70° wide-diameter rigid telescope using local anaesthesia if necessary but it may not be possible to see clearly the subglottic region, the laryngeal ventricles or the posterior glottic region. If there is doubt about the presence of papillomas, either in a new patient or in a patient thought to be in remission after previous treatment, examination under general anaesthesia is justified.

Radiology

Conventional plain, high-kilovoltage and beam filtration radiography or, in selected cases, computerised tomography (CT) may show the size and site of papillomas which impinge on the airway (Fig. 22.10) and may assist in the preoperative assessment of airway compromise. Chest films, including CT scanning, are used to detect pulmonary involvement (Fig. 22.5). It is not possible to rule out the presence of papillomas by radiological imaging.

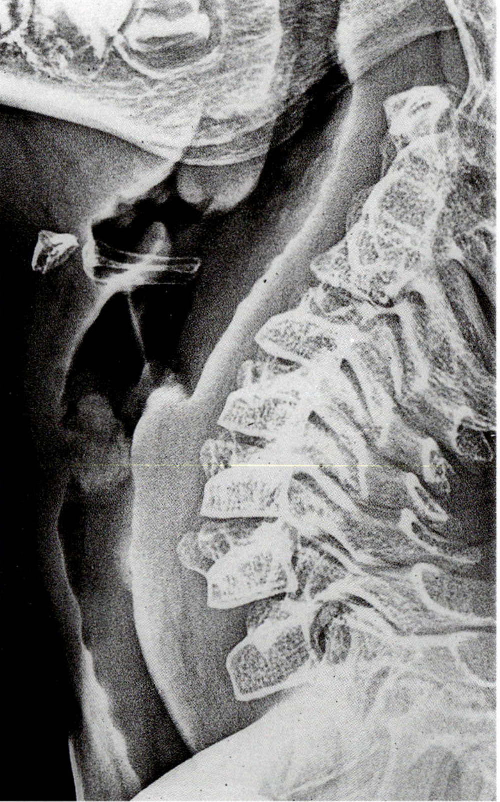

Figure **22.10**
Large masses seen on xerogram. Lateral view shows large supraglottic, glottic and subglottic masses representing laryngeal papillomas causing airway obstruction.

Anaesthesia for endoscopy

General anaesthesia is always used for endoscopic evaluation, for microlaryngoscopy and carbon dioxide

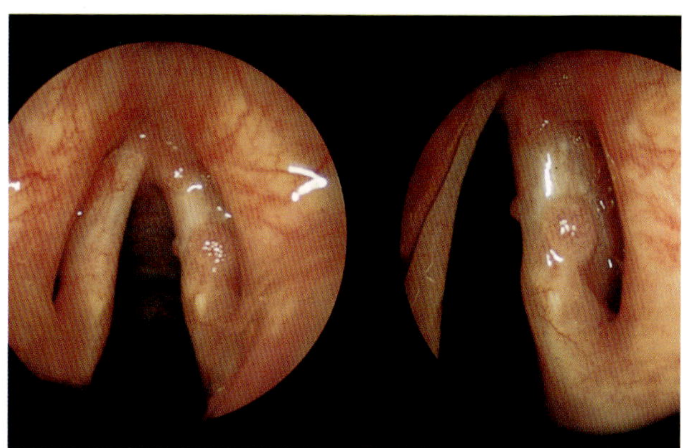

Figure **22.11**
View into the ventricle with 30° telescope. Scattered papillomas on the right vocal cord are seen more clearly when viewed with a 30° telescope to show the recess of the laryngeal ventricle.

laser surgery. The anaesthetic technique must ensure safety and allow maximum visual and surgical access. For adults anaesthesia is usually a relaxant technique with controlled ventilation and for infants and children it is a spontaneous respiration technique with inhalational anaesthesia; in all patients the general anaesthesia is supplemented by application of a measured amount of topical anaesthetic solution applied to the larynx and upper trachea. (See chapter 5 for detailed description of anaesthesia techniques.)

Endoscopic assessment

Direct examination with the naked eye through a hand-held open tube laryngoscope is the preliminary diagnostic procedure before further systematic evaluation for the presence of papillomas elsewhere. A more detailed assessment using 0° and 30° rigid telescopes (Fig. 22.11) follows, usually after suspension of the laryngoscope. External pressure on the neck and gentle repositioning of the laryngoscope will allow various areas to be more prominently displayed. One or other vocal fold can be rolled (Fig. 22.12) using a beaded sucker or other blunt instrument to reveal papillomas in the subglottic region. The false cord can be pushed aside and a 30° telescope used to visualize more of the upper surface of the vocal fold and the recesses of the laryngeal ventricles.

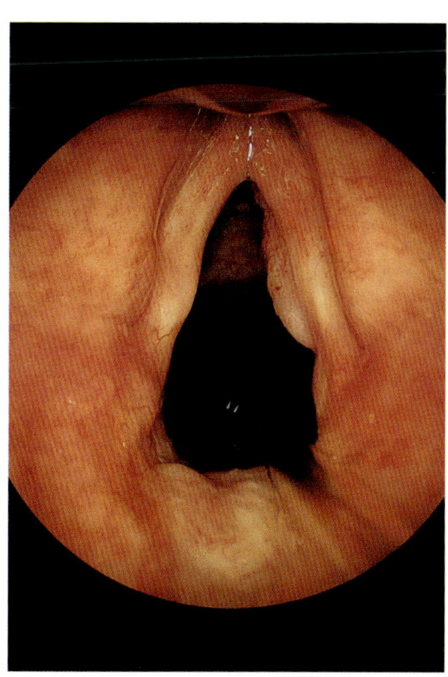

(a)

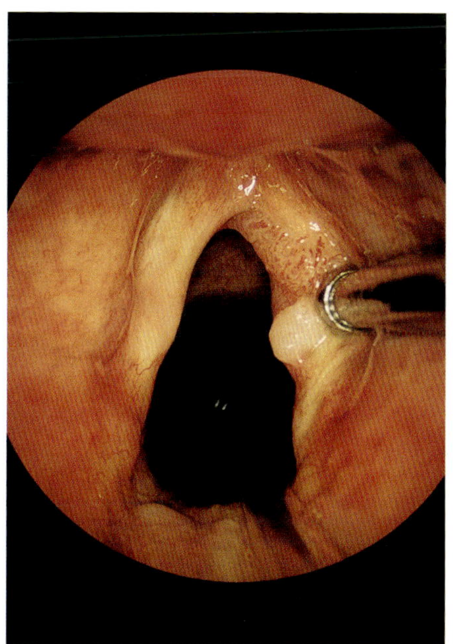

(b)

Figure **22.12**
Technique of 'rolling' the vocal fold. A sucker with a round beaded tip is used to display papilloma on the edge and undersurface of the vocal cord prior to direct laser treatment. As an alternative the laser beam can be bounced under the vocal fold by means of a metal mirror.

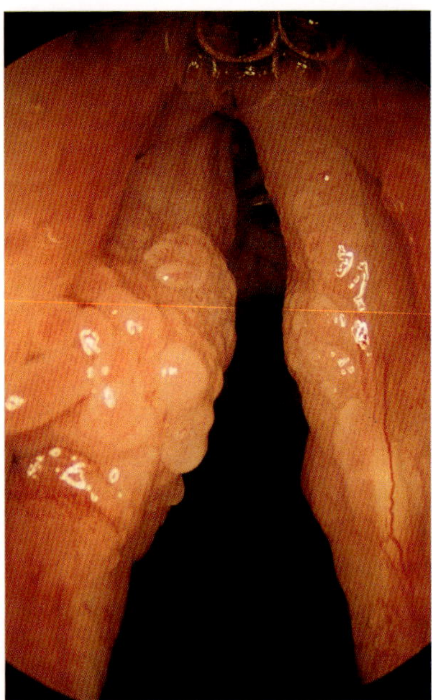

Figure **22.13**
Papillomas on both vocal folds. This is a typical appearance of a mass of papillomas on the left vocal fold and a less papilliferous mass covering the right vocal fold.

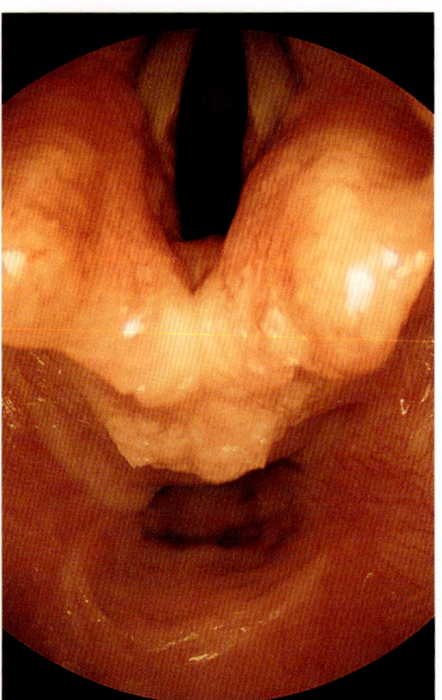

Figure **22.14**
Postcricoid papillomas. The 'laryngeal lift' has been performed to expose the postcricoid region and a small area of papillomas. There were no papillomas in the oesophagus.

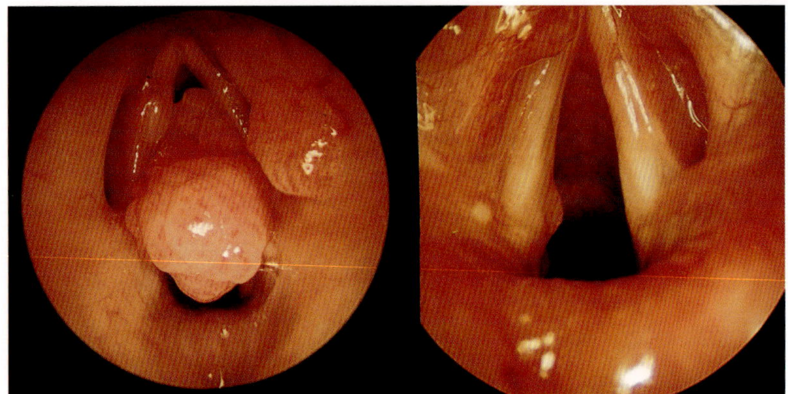

Figure **22.15**
Large mass of obstructing papillomas in a child. The large masses (left) were removed with forceps and scissors. Four weeks later (right) there is no further airway obstruction and the remaining scattered papillomas can be precisely treated with the laser.

Endoscopy of a patient being examined for the first time should include the nasal cavities, naso- and oropharynx, trachea, main bronchi and the upper oesophagus using appropriate endoscopes and telescopes for each anatomical site.

Rigid telescopes provide precise and comprehensive evaluation of the distribution of papillomas (Figs 22.13–22.18). Telescopes allow more extensive and complete examination than is possible with microlaryngoscopy. Once a laryngoscope has been fixed in position, if the microscope only is used, examination of the upper airways other than the larynx is limited. The most difficult areas in which to detect papillomas are: the ventricles (Fig. 22.19); the extreme anterior

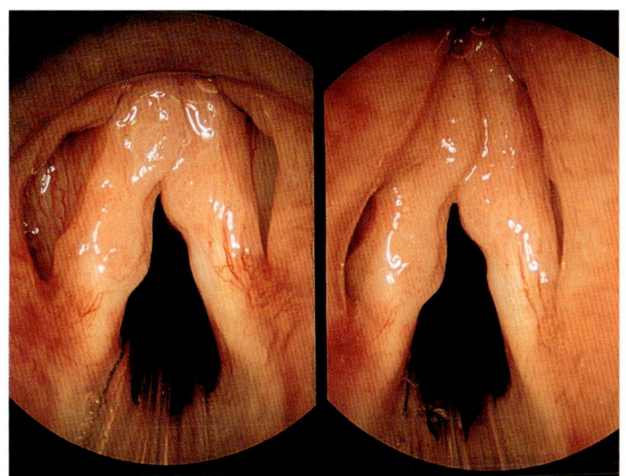

Figure **22.16**
Difficulty in exposure. Visualization of the lesions at the anterior commissure can be difficult (left). With a different laryngoscope (right) an improved view is obtained but care is needed to prevent formation of an anterior web.

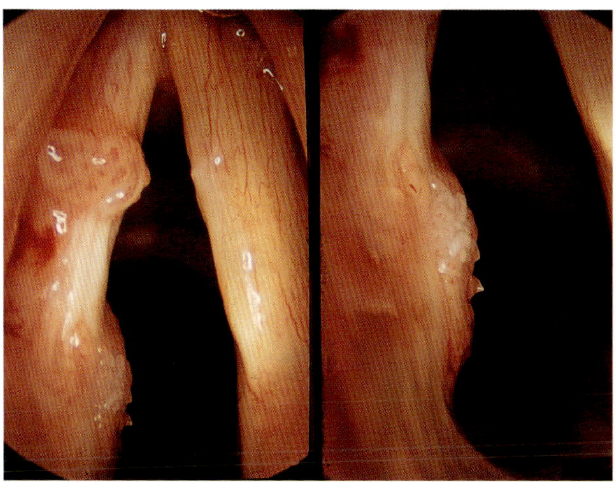

Figure **22.17**
Papilloma masses on the left vocal cord. An irregular mass on the upper surface of the left membranous vocal fold and a mass on the medial aspect near the vocal process (left); seen close-up (right).

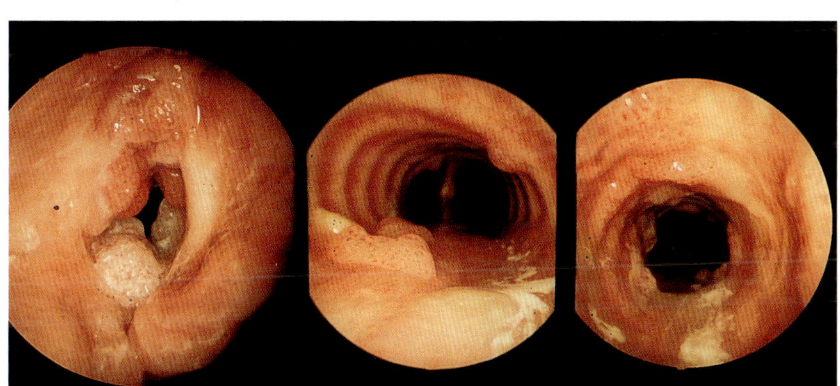

Figure **22.18**
Papillomas in larynx and trachea. Multiple masses making the larynx almost unrecognizable (left). Scattered papillomas in the mid-trachea (centre) and in the upper trachea (right).

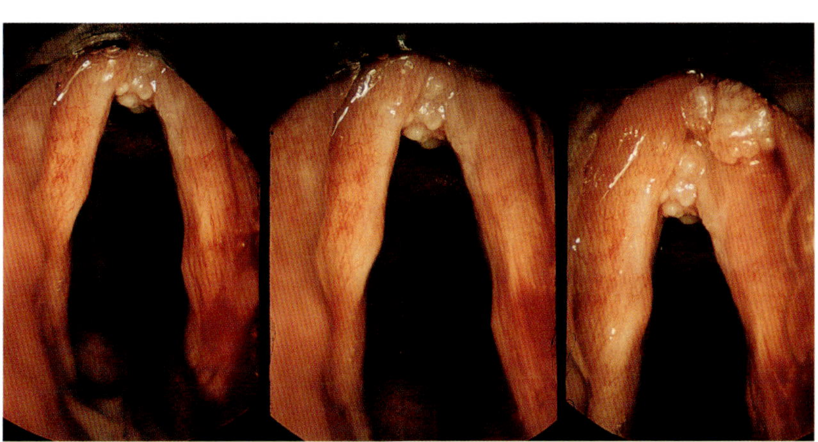

Figure **22.19**
Patient repositioning of the laryngoscope blade together with external pressure on the neck improves exposure of these papillomas at the anterior commissure and in the anterior recess of the right ventricle. Even so, access remains incomplete.

commissure and below it; under an already present laryngeal web; and in a distorted larynx which has been scarred by previous treatment.

TREATMENT

Medical treatment

Because of surgical frustration with recurrence and persistence of the disease, many forms of adjunctive therapy have been tried but none of these have proven to be beneficial over the long-term.

Autogenous papilloma vaccine and, at one stage, bovine wart vaccine have been used without success. Agents which have been applied topically to the papillomas include caustics, alcohol and podophyllin. Oestrogens have been injected. Systemic medications have included tetracyclines, arsenic, bismuth, potassium iodine compounds and androgens. Other treatments have included use of BCG vaccination, ultrasound, photodynamic therapy and radiation therapy. The cytotoxin, methotrexate, has been used without success.

Administration of interferon seems to have a beneficial effect in some patients and to have no effect in others. It appears that there may be accelerated growth of papillomas in some patients once the course of treatment is completed. Interferon therapy is expensive, it is difficult to be sure of the optimal dose, there is significant morbidity from side-effects, and unfortunately its early promise of producing remissions has not been fulfilled.

Principles of surgical treatment

With the exception of asymptomatic solitary papillomas on the mucosa of the soft palate, uvula or tonsillar pillars, papillomas in the pharynx, larynx and upper airways require treatment. The only effective treatment is repeated removal, regarded as the best palliation while awaiting remission. The carbon dioxide laser has no intrinsic curative property.

Because of unpredictable recurrences, sometimes after many years of apparent freedom from disease, it is prudent not to talk of 'cure'. We have patients whose growths seemed to be controlled with no sign of papillomas for 5, 10, 20 or even 25 years, and yet they reappeared. It is wiser to talk in terms of 'control' of the disease, arbitrarily defined as no evidence of disease for at least 12 months.

Aims of treatment

Maintain a clear airway
Improve and preserve voice
Avoid tracheotomy
Achieve 'control'

At the first examination precise and comprehensive pan-endoscopic assessment of the upper aerodigestive tract is necessary to ascertain the location, size and distribution of papillomas. In advanced cases where airway obstruction is severe (Fig. 22.15) substantial amounts of papilloma must be removed, usually with large cupped forceps, on one side only (to prevent adhesion) for both histological proof of the diagnosis and airway improvement. Precise removal of residual or recurrent papillomas is undertaken at subsequent operations.

Due care must be taken during induction and maintenance of anaesthesia in patients, especially infants and children, with potential airway obstruction. Facilities should be readily at hand for intubation or passage of a bronchoscope should severe obstruction occur.

The object of treatment for laryngeal airway obstruction is to provide and maintain a clear airway, at the very least sufficient to avoid tracheotomy; in some children with rapidly growing lesions operations are required every few weeks. The object of treatment in non-obstructive cases is to improve and preserve the voice and to achieve 'control'. Patients may require operations every few months but the rate of growth and the frequency of operations are variable not only from patient to patient but also, over time, for the individual patient.

Technique of papilloma removal

Maintain airway during induction of general anaesthesia
Choose laryngoscope providing best exposure
Assess with telescopes
Ventricles and subglottis are difficult areas
CO_2 laser with or without cupped forceps
Technique to minimize web formation
Frequency depends on recurrence rate
Treatment is palliative awaiting remission
The CO_2 laser has no curative powers

Various surgical treatments

Surgical treatment has included physical removal with cupped forceps, electrocautery, cryosurgery and carbon dioxide laser treatment. The latter is the treatment most commonly used as the laser is precise, attended by minimal bleeding, causes little pain and unlike electrocautery or cryosurgery, the zone of tissue injury does not extend much beyond the immediate area which has been treated.

Thyrotomy with laryngofissure and vein graft or skin graft onto the denuded vocal cord areas was advocated in the 1960s, but resulted not only in poorly vibrating vocal folds but also recurrence of the papillomas; the operation was abandoned.

Techniques of endoscopic treatment

Optimum exposure and visualization depends on good anaesthetic and surgical technique, using a laryngoscope whose design clearly displays the area to be treated and allows safe use of the laser (Figure 22.16), i.e. the laryngoscope should have a wide proximal opening, preferably one of the Lindholm operating laryngoscopes. In an adult whose larynx is difficult or impossible to visualize with standard laryngoscopes the Benjamin slimline laryngoscope is used as it allows binocular viewing for microlaryngoscopy and laser surgery. Under suspension laryngoscopy we proceed from examination with telescopes (Figs 22.16, 22.17) to operation using the microscope with a 400-mm objective lens.

It is clear that the operating microscope is advantageous in papilloma removal. The laser is used in almost every patient, sometimes in conjunction with angled cupped forceps. The surgeon, the patient and the parents should accept the need for repeated procedures when the tumours cannot be completely removed at one operation. It is prudent not to perform 'too much' surgery at one operation.

The use of cupped forceps alone will provoke troublesome, nuisance bleeding in the operative field so that after the initial removal it is difficult to visualize the remaining lesions. The carbon dioxide laser is therefore advantageous in allowing precise removal of multiple lesions at one operation.

Laser surgery

For microlaryngeal laser surgery the operating microscope has the laser attached to it by means of a micro-manipulator, positioned so that the laser beam has clear access through the proximal mouth of the laryngoscope. Accessory instruments for laser surgery include metal mirrors, metal anterior commissure protector 'paddles', moist cottonoids, and suction evacuators for moisture, steam and laser plume. For an anatomic site with difficult access such as a laryngeal ventricle, the subglottic region or the undersurface of an anterior web, the laser beam can be reflected onto the lesion using a small metal mirror. Metal protector 'paddles' are used to protect one vocal cord at the anterior commissure while performing laser treatment on the other side. The blunt tip of a beaded suction tube can be used as a probe to retract the false cord or to 'roll' the true cord (Fig. 22.12). External counter-pressure from a finger on the neck can improve exposure of the subglottic region and facilitate laser treatment.

Multiple sites can be treated at one operation with due care to prevent scarring and web formation.

Papillomas are vaporized using the micro-manipulator for constant visual control of the direction of the beam. Cupped forceps angled left, right or upwards are sometimes required after laser surgery or in conjunction with it to remove residual papillomas from areas where visualization and access are limited.

To minimize thermal injury to the surrounding tissues the tip of the suction tube should be held close to the site of laser surgery to remove smoke and vaporized steam so that the latter will not cause a secondary burn of nearby mucosa. Laser energy is used in short rather than prolonged bursts to allow cooling and to prevent unwanted heat coagulation. Gentle technique, avoidance of excessive endoscopic or laser trauma and, in selected cases, use of a postoperative moist air atmosphere minimizes stridor and respiratory distress. Small, wet neurosurgical cottonoids are used to protect adjacent tissues, the subglottic region and the surface of an anaesthetic tube if one is in use. Due precautions must be taken when the laser is being used to prevent tube ignition; more details are available in chapter 5 and chapter 9 on the use of the laser during anaesthesia.

Pedunculated masses or clumps on a narrow base can be excised from the underlying normal tissue using a small spot-size beam and the mass can be submitted for histopathologic examination.

Care must be taken to avoid injury to normal structures, especially at the anterior commissure where the potential for web formation is high, particularly if the operator is inexperienced. Techniques to minimize web formation include strict limitation of surgery to one side at the anterior commissure, use of small cupped forceps which allow a 'feel' of the underlying tissues which is not obtained with laser surgery and use of a laryngoscope to separate the false cords, and to some extent the true cords, to allow more precise surgical removal.

Subglottic and upper tracheal papillomas are lasered, if possible using a subglottiscope for direct visualization. The bronchoscopic laser coupler is essential for removal of papilloma in the mid or lower trachea and bronchi.

Recurrences

The mildest form of disease could be regarded, for example, as an adult with one, or perhaps two, distinct papillomas confined to the larynx which can be completely removed by one operation and which show no sign of recurrence. The most severe form of benign disease, on the other hand, might be a small child who presents with stridor and a husky, weak cry and who has multiple, uncountable areas of papillomas in the supraglottic larynx, on the vocal folds and in the subglottic region. Papillomas require removal at repeated operations under general anaesthesia; in some children operations are necessary every 2–3 weeks to maintain a clear airway for safe anaesthesia.

Between the two ends of this spectrum of the disease are many variations where patients have remissions and exacerbations at indeterminate and irregular intervals, which introduces an unfortunate element of uncertainty into their lives.

When there is persistent recurrence of disease, patients have been recorded as having required over 100 or even 200 operations. Tracheotomy although best avoided is an ever present possibility in these cases.

Complications

Web formation
'Seeding' of the tracheotomy
Spread to trachea, bronchi and lungs
Laryngocoele
Malignant transformation

Complications

The complications are those due to the disease itself and those due to the untoward results of treatment.

Complications of the disease include downward seeding and spread of the papillomas to the trachea (Fig. 22.18), at the carina (Fig. 22.20), in the main bronchi and sometimes in the lung parenchyma (see Fig. 22.5).

Tracheobronchoscopy should be performed at regular intervals in all patients requiring repeated

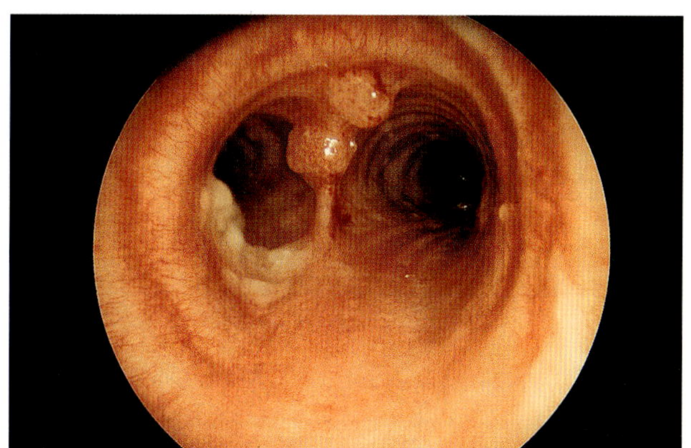

Figure **22.20**
Papillomas at the carina. Two distinct lesions at the carina. There were also laryngeal papillomas.

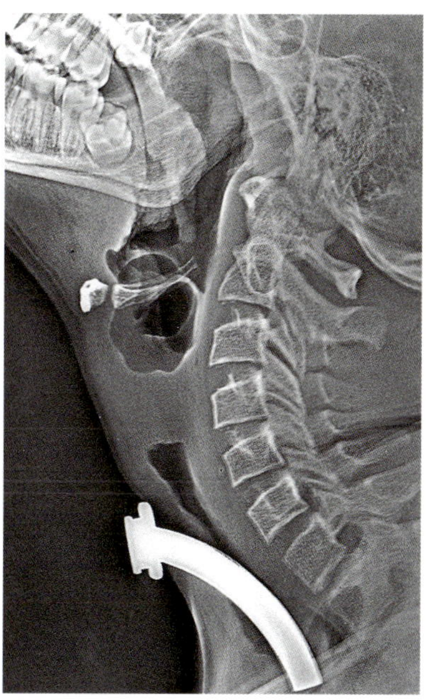

Figure **22.21**
Air-containing laryngocoele secondary to laryngeal papillomas. Xerogram showing obliteration of the glottic anatomy and an irregular air-containing laryngocoele secondary to obstruction of the saccular duct by papillomas.

operations, using a slim telescope passed through a laryngoscope in suspension; the telescope gives a clear view of the trachea, carina, bronchi and segmental openings. Spread can occur further than the bronchi until the lung parenchyma is affected; this will usually show first on a chest X-ray or preferably a CT scan (Fig. 22.5). We perform CT scans at approximately yearly intervals in patients with recurring, unremitting tracheobronchial disease. Scattered small or large nodules will be seen with adjacent cystic spaces. There is no known effective treatment for this stage of the disease.

Occasionally papillomas in the anterior ventricle obstruct the opening of the laryngeal saccule with formation of a secondary laryngocoele (Fig. 22.21).

Malignant change was thought to occur only in those individuals who had been treated previously with radiotherapy but change can occur in others. Smoking may be a factor in the malignant transformation but an occasional patient develops squamous cell carcinoma for unknown reasons. Such a change might be suspected if there are more severe symptoms, if excision is necessary more often than previously, if the disease is growing aggressively and spreading (Fig. 22.22), if there is limitation of vocal fold movement and if there is excessive bleeding at the time of excision.

Complications of the treatment are related to scar formation and stenosis. Scar formation at the anterior

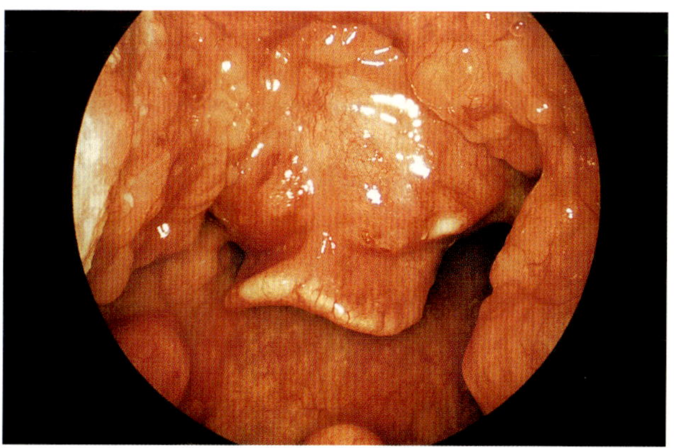

Figure **22.22**
Papillomas which developed malignant characteristics. Biopsy of the papillomas on the posterior surface of the epiglottis did not show any malignant changes but deep biopsy obtained by laser incision into the mass between the epiglottis and the base of the tongue revealed squamous cell carcinoma.

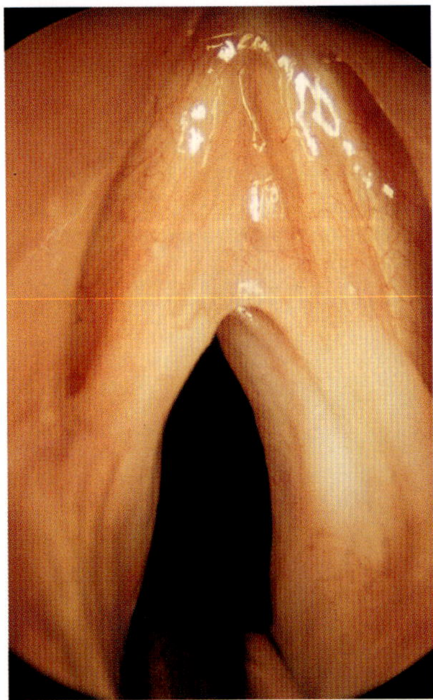

Figure **22.23**
Acquired laryngeal web. Moderate-sized, acquired, anterior glottic web after many operations for removal of papillomas. There were no recurrences of papillomas for 2 years, and a 'flag' operation was performed with an excellent voice result.

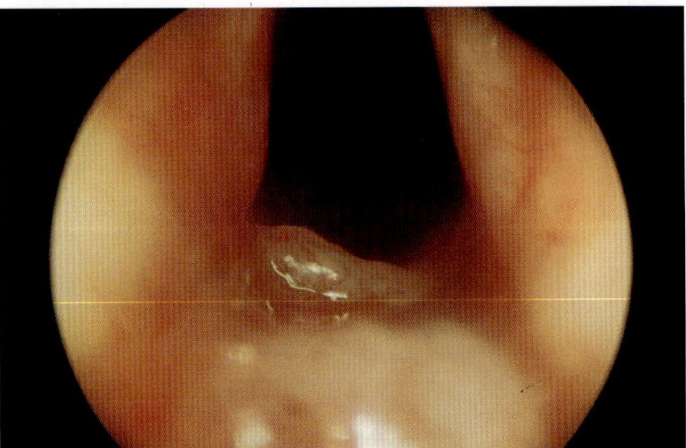

Figure **22.24**
Papillomas in posterior glottic space. This is a very unusual site for papillomas. In this adult female patient there were no other papillomas in the larynx.

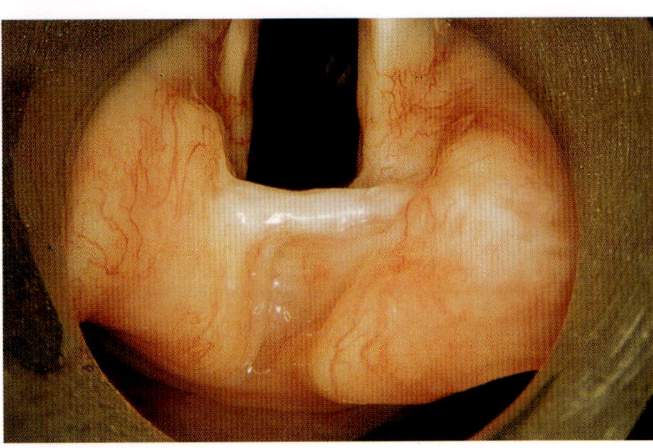

Figure **22.25**
Posterior glottic stenosis following repeated removal of papillomas. This patient had several operations to remove papillomas in and above the posterior glottic space and developed a transverse stenotic area which did not cause any airway symptoms.

commissure is sometimes inevitable because eventually papillomas have to be removed from the commissure itself and an anterior glottic web may form (Fig. 22.23). Some webs are small and visible only when viewed with the telescope under general anaesthesia; these webs do not cause significant symptoms. A few patients develop webs that occupy 20–30% of the anterior glottic opening. These can be seen at indirect laryngoscopy and produce a permanent change in the voice.

Large post-surgical webs which cause vocal disability should not be considered for treatment until there has been well-documented control of the papillomas for at least 1 year. This type of surgery should be delayed as long as possible and treatment should be undertaken only for serious dysphonia. There is a possibility that division of the web and the underlying tissues may lead to recurrence by reactivation of the dormant virus.

Removal of papillomas from the surface, the posterior edge and particularly the undersurface of an existing web is always attended by the possibility of causing more scar tissue and worsening the web itself.

Fortunately papillomas are unusual in the posterior glottic space (Fig. 22.24), but repeated surgical or laser treatment in this area has led to scarring and posterior glottic stenosis in several patients, although in our experience not to the point of causing airway obstruction (Fig. 22.25).

The most serious complication of the disease could be regarded as relentless, unremitting and persistent recurrence.

BIBLIOGRAPHY

Benjamin B, Parsons D (1988) Recurrent respiratory papillomatosis: a 10 year study. *JLO* **102**: 1022–8.

Benjamin B, Gatenby P, Kitchen R et al (1988) Alpha-Interfon (Wellferon) as an adjunct to standard surgical therapy and recurrent respiratory papillomatosis. *Ann Otol Rhinol Laryngol* **97**: 376–80.

Doyle D, Henderson L, Le Jeune F, Muller R (1994) Changes in human papilloma virus typing of recurrent respiratory papillomatosis progress into malignant neoplasm. *Arch Otolaryngol-Head Neck Surg* **120**: 1273–6.

Harries M, Juman S, Bailey C (1995) Recurrent respiratory papillomatosis in the larynx: re-emergence of clinical disease following surgery. *Ped Otorhinolaryngol* **31**: 259–62.

Healy GB, Gelber RD, Frawbridge AL, Grundfast KM, Ruben RJ, Price KN (1988) Treatment of recurrent respiratory papillomatosis with human leukocyte interferon. *N Engl J Med* **319**: 401–7.

Jackson C, Jackson CL (1942) *Diseases and injuries of the larynx* (New York: Macmillan) 346.

Kashima H, Mounts P, Leventhal B, Hruban R (1993) Sites of predilection in recurrent respiratory papillomatosis. *Ann Otol Rhinol Laryngol* **102**: 580–3.

Mackenzie M (1871) *Essays on growths in the larynx* (London: J & A Churchill).

Yoshpe N (1995) Oral and laryngeal papilloma: a pediatric manifestation of sexually transmitted disease? *Ped Otorhinolaryngol* **31**: 77–83.

23 Dysplasia and malignancy

BASICS

In keeping with the title and theme of this text only neoplastic lesions within the intrinsic larynx (sometimes called the endolarynx) will be discussed as lesions 'outside' the larynx are seldom amenable to endoscopic or microsurgical techniques.

Cancer of the larynx is the next most common malignancy of the head and neck after cancer of the oral cavity and tongue. These cancers are mostly diseases of middle-aged and older men who smoke. Depending on the extent of the laryngeal cancer at the time of diagnosis, there is a fairly favourable long-term outlook with an overall 5-year survival rate of 65–70%.

Cancer of the larynx

One of the common head and neck malignancies
Mostly affects men who smoke, 50–70 years old
Five times more common in males than females
Favourable 5-year outlook, depending on extent at diagnosis

The current concepts of treatment depend mostly upon the site and size of the primary lesion which is assessed not only by indirect and direct laryngoscopy but also by imaging studies. Clinical examination of the neck for direct spread or for nodal metastases, complete physical examination for the presence of distant metastases and histopathological analysis of biopsy specimens complete the evaluation.

Historical aspects of treatment

It is interesting to review historical aspects of treatment, especially the development of surgical procedures. Diagnosis, of course, depends almost entirely upon the ability to perform indirect laryngoscopy which was first introduced by Bozzini in 1807 but was not accepted until Manuel Garcia, a Spanish singing teacher, presented his own work in 1855. Not long after, in 1858, Rudolf Virchow's work *Cellular-Pathologie* dealt the final death blow to the outmoded 'humoral' theory of pathology and ushered in the era of diagnostic histopathology based on microscopic changes in biopsy material. Accurate laryngoscopic and histologic assessment had become possible, the more so since Horace Green had performed direct examination of the laryngeal introitus in 1852. The first laryngofissure for cancer was performed in 1851 by Gordon Buck, in the United States, but results were poor and it was abandoned until 'rediscovered'. Twenty years later the first complete excision of the larynx was performed by Theodore Billroth but was not well accepted because it involved leaving the patient with an open laryngotracheal defect.

By 1878 Billroth performed a vertical partial laryngectomy, an operation which was subsequently popularized by others including Felix Semon. Later a pharyngotomy approach was used for resection of supraglottic malignancy by Von Langenbeck and others, but it was not until Trotter (1913) described lateral pharyngotomy that this operation became the accepted procedure for partial laryngopharyngectomy. Meanwhile Thermistokles Gluck developed vertical partial laryngectomy and later the technique and indications for supraglottic partial laryngectomy were developed by Justo Alonso of Uruguay. From 1960 to 1980 Joseph Ogura, Max Som and others refined the techniques so that voice conservation procedures could be applied to more cases.

From its beginnings in the 1920s, radiation therapy used in fractionated doses was recognized as an effective and accepted treatment option which could preserve the voice. By the 1950s, radiation techniques had improved further with the advent of cobalt-60. Soon it was realized that radiation of all cases for possible cure might preserve the larynx, with the option of proceeding to salvage laryngectomy for radiation failures. At present, radiation is curative for early cancer with good preservation of voice. In more extensive tumours, radiation may be offered, together with chemotherapy, reserving surgery for non-responders or recurrences. However, even after years of evaluation, the effectiveness of deliberate, pre-planned combination radiation and surgery for advanced cancer remains undetermined.

Recent success with laryngeal transplantation in animals has not been followed by application to humans; despite the advances in renal, cardiac and liver transplantation, laryngeal transplantation after laryngectomy for cancer has not yet become a reality.

Increased risk

Tobacco
Alcohol
Previous irradiation

Epidemiology

Incidence

Cancer of the larynx is about five times more common in males than females. The peak incidence is in patients from 50–70 years old. In the USA it occurs more in black than white people. It accounts for more than 1% of all cancer diagnoses, but less than 1% of all cancer deaths.

An apparent increased incidence of laryngeal cancer noted in the last few decades is probably partly due to better diagnosis and partly due to increased exposure to environmental and occupational carcinogenic factors.

Geographic distribution

There is a great variation world-wide. For example, there is an 8–10 times higher incidence in India than elsewhere, and a higher incidence in the Basque country, apparently due to the use of 'black' tobacco with a high level of tar and aromatic amines. The age-standardized incidence rate per 100 000 people in Australia is 5.8 for males and 0.5 for females, a recent increase in females reflecting a world-wide trend. There is also a geographic difference in the distribution of the anatomic site of cancer which varies with race, gender and age of the patient. There is no known reason why glottic and supraglottic tumours occur about equally in black men whereas in white men glottic tumours are twice as common as supraglottic tumours. Supraglottic malignancies are commoner in females, especially black females.

Aetiologic studies

Aetiologic studies have identified three major predisposing factors: tobacco, alcohol and previous irradiation. There is an increasing incidence with increasing daily consumption of tobacco, not only in cigarette smokers but also in pipe and cigar smokers, snuff takers and those who chew tobacco. Pipe and cigar smokers tend to get cancer of the larynx more than cancer of the lung. There is a relative decrease in incidence in areas where 'blond' tobacco is used, and in smokers who use filter cigarettes. The risk decreases not only when cigarette smoking is stopped but it also decreases more the longer the time has been from cessation of smoking. Thus, to some extent cancer of the larynx can be considered 'preventable'. It is rare to see cancer of the larynx in either men or women who do not smoke.

There is a higher risk in alcoholics and in hard liquor drinkers, and there is evidence that tobacco and alcohol may act synergistically.

A deficient diet and malnutrition are significant in carcinogenesis. There is a possible protective effect not only by vitamins A, C and E but also by zinc, carbohydrates, dietary fibre, fresh food and vegetables. It is difficult to identify increased risk (allowing for tobacco and alcohol consumption) according to occupation, but evidence suggests an increased incidence from exposure to asbestos, in textile and construction workers and in workers exposed to substances such as cement dust, dyes, coal, tar, oil, grease, gasoline, paints and pigments.

Although the cause is multi-factorial, there is strong and constant evidence that exposure to tobacco and alcohol is a major cause. Therefore, avoidance of tobacco, controlled alcohol consumption and a healthy and nutritious diet are currently the most effective means for an individual to decrease the risk of developing laryngeal cancer.

Host factors

Immunologic response

The immunologic response of an individual patient may prevent or discourage the development of malignancy; both humoral and cell-mediated immune status are important. Suppression of the immune response is certainly more common in patients with cancer of the head and neck than in patients with cancer elsewhere in the body.

Immunoglobin A (IgA) has been demonstrated to decrease the ability of the host to destroy tumour – the tumour inhibiting response. On the other hand immunoglobin E (IgE) assists the body's defences; the level of serum IgE has been shown to increase in patients with head and neck cancer who have a recurrent tumour or metastases even before there is any clinical evidence of disease. Patients with a positive skin test to recall antigen, indicating the capability of responding well to antigen, appear to have an improved prognosis. Patients with head and neck cancer have depressed T-cell levels but the prognostic implications of these lowered levels are unclear.

Other possible aetiological factors involved in immunosuppression in laryngeal carcinoma may include viruses, e.g. herpes simplex virus and Epstein–Barr virus. In addition, association of laryngeal carcinoma with the human papilloma virus and *ras* oncogene activation has been suspected. Alcoholism, malnutrition, ageing, certain treatment modalities such as radiation and cytotoxic therapy, and even the effects of surgery and anaesthesia are immunosuppressives to some extent. This altered immune state may explain the relatively high association of carcinoma of the larynx with synchronous or metachronous primary malignancies of the lung, oral cavity and oesophagus.

Genetic factors

Genetic factors or some other factor causing impairment of the immune mechanism may be involved but have not been proven. Although patients with laryngeal cancer may have a family history of cancer elsewhere in the body, it is rare to have a family history of laryngeal cancer.

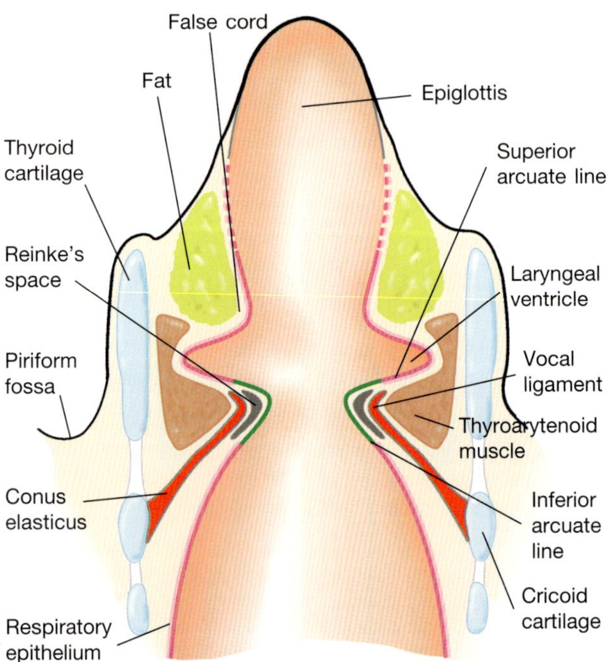

Figure **23.1**
Diagrammatic coronal cross-section of the normal larynx.

LARYNGEAL DYSPLASIA AND MALIGNANCY

Histology of the normal larynx

The vocal ligament and the medial thyroarytenoid (vocalis) muscle make up the substance of the vocal fold (Fig. 23.1) whose covering mucous membrane is normally non-keratinized squamous epithelium on the edge, undersurface (as far as the inferior arcuate line) and upper surface (as far as the superior arcuate line). The same non-keratinized squamous mucosa extends over the posterior surface of the epiglottis and the aryepiglottic folds. It may become keratinized in pathological states as a response to trauma or chronic irritation.

Nearby structures in the remainder of the endolarynx (Fig. 23.1) are normally covered by pseudo-stratified columnar, ciliated epithelium with goblet cells in the mucosa, typical of the respiratory tract. This respiratory epithelium can also undergo metaplasia in

Normal laryngeal epithelium

Non-keratinized squamous on vocal cord
Pseudo-stratified columnar, ciliated in the remainder of the endolarynx

response to trauma and chronic irritation, and sometimes malignant changes may eventually occur.

There has been, and still is, frustration for both clinician and histopathologist because of the confused nomenclature and the failure to define clearly the various epithelial changes which are likely to lead to malignancy. The natural history and malignant potential of these dysplastic changes remains uncertain. For optimum interpretation, the clinician should be familiar with the terminology used by the pathologist.

Leukoplakia and erythroplakia

Both are clinical terms describing an appearance seen at laryngoscopy and therefore should be used only by the laryngologist, not by the histopathologist.

- *Leukoplakia* is a descriptive term for a white patch, flat or raised, smooth or granular, localized or widespread, on a mucosal surface (Fig. 23.2). It is usually a sign of keratin, but a white patch might also be caused by adherent secretions or fungal infection.
- *Erythroplakia* (or erythroplasia) is a descriptive term for a red patch on a mucosal surface (Fig. 23.3); some laryngologists believe it carries an implication that carcinoma-in-situ is likely. It is caused by congested surface vessels, and biopsy might show malignancy, dysplasia or chronic inflammation.

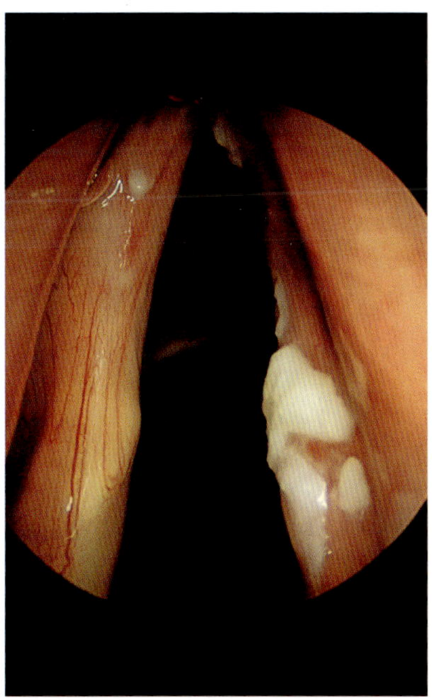

Figure **23.2**
Leukoplakia. Large white raised area posteriorly on the right vocal cord; other patches scattered anteriorly and one small area on the anterior surface of the left cord.

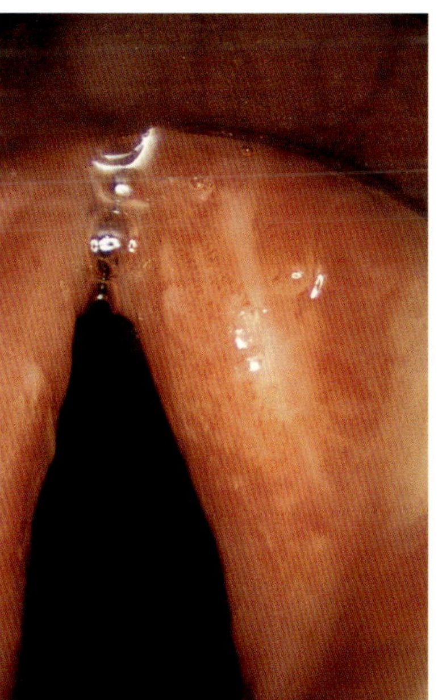

Figure **23.3**
Erythroplakia showing redness and congestion around the irregular lesion on the upper surface of the right vocal cord. Biopsy showed carcinoma-in-situ.

Hyperplasia, dysplasia and malignancy

A practical classification of alterations from the normal histologic pattern includes the changes of hyperplasia, dysplasia and squamous cell carcinoma.

- *Dysplasia* of the epithelium refers to a microscopic disorder in the cellular architecture with loss of normal maturation and stratification. It implies 'pre-malignancy' and is present in varying degrees in cases of keratosis with atypia but sometimes occurs independently of it.
- *Atypia* usually refers to abnormal variations in the size and shape of the cells without necessarily implying malignancy or pre-malignancy. Cellular atypia is always present to some degree in dysplastic epithelium, together with other changes such as keratinization, abnormal maturation and stratification of cells.

The changes commonly referred to by the histopathologist include:

- hyperplasia
- keratosis
- keratosis with atypia; usually designated mild, moderate or severe
- carcinoma-in-situ
- micro-invasive carcinoma
- invasive squamous cell carcinoma; usually described as well, moderately or poorly differentiated.

Hyperplasia, dysplasia and malignancy

Hyperplasia
Keratosis without atypia
Keratosis with atypia
  Mild
  Moderate
  Severe
Carcinoma-in-situ
Micro-invasive carcinoma
Invasive carcinoma

Histopathology of hyperplasia and dysplasia

The report of the histopathologist depends to some extent on subjective interpretation; different histopathologists, whose training and expertise may make them 'conservative' or 'aggressive' in their diagnoses, may differ in the grading of a particular specimen.

Changes (Fig. 23.4) which are the basis for categorization are discussed in the following sections.

Hyperplasia

Hyperplasia is not classified as a dysplastic change. There is thickening of the epithelial mucosa due mostly to an increase in the number of cells with little change in their character or maturation. This non-specific cellular proliferation is a response to chronic irritation caused by an external stimulus, and resolves when the stimulus ceases.

Keratosis without atypia

This is also sometimes called hyperkeratosis, usually a redundant term unless there are excessive areas of keratin. Keratosis may be defined as hyperplasia of the surface layer. The presence of keratin in the squamous epithelium of the larynx is always abnormal. It is a form of chronic laryngitis where the laryngeal mucosa becomes thickened in response to chronic irritation from noxious stimuli. Clinically it often occurs as raised white patches, localized or diffuse, on the true vocal cords, often bilaterally. The hyperplastic changes are first noted in the basal cell layer where the normal rectangular cells become cuboidal and are realigned. There is abnormal but fairly orderly epithelial maturation with excessive keratin on the surface. The cytologic features are bland and there may be no inflammatory reaction.

Pachydermia laryngis is a somewhat quaint otolaryngologic term for a cobbled, thickened appearance (Fig. 23.5) in the posterior glottis due to extensive keratosis.

Keratosis with atypia

There is epithelial dysplasia with moderate to severe nuclear pleomorphism so that some of the cells have features of malignancy. There are large atypical cells with large and small hyperchromatic nuclei and prominent nucleoli. There are increased numbers of

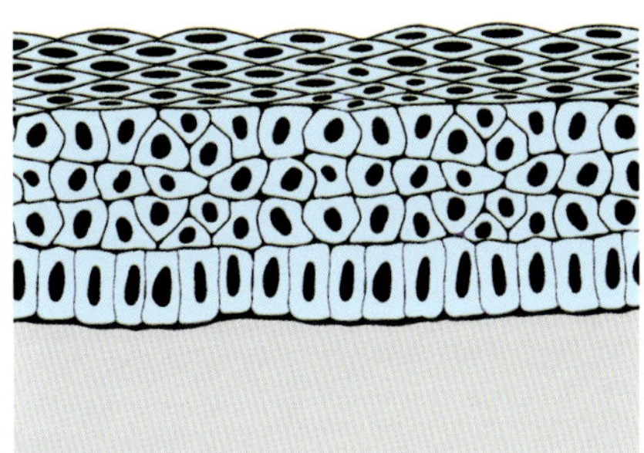

a. Normal.
Squamous epithelium. Non-keratinized columnar cells above the basement membrane.
Orderly maturation.

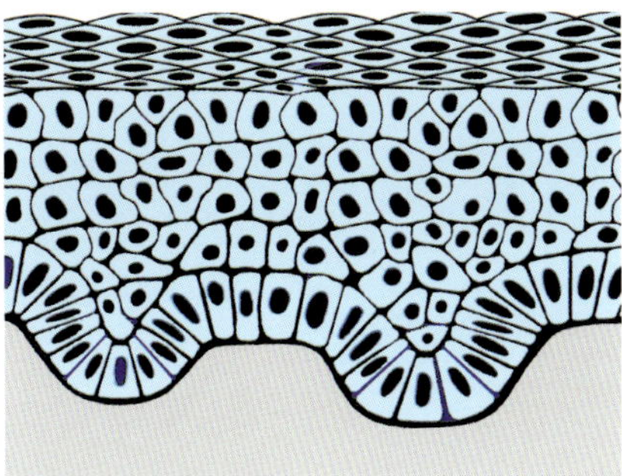

b. Hyperplasia.
Non-keratinized flat squamous cells.
Thickened squamous epithelium with proliferation of normal cells.
Some wrinkling of basement membrane.

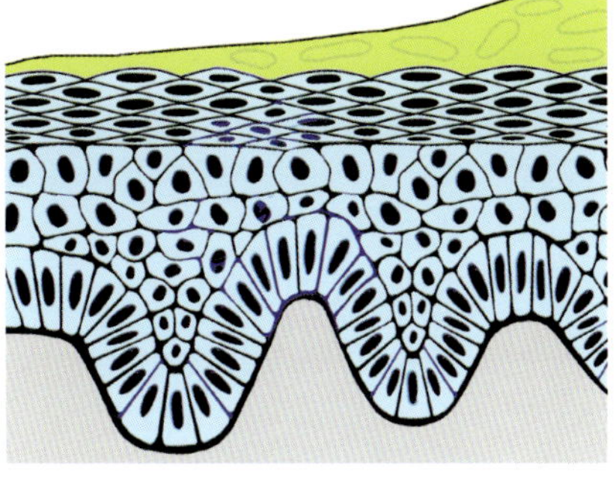

c. Keratosis without atypia.
Keratin formation.
Thickened epithelium.
Little change in cellular maturation.
No dysplasia.

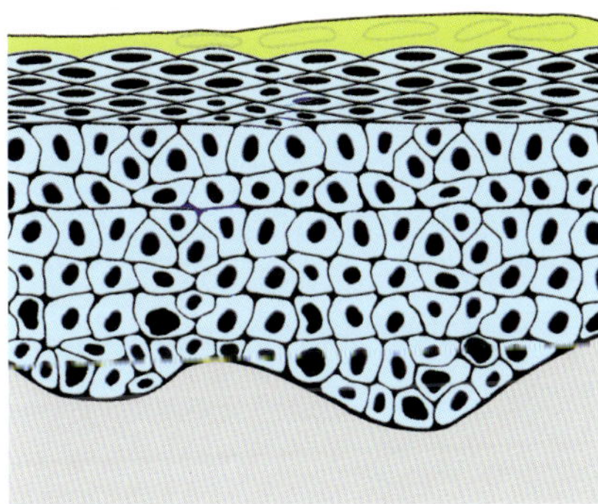

d. Keratosis with mild atypia.
Dyskeratotic changes.
Some dysplasia of cells in lower third.
Atypical cells.
Some irregular stratification.

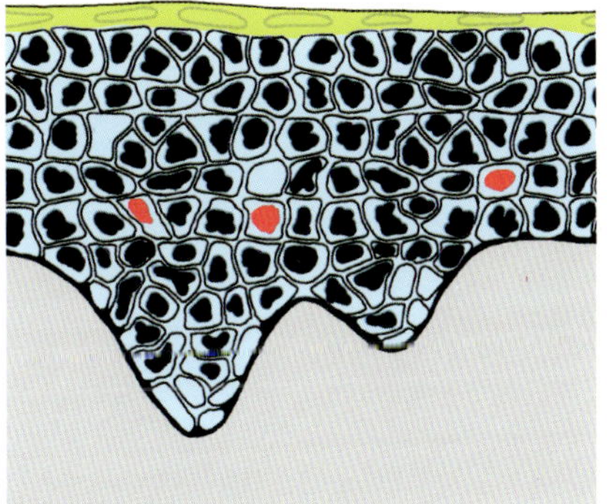

e. Carcinoma-in-situ (keratosis with severe atypia).
No surface squamous cells.
Cellular dysplasia of the whole thickness. Pronounced cellular pleomorphism. Basement membrane intact – no invasion.
Mitotic activity in middle and upper third.

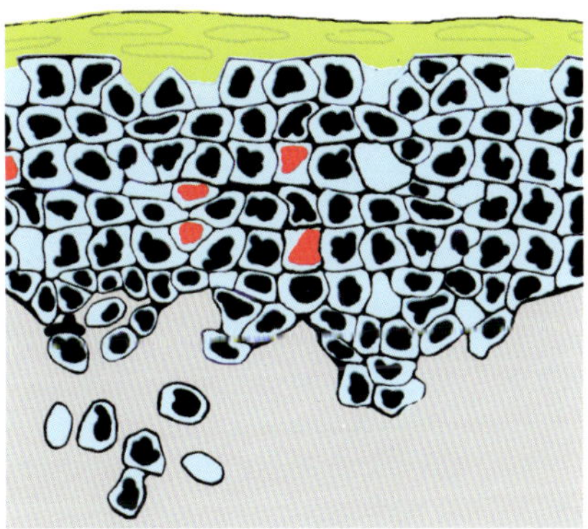

f. Microinvasive carcinoma.
Florid dysplasia.
Atypical cells reach beyond the basement membrane.
Early but very limited invasion.

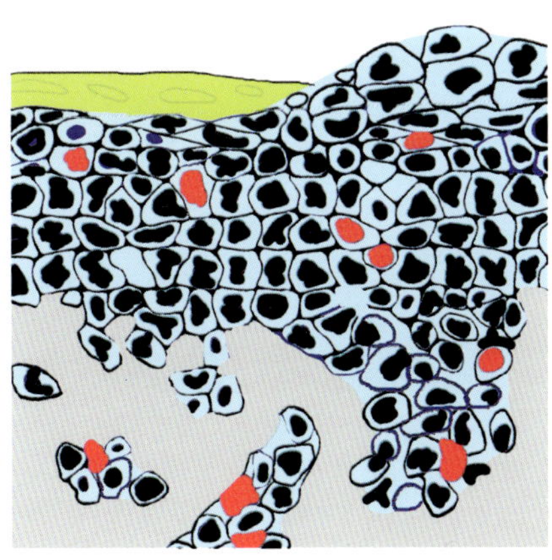

g. Invasive squamous carcinoma.
Extension through basement membrane.
Some features to identify squamous epithelium.
Retained features allow grading of degree of differentiation.

Figure **23.4**
Diagrammatic representation of normal vocal cord mucosa, hyperplasia, dysplasia and invasive carcinoma.

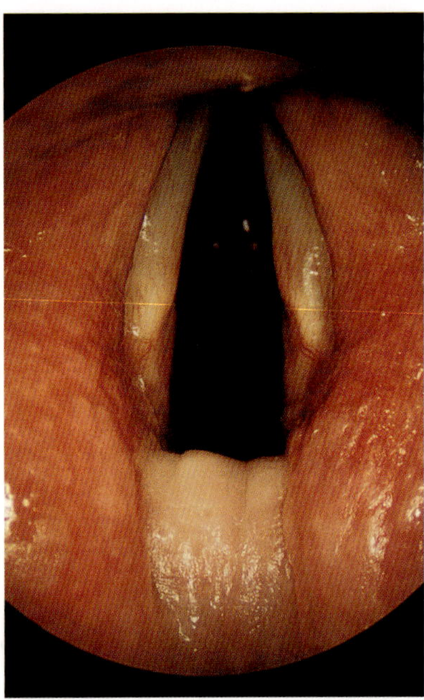

Figure **23.5**
Pachydermia in the interarytenoid region. Characteristic thickening of the squamous epithelium in the posterior glottis. It is not known why pachydermia occurs in the posterior glottis.

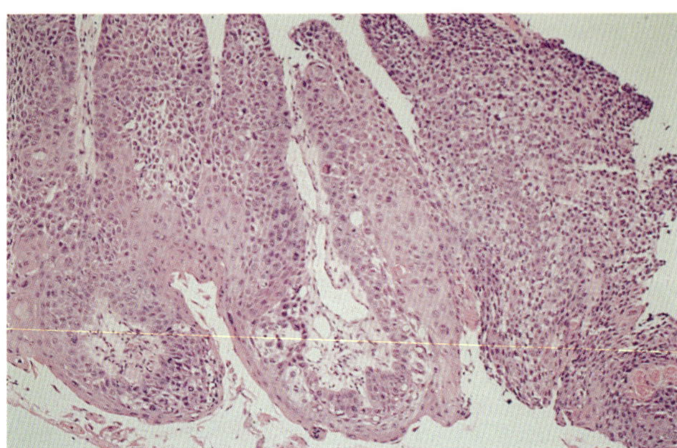

Figure **23.6**
Severe dysplasia in biopsy of laryngeal mucosa. Marked cellular pleomorphism and intact basement membrane.

abnormal mitoses in the middle or upper third of the mucosa; polarity of the cells is lost and irregular stratification disturbs the normal sequence of maturation (see Fig. 23.4). These findings allow grading of laryngeal biopsies. If the changes are confined to the basal third of the epithelial layer, atypia is described as mild. If the changes are more pronounced and extend more than two-thirds towards the epithelial surface (i.e. from the basal layer to just beneath the granular layer), atypia is said to be severe. Moderate dysplasia lies between mild and severe atypia with involvement of one-third to two-thirds of the epithelium.

Carcinoma-in-situ

Also known as intraepithelial carcinoma, non-invasive carcinoma or keratosis with severe atypia (Fig. 23.6).

Carcinoma-in-situ is the most florid form of epithelial dysplasia. When no normal cellular maturation can be seen, carcinoma-in-situ is present. Strict separation of carcinoma-in-situ and keratosis with severe atypia is sometimes not possible – there is very little difference.

There is cellular atypia of the whole thickness of the epithelium but no evidence of deep invasion to or beyond the basement membrane which maintains a sharp demarcation between the basal layer and the underlying stroma. The criteria of malignancy are present except for invasion – the changes are confined to the epithelial layer. There are irregularly arranged cells – atypical and immature with large darkly staining nuclei which vary in size and shape, and have large nucleoli and variable cytoplasmic keratinization. No normal flat squamous cells are seen on the surface. There is abnormal mitotic activity in the middle and upper third of the mucosa. Carcinoma-in-situ is a histologic diagnosis (see Fig. 23.4) not a clinical diagnosis. Carcinoma-in-situ in the larynx has not been proven to inevitably progress to invasive carcinoma.

Isolated carcinoma-in-situ is a relatively infrequent finding. Approximately 30% of biopsies showing carcinoma-in-situ (or keratosis with severe atypia) are associated with a co-existent invasive carcinoma 'nearby'. If more tissue was obtained by taking a larger biopsy or by stripping the lesion, it is likely that nearby areas of micro-invasive carcinoma would be found. The changes may be reversible if the causative irritant is identified and avoided.

Micro-invasive carcinoma

This is also known as carcinoma with superficial invasion. At this stage there is carcinoma-in-situ in the epithelium, *and* atypical epithelial cell groups reaching beyond the basement membrane, showing early but discrete and limited invasion. It is a histologic diagnosis and as the biological importance of micro-invasion is uncertain, is thought to carry the same prognosis as carcinoma-in-situ. Not all pathologists agree with the use of the term micro-invasive.

For squamous dysplastic changes in the laryngeal mucosa, there is neither general agreement on the natural history and malignant potential nor on the best form of treatment of these histopathologic changes. Long-term follow-up has shown that dysplastic mucosa has an increased chance of eventually developing into invasive carcinoma; the greater the dysplasia the greater the potential for progression to invasive carcinoma.

Important aggravating stimuli in the development of hyperplasia and dysplasia include smoking, alcohol, voice abuse, gastro-oesophageal reflux and various environmental irritants. Dysplasia occurs more often in men than in women, and is often more advanced in older patients.

Changes caused by smoking

There are consistent changes in the mucous membrane of the larynx that are most marked after prolonged smoking of tobacco which has high levels of tar and aromatic amines. Although the carcinogens are in different concentrations in the tobacco of different cigarettes, cigars and pipes and in tobacco which is chewed or taken as snuff, changes at the cellular level are similar. Compared to non-smokers the changes in the epithelial cells in the larynx have been shown to have similar alterations to those in the mucosa of the bronchi and the oesophagus. The surface epithelium becomes thicker due to excessive keratinization of the mucosa of the vocal folds and there is epithelial hyperplasia of both true cords and false cords and in the subglottic region. In habitual smokers there is squamous metaplasia, oedema and chronic submucosal inflammation. Eventually atypical nuclei appear in the cells and in more advanced cases there is a pattern of carcinoma-in-situ and finally invasive carcinoma. These changes in the mucous membrane occur predominantly in the true vocal cords and less often in the supraglottic region and false cord mucosa.

Thus, the carcinogens cause progressive changes in the mucous membrane. At any particular time any of the dysplastic changes may be taking place in different parts of the mucosa.

Premalignant lesions

The term premalignant or precancerous is generally taken to indicate a state where the cellular make-up is part way between normal and cancerous. Does it mean that given time and certain conditions the tissue *will* become malignant or does it mean that the changes in the tissue *may* become malignant or *may* be reversible? No unrelenting progression to malignancy in laryngeal lesions with severe dysplasia has been convincingly documented by repeated biopsies. Lengthy clinical evaluation suggests that laryngeal mucous membrane demonstrated by adequate biopsies to have keratosis with atypia or even carcinoma-in-situ but not to have invasive carcinoma may sometimes improve or even return to normal. Thus if the individual with premalignant laryngeal mucosa stops smoking there is a chance that invasive carcinoma may not follow.

There is an implication with the term 'premalignant' that there is an increased chance that the changes may progress to and result in invasive malignancy but there is also a chance they may be reversible. With this concept in mind it must always be remembered that severe dysplasia or in-situ-carcinoma often occurs adjacent to areas of infiltrating squamous carcinoma and the clinician must be prepared to obtain further biopsies in these cases. Biopsy results must always be correlated with the gross findings at laryngoscopy.

Lesions showing moderate or severe dysplasia, i.e. keratosis with moderate or severe atypia and carcinoma-in-situ, have a greater potential for malignant degeneration than lesions which show mild dysplasia. As the methods of grading dysplasia remain subjective there is still some doubt concerning the malignant potential in each grade. It is known to be higher in patients who continue to smoke, in men and in the aged.

Management of premalignant lesions

Cessation of tobacco and alcohol abuse is always a necessary part of treatment. Having graded the stage of premalignancy, the aims of therapy are to eradicate the disease. Prolonged regular follow-up should allow detection of residual, recurrent or progressive disease, which can be treated by surgical or laser removal.

In general, the size and appearance of the lesion and grade of dysplasia on biopsy suggests reasonable management strategies to the clinician:

- *Mild*. Regular observation by indirect laryngoscopy every 3–6 months. Biopsy if appearance changes.
- *Moderate*. Regular observation and repeat biopsy if no improvement or worse appearance.
- *Severe*. Repeat biopsy for possible invasive carcinoma. Removal of the dysplastic area by stripping and/or laser vaporization.

Regular follow-up is essential in each case.

Reasonable treatment for dysplasia

Mild	regular observation by indirect laryngoscopy
Moderate	regular observation for repeat biopsy
Severe	repeat biopsies; removal of lesion

Microsurgical procedures for laryngeal dysplasia

Biopsy	removal of part
Excision	removal of all of a proven lesion
Stripping	removal of all, plus surrounds, to enhance histopathological assessment

Biopsy is when part or, in some cases, all of a small lesion is removed for histopathologic examination. *Excision* is when all of a histopathologically proven lesion is removed. *Stripping* is when all of the lesion and surrounding margins are removed by precise microsurgical dissection, not, as previously advocated, by repeated punching out of irregular pieces or by tearing away the edge.

Histopathology of invasive squamous cell carcinoma

Almost all malignancies of the endolarynx arise from squamous epithelium. To be classified as a squamous cell carcinoma the tumour must have distinguishing features, seen at light microscopy, which identify stratified squamous epithelium, e.g. formation of extracellular or intracellular keratin and the presence of intercellular 'bridges' which are specialized junctional structures connecting the cytoplasmic borders of adjacent cells. The extent to which a malignancy retains these features and others, such as large polygonal cells with eosinophilic cytoplasm in a pavement pattern, allows assessment of the degree of differentiation from cells closely resembling normal squamous epithelium (i.e. well differentiated) to groups of cells showing no evidence of squamous epithelial origin (i.e. anaplastic).

Good differentiation is indicated in tumours by the presence of squamous epithelial 'pearls' which may show a central area of keratinization. All areas of the tumour section must be looked at carefully to identify differentiation. Squamous carcinomas may arise from mucosa lined normally by ciliated columnar epithelium which has undergone squamous metaplasia. Extension by malignant cells through the basement membrane into the underlying submucosal space of Reinke or thyroarytenoid muscle clearly confirms the diagnosis of invasive squamous cell carcinoma.

A typical early squamous cell carcinoma of the vocal cord (say 8–10 mm in diameter) may be a well-circumscribed, raised, nodular, papillary or sessile lesion whose central area is invasive, sometimes with surface ulceration, and whose periphery has an ill-defined border of dysplastic squamous mucosa or carcinoma-in-situ. It may spread sheetwise (the 'carpet' carcinoma described by Kleinsasser) by tongue-like extensions or it may extend to deeper structures by invasion.

Features of laryngeal cancer

Progressive hoarseness
Stridor from large obstructing tumour
'Something' in the throat
Referred pain in the ear (otalgia)
Lump in the neck
Advanced disease:
- Haemoptysis
- Dysphagia
- Halitosis
- Cachexia

Distant metastases

DIAGNOSTIC EVALUATION

Clinical features

Symptoms

The patient is often suspected of having laryngeal cancer before the history and examination have been completed. An elderly male smoker with progressive huskiness for some months is a likely candidate.

Progressive voice change, hoarseness or huskiness are the cardinal presenting symptoms caused by a tumour originating on or involving the vocal fold mucosa and causing interference with vibration. In more advanced cases with deeper infiltration, the vocalis muscle may be affected, the recurrent laryngeal nerve involved or, in supraglottic lesions, the voice may become muffled.

When there is a large obstructing tumour in the supraglottic or subglottic region there may be noisy breathing due to partial airway obstruction. The patient may complain of 'something' in the throat or throat discomfort, and in advanced cases with ulceration the patient may have halitosis or haemoptysis. The tumour may affect swallowing, causing dysphagia or odynophagia (pain on swallowing). Referred otalgia is a common symptom.

A mass in the neck may be due to regional nodal metastases or direct extension into the soft tissues through or around the laryngeal framework.

In advanced cases there may be malnutrition, weight loss, halitosis and symptoms from regional or distant metastases.

Signs

A husky, rough, change in the voice caused by a glottic mass, a muffled quality of the voice due to a supraglottic lesion, and partial airway obstruction due to a large supraglottic or subglottic tumour are often immediately evident, before examination of the upper respiratory tract begins.

Assessment for distant metastases includes a complete general physical examination.

Indirect laryngoscopy

Indirect laryngoscopy using a laryngeal mirror, a rigid telescope or a flexible laryngoscope is performed in

> **Indirect laryngoscopy**
>
> Small, raised, irregular lesion
> Large, exophytic or ulcerated tumour
> Reduced or absent vocal cord movement
> Assess airway for anaesthesia

the consulting room, office or clinic and usually allows the otolaryngologist to suspect malignancy, although only biopsy can be definitive.

In small lesions, stroboscopy may add to the suspicion of a mass interfering with vocal cord vibration but in most cases the mass has already been seen at indirect laryngoscopy. Photographic or video documentation can be performed at the time of indirect laryngoscopy.

Most lesions appear as raised, irregular, exophytic or ulcerated masses (Fig. 23.7) with surrounding erythroplasia and irregular vasculature. Symmetry and movement of each vocal cord are noted. Reduced or absent movement of one side may be due to an infiltrative mass, cricoarytenoid joint fixation or tumour involving the recurrent laryngeal nerve.

During examination, the degree of airway obstruction, its adequacy for anaesthesia, and the possibility of intubation difficulty should be determined (Fig. 23.8).

Neck examination

Examination and palpation of the neck for the presence, location and fixation of possible regional cervical node metastases is routine. Further information concerning the presence of nodal metastases may be obtained from axial computed tomography (CT) scans.

Laboratory tests

Tests such as a full blood count, immunoglobulin measurement and liver function studies add to the assessment of the patient's general state of health and nutrition; deficiencies can have a significant bearing on postoperative healing if surgical treatment is being considered.

Laryngeal imaging

The role of lateral X-rays, CT and magnetic resonance imaging (MRI) has been discussed in detail in

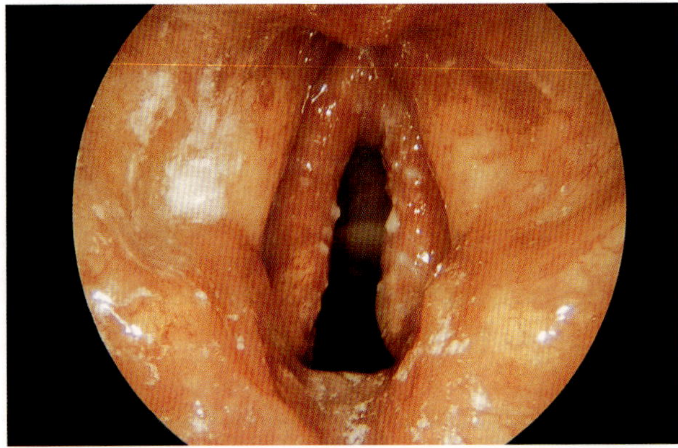

Figure **23.7**
Indirect laryngoscopy. Widespread chronic laryngitis and leukoplakia with severe congestion and irregular edges of the vocal cords. Repeated biopsies showed moderate dysplasia, but no invasive tumour.

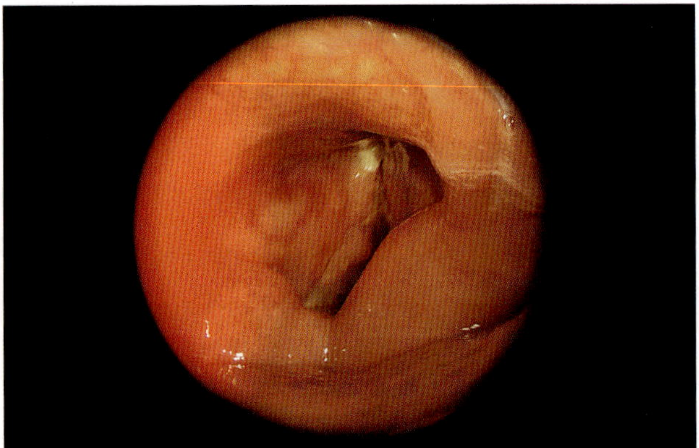

Figure **23.8**
Indirect laryngoscopy. Advanced carcinoma of the larynx causing moderately severe airway obstruction. Radiotherapy 12 months previously failed to control the disease.

chapter 3 on diagnostic imaging of the larynx. This rapidly advancing technology adds to the information obtained from indirect and direct laryngoscopy and helps build up a three-dimensional picture of the laryngeal mass. Unseen transglottic extension or deeper extension into the paraglottic region or subglottic area can be evaluated. Cartilage destruction, extension around cartilage or invasion through ligaments may be assessed, and axial CT or MRI studies may be more accurate than clinical evaluation for neck metastases, especially in the patient with a thick neck which is difficult to palpate.

Chest X-ray should be performed in every case, and further appropriate studies are necessary if bony or other metastases are suspected.

Thus, diagnostic imaging provides more accurate information to assist evaluation of the primary tumour, regional metastases and distant spread.

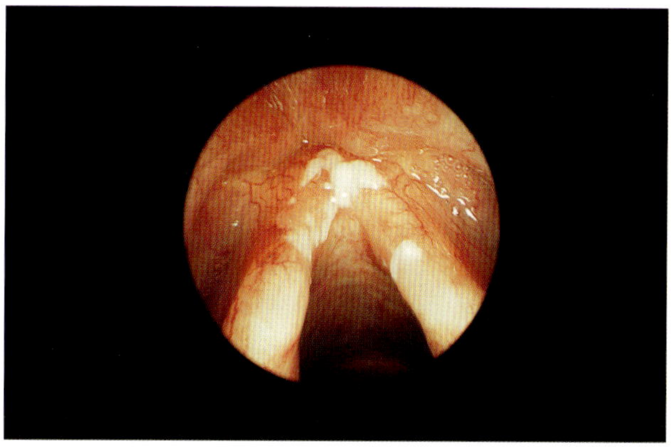

Figure **23.9**
View of the anterior glottis at direct laryngoscopy using a 50° telescope. The dysplastic changes and their relationship to the laryngeal ventricle and the anterior commissure are clearly seen.

Endoscopy and biopsy techniques

Peroral endoscopy under general anaesthesia is directed principally at the lesion seen at indirect laryngoscopy but pan-endoscopy including oesophagoscopy and tracheobronchoscopy are also performed to detect possible synchronous malignancy in the upper aerodigestive tract.

Chapter 5 on anaesthesia techniques and chapter 6 on direct laryngoscopy give details of the method. In summary, suspension laryngoscopy allows assessment with the naked eye, with rigid telescopes and with the operating microscope. The rigid telescopes – 0°, 30°, 50° and if necessary 70° – give the most comprehensive view (Fig. 23.9). Microlaryngoscopy allows carefully selected, multiple, generous biopsies to be taken. The anatomical site of each biopsy must be carefully recorded and the biopsy or biopsies from each specified area of mucosa sent in a separate labelled container to pathology. The histopathological results will allow 'mapping' of the surface aspects of the lesion so that, together with imaging assessment of any submucosal tumour spread, a reasonably accurate evaluation of the whole lesion can be obtained. Some surgeons advocate the use of a 'carcinoma gauge' for endoscopic measuring of laryngeal malignancies.

There are appearances which arouse suspicion of dysplasia or malignancy, namely asymmetry (Fig. 23.10), leukoplakia or erythroplakia (Fig. 23.11), prominent or atypical capillaries surrounding the lesion (Fig. 23.12), granularity, bleeding to the touch, thickening, irregularity, nodular ulceration and ulcerative or exophytic lesions (Fig. 23.13). The lesion may be difficult to visualize, e.g. in the ventricle (Fig. 23.14), in the posterior glottis (Fig. 23.15), or under a

Biopsy of laryngeal tumour

Single, from margin of clearly delineated small lesion
Multiple and generous from larger, irregular lesion
Leukoplakia, erythroplakia, asymmetry, bleeding are suspicious signs
Frozen section in selected cases

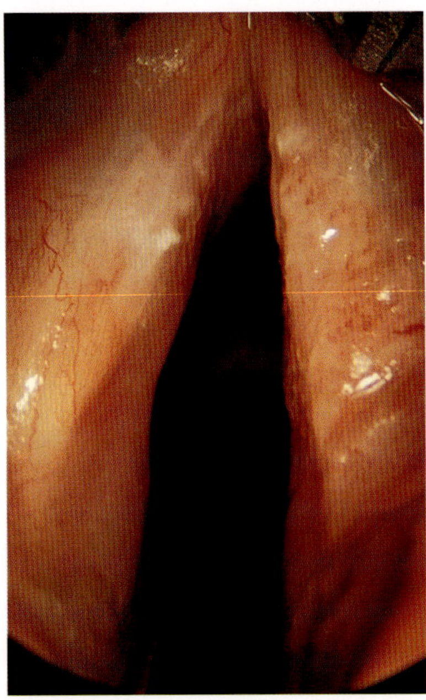

Figure **23.10**
Close-up of irregular right vocal cord of a 28-year-old female. Repeated biopsies over 12 months finally showed carcinoma-in-situ and the vocal cord was treated with the defocused carbon dioxide laser.

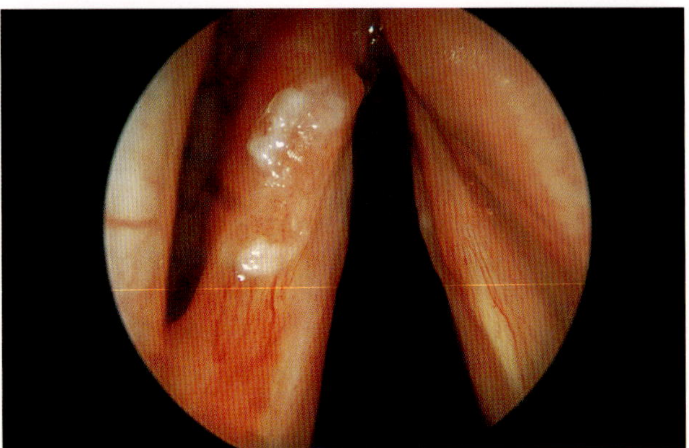

Figure **23.11**
Surface leukoplakia on a raised red lesion. Biopsy revealed carcinoma-in-situ and endoscopic laser treatment resulted in a relatively normal looking vocal fold. Subsequent biopsy showed no dysplasia.

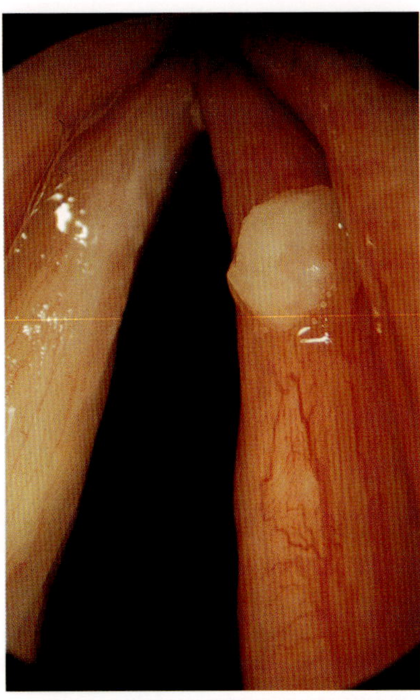

Figure **23.12**
Small raised lesion on the upper surface of the right vocal fold which is markedly different to the left. There are dilated vessels and there is mild oedema. Invasive squamous cell carcinoma.

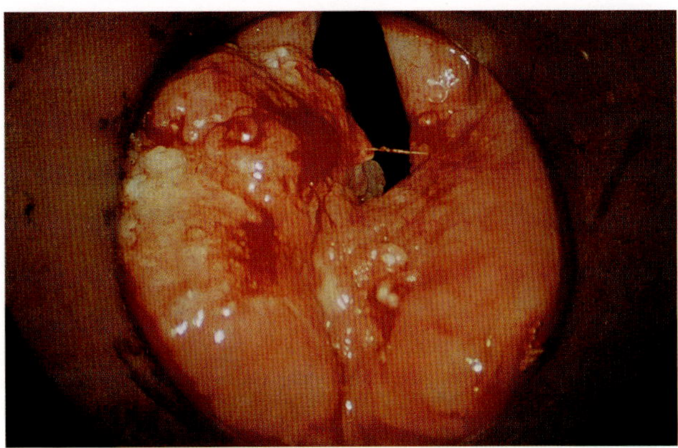

Figure **23.13**
Widespread grossly granular partly ulcerated malignancy in the posterior glottis and interarytenoid region. Bleeding to touch before biopsy. Squamous cell carcinoma.

web (Fig. 23.16). A biopsy must be taken from each area. Biopsies can be taken from areas that appear to be clear for better assessment of the microscopic extent of the lesion. The key to adequate biopsies depends on the knowledge of dysplastic or neoplastic mucosal multicentricity.

A single biopsy may be sufficient from the margin of a clearly delineated uniform lesion. It may be possible

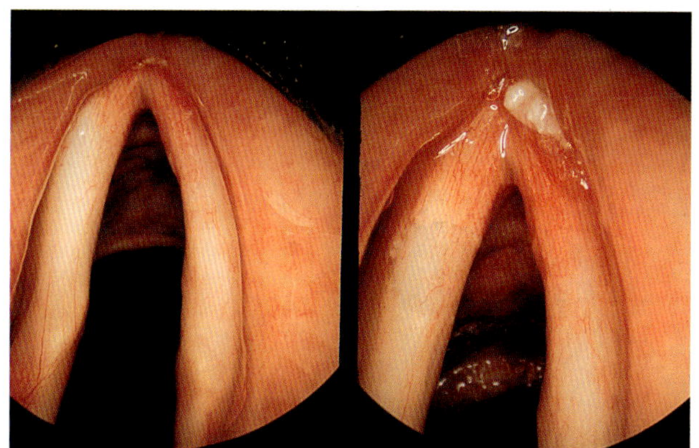

Figure **23.14**
Direct laryngoscopy shows only some mild erythema at the anterior end of the right vocal cord (left). After adjustment of the laryngoscope and use of a 30° telescope (right), quite a large lesion can be seen in the anterior end of the right ventricle. Carcinoma-in-situ.

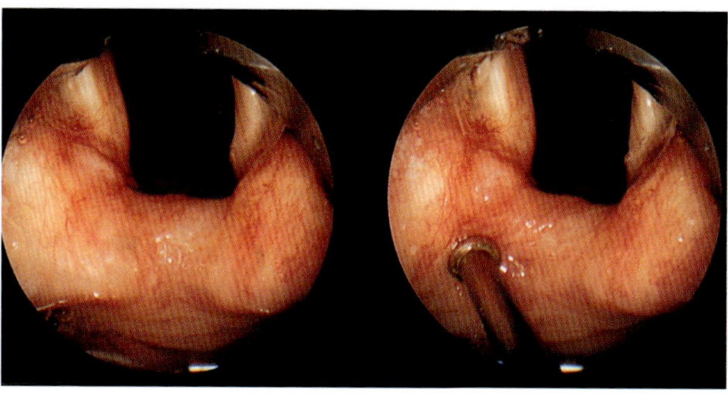

Figure **23.15**
Round, slightly raised area on left posterior glottic mucosa. Grasped with cup forceps and cleanly removed with scissors – mild dysplasia. Such a small lesion in this site might be missed when an endotracheal tube is in place.

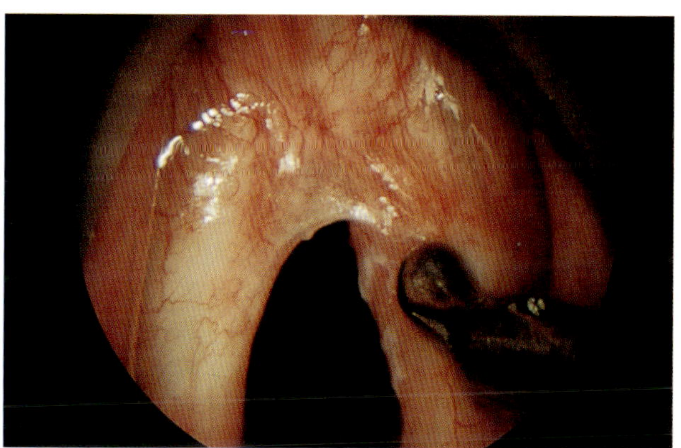

Figure **23.16**
Recurring dysplastic mucosa biopsied repeatedly over 12 years, leading to formation of an anterior glottic web. The technique of 'rolling' the tissues to reveal the leukoplakia patches is shown.

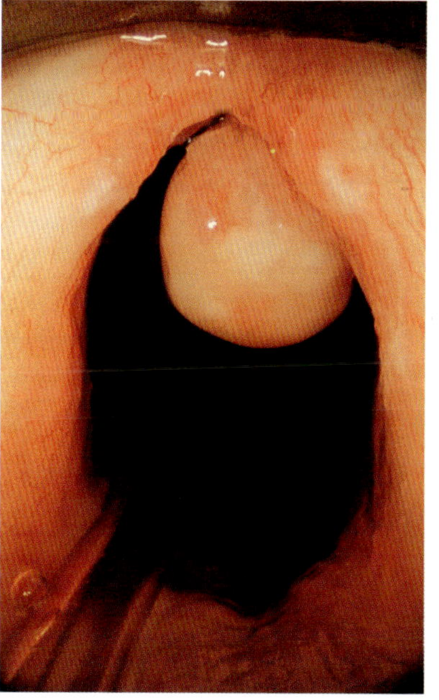

Figure **23.17**
Large round firm mass arising from a small pedicle under the anterior edge of the right vocal cord from an area previously biopsy proven to be dysplastic. A spindle cell variety of squamous cell carcinoma treated by radiotherapy, and free of disease for more than 5 years.

to attempt excision biopsy, e.g. a pedunculated lesion (Fig. 23.17), or complete removal with a surrounding margin of normal-looking tissue of a small lesion on the membranous vocal fold. Multiple, sizeable, representative, carefully labelled biopsies avoiding vital structures when possible are required from larger lesions.

Frozen section may be advisable in selected cases to be sure that adequate tissue to make a diagnosis

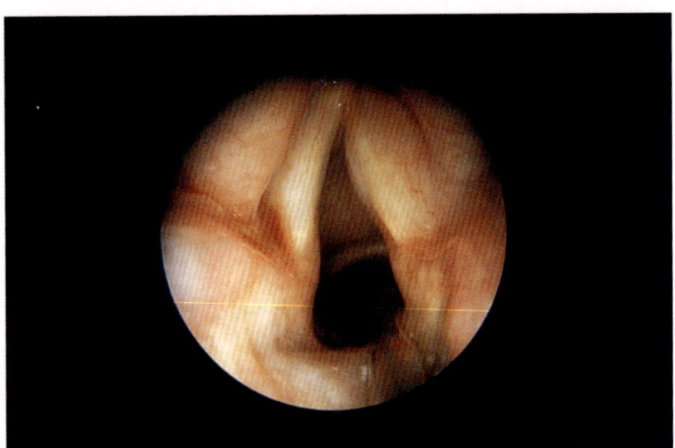

Figure **23.18**
Smooth mass evenly distending the right vocal fold. An incision was made for a deep biopsy which showed lymphoma.

Additional diagnostic procedures

Supravital staining
Photodynamic fluorescent examination
Contact endoscopy

has been obtained. In some cases frozen section is necessary for tissue diagnosis before proceeding immediately with laryngectomy.

It is occasionally necessary to make an incision through intact mucosa either with the laser or with cold instruments to gather a deep biopsy where no surface tumour or ulceration can be seen (Fig. 23.18).

Repeated, serial biopsies are taken from larynges with proven dysplasia and after surgical or radiation treatment in the search for residual or recurrent disease.

Supravital staining with 2% toluidine blue painted on the surface with an applicator has been used, without great enthusiasm, in an attempt to outline more accurately the dysplastic or malignant tissue. Squamous mucosa of the vocal fold does not normally stain, but areas of superficial carcinoma take up stain and define areas of biopsy. A new technique which appears to be more promising is 'photodynamic diagnosis' which has recently been used for early recognition of carcinoma of the bladder. Under general anaesthesia, a suitable tumour marker substance is instilled in the larynx. A special diagnostic fluorescent light is used for illumination and dysplastic or malignant areas fluoresce with a red colour. Further work will determine the place of this new diagnostic method.

Contact endoscopy during microlaryngoscopy has been advocated by Mario Andrea and others, and is described in chapter 6 on direct laryngoscopy in this book.

When there is a large tumour in the glottic or supraglottic region with oedema, ulceration or bleeding, maintenance of the airway for anaesthesia and laryngoscopic examination can be very difficult. The airway must always be secured before examination and biopsy. In some cases where a large tumour obstructs the airway, subtotal laser removal can be undertaken to improve the airway and to avoid tracheotomy.

The cricoarytenoid joints should be examined and probed on each side to assess mobility.

At the completion of the endoscopic evaluation, a drawing or sketch of the tumour showing its relationship to normal structures should be made together with photo or video documentation. In conjunction with CT scans and/or MRI, a final assessment is made so that treatment can be planned.

Anatomical classification

It is customary to divide the larynx into anatomical compartments to assist description of the site of origin of tumours and for staging and classification. The evidence to support what some investigators regard as artificial compartmentalization includes the results of dye injections in living and cadaver laryn-

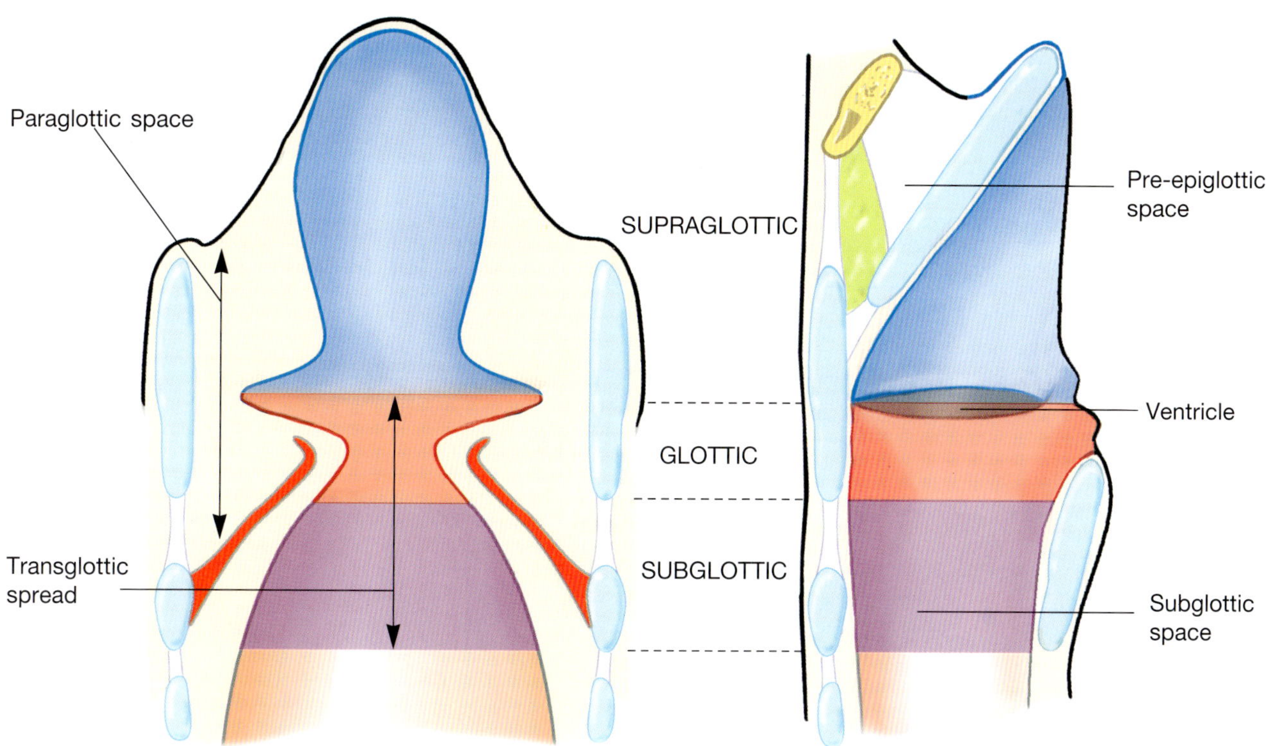

Figure **23.19**
Diagram showing regions, spaces and compartments of the larynx with reference to malignant disease.

ges, whole-organ serial sections, embryological studies indicating separate origin of the compartments and extensive and prolonged clinical observations. Although there is no universal agreement the following anatomical definitions are generally accepted:

- *Supraglottic region*. The lingual and laryngeal surface (Fig. 23.19) of the epiglottis, the laryngeal surface of the aryepiglottic folds and arytenoids, the false cords and the roof of the ventricles. Thus superiorly the boundary is the tip and lateral borders of the epiglottis and inferiorly a horizontal plane passing through the apices of the ventricles.
- *Glottic region*. This compartment is composed of both vocal folds (see Fig. 23.19), the vocal process of the arytenoid cartilages, the anterior commissure and the posterior glottic tissues at the glottic level. The inferior boundary is a horizontal plane 1 cm below the free edge of the vocal folds. This line is the boundary between the glottis and the subglottis (see later).
- *Subglottic region*. Extends from a horizontal plane 1 cm below the edge of the vocal folds inferiorly to the lower border of the cricoid cartilage (see Fig. 23.19). The definition of this region is not universally agreed upon. Some believe the superior border lies at the level of the edge of the vocal folds themselves – this concept would make the glottic region virtually two-dimensional.

In addition spread of cancer can be described as transglottic, paraglottic and pre-epiglottic as follows:

- *Transglottic carcinoma*. Describes tumours which have extended out of the glottic compartment to involve the larynx above the ventricle or in the subglottic region. These tumours have a tendency to invade the paraglottic space.

Anatomical compartments

Supraglottic region
Glottic region
Subglottic region
Transglottic spread
Paraglottic space
Pre-epiglottic space

Spread of laryngeal cancer

Diffuse superficial spread
Submucosal infiltration
Deeper invasion into muscle
Into and across anterior commissure
Transglottic spread
Pre-epiglottic and paraglottic spaces
Into the subglottic space
Through, around and beyond cartilage
Through thyrohyoid membrane

- *Paraglottic space*. Lies in the lateral hemilarynx and extends from the quadrangular membrane superomedially to the conus elasticus infero-medially. It is bounded laterally by the inner surface of the thyroid cartilage, medially by the laryngeal ventricle and posteriorly by the mucosa of the piriform sinus. It communicates superiorly with the space between the thyroid cartilage and the hyoid bone, anteriorly with the pre-epiglottic space and inferiorly with the space between the thyroid and cricoid cartilages.
- *Pre-epiglottic space*. The superior boundary is the hyo-epiglottic ligament (which assists in forming the valleculae) and the anterior boundary is the thyrohyoid membrane and ligament. Posteriorly the boundary is the anterior surface of the epiglottic cartilage and the thyro-epiglottic ligament. Laterally and inferiorly it is continuous with the upper part of the paraglottic space. The pre-epiglottic space contains fat and loose areolar tissue and carcinoma can spread directly into it through the perforations in the epiglottic cartilage.

Spread within the laryngeal anatomical compartments

The mode and direction of spread depends upon the location of the primary tumour and its relationship to nearby structures including the cartilaginous framework of the larynx. There may be diffuse superficial spread along the mucosal surfaces (the 'carpet' carcinoma), submucosal infiltration or deeper invasion into and beyond the underlying musculature.

With this latter spread, it is more difficult to assess the size of the infiltrating tumour even with the imaging techniques currently available. Cancer spread follows the planes of least resistance in the laryngeal compartments and, at least for a time, remains confined by the thyroid and cricoid cartilage and the conus elasticus. Later tumour invasion often occurs through areas in the cartilages that have undergone ossification; proteinases and other enzymes assist the degradation of the extracellular matrix. Spread will also occur through the thyrohyoid membrane where the superior laryngeal vessels and nerves pass.

Anteriorly, where the vocal ligaments are inserted into the posterior surface of the thyroid cartilage as Broyle's ligament, there are numerous vessels and lymphatics with an absence of a protective perichondrial or periosteal barrier. For these reasons tumour extension into the anterior commissure area, across the anterior commissure from one vocal fold to the other and into the thyroid skeleton is relatively common.

Posteriorly, submucosal spread along the upper surface of the cricoid cartilage can result in vocal cord immobility as the tumour encircles the arytenoid region and/or infiltrates the interarytenoid muscle (see Fig. 23.13). Other more common causes of limitation of movement of the hemilarynx are deep extension into the thyroarytenoid muscle or direct infiltration of the recurrent laryngeal nerve. Posterior spread can see tumour spill over the interarytenoid area and involve the postcricoid region. Superior extension is over the aryepiglottic folds or more anteriorly into the valleculae and base of tongue.

Inferior growth traverses the subglottis to the trachea and here a large tumour will cause airway obstruction. Extension outside the larynx occurs through the cricothyroid membrane, a vulnerable area just below the edge of the thyroid cartilage itself.

Transglottic extension and involvement of the paraglottic and pre-epiglottic spaces are common pathways of spread as outlined above.

Regional nodal metastasis and lymphatic infiltration

With the exception of the edge of the vocal folds themselves, the larynx is well supplied with lymphatics. The lymph vessels above the ventricles drain freely from one side to the other and flow into the superior and middle group of deep cervical jugular nodes. However, the lymphatics in the subglottic region behave more like those of the trachea, have little crossover and drainage is through the cricothyroid membrane to the middle and inferior jugular and the paratracheal groups of nodes.

Tumours in the supraglottis, where there is a rich lymphatic supply, metastasize earlier and, because they are often near the midline, contralateral or bilateral regional nodal metastases are not uncommon. Large supraglottic tumours have metastatic cervical spread in approximately 60% of cases.

Squamous cell carcinomas of the vocal fold seldom metastasize unless they are advanced and when they do it is usually to the same side of the neck. Carcinomas of the glottis, without fixation of the hemilarynx, have cervical metastases in less than 5% of cases; when the glottic disease is advanced the incidence rises to 20 or 30%.

Subglottic tumours spread to the prelaryngeal (Delphian) and paratracheal nodes in approximately 20% of cases; the spread is often silent and portends a poor prognosis.

The larger the tumour, the higher the rate of metastases. Similarly, contralateral spread implies a poor prognosis. CT and MRI have improved the detection of nodes previously not identified clinically. Extracapsular spread which may be macroscopic or microscopic is associated with a higher incidence of distant metastases.

Cervical metastases

Early glottic	less than 5%
Late glottic	20–30%
Large transglottic	50%
Supraglottic	up to 60%
Subglottic	20%

STAGING OF CARCINOMA OF THE LARYNX

The TNM (tumour-nodes-metastases) classification of malignant tumours is widely applied to squamous cell carcinoma of the larynx. It is not used for other malignant laryngeal tumours. It has been developed for end-stage reporting and need not be used to dictate treatment as each patient must be individually assessed. It has been pointed out (Ferlito et al 1995a,b) that cancer of the larynx can be staged at various times and under different circumstances with different results:

1 cTNM or *c*linical-diagnostic pretreatment classification based on physical examination and imaging;
2 sTNM or *s*urgical classification based on examination of the lesion after surgical exploration or treatment;

3 pTNM or *p*ostoperative pathologic classification based on the macroscopic and/or the microscopic findings;
4 rTNM or *r*e-treatment classification, necessary if the tumour recurs and requires further therapy;
5 aTNM or *a*utopsy classification, when the true extent of the tumour can be established.

The TNM classification has been reworked and refined by the UICC (International Union Against Cancer) and the AJCC (American Joint Committee on Cancer) (see Table 23.1) and, although it is the most widely used, it is not universally accepted. The TNM system is partly based on proven concepts and, like all classifications, it must have some compromises. For instance, there is controversy about the anatomical boundaries of the larynx and the division into the supraglottis, glottis and subglottis. The upper border of the subglottic region is arbitrarily defined and not universally agreed. The TNM classification fails to consider the severity of symptoms or the host's general state of health or their immune status. There is an unresolved problem defining the submucosal bulk of a tumour because the depth of invasion of a tumour is difficult to assess. Vocal cord 'fixation' and 'reduced mobility' are vague terms relying on subjective assessment. Clinical examination for regional lymph nodes, especially paratracheal and prelaryngeal nodes, is known to be unreliable. Nodes with metastatic disease may not be palpable, yet enlarged palpable lymph nodes do not necessarily contain tumour. The degree of differentiation of the tumour, the size and the rate of growth, which may not be related to the anatomical space in which it is growing, are important factors which influence outcome yet are not included in most staging systems. Pearson (1994) suggested simple division of laryngeal cancer into five groups: very early, early, intermediate, advanced and very advanced, and he proposed a new staging method which considered the biological factors in laryngeal cancer.

It is clear that small superficial cancers of the larynx, without suspicion of deep invasion, can be accurately staged by clinical examination but, as the cancer gets larger, clinical examination without imaging is often associated with significant underestimation of staging. For larger laryngeal and hypopharyngeal cancers a combination of clinical examination and CT and/or MRI leads to more accurate staging. Extension into the deeper tissues and infiltration outside the larynx is so difficult to evaluate that even with the best techniques the accuracy of staging may be poor; the true extent of disease may not be known until the larynx is examined after removal or at autopsy.

Nevertheless, there is a need for accurate staging of cancer. TNM staging is a concise method of describing tumour, is universally recognized, and offers a common language for comparing incidence, extent of disease and results of treatment. Although techniques such as CT and MRI assist the clinician, clinical staging is based mostly on the findings at indirect and direct laryngoscopy and from palpation of the neck for regional lymph nodes. The tumour in an individual patient can often be best described by a careful drawing to establish a tumour map supplemented by documentation using photography or video.

TREATMENT OF CARCINOMA OF THE LARYNX

General overview of treatment

All patients are strongly encouraged to stop smoking.

Advice on the management of premalignant and malignant laryngeal disease depends not only on the histopathology but also on the site, size and extent of the lesion as indicated by clinical findings, imaging evaluation with CT and MRI, assessment at microlaryngoscopy, host–tumour relationship, concomitant non-neoplastic disease and the wishes of the patient.

Treatment options include:

- no active treatment, but close follow-up for 5–10 years;
- repeat biopsy indicated by change in the appearance and progression of the lesion;
- endoscopic removal of affected mucosa by vaporization using the CO_2 laser, by incision removal or by vocal cord stripping using cold instrumentation for dissection;
- cordectomy, either by laryngofissure or by endoscopic technique;
- partial laryngectomy;

Table 23.1 Tumour classification according to AJCC and UICC

T. Primary Tumour

Tx Cannot be staged.
To No evidence of tumour.
Tis Carcinoma-in-situ.

Supraglottis
- T1 Tumour confined to one subsite of supraglottis, normal vocal cord mobility.
- T2 Tumour involves more than one subsite of supraglottis, normal vocal cord mobility.
- T3 Tumour limited to larynx with vocal cord fixation and/or involves postcricoid area, medial wall of piriform fossa or pre-epiglottic space.
- T4 Tumour invades thyroid cartilage or tissue beyond the larynx.

Glottis
- T1 Tumour limited to vocal cords. Normal mobility.
  - T1a One vocal cord.
  - T1b Both vocal cords
- T2 Tumour extends to supraglottis and/or subglottis and/or impaired vocal cord mobility.
- T3 Tumour limited to larynx, with vocal cord fixation.
- T4 Tumour invades thyroid cartilage or tissue beyond the larynx.

Subglottis
- T1 Tumour limited to subglottis
- T2 Tumour extends to vocal cord. Normal or impaired mobility.
- T3 Tumour limited to larynx with vocal cord fixation.
- T4 Tumour invades cartilage or tissue beyond the larynx.

N. Regional Nodes
- Nx Cannot be assessed.
- No No regional metastasis.
- N1 Metastasis in single ipsilateral node, less than 3 cm.
- N2 Metastasis in nodes less than 6 cm.
  - N2a Single ipsilateral node 3–6 cm.
  - N2b Multiple ipsilateral nodes less than 6 cm.
  - N2c Bilateral and contralateral node less than 6 cm.
- N3 Metastases in nodes greater than 6 cm.

M. Distant Metastases
- Mx Cannot be assessed.
- Mo No distant metastases.
- M1 Distant metastases.

Stage Groupings

Stage	T	N	M
O	Tis	No	Mo
I	T1	No	Mo
II	T2	No	Mo
III	T3	No	Mo
	T1–3	N1	Mo
IV	T4 or	N2–3 or	M1

- total laryngectomy;
- external beam radiotherapy;
- combination of surgery and radiotherapy;
- chemotherapy in combination with radiation or surgery or alone for palliation.

Because of these many options, a physician may develop strong opinions, not based on scientific evidence, which may be barriers to rational assessment of the value of different treatments and treatment combinations. These convictions may prevent presenting the patient with balanced information about the various treatment modalities available.

Treatment

No treatment; regular observation
Repeat biopsy; regular observation
Endoscopic removal of lesion
Cordectomy, endoscopic or by laryngofissure
Partial laryngectomy
Total laryngectomy
Radiotherapy
Chemotherapy, in combination or alone
Combination surgery and radiotherapy

NOTE: All patients require regular follow-up

Premalignancy

Discussion of treatment is made difficult because of the confusion over terminology among lesions such as keratosis with atypia, carcinoma-in-situ and microinvasive carcinoma. This situation is further complicated by the knowledge that detection of severe atypia or carcinoma-in-situ in laryngeal biopsies may indicate the presence nearby of invasive carcinoma. It is not easy to recommend definitive treatment options for 'early' lesions or 'premalignant' lesions, but close follow-up is always necessary. Biopsy findings should be correlated with the gross findings at indirect and direct laryngoscopy. For example, keratosis with severe atypia and several large irregular granular areas in the larynx with a short history may need more aggressive treatment and shorter follow-up review than a localized area also with a histological appearance of keratosis with severe atypia which has been observed for months or even a year or two.

Reasonable management of dysplasia in the laryngeal mucosa has already been outlined in the section on management of premalignant lesions in this chapter.

Some authorities recommend radiotherapy for widespread carcinoma-in-situ on one or both vocal cords, others prefer regular examination, repeat biopsy and cessation of tobacco and alcohol.

If the premalignant dysplastic mucosa proves on subsequent biopsy to have become invasive carcinoma, then laser treatment, surgical treatment or radiotherapy will be necessary.

Supraglottic carcinoma

Supraglottic carcinomas (Fig. 23.20) usually present later than glottic carcinomas. There is often a 'silent' period (Fig. 23.21) with few symptoms and, unlike glottic lesions, there is no cartilaginous framework to

Supraglottic carcinoma

Often a 'silent' symptomless period
No containing anatomical barriers
Rich bilateral lymphatic supply
Often presents late with neck metastases
50% present as T3 or T4 tumours

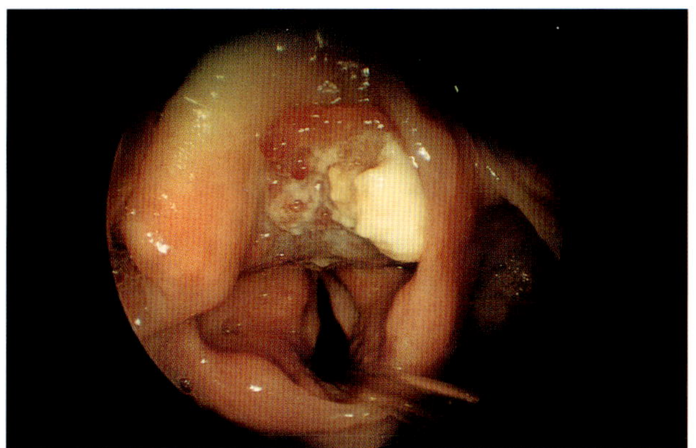

Figure **23.20**
Large supraglottic carcinoma on the posterior aspect of the epiglottis in an 83-year-old man who had been a heavy smoker. General anaesthesia using the Benjet tube; no airway problem.

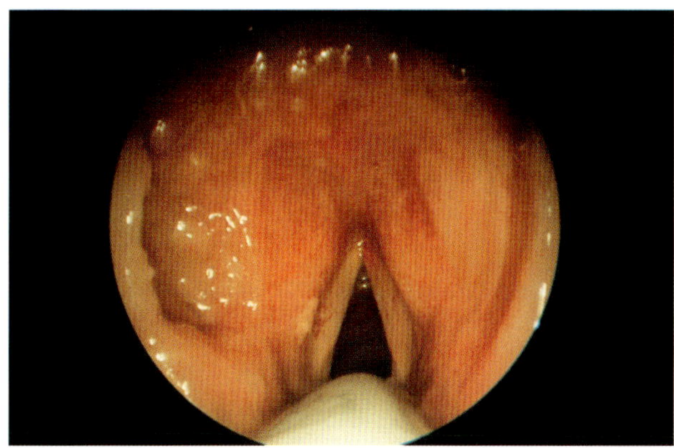

Figure **23.21**
Primary squamous cell supraglottic carcinoma on the medial aspect of the left aryepiglottic fold above the ventricular fold. The only symptom was referred pain to the ear.

act as a barrier to contain supraglottic tumour extension. In addition, the supraglottic region has a rich lymphatic supply distributed to both sides of the neck and node metastases are often present; a lump in the neck is a common presenting complaint. Over 50% of supraglottic carcinomas present as T3 or T4 lesions.

Location and spread of the tumour are major factors in considering treatment:

1 Tumours of the 'marginal zone' (which includes the lingual surface of the suprahyoid epiglottis and the edges of the aryepiglottic folds) tend to escape the larynx by spilling over into the valleculae, base of tongue, pre-epiglottic space and piriform sinuses, behaving like hypopharyngeal lesions and having a poorer prognosis.
2 Spread to the pre-epiglottic space from the laryngeal surface of the epiglottis occurs through fenestrae (small holes for blood vessels and fibrous tissue) in the epiglottis whose cartilage, unlike the thyroid and cricoid cartilage, does not ossify and therefore resists invasion. Tumour size may be underestimated because extension into the pre-epiglottic space is clinically silent; CT and MRI improve diagnostic localization.
3 Large ulcerative lesions may spread down via the ventricle so the tumour becomes transglottic and the voice becomes affected.
4 Spread tends to occur readily across the tendon at the anterior commissure where there is no inner perichondrium.

Location and spread

'Marginal zone' tumours escape the larynx
Pre-epiglottic space invasion may be underestimated
Paraglottic and transglottic extension
Spreads readily at anterior commissure
High incidence of lymph node metastases

5 The incidence of lymph node metastases in supraglottic cancer depends on the site, duration, spread and differentiation of the disease; it is reported to be found in approximately 50% of cases, and may be bilateral. Over 50% of early T1 and T2 supraglottic lesions have no clinically detectable (macroscopic) metastases and about half of these have occult (microscopic) disease. There is very little chance of long-term survival when lymph nodes are fixed and larger than 6 cm. The presence of neck node metastases becomes a critical factor in prognosis whether they are palpable clinically, found by imaging or proven histologically.

Treatment options for supraglottic carcinoma include:

- T1. A few early lesions limited to the laryngeal surface of the epiglottis can be excised endoscopically (preferably by laser), but conservative transoral removal should not allow management of neck disease to be neglected. If unsuitable for removal they can be irradiated.
- T2. More advanced, bulky lesions in a suitable patient with good pulmonary function can be treated by horizontal partial laryngectomy often combined with neck dissection (usually bilateral).

  Radiation of the primary and both sides of the neck is an alternative in a poor risk patient in whom dysphagia, aspiration and pneumonitis may cause postoperative morbidity. T1 and T2 tumours have a survival of about 70%.

  Recurrence after conservation surgery requires salvage laryngectomy.
- T3. Fixation of the vocal cord, spread to the pre-epiglottic space, piriform sinus or postcricoid area requires total laryngectomy. Neck dissection is often necessary.

  Planned combined radiotherapy and surgery has been reported as improving results but there is no convincing evidence of improved control of the primary tumour.

  Patients with T3 tumours have a 5-year survival of 30–50%.
- T4. Tumours invading the thyroid cartilage or extending into tissues beyond the larynx require total laryngectomy, usually bilateral neck dissection and possibly post-surgery radiation. The high incidence of neck metastases necessitates radical treatment of each neck. With large fixed nodes the prognosis is very poor.

Note: Tumours classified in the same T stage may require quite different treatment – once again the tumour and the patient must be considered together. Large volume tumours are less curable by radiotherapy and the presence or absence of neck nodes is a major factor in determining not only treatment but also prognosis.

Treatment options for supraglottic carcinoma

Endoscopic excision (laser)
Horizontal partial laryngectomy ± necks
Radiation primary and both necks
Total laryngectomy, neck dissection

The 'best' treatment must be carefully evaluated for each individual tumour and patient

Glottic carcinoma

T1 Carcinoma limited to the vocal cords

The TNM clinical staging system now separates T1a tumours limited to one vocal cord (Fig. 23.22) and T1b tumours which involve both vocal cords (Fig. 23.23). Previously there was dissatisfaction with this staging because tumours involving one or both vocal cords but with no extension and no loss of laryngeal

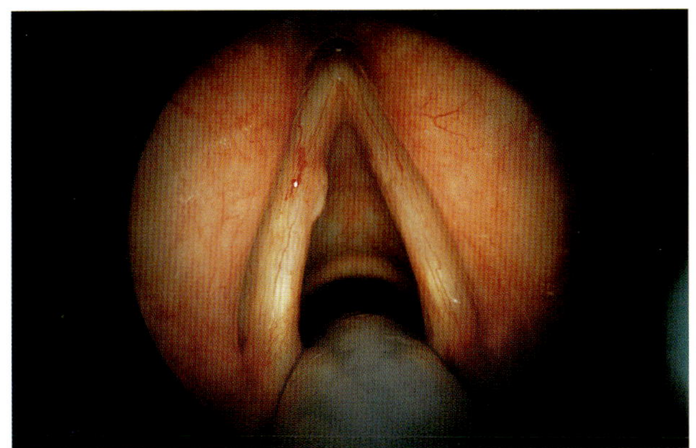

Figure **23.22**
Small primary squamous cell carcinoma in the centre of the left vocal cord, Stage T1a. Note the prominent vessels around the tumour.

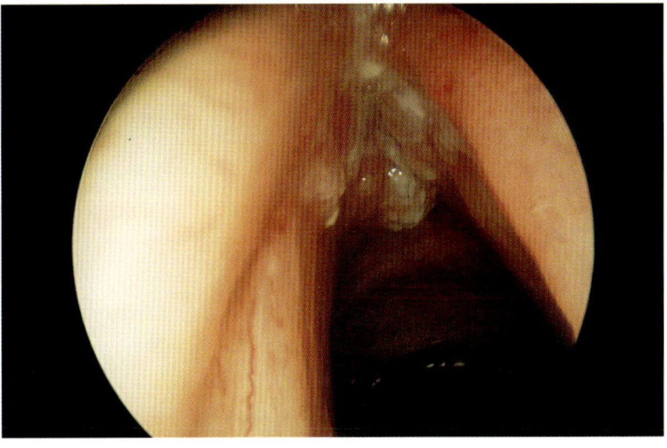

Figure **23.23**
Squamous cell carcinoma affecting the anterior end of both vocal folds and the anterior commissure and below. Stage T1b. Recurrence after anterior partial laryngectomy. Subsequent radiotherapy, further recurrence followed by laryngectomy.

mobility were placed in the same category (Fig. 23.24). There is growing evidence that greater involvement of the anterior commissure has a progressively worse outcome. For rational treatment decisions there must be evaluation of the involvement of the anterior commissure, the size and extent of the cancer including cord mobility, whether the tumour crosses sides at the anterior commissure, the depth of invasion and whether there is any spread to or beyond the thyroid cartilage. Lymph node metastases occur in less than 5% of cases.

Radiation therapy is often used and needs careful planning. Treatment takes some weeks. Tumour factors such as anterior commissure involvement and tumour bulk may be unfavourable indicators although results can be improved by use of hyperfractionation. Use of radiation for a relatively small laryngeal malignancy will preclude later radiation treatment of a subsequent primary malignancy in the irradiated field. Nevertheless radiation treatment gives very good results with about 90% 5-year survival.

Endoscopic carbon dioxide laser surgery also gives very good results, with the provisos that the vocal cord is mobile and that the larynx can be well

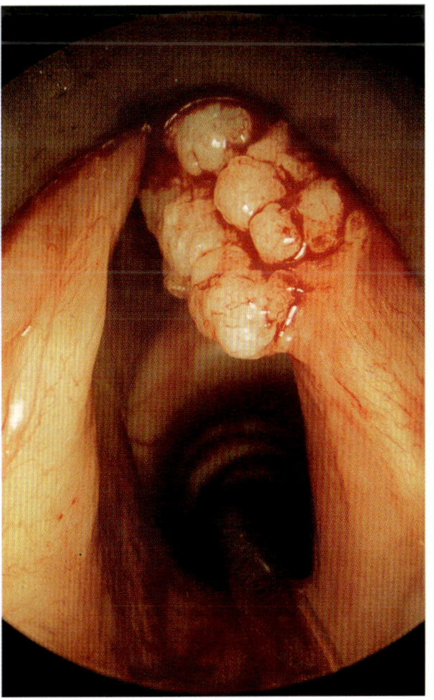

Figure **23.24**
Papilliferous squamous cell carcinoma with incomplete endoscopic exposure at the anterior aspect. A 70-year-old male with good vocal cord movement. Difficult to stage.

exposed so the tumour can be confidently removed with a normal margin; frozen section biopsies from the surgical margins are taken to confirm the adequacy of resection. Tumours involving both vocal cords are not readily treatable by laser excision, although Steiner (1993) has reported curative laser microsurgical treatment of relatively advanced laryngeal malignancies.

Laryngofissure and cordectomy for unilateral disease of the vocal fold is seldom indicated, unless, for example, there are no facilities for radiation available. Fronto-lateral partial laryngectomy, an extended operation for resection of the anterior commissure, anterior part of the vocal cords and the contiguous cartilaginous framework, can be effective in 90% of cases. Techniques of extended partial laryngectomy permit resection and immediate reconstruction of defects which may involve part or all of both membranous vocal folds.

Therefore the outlook for T1 tumours is good, with a 90% survival rate irrespective of the type of treatment. The voice is retained and although the quality may be affected, it remains good for everyday communication.

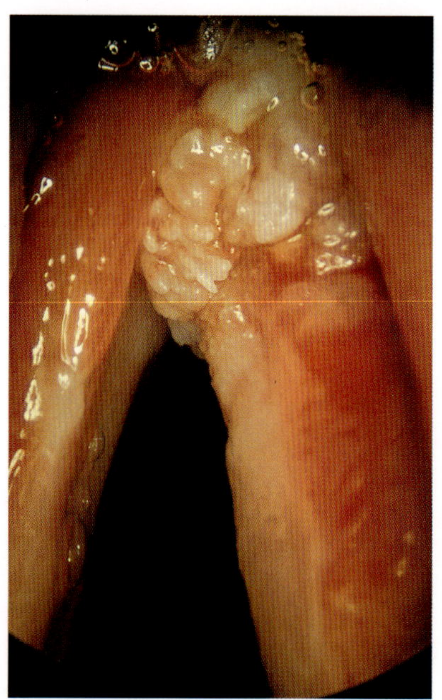

Figure **23.25**
More extensive squamous cell carcinoma of the anterior part of the right vocal cord, anterior commissure under the vocal fold and superiorly extending into the ventricle and undersurface of the ventricular fold. Transglottic tumour.

T2 Carcinoma extending to the supraglottis or subglottis with impaired mobility

Transglottic spread, involving superior spread, and/or inferior extension towards the subglottis (a T2 lesion on TNM staging) means a poorer prognosis but staging may be imprecise because of the uncertainty in evaluation of deep extension and infiltration (Fig. 23.25). It becomes more difficult to control both the primary tumour and the lymphatic spread with nodal metastases. Lesions causing impaired motion but not total fixation of the vocal cord have a 60% survival rate compared to T1 cancers which have a 90% survival rate.

The size of the lesion often correlates with spread from the primary site, e.g. lesions less than 2 cm seldom invade cartilage, lesions larger than 3 cm usually have tumour in the laryngeal cartilages and lesions larger than 4 cm have approximately 50% incidence of regional cervical metastases.

Downward spread into the subglottis carries a poor prognosis. Limited tumours with less than 1 cm of subglottic extension anteriorly can be treated by vertical partial laryngectomy and patients have an 85% survival but extension greater than 1 cm requires laryngectomy and the survival rate drops to about 60%.

It is difficult to state ‘best’ treatment. Primary radiotherapy is used for early lesions in most centres. Radiotherapy has the advantage of vocal preservation, fewer complications, lower cost, avoidance of hospitalization and easy follow-up. Salvage partial or total laryngectomy is required for radiation failures, depending upon the extent of the original tumour. In some centres transglottic tumours are treated with radiotherapy while in others transglottic T2 and T3 tumours are selected for hemilaryngectomy voice conservation surgery.

Laser excision of early lesions may be acceptable to surgeons who are aggressive with endoscopic laser excision.

It must be remembered that cervical metastases, which occur in 10–15% of T2 cancers, must be

Treatment options for glottic carcinoma

Endoscopic excision (laser or cold surgery)
Primary radiotherapy for T1, T2, some T3
Total laryngectomy for most T3, treatment failures or advanced lesions (+ neck dissection)
Radiotherapy or neck dissection for nodal metastases

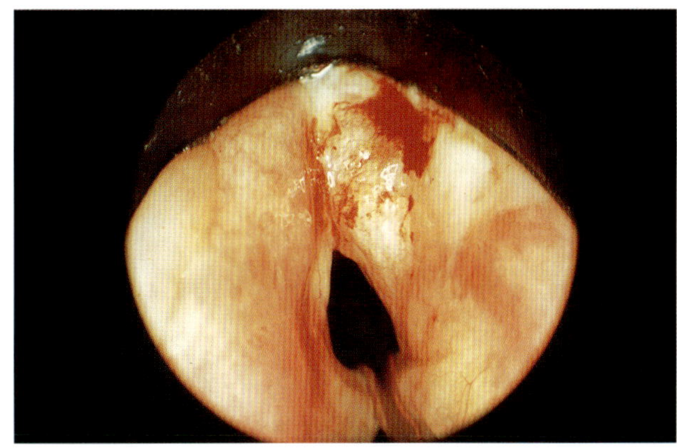

Figure **23.26**
Extensive squamous cell carcinoma of the right vocal cord which was fixed. No metastases in the neck.

treated, usually by radiotherapy together with the primary but sometimes by neck dissection.

T3 Carcinoma with a fixed cord

Deep tumour invasion causes the hemilarynx to be fixed (Fig. 23.26) and is often associated with cervical lymph node metastasis; the combination carries a poor prognosis. The cord may be fixed because of tumour extension into the thyroarytenoid muscle, invasion around the cricoarytenoid joint or spread in the perineural space of the recurrent laryngeal nerve. However, because spread is difficult to assess before surgery, partial laryngectomy may not be indicated.

Total laryngectomy is required for most patients with a T3 laryngeal cancer and overall there is approximately a 60% 5-year survival. Survival is less for undifferentiated tumours, histologically positive regional lymph nodes, subglottic extension and airway obstruction which requires a tracheotomy before operation.

Primary radiotherapy for T3 cancers has a 5-year survival rate of 50–55%; with subsequent surgical salvage the survival rate rises to approximately 70%. Radiation gives better results in older patients and in tumours that are not deeply invasive or obstructing the airway.

Combined therapy has been advocated for T3 tumours for many years but there is little proof that survival is improved. Preoperative radiotherapy carries a higher possibility of surgical complications such as infection, blowout of the carotid arterial system or a postoperative pharyngocutaneous fistula.

Nodal metastases are palpable in 30% of patients and are found as occult deposits in 10%. They must be treated at the time of initial surgery or postoperatively.

T4 Carcinoma invading thyroid cartilage or extending into tissues beyond the larynx

Regional cervical nodal metastases are found in up to 50% of this group, so aggressive treatment, usually total laryngectomy which is sometimes accompanied by resection of the hypopharynx or the cervical oesophagus, is required. The rate of cervical metastases has been quoted from 10% to 50% depending upon patient group and extent of disease.

Once the cancer has escaped the larynx there is usually pain and dysphagia; due to its size, the tumour often causes airway obstruction which may require emergency tracheotomy. Postoperative radiotherapy should be considered for nodal metastases found in tissue removed at surgery, for a poorly differentiated cancer and if tracheotomy is required as an emergency. When cervical metastases have been palpated clinically, neck dissection (unilateral or bilateral) can be followed by postoperative radiation.

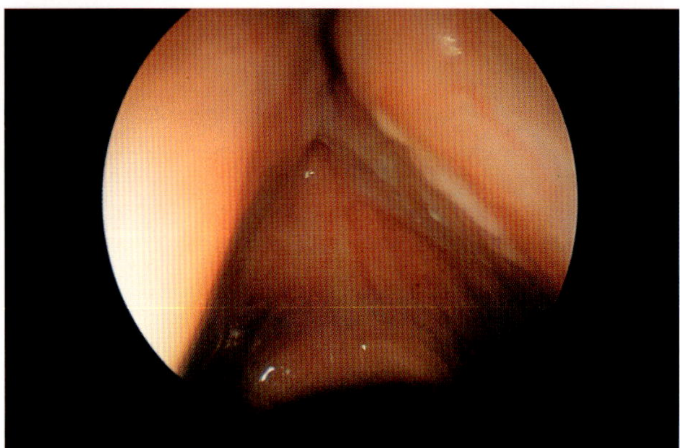

Figure **23.27**
Subglottic squamous cell carcinoma. A male aged 61 years; multiple biopsies over 7 years showed dysplasia but biopsy on this occasion showed invasive disease.

Description of surgical procedures for laryngeal carcinoma

Biopsy
Vocal cord stripping
Endoscopic laser microsurgery
Laryngofissure and cordectomy
Hemilaryngectomy
Fronto-lateral partial laryngectomy
Horizontal partial laryngectomy

A study of previously untreated advanced (Stage 3 and 4) squamous cell laryngeal carcinomas showed that induction chemotherapy followed by definitive radiation was effective in preserving the larynx in a high percentage compared to treatment by conventional laryngectomy and postoperative radiation; survival rates were equal.

Subglottic carcinoma

Subglottic cancer is rare, accounting for approximately 5% of all laryngeal cancers (Fig. 23.27). It tends to present in an advanced stage, often with cervical metastases. There is frequently invasion of the thyroid and cricoid cartilages with circumferential extension or upward extension to the vocal cords, sometimes with airway obstruction. CT may be helpful in delineating the extent of the cancer and the presence of cartilage destruction.

Treatment for most lesions is total laryngectomy and must include a substantial margin of trachea below the tumour, thyroid lobectomy and resection of the paralaryngeal and paratracheal lymph nodes.

Combination therapy for the more advanced lesions may reduce stomal recurrence, but comparative survival rates are not known because of the rarity of subglottic cancer.

SURGICAL PROCEDURES

Operative procedures for premalignant and malignant laryngeal disease range from simple biopsy to radical operations such as laryngopharyngectomy and bilateral neck dissection. Only the technique of biopsy and the commonly performed 'conservative' operations will be described.

Biopsy

Biopsy involves taking single or multiple specimens from areas with a suspicious appearance and sometimes from the surrounding mucosa even though it might appear 'normal' macroscopically. Histopathologic examination provides proof of disease and assists assessment of size and spread.

Excision biopsy of small carcinomas with cold instruments (Fig. 23.28) or the CO_2 laser is possible and if the margins of the resulting defect are found

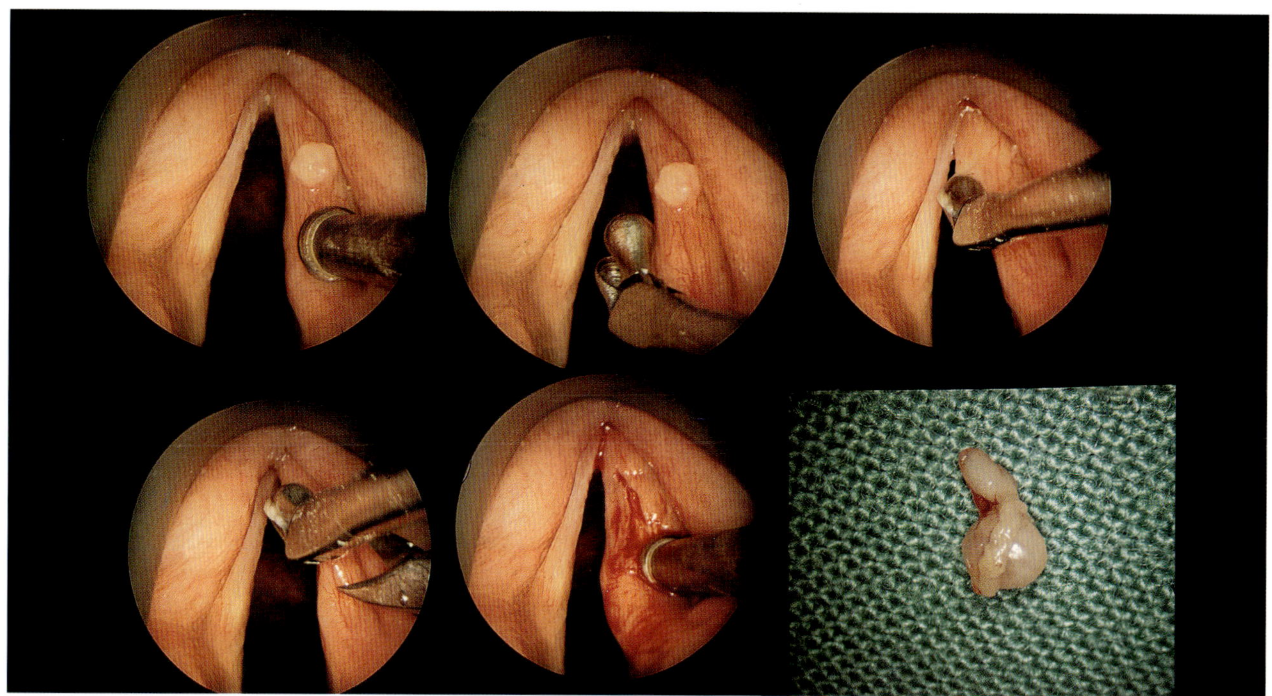

Figure **23.28**
Steps in excision biopsy of a suspicious mass on the upper surface of the right vocal fold. It is picked up with cupped forceps and removed with scissors. Further small biopsies from the edges of the wound showed no malignant change. Careful follow-up required.

to be clear no further immediate treatment is indicated, but long-term follow-up is mandatory.

The reader is referred to the subsection on endoscopy and biopsy techniques in the section on diagnostic evaluation earlier in this chapter for a fuller description of biopsy techniques.

Vocal cord stripping

Areas of mucosal dysplasia often co-exist with nearby micro-invasive or invasive carcinoma. Even though multiple biopsies are taken using supravital staining to identify suspicious areas, the histopathology might be inconclusive. Thorough microlaryngoscopy may indicate a need to submit a specimen of the mucosal edge of the vocal fold obtained by a 'stripping' technique. The edge and adjacent upper and lower surfaces of the vocal fold are grasped with wide forceps (such as Jako or Bouchayer) and meticulously dissected from the underlying vocal ligament as a strip of mucosa from the vocal process of the arytenoid forwards to the anterior commissure. The undersurface of the fold is displayed by 'rolling' the free edge with a blunt instrument, such as a sucker, in the lateral part of the ventricle. The specimen is correctly oriented on paper and immersed in fixative.

Repeated stripping or stripping after laser treatment or after radiotherapy is more difficult and may require removal of multiple piecemeal specimens.

Endoscopic laser microsurgery

Transoral microlaryngeal techniques with the laser are widely recognized as satisfactory treatment for dysplasia and limited invasive neoplasia. Results are excellent for well-defined carcinomas confined to the

Indications for endoscopic laser surgery

Proven dysplasia
Biopsy excision
Excision of proven carcinoma
Debulking of obstructive tumour to avoid tracheotomy
Palliation of untreatable tumour

mobile part of the vocal fold with good vocal cord movement; endoscopic exposure must be satisfactory to ensure accurate removal with a 2 mm margin around the carcinoma. There is a 90% control rate of carcinoma-in-situ and localized T1 carcinomas. Spread past the anterior commissure, involvement of the vocal process and extension into the lateral ventricle or subglottis are generally regarded as contraindications. Aggressive endoscopic laser removal of more advanced laryngeal carcinomas, with voice conservation, has been applied by Steiner (1995) to T2 and T3 lesions using specially made instruments; results are reported to be good.

With good access and exposure of the larynx, peroral suspension microlaryngoscopy for carcinoma-in-situ and T1 carcinomas should be as effective as other treatment options such as radiotherapy, laryngofissure, cordectomy, hemilaryngectomy and total laryngectomy.

The many endoscopic applications of the carbon dioxide laser in laryngeal malignancy include vaporization of proven dysplastic areas of mucosa, biopsy excision of a well-circumscribed lesion, excision of selected carcinomas, debulking of obstructive tumours to avoid tracheotomy before laryngectomy and, occasionally, to palliate otherwise untreatable tumours. In addition, laser removal of sufficient bulk of an overhanging ventricular fold will not only allow direct access to an otherwise hidden tumour in the ventricle but will also improve visualization for indirect laryngoscopy at follow-up.

For supraglottic carcinomas, laser excision can be safely used only for localized lesions on the superior edge of the laryngeal surface of the epiglottis.

Laryngofissure and cordectomy

Early carcinomas limited to the vocal fold are usually treated by radiotherapy; when this facility is not available or there is a recurrence after radiotherapy the disease can be managed by laryngofissure and cordectomy, i.e. opening the larynx for removal of tumour and the involved vocal cord.

A preliminary tracheotomy is usually performed but is not always essential. A horizontal or vertical skin incision or a small apron flap gives access to allow midline division of the perichondrium of the thyroid cartilage, if necessary using an oscillating saw. The cricothyroid membrane is opened below, and the incision widened to give interior access upwards to the anterior commissure; it is an advantage to have already divided the anterior commissure exactly in the midline at preliminary microlaryngoscopy. The incision is extended superiorly to the petiole of the epiglottis and the thyroid alae are spread apart.

The specimen consists of the involved vocal cord from the anterior commissure to the vocal process, the tumour, and the thyroarytenoid muscle, usually with the inner perichondrium laterally. The wound is drained and closed following haemostasis and suturing of the cut edges of the thyroid cartilage in the

Cordectomy specimen

Involved membranous vocal fold
Thyroarytenoid muscle
Tumour
Internal thyroid perichondrium

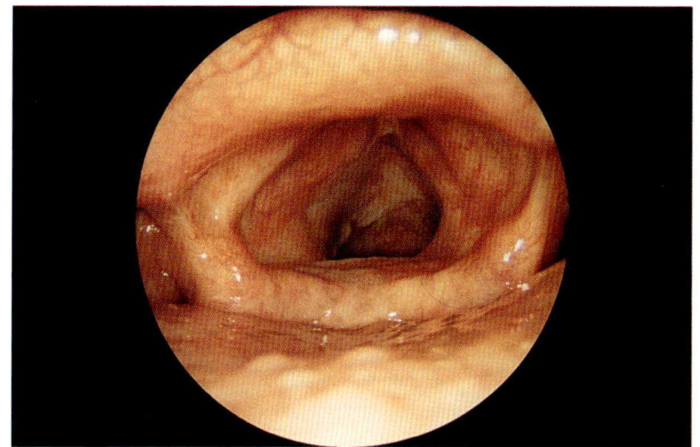

Figure **23.29**
Indirect laryngoscopy. Previous left cordectomy for squamous cell carcinoma 7 years before. The voice was very good but husky.

Hemilaryngectomy specimen

Involved vocal cord
Anterior margin of uninvolved cord
Vocal process of arytenoid
Ventricular fold and ventricle
Thyroarytenoid muscle
Cartilaginous thyroid ala
Tumour

midline. When fully healed, a pseudocord of scar tissue forms with a resultant husky voice (Fig. 23.29).

Hemilaryngectomy

Vertical partial laryngectomy (often referred to as hemilaryngectomy) is the surgical procedure for T2 and selected T3 glottic carcinomas. It is regarded as standard surgical treatment for lesions which involve the vocal process of the arytenoid or the anterior commissure. The basic operation has been extended to encompass tumours which spread beyond the vocal fold, e.g. complete removal of one arytenoid or of a few millimetres of the contralateral vocal fold. There are various reconstructive procedures for these expanded operations.

The procedure requires tracheotomy, skin incision and exposure of the thyroid cartilage as for laryngofissure. The anterior vertical perichondrial incision is extended backwards inferiorly and superiorly along the borders of the thyroid cartilage, and the perichondrium is elevated. Vertical thyroid cartilage cuts are made anteriorly 2 or 3 mm off the midline towards the uninvolved side and posteriorly anterior to the greater and lesser cornua sufficient to leave a vertical supporting strut of cartilage approximately 5 mm wide. Upper and lower cuts then allow mobilization and removal of the thyroid ala along with the soft tissues of the hemilarynx containing the tumour.

The specimen of removed tissue after a standard hemilaryngectomy therefore consists of the tumour and the involved vocal cord, the anterior commissure with a small margin of the contralateral vocal cord, the vocal process of the arytenoid, the ventricular fold and ventricle, the thyroarytenoid muscle and most of the ipsilateral ala of the thyroid cartilage. If the arytenoid is entirely removed, a pedicled sternohyoid muscle flap can be brought in to restore bulk posteriorly so the healed pseudocord will produce a satisfactory voice. There are also other methods to reconstruct the resected vocal cord after hemilaryngectomy.

The patient's general physical condition, especially pulmonary function, should be considered before hemilaryngectomy. Careful patient selection will minimize the incidence of postoperative aspiration and pulmonary complications. Complications of hemilaryngectomy include infection, laryngocutaneous fistula, persistent aspiration, pneumonitis with subsegmental collapse and later laryngeal stenosis. Failed hemilaryngectomy will require total laryngectomy.

Complications of hemilaryngectomy

Wound infection
Laryngocutaneous fistula
Aspiration and pneumonitis
Laryngeal stenosis
Need for later total laryngectomy

Contra-indications to hemilaryngectomy

Involvement of > 30% of contralateral cord
Extensive transglottic spread
Tumour in the posterior glottis
Thyroid cartilage involvement
Subglottic extension
Poor pulmonary function

Contraindications to hemilaryngectomy include one or more of the following: tumour involving not only one side, but also greater than 30% of the other cord; fixation of the hemilarynx; extensive transglottic spread; tumour in the posterior glottis; involvement of both arytenoids; invasion of the thyroid cartilage; and subglottic extension greater than 0.5 cm posteriorly and 1.0 cm anteriorly. Post-radiation failure is a relative contraindication, as is fixation of the hemilarynx.

Fronto-lateral partial laryngectomy

Removal of part or all of both membranous vocal folds is a radical extension of hemilaryngectomy for more widespread carcinoma and may require either a two-stage procedure or long-term laryngeal stenting to minimize laryngeal stenosis. The risk of postoperative aspiration is high; candidates for this procedure must be very carefully chosen. Specific reconstructive methods are required to prevent disabling aspiration and to assist in the production of an effective postoperative voice.

Horizontal partial laryngectomy

This voice conservation operation is for supraglottic carcinoma; neck dissection is frequently necessary. Voice, swallowing and nasal respiration are retained. The procedure is also known as supraglottic hemilaryngectomy or subtotal supraglottic laryngectomy.

The surgical specimen contains the epiglottis, tumour, pre-epiglottic space, ventricular folds, hyoid bone and superior half of the thyroid cartilage, usually with a neck dissection specimen. Tracheotomy is necessary and a cricopharyngeal myotomy is performed to decrease postoperative aspiration.

Complications such as persistent aspiration occur more often and may be more persistent than after vertical partial laryngectomy.

Other 'conservative' operations, including extended supraglottic laryngectomy, partial laryngopharyngec-

Horizontal partial laryngectomy specimen

Epiglottis
Pre-epiglottic space
Ventricular folds
Hyoid bone
Superior half of thyroid cartilage
Usually neck dissection
Tumour

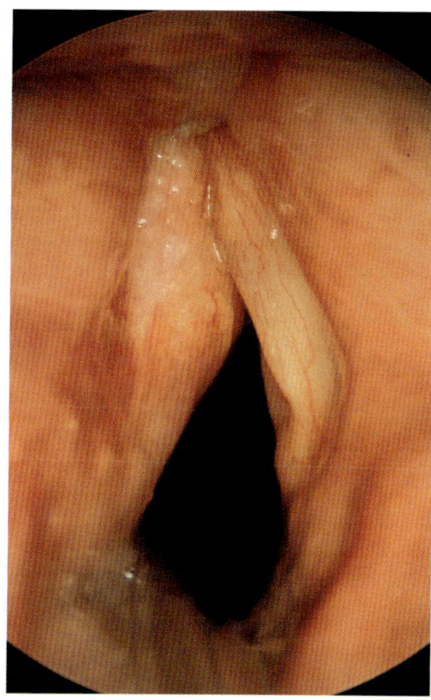

Figure **23.30**
Squamous cell carcinoma of the left vocal cord from the anterior commissure to the vocal process of the arytenoid in a 35-year-old pregnant female. Good vocal cord movement. Treated with radiotherapy and clear of disease for more than 3 years.

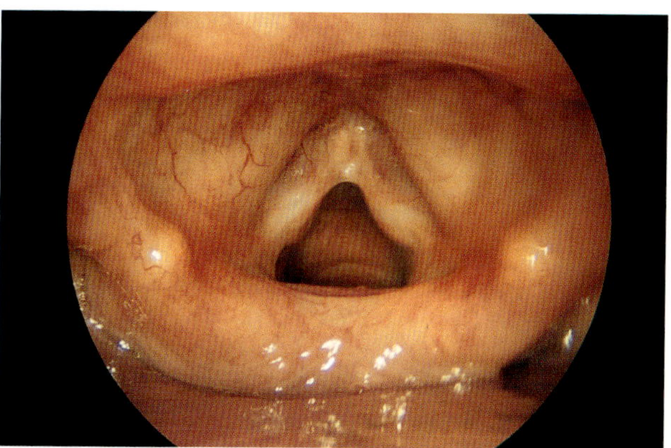

Figure **23.31**
Indirect laryngoscopy. Radiation 8 years previously for squamous cell carcinoma. Post-radiation anterior glottic web.

tomy, supracricoid partial laryngectomy and near total laryngectomy are seldom performed and will not be described, nor will total laryngectomy or laryngopharyngectomy.

Although conservation surgery with partial removal of the larynx interferes with laryngeal function to some extent, most patients have a serviceable voice sufficient for a normal conversation and many return to their usual work and lifestyle.

FURTHER TREATMENT AND POST-TREATMENT CONSIDERATIONS

Age

The survival rate for elderly patients with tumours is less than for younger patients irrespective of original site, extent of the tumour, degree of cellular differentiation, vocal cord fixation, extension in or outside the larynx, lymph node metastases or mode of treatment.

Older patients, even with advanced disease, can usually tolerate total laryngectomy, but partial laryngectomy has high morbidity including infection, poor healing and postoperative aspiration, more so if cardiovascular and pulmonary function are poor.

Carcinoma of the larynx does occur in patients (Fig. 23.30) under 40 years old and, very occasionally, in teenage patients. In this younger age group there is a male to female ratio of only 2 : 1 in contrast to the marked male preponderance in older patients. Further, it appears that smoking and alcohol exposure are less important causative factors. Surgery is well tolerated in younger patients and an aggressive approach is recommended for recurrence or for a second primary.

The post-irradiated larynx

There is morbidity after radiation treatment of laryngeal cancer both with a radical curative dose and pre- or postoperative combined radiation and surgery. The side-effects include skin reaction, mucositis with irritation, sore throat, formation of a small anterior web (Fig. 23.31), and difficulty swallowing. Oedema commences towards the completion of the course of therapy and often causes persistent symptoms.

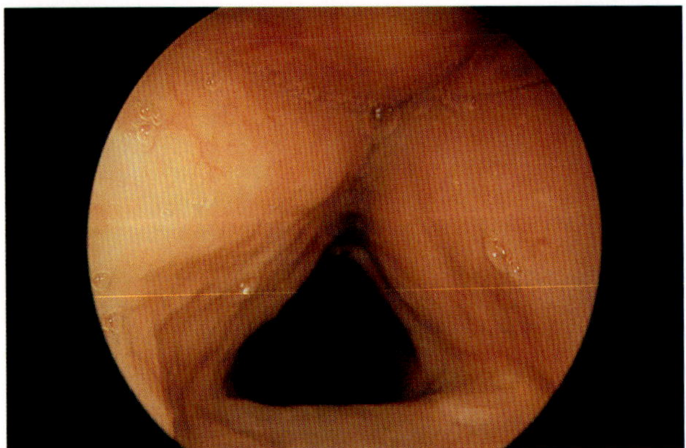

Figure **23.32**
Chronic post-radiation oedema in the glottic and supraglottic tissues.

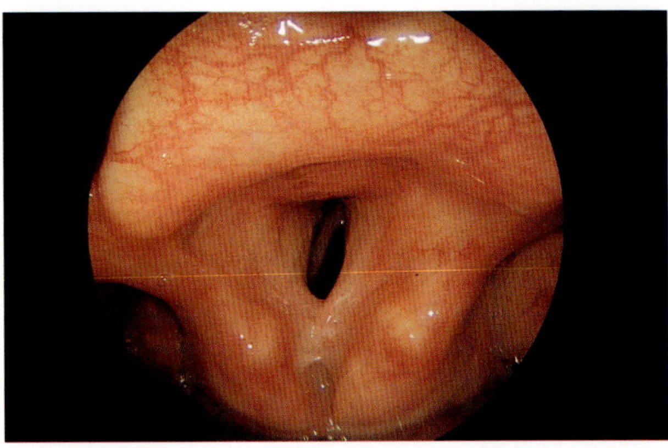

Figure **23.33**
Chronic post-radiation supraglottic stenosis. The patient becomes short of breath on exertion.

Oedema usually lasts for several months but may last for years (Fig. 23.32). The presence of chronic oedema may raise the question of hidden, residual or recurrent cancer, and in patients with severe pain the possibility of radionecrosis of cartilage or of perichondritis due to interference with the blood supply must be considered. Because oedema can obscure residual or recurrent tumour, biopsy or repeated biopsies may be necessary, especially if a vocal cord which was initially mobile becomes fixed in the post-irradiation period. In these circumstances it may be difficult to prove or disprove cartilage necrosis. Sometimes if there is intolerable persistent pain, total laryngectomy may be necessary and malignant disease may be found in the laryngectomy specimen.

Voice quality is usually good after radiotherapy although most patients complain of dryness in the mouth and throat due to diminished secretions.

Chronic laryngeal stenosis (Fig. 23.33) is another possible complication after radiation reaction and is usually very difficult to manage.

Irradiated tissue is more likely to develop malignancy than non-irradiated tissue, and some patients develop a malignancy in the irradiated field (Fig. 23.34). Such radiation-induced malignancy may take 10 years or more to develop, whereas recurrent or residual disease usually manifests itself in the first few months or years.

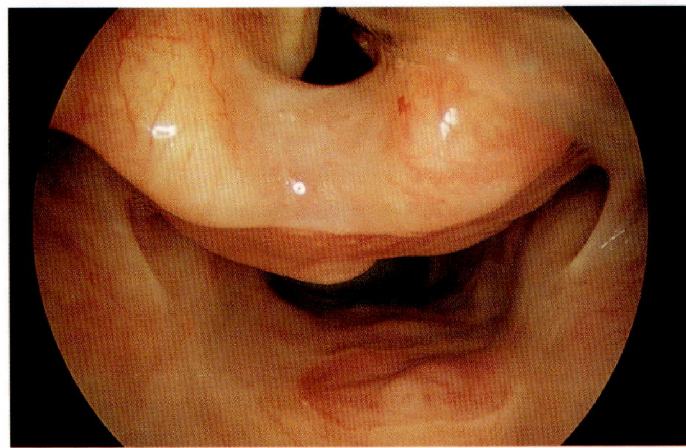

Figure **23.34**
Female patient treated 22 years before for squamous cell carcinoma of the right vocal cord. Suspicious areas in the hypopharynx and postcricoid region showed mild to moderate dysplasia.

Stomal recurrence

Cancer recurrence at the laryngectomy stoma is a serious problem which occurs in about 10% of laryngectomies. It presents as a nodule or nodules at the skin–mucosal junction, often with infection and ulceration and sometimes with deep extension. Radiotherapy is the usual treatment with about 20% 3-year survival.

Likelihood of stomal recurrence

Bulky transglottic tumour
Subglottic extension
Primary subglottic tumour
Paratracheal nodal involvement
Emergency or pre-operative tracheotomy

Measures to minimize stomal seeding should be taken, especially in high-risk patients such as those with carcinoma which is transglottic, has bulky subglottic extension, is primarily subglottic or when there is paratracheal lymphatic spread. A preoperative or emergency tracheotomy to overcome airway obstruction is associated with a higher incidence of stomal recurrence. For this reason 'emergency laryngectomy' has been advocated so long as there is histologic proof of carcinoma and the patient is prepared for immediate laryngectomy. Alternatives to avoid tracheotomy are to treat the airway obstruction by intubation and/or debulk the tumour with laser before laryngectomy. In high-risk patients, elective postoperative irradiation may be indicated.

Palliation of advanced disease

Even though advanced laryngeal tumours can be treated with approximately 50% 5-year survival, the other 50% of patients either do not respond to treatment or they have distant metastases so treatment of the primary tumour is not feasible. These patients require palliation with chemotherapy, radiotherapy or sometimes operative removal of obstructing masses. Generally, palliative treatment involves pharmacological pain relief, airway support, good nutrition and the provision of emotional and social support in the home for as long as possible.

Primary tumours

Index
Synchronous
Metachronous

Second primary tumours

- An *index* primary is the first diagnosed malignancy.
- A *synchronous* primary is a second malignancy diagnosed within 6 months of the index primary.
- A *metachronous* primary is a second malignancy diagnosed 6 months or more after the index primary.

The 'condemned mucosa syndrome' was proposed in 1953 by Slaughter et al who also coined the term 'field cancerization' referring to the multicentric origin of oral squamous cell carcinoma.

Although tobacco and alcohol are the major external carcinogens of head and neck cancer, it has been shown that there is an underlying predisposition to environmentally induced malignancy not only in patients with chromosome instability syndromes but also in others with defective DNA repair mechanisms. In addition, head and neck cancer patients may be found to be mutagen-sensitive using an assay which quantifies the number of chromosome breaks in lymphocytes after exposure to a mutagen such as bleomycin. Mutagen sensitivity plays a role in carcinogenesis of many tissues which have direct exposure to the environment such as the respiratory, digestive and integumentary systems.

Both host and environmental factors contribute to the formation of second primary malignancies. The underlying defect in DNA repair implies that there is an inability to prevent the final step in carcinogenesis. The exposure to carcinogen appears to activate an entire mucosa, i.e. 'field cancerization' as originally proposed.

There is a lack of agreement regarding the best methods for detection of the second primary malignancy, e.g. does chest X-ray performed regularly – say every 3, 6 or 12 months – substitute for screening bronchoscopy, or does barium swallow substitute for screening oesophagoscopy? The responsibility for these decisions lies with the clinician. Having diagnosed an index primary squamous cell carcinoma of the upper aerodigestive tract, there must be a constant awareness that a simultaneous primary can be found in approximately 10% of patients. A regular history, physical examination, and follow-up investigative radiography and endoscopy may be necessary. Abstention from tobacco and alcohol is extremely important in the prevention of the second malignancy although there is still some doubt that once activated, the process of field cancerization is reversible by avoiding these carcinogenic drugs.

Recent studies have strongly suggested a significant advance in decreasing the incidence of second primaries by using differentiation therapy employing retinoids to reverse cellular differentiation. Chemoprevention may reverse the process of leukoplakia, associated dysplasia and carcinoma-in-situ of the oral cavity. It may be that concentration on early diagnosis, removal of carcinogens and differentiation therapy will improve the outcome. Unfortunately present efforts at prevention, early detection and treatment have proved disappointing.

VERRUCOUS CARCINOMA

This highly differentiated variant of squamous cell carcinoma accounts for 2–4% of laryngeal carcinomas and may exhibit exuberant growth over a large area of the glottis and supraglottis (Fig. 23.35).

Verrucous carcinoma usually presents as a large clearly delineated, keratotic, papillomatous, exophytic, warty lesion exhibiting slow but inexorable growth and typically occurs in cigarette-smoking males over 50 years of age. The presenting symptom is usually hoarseness and sometimes airway obstruction caused by a bulky tumour.

The histologic appearance is of a papillary tumour with hyperkeratosis and epithelial hyperplasia due to proliferation of suprabasal cells with an intact base-

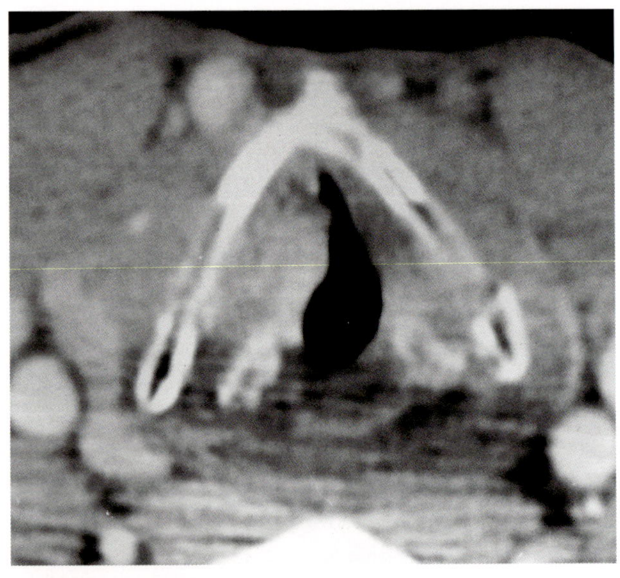

(a)

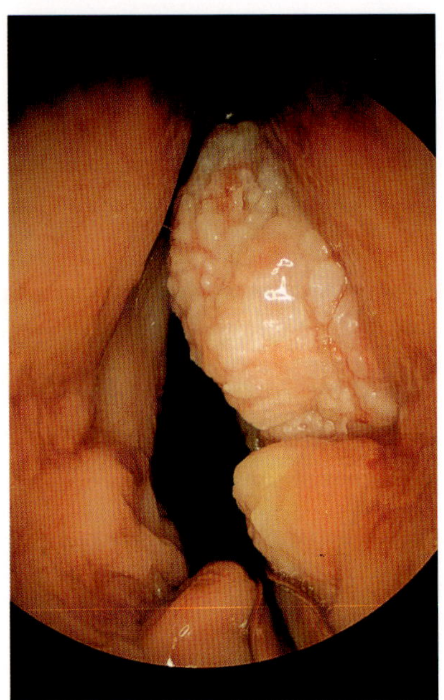

(b)

Figure **23.35**
Verrucous carcinoma. CT scan (a) shows irregular mass apparently replacing the right vocal fold. At endoscopy (b) a white papilliferous lesion proved to be verrucous carcinoma. It was removed by serial laser treatments.

ment membrane; there is minimal cytologic atypia, so the criteria for malignancy are minimal or absent. There are greatly thickened surface papillomatous exophytic folds of well-differentiated, keratinized squamous epithelium with an orderly maturation sequence from the active basal layer.

The tumour pushes aggressively into underlying tissues but has no infiltrating edge and rarely metastasizes. The diagnosis is difficult to make on small biopsies and a full-thickness biopsy is necessary to identify the basement membrane and to distinguish verrucous from invasive squamous cell carcinoma. It is said that 15–20% of verrucous carcinomas may have coexisting infiltrating squamous cell carcinoma, and serial sections are recommended.

Surgery is the treatment of choice and involves laser excision for small tumours, partial laryngectomy for selected larger tumours and total laryngectomy for the remaining 20–25% of more extensive tumours. Although some physicians report good results with radiotherapy, it is generally considered to be less effective than surgery, and has been shown to promote malignant behaviour with anaplastic transformation and to increase the incidence of regional cervical metastases.

OTHER MALIGNANT LARYNGEAL TUMOURS

Many unusual malignancies have been reported. A surprisingly varied number of rare tumours, each with distinctive features (Table 23.2) may derive from the different types of cell in the larynx: epithelium, mucous gland cells, neuroendocrine cells, and cells from supporting mesenchymal structures and lymphoreticular elements.

The salient features of some selected tumours will be described. For further information the reader is referred to a major textbook such as *The larynx*, edited by Marvin P Fried (1996), whose Ch. 40 has an exhaustive list of references.

Table 23.2 Histopathological types of rare laryngeal malignancies

Squamous cell variants (of epithelial origin)
- Pseudosarcomatous carcinoma (spindle cell carcinoma)
- Basiloid-squamous carcinoma
- Lymphoepithelioma (undifferentiated carcinoma of lymphoepitheliomatous type)

Adenocarcinomas (of glandular origin)
- Adenocarcinoma
- Adenoid cystic carcinoma
- Mucoepidermoid carcinoma (and its variant adenosquamous carcinoma)
- Giant cell and clear cell carcinomas
- Mucous gland carcinoma
- Acinic cell carcinoma

Carcinomas of neuroendocrine origin
- Carcinoid carcinoma (well-differentiated)
- Atypical carcinoid carcinoma (moderately-differentiated)
- Small (or oat) cell carcinoma (poorly-differentiated)

Sarcomas (of structural element origin)
- Chondrosarcoma
- Fibrosarcoma
- Osteosarcoma
- Rhabdomyosarcoma
- Liposarcoma
- Other very rare tumours: osteosarcoma, synovial sarcoma, leiomyosarcoma, etc.

Tumours of lymphoreticular origin
- Malignant lymphoma
- Plasmacytoma
- Mycosis fungoides
- Malignant fibrous histiocytoma

Metastases to the larynx
- Melanoma
- Renal carcinoma
- Many other organs, all very rare

Pseudosarcomatous carcinoma

The histologic elements appear to be simultaneous squamous epithelial malignancy and spindle cell sarcomatous tissue. Although both components have been found in metastatic foci, some controversy remains about whether the tumour should be considered a variant of squamous cell carcinoma.

Lymphoepithelioma

This is another variant of squamous cell carcinoma which usually occurs in the lymphoid tissue of Waldeyer's ring. In the larynx, it has been found arising among the lymphocytes of the ventricle.

Adenocarcinomas

These arise from seromucinous minor salivary glands in the supraglottic or subglottic areas. They are usually present in elderly males as a large bulky tumour with regional, even distant, metastases and consequently they have a dismal prognosis. Adenoid cystic carcinoma is the common subtype, then mucoepidermoid carcinoma and other much rarer subtypes.

Carcinomas of neuroendocrine origin

Carcinoid, atypical carcinoid and small cell carcinoma are thought to arise from Kulchitsky cells; intracellular neurosecretory granules are identified by the electron microscope. Because of frequent spread to cervical nodes and distant metastases, prognosis is usually poor. Carcinoid, the rarest form, has the lowest grade of activity and small cell carcinoma has the highest.

Sarcomas

Whether cartilaginous tumours are classified as chondromas or low-grade chondrosarcomas is often controversial. Chondrosarcomas arise more often from the cricoid than the thyroid cartilage and usually cause airway obstruction. Poorly differentiated tumours recur quickly and have distant metastases early.

Fibrosarcomas arise from fibroblasts in the anterior larynx and tends to recur and metastasize regionally and distally.

Others

Non-Hodgkin's lymphoma and extramedullary plasmacytoma present very rarely as isolated lesions confined to the larynx. Long-term follow-up for systemic involvement is imperative.

Because of the great rarity of non-squamous cell malignancies of the larynx, there is little substantial information about treatment other than surgical removal and there are few reports about outcomes.

BIBLIOGRAPHY

American Joint Committee on Cancer (1992) *Manual for staging of cancer*, 4th edn (Philadelphia: JB Lippincott).

Batsakis JG (1974) 'Leukoplakia', 'keratosis' and intraepithelial squamous cell carcinoma of the head and neck. In: Batsakis JG, ed., *Tumours of the head and neck* (Baltimore: Williams and Wilkins); 68–75.

Blackwell KE, Calcaterra TC, Fu Y-S (1995) Laryngeal dysplasia; epidemiology and outcome. *Ann Otol Rhinol Laryngol* **104**: 596–602.

Ferlito A, Harrison DFN, Bailey B, De Santo L (1995a) Are clinical classifications for laryngeal cancer satisfactory? *Ann Otol Rhinol Laryngol* **104**: 741–7.

Ferlito A, Rinaldo A, Devaney KO (1995b) Malignant laryngeal tumors: phenotypic evaluation and clinical implications. *Ann Otol Rhinol Laryngol* **104**: 587–9.

Fried, MP (ed.) (1996) *The larynx* (St Louis: Mosby) 473–85.

Gray SD, Hammond E, Hanson DF (1995) Benign pathologic responses of the larynx. *Ann Otol Rhinol Laryngol* **104**: 13–18.

International Union Against Cancer (1992) *TNM classification of malignant tumours*, 4th edn, 2nd revision (Berlin: Springer).

Michael L (1987) *Ear, nose and throat histopathology* (Berlin: Springer); 374–81.

Pearson B (1994) A new TNM proposal (abstract). *Second World Congress on Laryngeal Cancer, Sydney, Australia, 1994*.

Slaughter DP, Southwick HW, Smejkal W (1953) 'Field cancerization' in oral stratified squamous epithelium. *Cancer* **6**: 963–8.

Sllamniku B, Bauer W, Painter C, Sessions D (1989) The transformation of laryngeal keratosis into invasive carcinoma. *Am J Otolaryngol* **10**: 42–54.

Steiner W (1993) Results of curative laser microsurgery of laryngeal carcinomas. *Am J Otolaryngol* **14**: 116–12.

Sturgis EM, Miller RH (1995) Second primary malignancies in the head and neck cancer patient. *Ann Otol Rhinol Laryngol* **104**: 946–54.

The Department of Veterans Affairs Laryngeal Cancer Study Group (1991) Induction chemotherapy plus radiation compared with surgery plus radiation in patients with advanced laryngeal cancer. *N Engl J Med* **324**: 1685–90.

VI CONGENITAL ABNORMALITIES

24 Laryngomalacia

INTRODUCTION

Laryngomalacia has also been called 'floppy larynx', a rather appropriate descriptive term.

Both names imply a weakness of the supraglottic tissues which allows collapse and partial airway obstruction with inspiration (Fig. 24.1). The features of laryngomalacia are:

- intermittent inspiratory stridor
- signs of upper airway obstruction
- a normal cry
- general health and development which is usually (but not always) normal.

The cause of the exaggerated floppiness and instability of the supraglottic structures is not known.

A confident diagnosis of laryngomalacia can be made after confirming the abnormal dynamic changes during respiration at laryngoscopy, either direct laryngoscopy with rigid instruments under general anaesthesia or indirect laryngoscopy using a flexible fibreoptic laryngoscope without general anaesthesia. Although laryngomalacia is classified as a congenital condition, some authorities point out that it can hardly be regarded as a true malformation when the laryngeal dysfunction is usually self-correcting as the child grows and the larynx becomes more stable. Most infants thrive despite the stridor which is often more distressing to the parents and other observers than to the child.

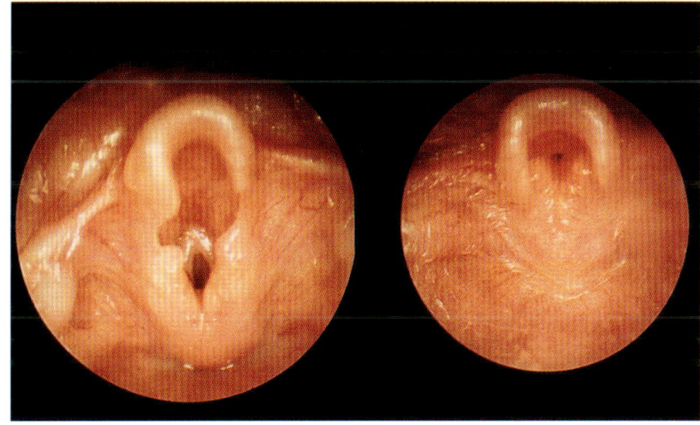

Figure **24.1**
Clear expiratory airway (left) but severe supraglottic inspiratory obstruction (right). The laryngoscope prevents collapse of the epiglottis by pressure on the glotto-epiglottic ligament.

CLINICAL FEATURES

The stridor starts in the first days or weeks of life and persists as a variable, intermittent, harsh, inspiratory,

Features of laryngomalacia

Commonest cause of stridor in infants
Starts soon after birth
Variable intermittent inspiratory stridor
Normal cry
Usually well and thriving
Confirmed by endoscopy
Rarely warrants surgical treatment
Cause unknown

crowing noise, sometimes described as low-pitched and fluttering. Often, when the stridor is loud, a palpable vibration can be felt by placing a hand on the chest. Some infants are described as 'mucousy' but aspiration of the pharynx does not relieve the noisy breathing. Symptoms are intermittent, being worse when the infants lie on their back; most patients seem more comfortable, or at least less noisy, when lying prone. The stridor is usually worse with crying, feeding, during periods of excitement and activity or when the child lies supine or has the head flexed; at other times the patient sleeps quietly and the noise is scarcely noticeable or is absent. Observation and re-examination over a period of days or weeks may be helpful. Persistent airway obstruction over a long period may be followed by deformity of the chest and a few patients develop pectus excavatum.

Cyanotic attacks are uncommon and if they occur, the presence of other causal pathology should be suspected. Similarly, although feeding may be slow and noisy, if persistent dysphagia is present, especially if it is associated with aspiration, the clinician should be alerted to the possibility of a condition other than laryngomalacia.

Most infants with laryngomalacia gain weight and progress normally with satisfactory general development. Although the noisy breathing may be distressing to the parents, once a firm diagnosis has been made by endoscopic examination, concern will be allayed and there will usually be no necessity for treatment. Regular observations should be made until the symptoms subside in the knowledge that the stridor is self-correcting with further growth, usually resolving entirely by the third year of life. Very occasionally it persists for years, even into early teenage.

EPIDEMIOLOGY

Laryngomalacia occurs world-wide and is the commonest cause of stridor in an infant. About two-thirds of the children are male, a ratio consistent with the incidence of other congenital laryngeal anomalies. An association has been suggested, but is not always present, with micrognathia and also with gastro-oesophageal reflux. Stridor similar to that in laryngomalacia is seen occasionally in older children with exercise-induced dyspnoea and inspiratory stridor which resolves promptly as the degree of exertion is decreased. Rare cases of familial laryngomalacia have been described.

PATHOLOGY

Chen and Holinger (1994) pointed out that a number of abnormalities have been observed as the cause of obstruction and they described six mechanisms:

1 inward collapse of the aryepiglottic folds, primarily the cuneiform cartilages (Figs 24.1, 24.2);
2 an elongated epiglottis that curls upon itself and contributes to obstruction during inspiration (Fig. 24.3);
3 anterior and medial collapsing movements of the arytenoid cartilages to occlude the laryngeal inlet during inspiration (Fig. 24.2);
4 postero-inferior displacement of the epiglottis;
5 short aryepiglottic folds;
6 an overly acute angle of the epiglottis at the laryngeal inlet.

Naturally two or more of these mechanisms often occur together.

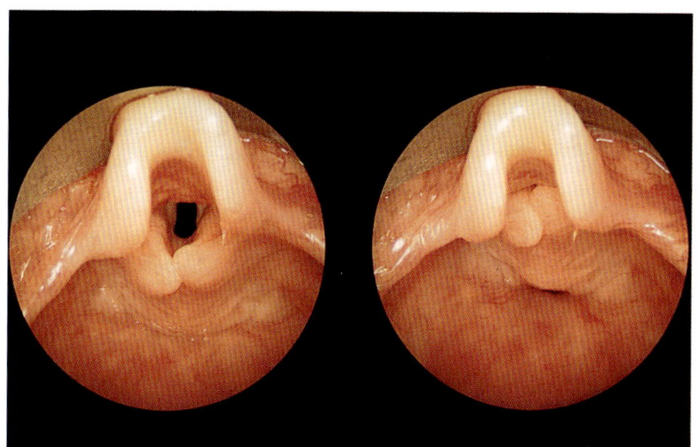

Figure **24.2**
Larynx during expiration (left). Anterior movement of the cuneiform and arytenoid cartilages during inspiration (right).

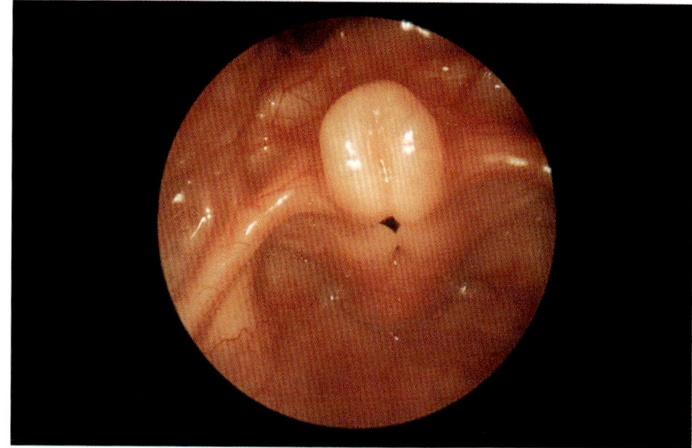

Figure **24.3**
Elongated, omega-shaped, curled epiglottis, a major factor in obstruction.

The aetiology is unknown and although most theories suggest an intrinsic anatomical abnormality of the supraglottic larynx, there is no agreement as to the pathophysiology and detailed studies are lacking. There is no known gross or microscopic evidence of weakness, immaturity or other abnormality of the laryngeal cartilages. Some claim that associated neurologic findings including central and obstructive apnoea indicate that laryngomalacia may be a manifestation of delayed neuromuscular control.

RADIOLOGY

No consistent or reliable radiological diagnostic features on the plain X-rays have been described, but the lateral airways film will assist in excluding the presence of a laryngopharyngeal mass or cyst, subglottic stenosis or narrowing of the intrathoracic trachea. Fluoroscopy from the lateral aspect may show anterior prolapse of the aryepiglottic folds, but it is unreliable as a diagnostic study.

ENDOSCOPIC INVESTIGATION

For a confident diagnosis of laryngomalacia, indirect laryngoscopy with a flexible laryngoscope or direct examination of the pharynx, larynx, trachea and bronchi under general anaesthetic is necessary. Oesophagoscopy, and if necessary biopsy, is indicated if there is a likelihood of gastro-oesophageal reflux, vascular ring or other congenital anomaly affecting the oesophagus. Flexible laryngoscopy does not exclude tracheo-bronchial or oesophageal pathology. Complete endoscopic examination not only positively confirms the diagnosis of laryngomalacia beyond doubt but will also detect associated abnormalities, e.g. subglottic stenosis or inominate artery compression, which are found in approximately 10% of patients. The endoscopist requires considerable experience and judgement to identify the diagnosis and to rule out other congenital lesions.

Indications for direct endoscopy

Not every infant with inspiratory stridor that is suspected of being due to laryngomalacia requires endoscopic assessment. Selection can be made on the basis of the severity and persistence of the stridor, the presence of other associated symptoms, a significant radiological abnormality of the trachea or lung fields and the degree of anxiety in the parents or attending physician. On the other hand, some paediatric endoscopists advise endoscopic assessment of all infants with stridor on the basis that the cause cannot be identified unless diagnostic examination is performed.

Indications for endoscopy

Severe or progressive stridor
Cyanotic or apnoeic attacks
Coexistent radiologic lesion
Other symptoms, e.g. aspiration, failure to thrive
Undue anxiety

Endoscopic findings

Epiglottis usually tall and curled
Supraglottic structures thin and pliable
Sucked in during inspiration
Blown out during expiration
Normal glottis, subglottis and trachea

Findings at endoscopy

The changes are in the supraglottic tissues, namely the epiglottis, aryepiglottic folds, cuneiform and arytenoid cartilages. The base of tongue, pharyngeal walls, glottic opening, vocal folds and subglottic region show no changes, unless there is a second anomaly, e.g. subglottic stenosis.

When stridor is present during induction of general anaesthesia, gentle positive pressure ventilation applied with a face mask to assist respiration and increase the depth of anaesthesia may improve or even completely abolish the stridor. Holding the chin forwards may alleviate it. The characteristic supraglottic changes of laryngomalacia may be seen during initial laryngoscopy. The altered dynamics are identified best when muscular tone returns at the end of the procedure after anaesthesia has been discontinued.

The epiglottis is often tall, narrow and folded upon itself (Fig. 24.3) so that its lateral margins lie close together posteriorly giving a tubular appearance when viewed from behind with a 30° telescope (Fig. 24.4). Although often omega-shaped, it may be narrow and short or elongated on a broad base. These findings of altered epiglottic shape are seen in normal infants without stridor and cause and effect has not been clearly established. The aryepiglottic folds and arytenoids are thin, pale and flaccid so that there is an appearance of laxity; redundant tissues are sucked into the larynx on each inspiration (Fig. 25.5) resulting in the inspiratory stridor. During expiration the tissues are blown outwards so that there is an uninterrupted outflow of air (Fig. 25.5). The aryepiglottic folds, cuneiforms and arytenoids can be 'opened' and held outward by placing a laryngoscope blade behind the epiglottis on its laryngeal surface but above the vocal cords to prevent collapse of the airway. The stridor and obstruction are thus immediately corrected by providing an unimpeded airway.

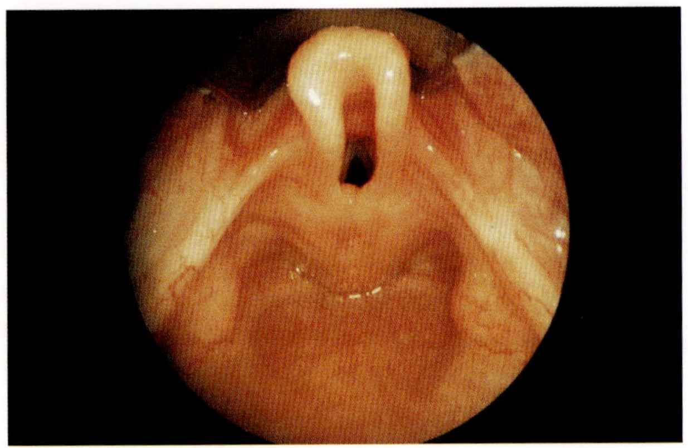

Figure **24.4**
Tall, curled, 'tubular' epiglottis viewed with a 30° telescope.

The distal tip of the laryngoscope blade must be placed at the base of the tongue in front of the epiglottis while awaiting the return of muscular tone and movement, so as not to prevent or distort the supraglottic changes which are observed as anaes-

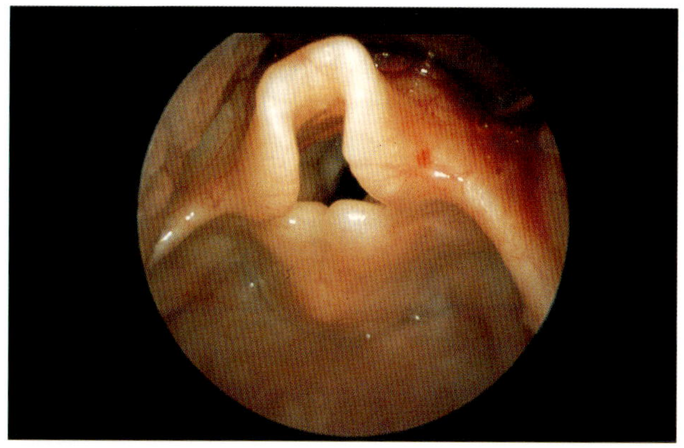

(a)

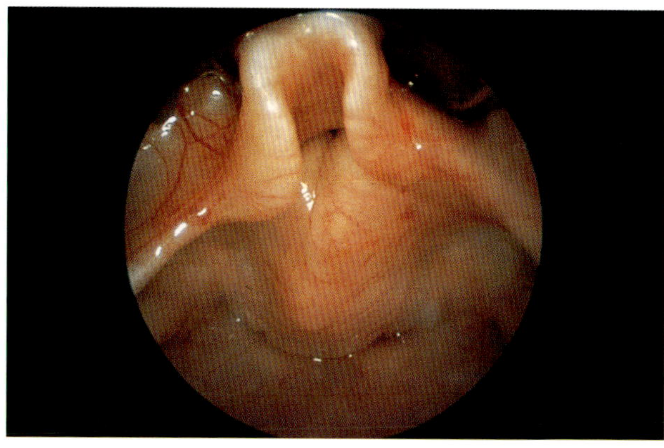

(b)

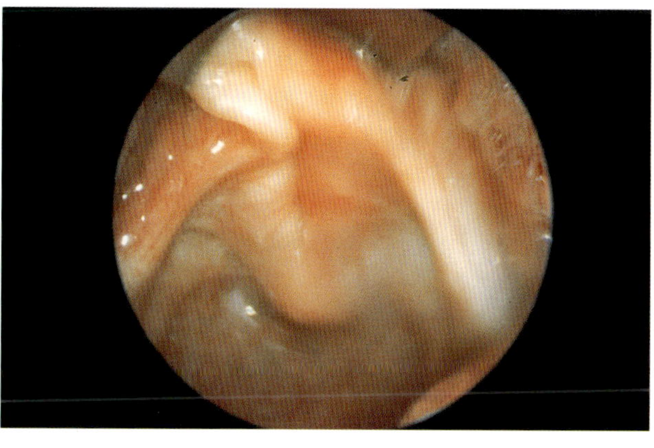

(c)

Figure **24.5**
The dynamic changes in one respiratory cycle are shown dramatically in these three views. Expiration is unimpeded (a) but with inspiration the floppy tissues obstruct (b). A violent inspiratory effort distorts the supraglottic tissues (c).

thesia is discontinued and oxygen is administered via a small tube introduced into the oropharynx. This technique ensures ample time to examine the dynamics of the supraglottic structures and assess vocal cord movements as they return.

TREATMENT

Few patients need treatment. A conservative approach for a condition which is usually self-limiting is appropriate for most infants but a few with severe obstruction may require surgery. Holinger and Koniov (1989) reported that 1 in 305 patients in one series and 4 of 1415 patients in another required a tracheotomy. It seems difficult to reconcile the very few patients requiring surgical treatment in these series reported some years ago with the many children treated surgically in more recent series; one report is of 115 patients treated operatively over 7 years.

Indications for surgery

Indications for operation include severe stridor with failure to thrive, obstructive apnoea, weight loss, chest deformity, cyanotic attacks, pulmonary hypertension, cor pulmonale, and desaturation found by studies in hospital documenting hypoxaemia and hypercapnoea.

In exceptional cases there is severe airway obstruction associated with pectus excavatum and failure to thrive; if the clinician ensures there is no unrecognized coexistent cause of airway obstruction, then surgical treatment is indicated. When treatment is reserved for severe cases the results are good, although rarely

Indications for surgery

Severe, persistent stridor ± apnoea
Failure to thrive
Respiratory decompensation
Chest deformity

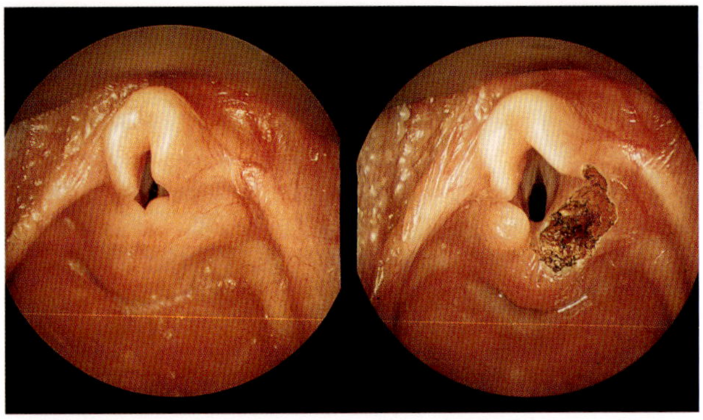

Figure **24.6**
Endoscopic laser aryepiglottoplasty to remove excess obstructing floppy tissue on the right side.

patients do not respond satisfactorily and a tracheotomy may finally be necessary.

Surgical procedures

Procedures which have been advocated include laser division of the aryepiglottic folds, partial amputation of the epiglottis, epiglottopexy with glosso-epiglottic adhesion, removal of redundant supra-arytenoid mucosa and the lateral borders of the epiglottis, removal of the corniculate and cuneiform cartilages and surrounding mucosa, and lastly tracheotomy.

The treatment of choice appears to be endoscopic trimming and removal of the prolapsing aryepiglottic fold and division of tight, short aryepiglottic folds preferably with the carbon dioxide laser (Fig. 24.6). Excess mucosa contributing to obstruction is removed, namely the redundant supra-arytenoid mucosa including the cuneiform cartilage. Some writers advocate epiglottopexy, suturing the anterior surface of the epiglottis to the base of the tongue. Others believe that identifying and treating gastro-oesophageal reflux is an important part of treatment.

Kelly and Gray (1995) reviewed the complications of these procedures including posterior stenosis caused by simultaneous bilateral supraglottoplasty. They recommend unilateral operation in the knowledge that a second procedure on the other side may be required later for complete relief of symptoms.

BIBLIOGRAPHY

Belmont JR, Grundfast K (1984) Congenital laryngeal stridor (laryngomalacia): etiologic factors and associated disorders. *Ann Otol Rhinol Laryngol* **93**: 430–5.

Benjamin B (1994) Airway obstruction. In: Freeman NV, Burge DM, Griffiths DM, Malone PSJ, eds; *Surgery of the newborn* (London: Churchill Livingstone) 409–30.

Chen J-C, Holinger LD (1994) Congenital laryngeal lesions: pathology study using serial macrosections and review of the literature. *Pediatr Pathol* **14**: 301–25.

Holinger LD, Koniov RJ (1989) Surgical management of severe laryngomalacia. *Laryngoscope* **99**: 136–42.

Hui Y, Gaffney R, Crysdale W (1995) Laser aryepiglottoplasty for the treatment of neurasthenic laryngomalacia in cerebral palsy. *Ann Otol Rhinol Laryngol* **104**: 432–6.

Kelly SM, Gray SD (1995) Unilateral supraglottic epiglottoplasty for severe laryngomalacia. *Arch Otolaryngol Head and Neck Surg* **121**: 1351–4.

Roger G, Denoyelle F, Triglia J, Garabedian E (1995) Severe laryngomalacia: surgical indications and results in 115 patients. *Laryngoscope* **105**: 1111–17.

Smith R, Bauman N, Bent J, Kramer M, Smits W, Ahrens R (1995) Exercise-induced laryngomalacia. *Ann Otol Rhinol Laryngol* **104**: 537–42.

Zalzal GH, Anon JB, Cotton RT (1987) Epiglottoplasty for the treatment of laryngomalacia. *Ann Otol Rhinol Laryngol* **96**: 88–92.

25 Congenital webs

Laryngeal webs are uncommon congenital anomalies. Web, atresia and subglottic stenosis are thought to result from different degrees of failure of resorption of the actively proliferating epithelium which temporarily obliterates the developing laryngeal opening during the seventh and eighth week of intrauterine development. Normally the lumen of the laryngotracheal groove is re-established and the vocal cords appear separately on each side.

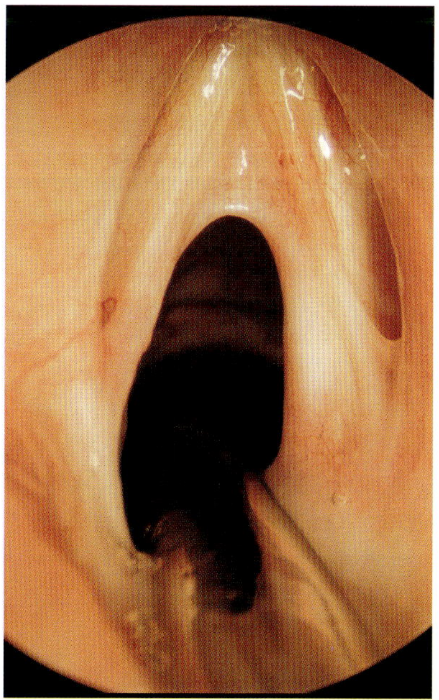

Figure **25.1**
Acquired web following injudicious surgery. Must be differentiated from congenital web.

CLASSIFICATION

The most common laryngeal webs occur at the glottic level (Fig. 25.1). Classification is according to anatomical site:

- supraglottic webs (Fig. 25.2) are very rare and difficult to recognize and treat;
- glottic webs are the commonest;
- interarytenoid webs are next most common;

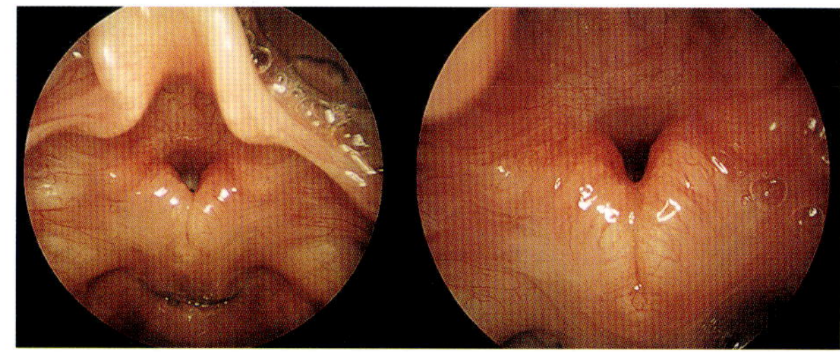

Figure **25.2**
Congenital supraglottic web. The narrowing is at the level of the false cords and above. There is also a moderate-sized anterior glottic web and a subglottic stenosis.

Classification of webs
Supraglottic Glottic Interarytenoid Subglottic

Clinical features
Abnormal cry or voice Varying degree of obstruction Recurrent 'croup' Other congenital anomalies

- subglottic webs are rare; they may be difficult to distinguish from subglottic stenosis or inferior extension of a glottic web.

GLOTTIC WEBS

Small webs are thin and lie between the anterior end of the vocal folds. Large webs are thicker anteriorly, have a thin, crescentic posterior edge and according to their size occupy more or less of the glottic opening.

Clinical features

All but the most minor glottic webs affect vocalization to some degree. The cry of an infant may be weak, abnormal or even absent; older children have a husky voice.

Large, obstructing webs cause varying degrees of stridor, and respiratory distress or dyspnoea on exertion in older children. Recurrent or atypical episodes of 'croup' occur in some patients, especially those whose web is associated with subglottic stenosis.

Severe cases may have cyanotic attacks and require tracheotomy at or shortly after birth to provide an airway and to permit thorough assessment of the abnormality.

There is about one chance in three of having a further anomaly of the respiratory tract. Congenital subglottic stenosis is a common association when the glottic web is severe; a lateral X-ray of the larynx (Fig. 25.3) may provide valuable information about the anterior thickness of the web and the presence of subglottic stenosis.

Congenital anomalies of other organ systems are common in patients with laryngeal webs but there is no regular pattern to the abnormalities of those organs which are not in the respiratory system. Some major cardiac abnormalities are incompatible with life. Abnormalities have also been reported in the musculoskeletal, gastrointestinal, reproductive and endocrine systems.

Endoscopic diagnosis

Confirmation and precise assessment are made under general anaesthesia; endoscopy includes a search for abnormalities of the tracheobronchial tree, e.g. tracheobronchomalacia, tracheal stenosis.

Using telescopes and the microscope it is essential to inspect and palpate the web to assess not only its size but also the thickness at and below the anterior commissure. The size of the web can be expressed, by visual assessment, as an approximate percentage of the glottic opening. The presence and severity of congenital subglottic stenosis is best assessed by a combination of endoscopic examination and radiological study.

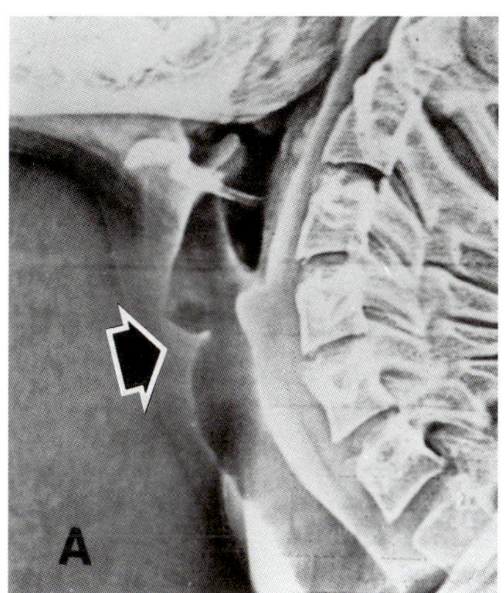

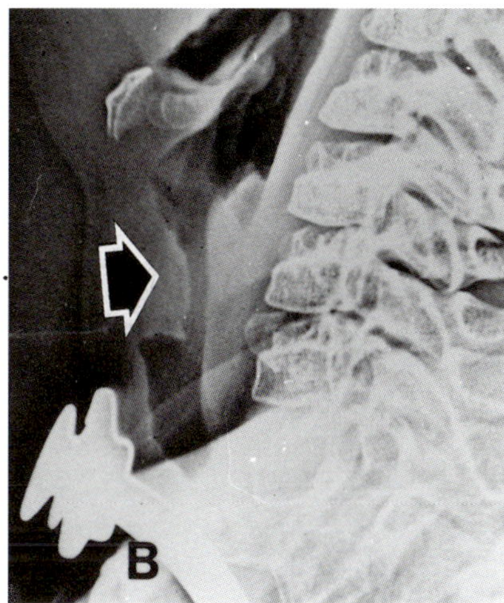

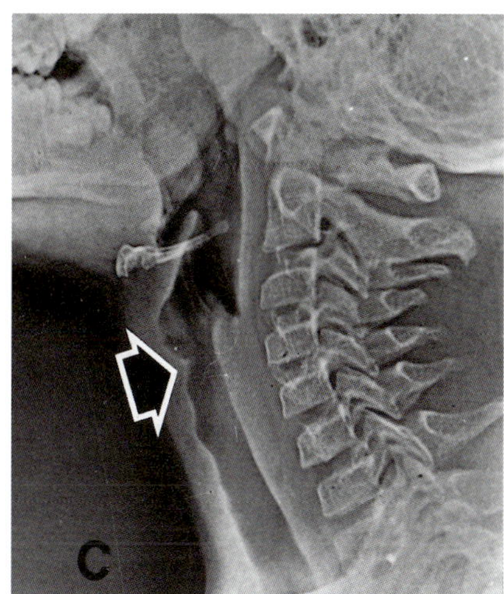

Figure **25.3**
Lateral xeroradiographs of congenital webs. A. Thick at the anterior commissure, thin posterior edge. B. Large glottic web with severe subglottic stenosis. C. Congenital subglottic web.

Endoscopic diagnosis

Size
Anterior thickness
Subglottic extension
Other respiratory tract abnormalities

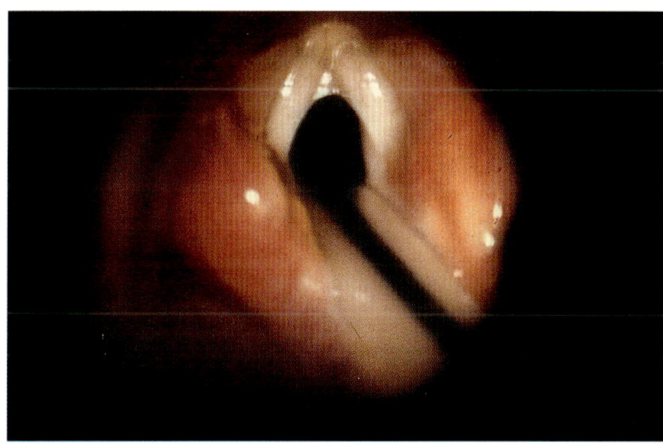

Figure **25.4**
Thin glottic web. Small, membranous, transparent, anterior web.

There may be only a small, thin membrane (Fig. 25.4) or there may be a large thick web (Fig. 25.5) causing life-threatening obstruction. The free posterior edge of the web is thin, concave backward and sharply outlined (Fig. 25.6) while the anterior part is thicker. The undersurface, seen obliquely with a 30° or 70° telescope, is concave downwards.

Treatment

The need for treatment depends on the clinical features, the extent of the web and the severity of any associated subglottic stenosis. Some require no treatment, e.g. in infants unlikely to survive other major abnormalities or those with a tiny, relatively asymptomatic web. In severe cases with airway obstruction and cyanosis it is necessary to provide an artificial airway. In an emergency, introduction of a small-diameter endotracheal tube, stiffened by an introducer, is usually possible whether or not a web

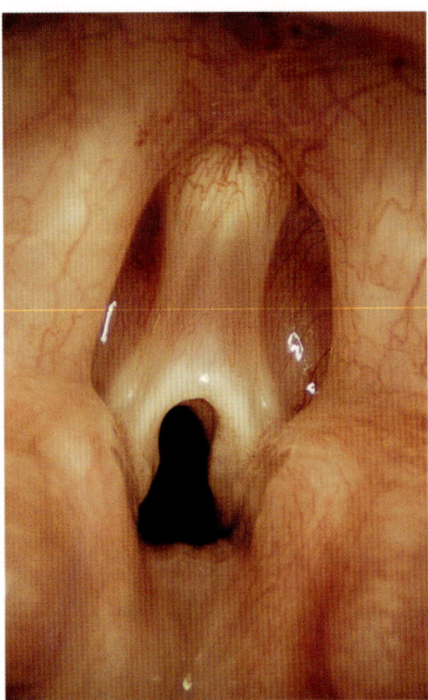

Figure **25.5**
Severe congenital web. The outline of the vocal ligaments can be seen. The glottic lumen is greatly reduced.

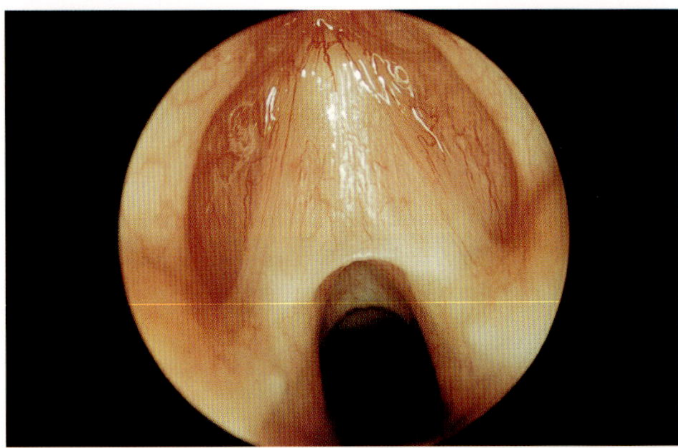

Figure **25.6**
Medium-sized congenital glottic web. Infant with a weak cry but no airway obstruction. This photograph with a 30° telescope shows the associated subglottic stenosis.

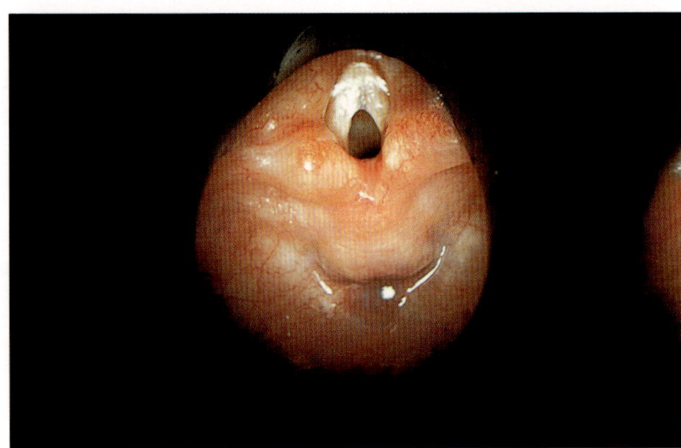

Figure **25.7**
Small congenital web divided using scissors. Thin anterior web in a baby who was aphonic. After simple division with microlaryngoscopy scissors and recovery from anaesthesia the cry was normal.

has been defined as the cause of the obstruction. At times, an unrecognized thin web may be ruptured by the passage of an endotracheal tube or a bronchoscope, so that subsequently it cannot be identified. In severe cases the airway must be maintained by a tracheotomy.

Many forms of treatment have been advocated:

- simple microsurgical division with scissors followed by 'dilatation';
- microcauterization;
- laser treatment;
- laryngofissure to allow removal of redundant soft tissue or cartilage in the subglottic region and accurate trimming and repair of the web with or without use of a stent or keel.

There is no obviously superior form of treatment; it is seldom possible to relate the form of treatment to any specific web. The following procedures are recommended:

- Thin, membranous glottic webs respond well to simple incision or rupture using a bronchoscope or dilator (Fig. 25.7).
- Medium webs can be improved by precise endoscopic excision of the triangular membranous web and insertion of a Lindholm 'flag' to minimize adhesions and reformation of the web. A thin, shaped piece of silastic sheeting is held in place between the cut edges by threads anchored to the

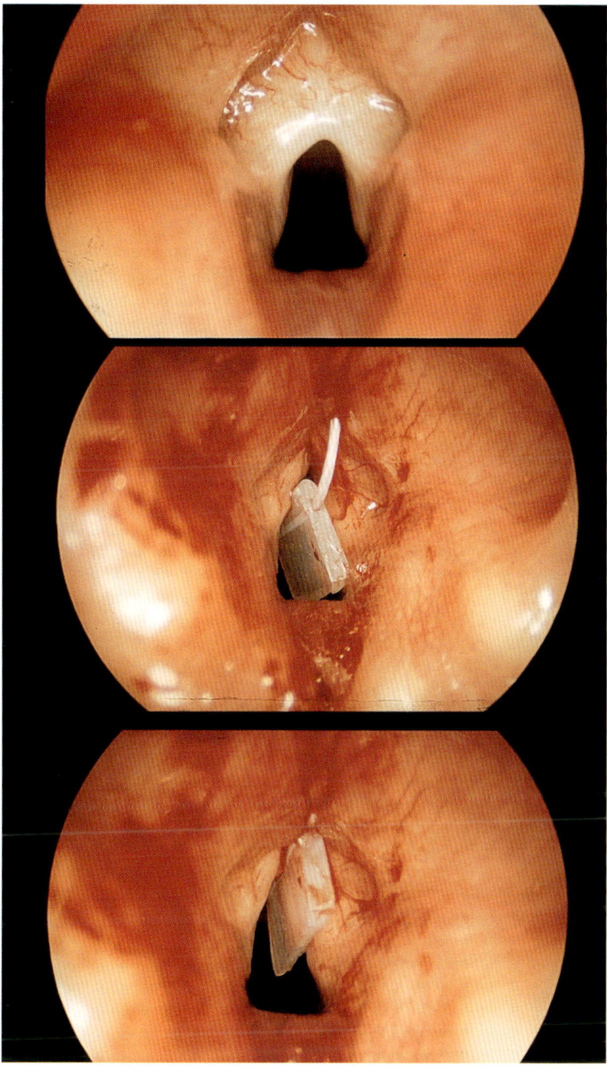

Figure **25.8**
Lindholm flag. Moderate web (top). Divided web and flag, which is silastic sheet doubled over a thread, being placed (centre). Flag pulled forward into final position (bottom).

Recommended treatment

Incision or rupture of thin web
Lindholm 'flag' for medium web
Laryngoplasty for severe web

skin of the neck both above and below the glottis for about 10 days (Fig. 25.8).

- Thick webs with obstructing subglottic stenosis require laryngofissure when the child is at least 4 or 5 years of age.

  The operation commences with microlaryngoscopy for accurate placement of an incision on one side, along the presumed edge of the vocal fold medial to the line of the vocal ligament. A transverse skin incision allows the larynx to be opened in the midline. The abnormal cricoid cartilage and the soft tissue of the web are resected submucosally preserving as much mucosa as possible to repair the edge and underface of one vocal fold. An anterior graft of rib cartilage may be necessary to augment the subglottic diameter.

Results

Voice improvement with medium or thick webs may not be satisfactory, e.g. web excision and use of the keel may achieve a better-looking glottis, and although the voice may be improved, vocal fold vibration remains limited.

Voice improvement is difficult with webs which are thick and those associated with subglottic–cricoid abnormality.

In general, the smaller the web and the simpler the treatment, the better the voice result.

INTERARYTENOID WEBS

The distinctive feature of this rare anomaly is a band of tissue joining the postero-medial surfaces of the arytenoid cartilages with restricted abduction of the vocal cords.

Embryology

During embryogenesis of the larynx, large arytenoid swellings form on each side of the sagittal laryngeal cleft and by the fifth week epithelium between the medial aspects of the arytenoid swellings fuses to form the epithelial lamina which normally dissolves to reopen the sagittal cleft. It appears that failure of

Features of interarytenoid web

Inspiratory stridor
Cyanotic attacks
Repeated aspiration
Other, non-airway anomalies

resorption leads to congenital interarytenoid web. Since the arytenoid and cricoid are derived from the same brachial arch, an arrest in arytenoid development may be associated with cricoid maldevelopment, such as congenital subglottic stenosis.

Clinical features

The major presenting feature is inspiratory stridor. Other features include obstructive cyanosis at birth and in the neonatal period, unexplained airway obstruction and episodes of apnoea or cyanosis that require immediate intubation or even tracheotomy before further assessment can be safely undertaken.

Endoscopic diagnosis

Interarytenoid web restricting abduction
± Large arytenoids
± Subglottic stenosis
Difficulty exposing the larynx
Difficulty maintaining the airway
Use special-purpose slim laryngoscopes
No endotracheal tube

Older infants may present with recurrent or atypical 'croup'. There is no abnormality of cry or voice. Many infants have repeated aspiration during feeding but the reason for this is not known.

More than half the patients have non-airway anomalies which are not confined to any particular organ system.

Endoscopic diagnosis

Definitive diagnosis requires laryngoscopy and bronchoscopy under general anaesthesia. In many cases other associated laryngeal anomalies, notably

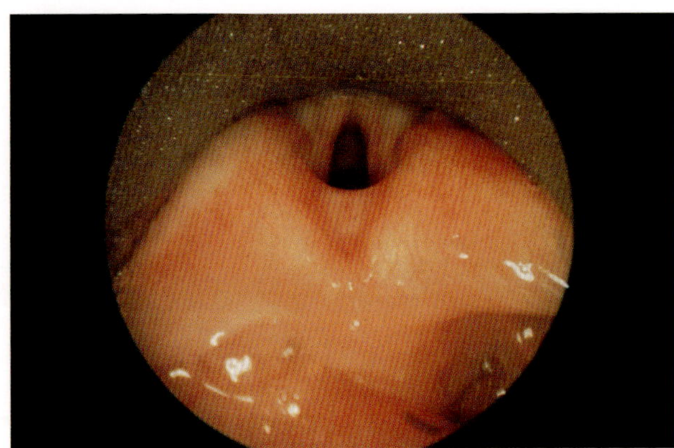

Figure **25.9**
Laryngoscopy for congenital interarytenoid web. Exposure of the larynx is difficult. The arytenoids are large and the web is stretched between them.

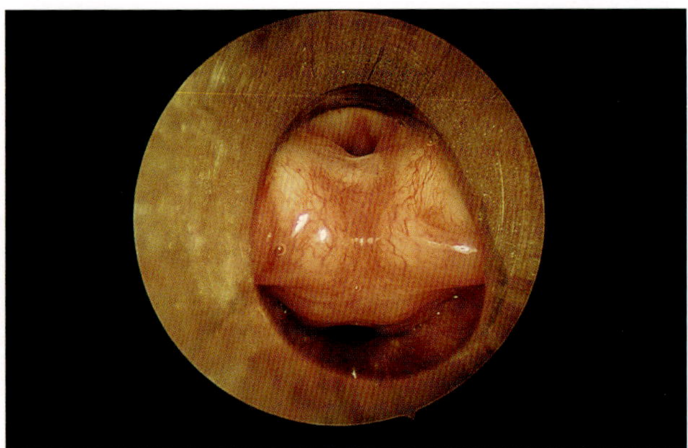

Figure **25.10**
Holinger laryngoscope in the posterior glottis. The slim barrel of the Holinger anterior commissures laryngoscope is used to spread the posterior supraglottic tissues to display the interarytenoid web.

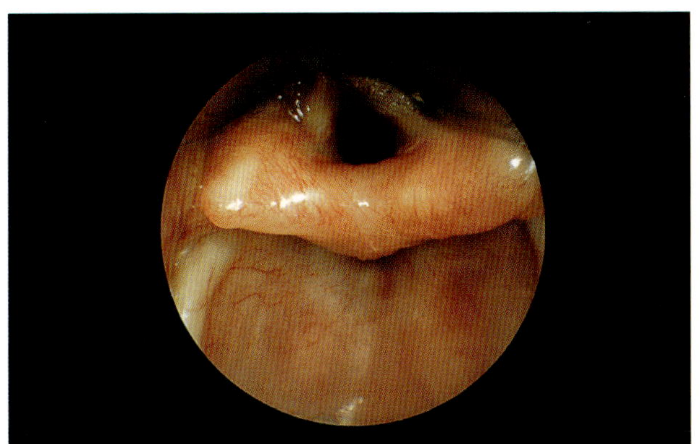

Figure **25.11**
Interarytenoid web. Thick tissue tethers the arytenoids to one another.

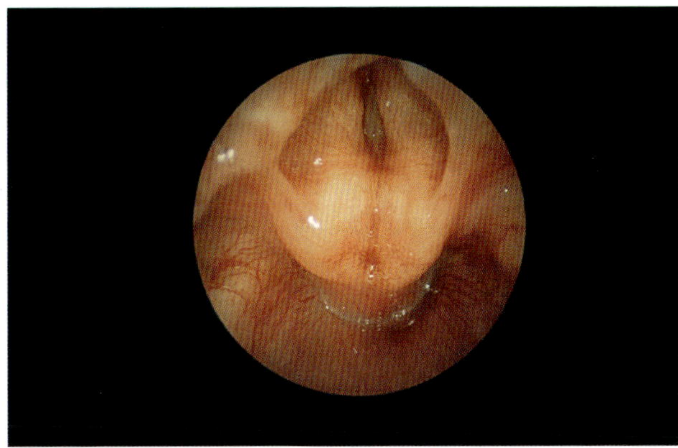

Figure **25.12**
Laryngeal atresia. Attempted intubation at birth was not successful and life was maintained for about 20 minutes by ventilation via coexistent H-type tracheo-oesophageal fistula until a tracheotomy was performed. A rudimentary outline of the glottis is visible.

large, bulky arytenoids and congenital subglottic stenosis, can be identified at direct endoscopy.

At endoscopy it is difficult to expose and visualize the larynx (Fig. 25.9) and it is also difficult to maintain a good airway under anaesthesia because of the obstructive anomalies and the abnormal position and anatomy of the larynx. The arytenoids are often large, a finding difficult to quantify and describe in detail.

The posterior larynx must be examined without the presence of an endotracheal tube. Direct inspection presents difficulty in every case and special-purpose hand-held slim laryngoscopes (Fig. 25.10), such as the Holinger anterior commissure laryngoscope or the Holinger–Tucker–Benjamin infant laryngoscope and subglottiscope (see Fig. 6.8) should be used. This technique allows unhurried and comprehensive evaluation and includes palpation of the extent and thickness of the web by separating the arytenoids (Fig. 25.11), testing of crico-arytenoid joint mobility, calibration of the subglottis and assessment of vocal cord movement as anaesthesia is discontinued.

Treatment

The definitive management of congenital interarytenoid web has not been established. The timing of tracheotomy depends on the severity and progressive nature of laryngeal obstruction. Those with significant subglottic stenosis or other congenital anomaly such as dysmorphic facies or midface hypoplasia contributing to upper airway obstruction need long-term tracheotomy. Decannulation in 3–5 years is usually possible and there is a good long-term prognosis. Infants without subglottic stenosis tend to have minor obstructive features and usually do not require intubation or tracheotomy. Parents can be assured that the airway will improve with age.

CONGENITAL LARYNGEAL ATRESIA

Total atresia is extremely rare and fatal (Fig. 25.12), unless an emergency tracheotomy is performed immediately after birth.

The presence of an associated upper pouch H-type tracheo-oesophageal fistula can allow sufficient air exchange by positive pressure ventilation while preparations are made for endoscopy to confirm the diagnosis prior to tracheotomy.

BIBLIOGRAPHY

Benjamin B (1983) Congenital laryngeal webs. *Ann Otol Rhinol Laryngol* **92**: 317–26.

Benjamin B, Mair EA (1991) Congenital interarytenoid web. *Arch Otolaryngol Head Neck Surg* **117**: 1118–22.

Cohen SR (1985) Congenital glottic webs in children. *Ann Otol Rhinol Laryngol* **94** (Suppl 121): 1–16.

26 Congenital clefts

CLASSIFICATION

Congenital clefts are rare midline anomalies characterized by a deficiency which is almost always in the posterior larynx sometimes extending inferiorly into the tracheo-oesophageal wall. The types of clefts (Benjamin and Inglis, 1989) include:

- *Anterior laryngeal cleft*. Occurs at the anterior commissure and is extremely rare.
- *Posterior laryngeal cleft*. Occurs when the normal medial fusion between the larynx and the hypopharynx is arrested.
- *Laryngotracheo-oesophageal cleft*. This is the correct descriptive term for a deficiency which extends inferiorly into the cervical trachea or further into the thoracic trachea creating a common lumen for the trachea and oesophagus. A tracheo-oesophageal cleft is often associated with major anomalies of other organs and is usually fatal.

Posterior laryngeal and laryngotracheal clefts can be classified into four types according to the extent of the cleft (Fig. 26.1). This classification relates to the anatomical anomaly, symptoms and treatment and allows for the recognition of minor clefts.

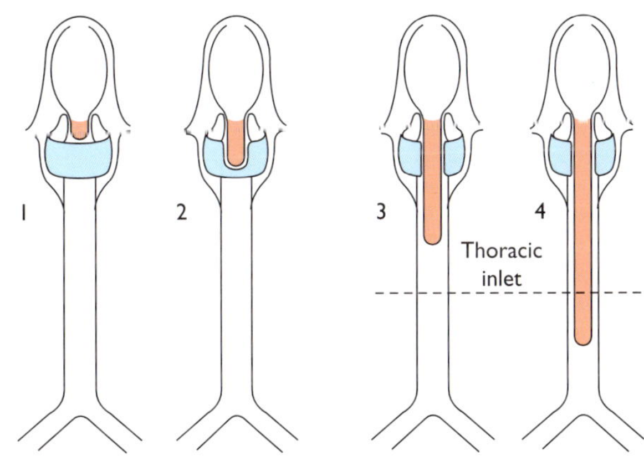

Figure **26.1**
Classification of clefts. Diagram illustrating classification into four types, depending on the extent of the cleft.

Type 1. Supraglottic membranous interarytenoid cleft, above the level of the vocal cords (Fig. 26.2).

Type 2. Partial cricoid cleft, extending below the level of the vocal cords and partly, but not completely, through the posterior lamina of the cricoid, i.e. partial posterior cleft of the cricoid cartilage (Fig. 26.3).

An occult or submucous cleft occurs when the deficient part of the cricoid cartilage and interarytenoid muscle is covered by intact mucous membrane.

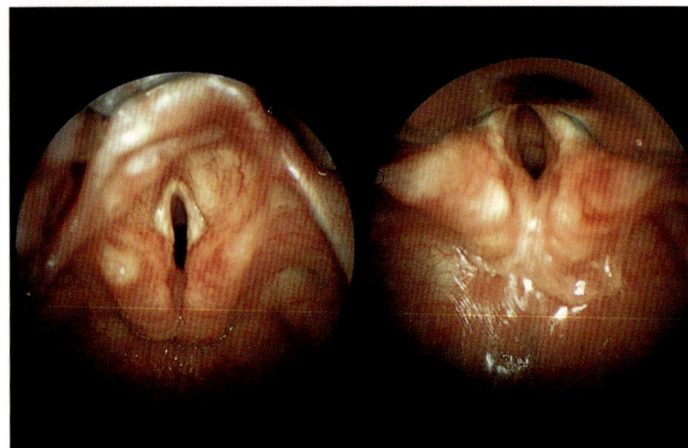

Figure **26.2**
Type 1 cleft. Cleft does not extend past the level of the glottis. The larynx has a near normal appearance (left) until the posterior structures are spread apart (right).

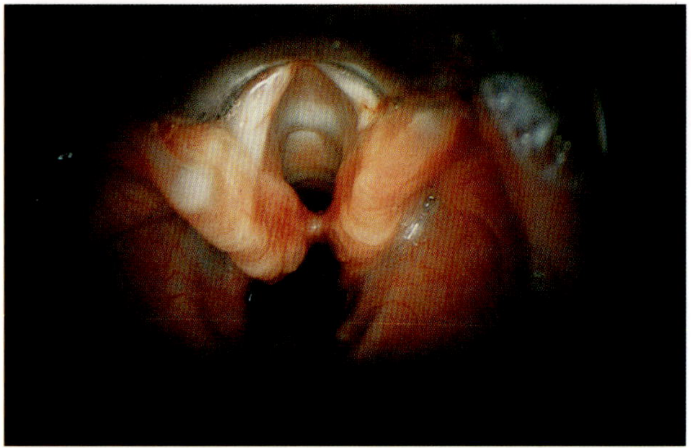

Figure **26.3**
Type 2 cleft. Extends past the glottis level and partly through the lamina of the cricoid cartilage.

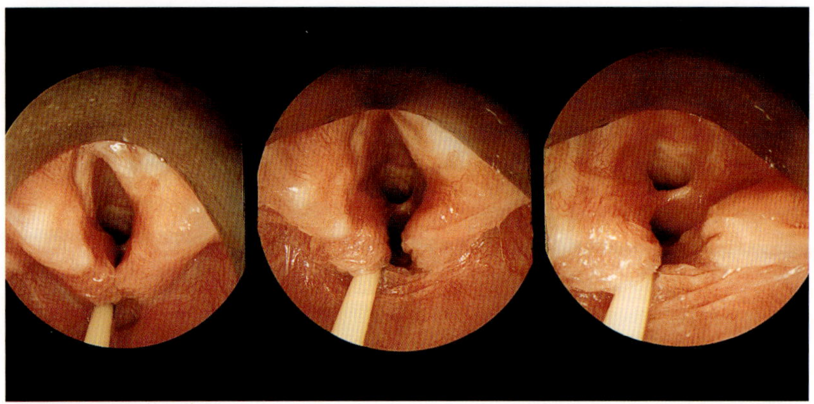

Figure **26.4**
Type 3 cleft. As the tissues are separated the cleft is seen to extend past the cricoid and into the cervical tracheo-oesophageal wall.

Type 3. Total cricoid cartilage cleft extending completely through the cricoid cartilage with or without further extension into part of the cervical tracheo-oesophageal wall (Fig. 26.4).

Type 4. Extensive cleft into part or all of the thoracic tracheo-oesophageal wall to the carina or, very rarely, into a main bronchus.

EMBRYOLOGY

During development of the larynx, the trachea and oesophagus at first share a common lumen which becomes separated into two by the tracheo-oesophageal septum, normally completed by 35 days gestation. Failure of the interarytenoid tissues or cricoid cartilage to fuse produces a laryngeal cleft.

Partial or complete failure of formation of the tracheo-oesophageal septum results in a more extensive laryngotracheo-oesophageal cleft.

Minor supraglottic Type 1 clefts are due to absence of the interarytenoid soft tissues and musculature. The embryological mechanism of failure of fusion of the cricoid cartilage is controversial and confused by the fact that a common tracheo-oesophageal tube with an intact cricoid above has been observed on very rare occasions.

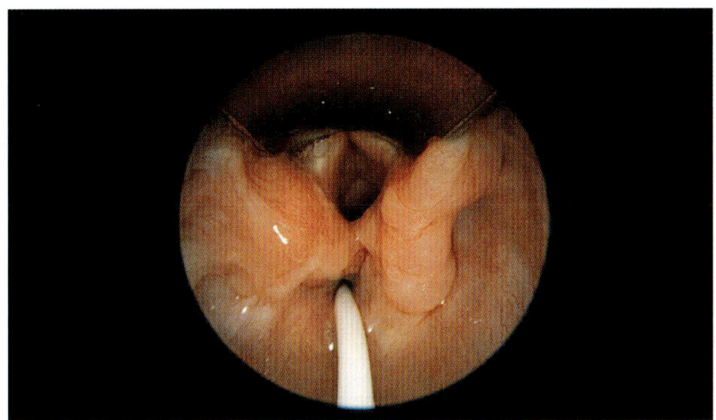

Figure **26.5**
Cleft with lymphangioma. Mass of lymphangioma behind right arytenoid was a contributory factor in causing moderate inspiratory stridor.

Stridor due to partial obstruction of the larynx may be one of the presenting symptoms, especially in infants with Type 1 or Type 2 clefts. Inspiratory collapse of the redundant mucosa of the unstable, incompletely formed posterior laryngeal framework or of an associated bulky hamartomatous lesion partly occludes the lumen (Fig. 26.5). This explains why an erroneous diagnosis of laryngomalacia may be made.

CLINICAL FEATURES

Aspiration may be intermittent and variable with Type I cleft. All patients with Types 2, 3 and 4 clefts have persistent aspiration into the tracheobronchial tree and lungs and some have partial airway obstruction.

Aspiration manifests as coughing, choking and cyanotic episodes precipitated by feeding. Sometimes between feeds there may be aspiration of pharyngeal secretions. There may be recurrent respiratory infections and aspiration pneumonitis showing as segmental or subsegmental collapse on chest X-ray.

Some infants have a weak abnormal cry; in others the cry is normal.

ASSOCIATED ANOMALIES

Over half the patients with clefts have other abnormalities; oesophageal atresia with or without tracheo-oesophageal fistula and gastro-oesophageal reflux are the most common. Evans et al (1995) reported that 37% of 44 patients with laryngeal clefts also had tracheo-oesophageal fistula with or without oesophageal atresia. Other associated defects include cleft lip and palate, congenital cardiac defects, gastrointestinal abnormalities (particularly of the anus), genitourinary anomalies (particularly hypospadias), the VATER syndrome and other tracheobronchial abnormalities. Laryngeal cleft is likely to occur in Opitz–Frias syndrome (or G syndrome) and Pallister–Hall syndrome. Laryngeal cleft can be familial, and if so the inheritance pattern is autosomal dominant.

Clinical features

Aspiration, especially Types 3 and 4
Stridor, especially Types 1 and 2
Weak, abnormal cry
Associated anomalies in over 50%

DIAGNOSIS

The cardinal presenting feature is aspiration whose severity depends, to some degree, on the extent of the cleft. Other features include respiratory distress and intermittent inspiratory stridor.

Direct endoscopy should be part of the investigation in every child with persistent aspiration, specifically searching for cleft larynx and other causes of aspiration such as vocal cord paralysis, H-type tracheo-oesophageal fistula and gastro-oesophageal reflux. Incoordinate swallowing is another common cause of aspiration and is best demonstrated on contrast oesophageal swallow studies. In cleft larynx, aspiration of contrast material can represent a hazard; it is safer to proceed initially to endoscopy when a cleft is suspected.

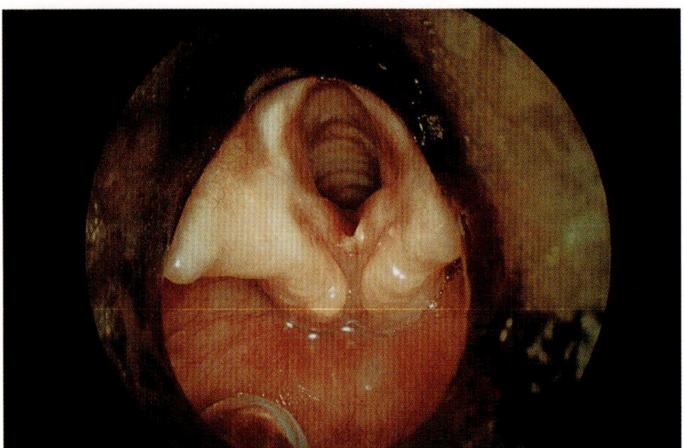

Figure **26.6**
Laryngoscopic technique. The barrel of a Holinger laryngoscope separates the vocal cords and allows confirmation of a minor posterior cleft.

Endoscopic diagnosis

Direct laryngoscopy
General anaesthesia
Various techniques
Laryngoscope to splay posterior glottis
Can be mistaken for laryngomalacia

Various specific endoscopic diagnostic techniques have been described including:

- Examination of the postcricoid and upper oesophageal region with a large endotracheal tube placed to spread the posterior laryngeal tissues.
- Probing the interarytenoid region and posterior glottis with an instrument in each hand while the larynx is in suspension.
- Measurement of the height of the interarytenoid notch.
- The most reliable method is direct inspection under general anaesthesia, either naked eye or using a 0° telescope, with a suitably chosen laryngoscope such as a Holinger anterior commissure paediatric instrument. The distal beak is used to deliberately separate and splay the posterior glottis for careful inspection (Fig. 26.6) taking care that redundant mucosa does not fill the cleft to disguise its presence. The size of the cleft is assessed, especially its lower extent in relation to the level of the vocal cords and cricoid cartilage.

With increased awareness and improved endoscopic techniques minor laryngeal clefts, especially Type 1, are now recognized more often. These patients have a good prognosis and the surgical approach for closure is less complicated than for major clefts.

It must be emphasized that, although the clinical features of a supraglottic interarytenoid cleft may suggest laryngomalacia, definitive diagnosis of the anomaly can be made only by careful examination of the interarytenoid and posterior glottic region.

Any child with a tracheo-oesophageal fistula and persistent aspiration should be suspected of an undiagnosed cleft until it is excluded by endoscopic examination.

TREATMENT

Stabilization

Resuscitation, ventilation and minimization of contamination of the lung are the first priorities in a newborn once the diagnosis of laryngeal or laryngotracheal cleft has been confirmed. Oral feeding must be avoided, and if necessary ventilation is assisted by endotracheal intubation. Extracorporeal membrane oxygenation may be required for operative treatment and postoperative maintenance when it is judged that an attempt at major transthoracic operative closure is indicated for complete laryngotracheal cleft. The ultimate prognosis is often poor.

Tracheotomy is now seldom necessary.

With Type 1, 2 and 3 clefts which do not extend past the thoracic inlet, operative treatment is usually not urgent; the infant can be stabilized and other organ systems checked for abnormalities. Gastro-oesophageal reflux often complicates the problem. It must be recognized and treated medically if possible, but fundoplication is often required and will improve the chance of successful repair of the cleft.

It seems that patients with minor clefts (Types 1 and 2) do not require assisted ventilation, should initially be tube fed to reduce aspiration, have a good prognosis and can usually be managed conservatively by thickened feedings and feeding in the upright position. If aspiration continues to be a significant problem, endoscopic microsurgical repair is the method of choice for Type 1 and possibly Type 2 anomalies. On the other hand, some Type 2 clefts which include part of the cricoid and Type 3 (which include part of the tracheo-oesophageal wall), require open surgical techniques.

Treatment

Stabilization
Endoscopic repair
Open repair
Always control reflux

Endoscopic repair

Patients with Type 1 and Type 2 clefts, who do not 'outgrow' their aspiration are usually suitable for endoscopic microsurgical repair under general anaesthesia. With the larynx in suspension, using 18-cm long paediatric instruments, including a small needle holder, the edges of the mucosal margins of the cleft are excised and, if possible, closed in two layers with fine sutures. Tracheotomy is unnecessary, but endotracheal intubation for several days after operation may be desirable if stridor had been a preoperative problem.

A nasogastric feeding tube which might cause pressure erosion on the suture line should be avoided.

Open repair

Open surgical approaches include anterior laryngofissure and lateral pharyngotomy for Type 3, some Type 2 and revisions. A lateral thoracotomy or anterior median sternotomy is used for Type 4 clefts.

The anterior laryngofissure approach is recommended for smaller clefts. Access is direct and midline, with good exposure, and there is no risk to the recurrent laryngeal nerve. A low tracheotomy away from the operative site is usually necessary. Laryngofissure is extended superiorly and inferiorly sufficient for adequate exposure to allow excision of the cleft margins and closure in two layers. Prescott (1995) has recommended repair of the defect in the posterior lamina of the cricoid cartilage using a costal cartilage graft for an improved postoperative contour of the subglottic region.

A lateral pharyngotomy approach has been recommended but endangers the recurrent laryngeal nerve, requires rotation of the larynx and, compared to the anterior approach, gives limited surgical access.

Revisions

It is not uncommon for revision surgery to be required for partial or complete breakdown of the repair site after one or even two attempts at repair. Difficult Type 2 cases may need open repair. Gastro-oesophageal reflux must always be adequately treated.

BIBLIOGRAPHY

Benjamin B, Inglis A (1989) Minor congenital laryngeal clefts: diagnosis and classification. *Ann Otol Rhinol Laryngol* **94**: 627–30.

Evans KL, Courteney-Harris R, Bailey CM, Evans JNG, Parsons DS (1995) Management of posterior laryngeal and laryngotracheo-oesophageal clefts. *Arch Otolaryngol Head Neck Surg* **121**: 1380–5.

Holinger LD (1997) Congenital laryngeal anomalies. In: Holinger LD, Lusk RP, Green CG (eds) *Paediatric laryngology and bronchoesophagology* (Philadelphia–New York: Lippincott–Raven); 157–8.

Prescott CAS (1995) Cleft larynx: repair with a posterior cartilage graft. *Int J Paediatr Otorhinolaryngol* **31**: 91–4.

27 Rare conditions

ABNORMALITIES OF THE EPIGLOTTIS

CRI-DU-CHAT SYNDROME

FOURTH BRANCHIAL CLEFT CYST

GASTRIC HETEROTOPIA

PLOTT'S SYNDROME

BENIGN JUVENILE XANTHOGRANULOMA OF THE LARYNX

ARTHROGRYPOSIS MULTIPLEX CONGENITA

A variety of abnormalities of the larynx are possible during development of the embryo and may affect laryngeal function in the newborn infant. Many rare and unusual anomalies have been reported but, as an exhaustive analysis is beyond the scope of this text, only a few will be briefly described.

ABNORMALITIES OF THE EPIGLOTTIS

Hypoplasia (Fig. 27.1), complete absence and bifid epiglottis have been described. They usually occur in association with congenital anomalies of other organ systems.

The clinical features include stridor, aspiration and an obstructive sleep pattern. Aspiration may slowly improve with time or may require gastrostomy and/or fundoplication. Airway obstruction may necessitate tracheotomy.

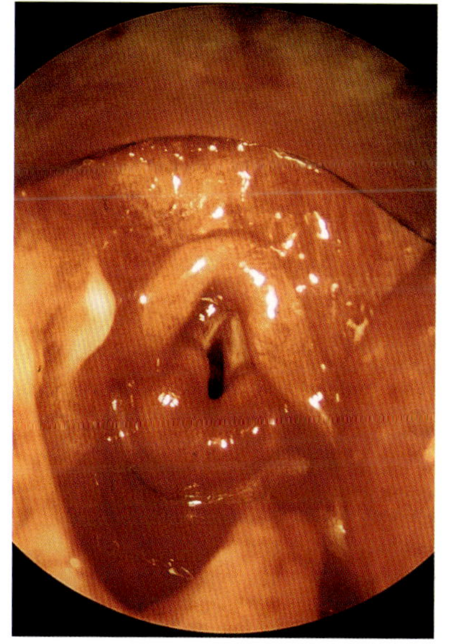

Figure **27.1**
Hypoplasia of the epiglottis. Endoscopic photograph, on the first day of life, showing the hypoplastic epiglottis, large arytenoids and short aryepiglottic folds. Respiratory distress, cough and stridor developed 30 minutes after birth.

CRI-DU-CHAT SYNDROME

This chromosomal disorder is due to partial deletion of the short arm of chromosome 5. The infant has a characteristic congenital high-pitched stridor with a cry which may be quite similar to the meowing sound of a cat. Endoscopic abnormalities similar to the changes in laryngomalacia and an 'open' posterior part of the larynx have been described. In one case (Fig. 27.2) we found virtual absence of the false cords.

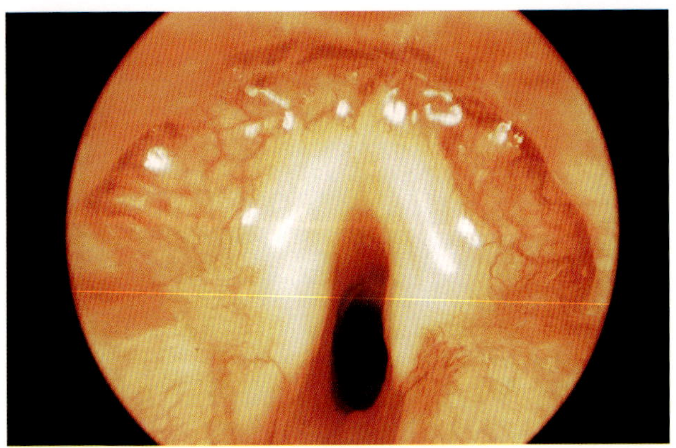

Figure **27.2**
Larynx in cri-du-chat syndrome. The vocal folds appear to be somewhat hypoplastic but the striking abnormality is the near absence of ventricular folds, allowing direct visualization of the ventricles on each side.

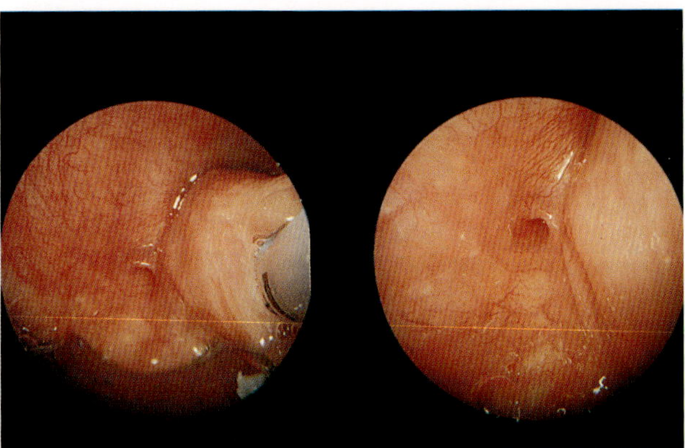

Figure **27.3**
Fourth branchial cleft opening. A small opening is seen beside the larynx in the apex of the left piriform fossa (left). A close-up view (right) shows the opening which can be catheterized to assist identification of the sinus during removal.

Associated abnormalities include microcephaly, hypertelorism, generalized hypotonia, mental retardation, low slung ears and a beak-like profile. In general, the prognosis is poor.

FOURTH BRANCHIAL CLEFT CYST

On rare occasions an anomaly of a fourth branchial arch forms a sinus whose apex is in the piriform fossa (Fig. 27.3); all reported cases have been on the left side. There are arguments for regarding it as part of either a third or more likely a fourth branchial arch. In any case infants, older children or adults can present with repeated infections or suppuration in the sinus tract and the surrounding soft tissues of the neck, with retropharyngeal cellulitis or thyroiditis. A thyroid scan in an adult will frequently show a hypofunctioning left thyroid lobe.

Diagnosis is made by a contrast swallow study together with careful endoscopy to identify the mouth of the sinus, which can be catheterized at the time of laryngoscopy for the instillation of methylene blue to trace the extent of the lesion. Surgical treatment requires removal of the entire tract in a period between episodes of inflammation. In infants, an acute abscess can cause life-threatening airway obstruction, which can be relieved by opening the abscess in the neck.

GASTRIC HETEROTOPIA

Gastric heterotopia describes a specific choristoma, i.e. an extragastric collection of normal gastric mucosa, an anomaly which has been reported in rare cases in the head and neck region. Gastric heterotopia in the upper oesophagus is occasionally an incidental endoscopic finding; the oesophageal lesions are virtually always longitudinal flat patches of mucosa only. Rarely exceeding 5–6 mm in extent, they differ from hypopharyngeal lesions in size and architecture.

In the hypopharynx these lesions may be large enough to impinge on the larynx and cause airway obstruction (Fig. 27.4). A diagnosis of gastric heterotopia might be suspected from the macroscopic appearance because of the similarity of the folds to normal gastric mucosa, but biopsy is essential to prove the diagnosis.

Biopsy shows gastric mucosa, submucosa and muscularis propria containing ganglionated nerve plexuses similar to that of normal stomach.

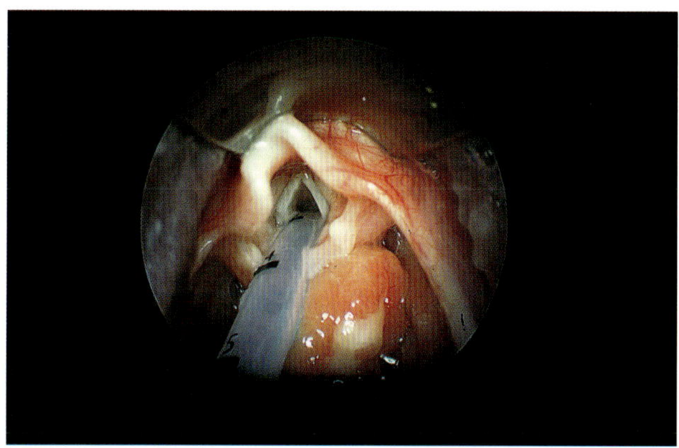

Figure **27.4**
Gastric heterotopia in the hypopharynx. Radiological study had revealed a mass in the hypopharynx as the cause of variable inspiratory stridor and failure to thrive at 4 months. The mass was removed endoscopically from the surface of the constrictor muscle using the carbon dioxide laser.

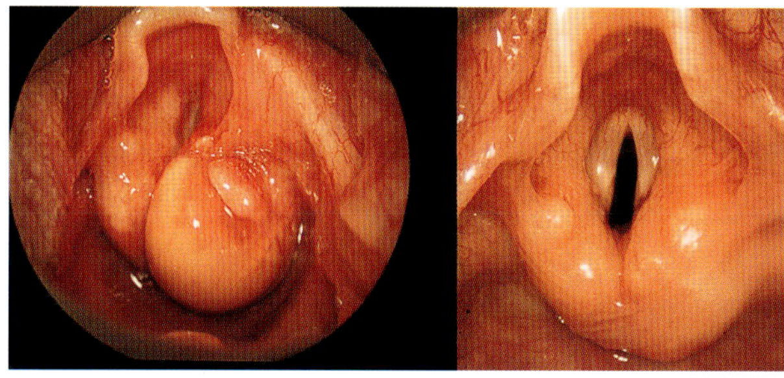

Figure **27.5**
Benign juvenile xanthogranuloma of the larynx. Bilateral swellings, larger on the right side than the left, almost filling the supraglottic larynx at the time of diagnosis (left) in a 5-month-old infant. There was almost complete resolution, without treatment (right), 10 months later. The tracheotomy was removed the day after this photograph was taken.

Treatment requires complete removal; the Lindholm laryngoscope gives excellent access for laser excision.

PLOTT'S SYNDROME

This hereditary neuromuscular disorder features congenital laryngeal adductor paralysis. The condition is X-chromosome linked and is associated with mental retardation. The prognosis for life is poor.

BENIGN JUVENILE XANTHOGRANULOMA OF THE LARYNX

Benign juvenile xanthogranuloma is one type of histiocytosis, a term referring to a group of non-inflammatory proliferative disorders of the monocyte/macrophage and dendritic cell systems. It is a normolipaemic, self-limiting condition usually presenting with cutaneous, orbital or occasionally with visceral lesions.

Very rarely it can occur in the larynx (Fig. 27.5), causing airway obstruction and may require a tracheotomy. The expectation is for spontaneous resolution over many months although laser treatment to remove the bulk of the mass can be considered.

ARTHROGRYPOSIS MULTIPLEX CONGENITA

This uncommon congenital disorder, which is sometimes familial, is characterized by multiple joint deformities and other congenital defects such as facial diplegia (Möbius' syndrome), difficulty in swallowing and other central nervous system abnormalities.

There may be Pierre Robin-like features (micrognathia, glossoptosis, cleft palate), dysphagia, aspiration, changes in the cry, vocal cord paralysis, supraglottic changes similar to those of laryngomalacia and hypertrophy of the cricopharyngeus muscle.

Central nervous system dysfunction rather than simple peripheral muscle weakness accounts for the dysphagia and respiratory difficulty. A tracheotomy and feeding gastrostomy may be part of the management but the long-term prognosis is poor.

VII ACUTE INFLAMMATORY AIRWAY OBSTRUCTION

28 Acute inflammatory airway obstruction

CLASSIFICATION

Acute infectious diseases of the upper respiratory tract which cause airway obstruction include:

Oropharynx
- acute bacterial or viral infection causing obstructive hypertrophy of the tonsils and adenoids
- infectious mononucleosis causing obstructive hypertrophy of the tonsils and adenoids
- peritonsillar abscess
- retropharyngeal abscess
- parapharyngeal abscess
- Ludwig's angina

Larynx
- acute laryngotracheobronchitis

- spasmodic croup
- bacterial tracheitis
- acute supraglottitis (epiglottitis)
- diphtheria.

The latter five infectious diseases of the larynx will be discussed in detail in this chapter. These illnesses can be severe enough to cause life-threatening airway obstruction in infants, in children and sometimes in adults. Successful treatment requires interdisciplinary co-operation among paediatricians, physicians, anaesthesiologists, intensivists and nursing personnel to minimize mortality and morbidity. There is no other area of medicine or surgery where skilled care contributes more to patient welfare. Each of these diseases causes respiratory distress and, at times, can progress to total respiratory obstruction. Clinical differentiation between them is critical for early recognition, appropriate medical management, provision of an artificial airway and optimal intensive care with a minimum of complications.

Infants and children with airway obstruction can quickly become cyanotic and hypercarbic. It has been estimated, for example, that in a 9-month-old with a normal subglottic diameter of 6 mm, just 1 mm of subglottic mucosal oedema reduces the cross-sectional area by over 50% causing an 80% decrease in airflow. Inflammatory oedema, cellular tissue response and release of chemical mediators in the subglottic mucosa within the cricoid in severe cases of croup can cause obstruction at the most critical site in the airway.

HISTORICAL BACKGROUND

Before the twentieth century, in most parts of the world and especially in Europe, a diagnosis of croup meant the probability of death because *diphtheria* was the only recognized cause and most cases were fatal.

About 100 years ago, O'Dwyer from New York introduced a set of different-sized brass tubes which were passed over the back of the tongue into the larynx with a special introducer. They were widely used to relieve airway obstruction due to diphtheritic laryngitis until tracheotomy became the treatment of choice. Since antitoxin and then diphtheria immunization became available in the mid-1920s, the incidence of diphtheria has dramatically reduced although sporadic cases are still seen. The disease remains an endemic threat to life in many Third World nations.

Acute laryngotracheobronchitis or 'croup' was described as a distinct disease entity by Baum (1928) and by the mid-1950s the causal association with para-influenza virus had been reported.

At the end of the eighteenth century, Mainwaring presented the first clear description of obstructive *acute epiglottitis* describing the epiglottis as 'thickened and standing erect' and although the clinical features resembled croup he considered it to be a different disease. Little more was known until the first modern report of acute epiglottitis in 1926 and finally Sinclair's historic paper in 1941 described 10 children with acute epiglottis and established it as a separate disease.

Advances in the management of acute obstructive diseases have involved the use of nebulized racemic epinephrine and the administration of steroids for viral acute laryngotracheobronchitis, the change from tracheotomy to intubation to secure an artificial airway, the use of more powerful and effective antibiotics and, most recently, immunization with *Haemophilus influenzae* Type B vaccine.

Important advances in treatment

Diphtheria antitoxin
Diphtheria immunization
Effective antibiotics
Intubation instead of tracheotomy
Racemic epinephrine for croup
Steroids for croup
Hib vaccine

DIFFICULTIES AND DILEMMAS

Problems in the management of severe upper airway obstruction arise from confusion with differences in nomenclature, difficulty making a diagnosis, confusion over the value of investigations, uncertainty in assessing the need for an artificial airway, and unexpected or rapid deterioration to respiratory obstruction. It has become obvious that each hospital should have a clear protocol to manage a child presenting with airway obstruction, depending upon the facilities and the skills available in that particular hospital (see Fig. 28.6). The concept of a management plan to direct the care of the patient, to confirm the diagnosis and to institute appropriate therapy according to an orderly sequence of events involves having a team consisting of members from the emergency department, resident staff, intensive care physicians, paediatricians, otolaryngologist, anaesthesiologist and intensive care nursing staff.

Patients with severe airway obstruction, imminent respiratory collapse, suspected supraglottitis or suspected foreign body inhalation are directed immediately to the operating theatre. Under general anaesthesia direct examination by laryngoscopy and bronchoscopy will determine the diagnosis and an airway can be secured.

Patients who present with signs of respiratory tract obstruction but who are coping adequately are transferred to the intensive care ward where monitoring of the airway obstruction can be continued with immediate transfer to the operating theatre if obstruction increases.

Each of the laryngeal diseases will be described in detail and management principles for patients presenting to hospital with moderate or severe upper airway obstruction will be examined.

ACUTE LARYNGOTRACHEITIS

Also known as acute viral laryngotracheobronchitis, subglottic laryngitis and, most commonly, 'croup'.

Epidemiology

Croup is a common infection of the middle and lower respiratory tract and is the most common cause of airway obstruction in infants and children. From 3 to 5% of children have at least one episode of croup and it recurs in about 5% of these.

It occurs most often in the cooler months of autumn and early winter with a peak incidence corresponding to outbreaks of parainfluenza virus and respiratory syncytial virus. Parainfluenza virus Types 1, 2 and 3 and respiratory syncytial virus (RSV) are the main causes of croup but influenza virus Type A causes the most severe symptoms. Influenza virus Type B, myocoplasma pneumoniae, herpes simplex and other viruses are less commonly implicated aetiological agents. The disease is often complicated by secondary bacterial infection of the lower airways and possibly precipitates bacterial tracheitis (which will be discussed later).

Management difficulties

Confusion with nomenclature
Diagnostic difficulty
Inappropriate investigations
Uncertainty about intubation
Unexpected deterioration

Acute viral laryngotracheitis

Usually in autumn and winter
Commonest 6–48 months of age
Commoner in boys
Parainfluenza virus and RSV

Boys are affected more often than girls in a ratio of almost 2 : 1. Croup is most common between 6 months and 4 years of age with a peak at 1–2 years. It is seldom seen in children over 5 years of age. A diagnosis of croup in an infant younger than 3 months should be viewed with suspicion as it raises the possibility of an underlying anatomical abnormality such as congenital subglottic stenosis or congenital subglottic haemangioma. Similarly, atypical or recurrent croup in an infant or older child may require radiological investigation and endoscopic evaluation for a laryngeal abnormality, inhaled subglottic foreign body or tracheal narrowing.

Clinical features

Onset with URT symptoms
Harsh, barking, 'croupy' cough
Variable inspiratory stridor
Usually lasts 1–3 days
A few need hospitalization

Pathogenesis

The reason why the incidence of croup varies dramatically from year to year in a community is not known. It follows the prevalence of parainfluenza and other causative viral agents which are highly contagious and spread directly from infected droplets which can survive on environmental surfaces for 5–6 hours. The offending virus reaches the nasal or pharyngeal mucosa, causes nasal congestion and sore throat and spreads to the larynx and trachea where local cellular defences and ciliary function are inhibited. In the larynx and subglottic tissues the result is intense erythema and inflammatory oedema with thick secretions which become purulent with secondary bacterial infection. Often the mucosal cells of the bronchi and bronchioles are also involved and fibrinous exudate further obstructs these airways with atelectasis and mucous plugging also impairing gas exchange.

There is increasing evidence that allergy may play a contributing role; children with a history of croup often have hyperreactive airways and an increased incidence of allergic problems. Patients with recurring croup may have an underlying abnormality of their airways. It is thought that laryngotracheobronchitis is rare in the first few months of life because of passive transfer of maternal virus-specific immunoglobulins.

It has been postulated that spasmodic croup, which shows many differences from the usual viral croup, may be caused by an allergic reaction to viral antigens, but this has not been proven.

Clinical features

The common initial presentation of viral laryngotracheobronchitis is in autumn or winter with typical manifestations of an upper respiratory tract infection (URT): rhinorrhoea, sore throat, 'mucousy' cough and a low-grade fever. Within 24 hours the infection involves the larynx and trachea producing a harsh, barking or brassy cough, frequently hoarseness and variable inspiratory stridor, which is usually worse in the evening and at night. Adenovirus and influenza virus infections cause more severe manifestations with headache, myalgia and soreness or pain on swallowing.

The illness is self-limiting and usually lasts between 1 and 3 days. Some patients have a protracted course with greater airway obstruction, more toxicity and physical signs such as lethargy, tachycardia, sternal retraction and even cyanosis. Physical examination confirms findings associated with the above symptoms and allows assessment of severity for possible hospitalization, observation and, in cases with severe airway obstruction, provision of an artificial airway. Auscultation of the lungs may detect rales, wheezing and even areas of atelectasis with decreased air entry. Children with severely obstructed airways become agitated, restless, develop severe stridor, fatigue and increased tachycardia. They progress to hypotonia, cyanosis or extreme pallor and, finally, cardiopulmonary arrest.

Diagnosis

Assessment of croup is subjective and may be difficult. There are no laboratory measurements of the degree of severity. The diagnosis is based primarily on clinical evaluation by an experienced observer without the need for tests such as X-rays, blood gases or sputum cultures. Usually it is not difficult to differentiate croup from acute supraglottitis, spasmodic croup or diphtheria but, as the illness progresses, if the child becomes more toxic and more obstructed, features suggesting bacterial tracheitis may be recognized, a diagnosis which cannot be suspected early in the course of the illness.

Most children settle at home and are not sufficiently unwell to require medical attention. Of the 1–2% of children who require hospital admission, most are observed while breathing moist air and do not need any other treatment. However, for reasons that are not clear, a few children progress to moderate or severe airway obstruction and need close observation in the intensive care ward. They may require medical treatment or, in severe cases, provision of an artificial airway by nasotracheal intubation under general anaesthesia.

Other diagnostic tests

Imaging by lateral or antero-posterior radiographs is seldom necessary but when performed, in severe cases may show haziness or narrowing of the subglottis with air distending the hypopharynx above the obstruction. Although X-ray may not be able to confirm the diagnosis of croup the appearance of a normal epiglottis certainly lessens the possibility of acute supraglottitis. Children with typical, mild or even moderate clinical features do not usually need radiographic studies.

Laboratory examination of blood is seldom useful, the white blood cell count is usually normal and blood gas changes occur late in the sequence of airway obstruction. Venipuncture is usually an unnecessary disturbance in a child with severe croup.

Microbiological tests may be indicated in some hospitalized patients. Indirect fluorescent antibody tests or enzyme immunosorbent assays are available for most common pathogens, but the results take time for completion and are irrelevant in the clinical management.

Table 28.1 Severity and treatment of croup

Severity and symptoms	*Treatment*
Mild	
• barking cough	Home
• inspiratory stridor when the child is upset	No specific treatment
• no sternal or suprasternal recession	Moist air
Moderate	
• inspiratory stridor	Home/hospital observation
• suprasternal, sternal retraction in inspiration	?nebulized budesonide
	Moist air
Severe	
• inspiratory and expiratory stridor	Hospital – IVI fluids
• marked sternal, suprasternal retraction	Steroids
• restlessness (indicative of hypoxia)	Nebulized adrenaline
• pallor; cyanosis; fatigue	Oxygen
	Intubation for <1% of hospitalized patients

Management

Medical

Supportive treatment and observation with no specific therapy is all that is required for most patients hospitalized for croup (Table 28.1).

Those warranting **admission to the intensive care unit** should be managed according to the hospital protocol. If there is moderate to severe airway obstruction, close monitoring of respiratory rate, pulse oximetry and transcutaneous carbon dioxide monitoring are indicated. The patients should be disturbed as little as possible; they are often most comfortable in their mother's arms.

Intravenous fluids are administered to those who may become dehydrated.

The inspired air can be humidifed but only if the child is comfortable in a mist tent; some children are frightened by enclosure.

Sedation does not have universal support because it may decrease restlessness which can be an important sign of airway obstruction or hypoxia. Sedatives should not be given to a patient with signs of respiratory failure.

Oxygen is not given routinely but is used in those who show signs of hypoxia, worsening airway obstruction or those being transported to the operating theatre for anaesthesia, endoscopy and intubation.

Topical vasoconstrictors, such as nebulized racemic epinephrine are usually beneficial, at least in the short-term, apparently by lessening mucosal oedema. There is the possibility of a rebound effect – after an initial improvement for 30–60 minutes, symptoms return to the pretreatment level or worse. Children treated by inhalation of racemic epinephrine should not be sent home for a minimum of 6 hours, and some hospitals insist that these children be admitted overnight. The α-adrenergic effect of the drug causes mucosal vasoconstriction, reduces oedema and possibly produces some temporary bronchodilatation. Recent reports suggest that nebulized budesonide may be a treatment option in moderate croup.

Steroid administration has been controversial until recent overwhelming evidence in favour of intramuscular and/or intravenous use. Dexamethasone (0.6 mg/kg) is used either as a single dose or in divided doses for 2 to 3 days. However, the usual time for the drug to be effective in lessening the need for intubation yet devoid of side-effects is 2 or 3 days. There is a significant clinical improvement in steroid-treated intubated patients in the first 24 hours, with not only reduced duration of intubation but also reduced risk of re-intubation. Because most cases of acute laryngotracheobronchitis are uncomplicated, self-limiting and require no treatment, steroid treatment should be considered only in moderate or severe cases.

Antibiotics are not given for uncomplicated laryngotracheobronchitis but are warranted for bacterial superinfection, ideally after a culture of sputum or tracheal secretions.

> **Treatment**
>
> Most require observation only
> Moist air
> Nebulized racemic epinephrine
> Dexamethasone
> < 1% need nasotracheal intubation

Intubation

Provision of an artificial airway by endotracheal intubation is required in very few of those seeking medical attention. Elective intubation has been reported as necessary in 1–7% of patients admitted to hospital and is the only therapy for otherwise intractable progressive airway obstruction.

The decision for intubation should be made on clinical grounds, not on the basis of blood gases or X-rays. Indications for intubation include progressive obstruction, respiratory distress causing worsening fatigue, decreased respiratory effort, hypoxaemia and increased oxygen requirements, acidosis, agitation, restlessness, and poor response to repeated treat-

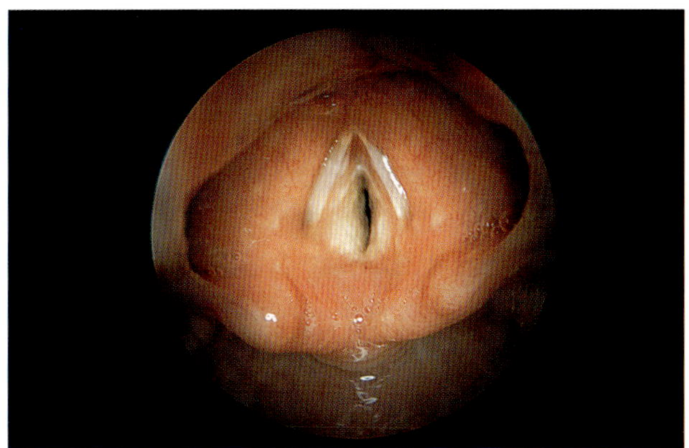

Figure **28.1**
Acute laryngotracheitis. Endoscopic photograph under general anaesthesia immediately before intubation. Severe subglottic oedema with a fibrin-like surface has narrowed the airway to an antero-posterior slit.

ment with racemic epinephrine. Preparations for 'elective' intubation should be commenced before more severe features such as extreme pallor, cyanosis, decreased consciousness, marked upper airway obstruction and impending respiratory failure develop.

Endoscopy reveals a firm bilateral subglottic inflammatory swelling narrowing the airway to an antero-posterior slit (Fig. 28.1). Details of the technique of anaesthesia and intubation are given later in this chapter.

Extubation

In laryngotracheobronchitis, extubation is performed when there is a leak around the tracheal tube, the child is afebrile and there are minimal, loose secretions. If these indications are not present after 7 days, elective extubation is attempted. If extubation fails, the child is re-intubated and diagnostic endoscopy arranged. If endoscopy shows necrosis or ulceration in the larynx due to prolonged intubation, a tracheotomy is usually necessary. If severe intubation changes are not present, the child is re-intubated, preferably with a tube of smaller diameter, for a further 1 or 2 days before extubation is again attempted.

Extubation

Child well, afebrile
Leak around the tube
Minimal tracheal secretions
7th day if not before

Complications of intubation

Children intubated for obstruction due to acute laryngotracheobronchitis are often relatively easy patients to nurse in a paediatric intensive care unit but complications are possible. They include blockage or displacement of the endotracheal tube, the use of excessive sedation and psycho social stresses for both the parents and the child. The most serious complications are cerebral hypoxia causing brain damage and laryngeal trauma from prolonged intubation. The incidence of acquired subglottic stenosis after intubation for croup was 2.4% in the series of McEniery et al (1991), but has been reported as much higher.

Complications

Blocked tube
Displaced tube
Excessive sedation
Psycho-social stress
Cerebral hypoxia
Laryngeal intubation trauma

ACUTE SUPRAGLOTTITIS

Acute supraglottitis has been known as acute epiglottitis for many years and, although there is a trend to use the former, more appropriate name, the latter remains firmly entrenched in the literature. This fulminating localized infection is a cellulitis of the soft tissues surrounding the epiglottis, arytenoid cartilages and aryepiglottic folds due to *Haemophilus influenza* Type B. It occurs in infants, children and sometimes in adults. It is the most frightening of paediatric infectious obstructive airway emergencies and if untreated death can occur within hours due to gross swelling of the supraglottic tissues, notably the epiglottis and the aryepiglottic folds. The prognosis depends on early diagnosis and effective treatment.

Acute supraglottitis

Occurs throughout the year
Usually 1–5 years of age
Occurs in infants and adults
Commoner in males
Haemophilus influenzae Type B
Usually positive blood culture

Aetiology and pathophysiology

The causal agent in infants and children is usually *Haemophilus influenzae* Type B which is found in blood culture in approximately 90% and in culture from secretions on the epiglottis in about 50%. In adults and immunocompromised patients, other organisms such as *Streptococcus pneumoniae*, *Staphylococcus aureus*, *Streptococcus* Group A, B and C, and other less common organisms can be isolated.

Local invasion of the supraglottic mucosa results in fulminating, dense, inflammatory infiltration by polymorphonuclear leukocytes, blood and oedema. Micro-abscesses or occasionally macro-abscesses are sometimes found in post-mortem specimens. Enlargement of supraglottic tissues including the epiglottis, aryepiglottic folds, ventricular folds and soft tissues around the arytenoids creates a ball-valve effect which is made worse by thick secretions which the patient finds difficult to clear because of extreme pain on swallowing. Strangely, the acute localized infection seldom spreads to the glottis or subglottis or far into the base of the tongue. The peak incidence is in the 2- to 4-year-old age group, but acute supraglottitis occurs at any age from 6 months to the elderly. Boys are slightly more at risk than girls. There is little seasonal variation.

Mortality was high before modern treatment with antibiotics and use of an artificial airway. Deaths are now uncommon. Children who die of the disease usually arrive at hospital deeply comatosed or intubated and ventilated, having already suffered brain damage.

Clinical features

Acute supraglottitis has a rapid onset. A healthy child may develop non-specific symptoms of an upper respiratory tract infection such as sore throat, mild fever and cough. These symptoms progress rapidly, in a few hours, to painful sore throat, difficulty swallowing, often with drooling, fever up to 38° or 39° C and increasing respiratory distress leading to airway obstruction within 12–24 hours. Exquisite pain on swallowing is the most distinctive feature and causes drooling in most patients. The older child characteristically sits upright leaning on outstretched arms, mouth open, jaw thrust forward in a position to 'splint' the airway, looking anxious and breathing with shallow inspiratory stridor. The jaw is protruded to maximize the lumen of the airway. The voice may be muffled or normal but the patient is reluctant to talk. This dramatic clinical picture should alert the physician to acute supraglottitis. The child may refuse to eat or drink and may refuse to sleep.

Clinical features

Rapid onset
Painful sore throat
Odynophagia
Drooling
Older child sits up
Muffled voice
Shallow inspiratory stridor

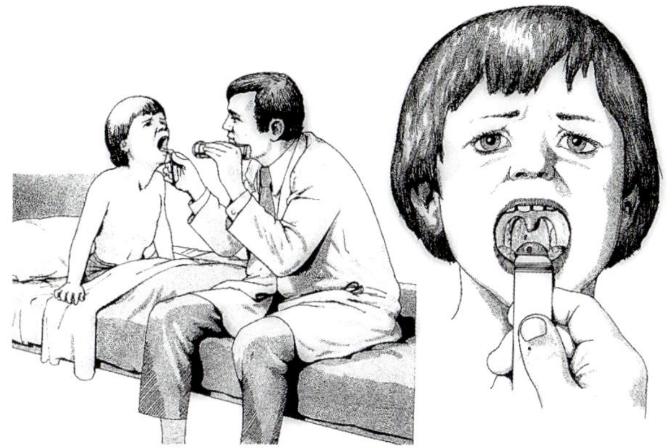

Figure **28.2**
Technique used for examination of the oropharynx for suspected acute supraglottitis when airway obstruction is not severe. Facilities for mask ventilation and intubation should be readily available.

Atypical or unusual presentations may be confusing. Septicaemia can lead to meningitis, pericarditis or distant infection such as perinephric abscess or joint abscess. Some patients present to the emergency room intubated and ventilated because they have become comatose in another hospital without a diagnosis having been made.

On physical examination, the clinician may encounter a frightened, anxious, pale, irritable child who is breathing slowly and cautiously. A younger child may be quiet and if respiratory distress seems to lessen it may be an ominous sign caused by extreme fatigue indicating that respiratory and cardiac arrest are imminent.

There is a continuing controversy about clinical examination of the oropharynx with a tongue depressor as this interference may precipitate serious obstruction. On the other hand, physical examination of the oral cavity and oropharynx can be undertaken except in advanced cases where there may be a danger of causing complete obstruction. Laryngospasm may precipitate obstruction but it is likely that the patient can be resuscitated by using 100% oxygen for assisted ventilation with a face mask.

Forcing a child to lie down against his wishes may also be dangerous and precipitate obstruction and asphyxia; a good guide is that a child who is able to lie down without increased respiratory distress can have direct examination with little fear of worsening the situation. A brief examination of the oropharynx will eliminate other possible causes of acute inflammatory airway obstruction such as inflamed, grossly enlarged tonsils (sometimes caused by infectious mononucleosis), peritonsillar abscess, retropharyngeal abscess and the rare, but vitally important, case of diphtheria. It is helpful to use an angled, metal tongue depressor and a bright light from a head mirror or a powerful torch; the dorsum of the tongue is momentarily but firmly depressed allowing the epiglottis to be seen (Fig. 28.2). A large, swollen, red epiglottis and surrounding tissues with mucopurulent secretions confirms the diagnosis although occasionally the epiglottis itself is less involved and the airway is obstructed by swelling of the aryepiglottic folds, arytenoids and false cords, hence the preference for the name acute supraglottitis. Examination of the oropharynx should be performed only where there is equipment and facilities for provision of an artificial airway. Once a positive diagnosis is made there should be no further examination and X-ray is not required. In a co-operative older child, and certainly in an adult, pernasal indirect flexible laryngoscopy should be undertaken and will confirm the diagnosis.

The diagnosis of acute supraglottitis is readily made when the classic clinical features are present, but it may be misdiagnosed in younger patients with an atypical presentation if a high index of suspicion is not maintained.

Diagnostic imaging

Lateral X-ray of the neck is performed only when there is substantial doubt about the diagnosis and when the X-ray can be taken in or near the intensive care unit or operating theatre. The film must be read by an experienced clinician or radiologist or the findings may be misinterpreted. The pharynx and hypopharynx are ballooned and dilated by air above the grossly swollen rounded epiglottis and thickened aryepiglottic folds (Fig. 28.3).

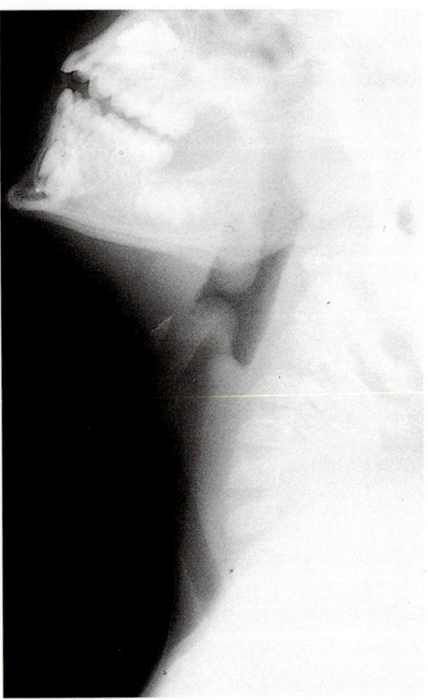

Figure **28.3**
Acute supraglottitis. Lateral airways X-ray. Severe swelling of the supraglottic tissues is obvious against the contrast of air, ballooned in the laryngopharynx. Care must be taken during the X-ray procedure that extension or manipulation of the neck does not worsen the respiratory obstruction.

Management

The treatment of acute supraglottitis has changed during the last 25 years. Tracheotomy has been replaced by pernasal intubation, more powerful and effective antibiotics are available, new technology and dedicated nursing is available in paediatric intensive care units and the development of an effective Hib vaccine has dramatically reduced the incidence of systemic *H. influenzae* Type B infections.

Maintenance and restoration of the airway is essential. Most authorities recommend placement of an endotracheal tube under controlled conditions in all infants and children once the diagnosis has been made. In adults, however, the progress of the disease is not so dramatic nor necessarily so relentless; observation in an intensive care unit with the option of 'elective' intubation if the airway deteriorates is usually reasonable.

Tracheotomy provides an equally safe airway if the patient is to be cared for in a hospital which does not have intensive care facilities for intubated patients. Orderly completion of a tracheotomy usually requires prior passage of an endotracheal tube or bronchoscope under general anaesthesia.

In infants and children, once a diagnosis of acute supraglottitis has been established or suspected, immediate arrangements are made for anaesthesia and intubation in an operating theatre, with an otolaryngologist in attendance. Should intubation with an anaesthetic tube be difficult or fail, intubation with a bronchoscope is usually possible or, very occasionally, an urgent 'crash' tracheotomy will become necessary.

Treatment

Admit to ICU
Pernasal intubation
Intravenous antibiotics
Extubation within 36 hours

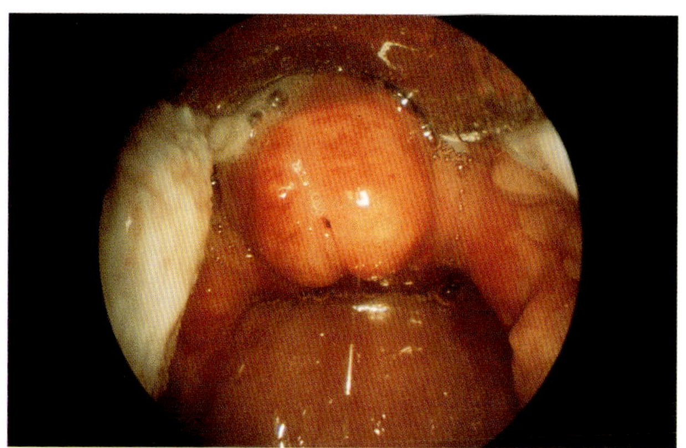

Figure **28.4**
Acute supraglottitis. Endoscopic photograph immediately before intubation under general anaesthesia. There is only a tiny opening representing the airway.

Extubation

Afebrile, no signs of toxicity
Minimal tracheal secretions
Able to sip fluids
Resolution of swelling at laryngoscopy

In some cases, where the cause of airway obstruction is doubtful, diagnostic laryngoscopy and bronchoscopy is required. Endoscopy quickly reveals the dramatic obstructive swelling of the supraglottic tissues (Fig. 28.4). Details of the technique of anaesthesia and intubation are given later in this chapter.

Antibiotics

Antibiotics to treat septicaemia and systemic infection are of vital importance and a third-generation cephalosporin is now recommended. Cefotaxime (100–180 mg/kg/day in 4 divided doses) or ceftriaxone (100 mg/kg/day as a single daily dose) is currently the treatment of choice.

Steroids

The use of steroids has little support.

Extubation

Various opinions have been expressed on the subject of 'when to extubate'. Some believe it can be safely done within 12–24 hours while others leave the tube in place for 3–4 days. All warn of the danger of accidental extubation and the need for emergency re-intubation.

It seems reasonable to consider extubation when there are no longer signs of toxicity, when there are minimal tracheal secretions on suctioning and when examination of the supraglottic tissues, either by direct or by fibreoptic laryngoscopy, shows resolution of the swelling. A useful test is the ability of the child to sip fluids. Using these criteria extubation can usually be safely accomplished within 36 hours. The antibiotics should be continued for 7–10 days.

Differential diagnosis

Acute viral laryngotracheitis is much more common than either acute supraglottis or bacterial tracheitis. The clinical features usually allow diagnosis before endoscopy (Table 28.2)

Complications

The most serious complication of acute supraglottitis is acute respiratory obstruction leading to serious brain damage or death. Before modern, aggressive treatment the mortality rate was very high, but it is now approximately 1%.

Tube obstruction and accidental extubation are the important complications of treatment. Re-intubation can be necessary either after accidental removal of the tube during the treatment period or after 'elective' extubation has been performed but airway obstruction persists or recurs.

Table 28.2 Differential diagnosis of acute inflammatory airway obstruction

Feature	*Viral laryngotracheitis ('croup')*	*Bacterial tracheitis*	*Acute supraglottitis*
Age	6–48 months	Children of any age; uncommon	1 to 5 years Less common in adults
Cause	Parainfluenza virus and Respiratory syncitial virus	*Staphylococcus aureus*	*Haemophilus influenzae* B
Obstruction	Subglottic oedema	Tracheal secretions, membranes	Supraglottic swelling
Onset	Slow, 24–48 hours	More rapid, 12–24 hours	Rapid, 6–12 hours
Stridor	Inspiratory	Inspiratory and expiratory	Inspiratory, shallow
Voice	Hoarse	Hoarse	Muffled
Swallowing	Normal	Normal	Painful, drooling
Cough	Croupy	Barking	None
Previous attacks	Common	None	None
X-ray	Subglottic swelling	Irregular tracheal membranes	Grossly swollen supraglottis
Treatment	Moist air, steroids, racemic epinephrine	Antibiotics, bronchoscopic toilet, removal of crusts	Antibiotics intravenously
Intubation	Sometimes	Usually Sometimes tracheotomy	Always, in infants and children

Unlike prolonged intubation for acute laryngotracheobronchitis where the tube has been passed through a grossly abnormal subglottic area and remains in situ for 5–7 days, there is little chance of laryngeal injury from intubation for supraglottitis.

Simultaneous meningitis, pericarditis or other localized suppurative complications of septicaemia are possible.

Prevention

It has been said that 1 child in 200 is likely to suffer a serious *Haemophilus influenzae* infection in their first few years, but studies have already shown a significant drop in the incidence of acute supraglottitis in populations which have started routine vaccination. The polysaccharide–protein conjugate vaccine has good immunogenicity and immunologic memory, and it is conceivable that acute supraglottitis will become a medical rarity in the same way that diphtheria is now seldom seen.

BACTERIAL TRACHEITIS

Bacterial tracheitis is also known as bacterial laryngotracheobronchitis, membranous laryngotracheobronchitis, pseudo-membranous laryngotracheobronchitis and bacterial croup. It is a relatively rare infection somewhat similar to acute supraglottitis in its severity and threat to life. There is acute inflammation of the subglottic larynx and trachea accompanied by adherent mucopurulent pseudo-membranes. The disease is either being recognized more often or is actually increasing in incidence and now must be considered in the differential diagnosis of all children presenting with acute inflammatory airway obstruction.

Epidemiology

It is a relatively rare but serious infection affecting males more than females in a ratio of about 2 : 1. There is a wide age range from a few weeks old into adulthood with a mean age of 4–5 years.

Aetiology and pathophysiology

Bacterial tracheitis is an acute bacterial infection involving not only the subglottic larynx and trachea but also the bronchi and the lung parenchyma. *Staphylococcus aureus* is by far the most frequent pathogenic bacterium isolated but others include *H. influenzae*, *Streptococcus pneumoniae*, alpha-haemolytic streptococcus and others. Although the exact aetiology remains uncertain, it seems likely that bacterial tracheitis may be a super-infection by a bacterial pathogen on a primary viral infection, i.e. a bacterial complication of viral laryngotracheobronchitis in which favourable conditions exist for bacterial colonization and formation of a mucopurulent membrane. Circumstantial evidence for this includes the fact that most children have an antecedent viral respiratory illness, that the attacks occur during the cold months and that viruses are sometimes isolated as well as the bacterial pathogen.

Clinical features

The presentation is often initially similar to acute laryngotracheobronchitis with symptoms of runny nose, sore throat, fever and cough followed by hoarseness, wheezing, respiratory distress and stridor. The clinical features depend upon the stage of the disease; later presentation is with general deterioration, high fever, more severe obstruction, increased toxicity and diminished response to supportive therapy such as racemic epinephrine. Children presenting late will be near to cardiopulmonary arrest.

As there may be few distinguishing features from acute laryngotracheobronchitis or even acute supraglottitis, bacterial tracheitis may not be suspected until a surprise diagnosis is made at direct examination. After intubation copious purulent secretions and scattered membranes are found in the subglottic larynx and trachea.

Diagnostic imaging

Lateral X-rays may be helpful but must be performed with caution in any child with airway obstruction; the film may show radio-opaque material in the tracheal lumen, which sometimes raises concern about the possibility of an inhaled foreign body. The appearance represents the partly detached pseudo-membrane and thick intraluminal secretions. Subglottic narrowing is likely to be seen on the lateral X-ray. Chest X-ray may show pulmonary infiltrates consistent with pneumonia.

Bacterial tracheitis

Any age in childhood
Commoner in boys
? increasing in incidence
Virulent *Staph. aureus* infection
Initial URT infection symptoms
Later toxicity, severe obstruction
May be radio-opacities in trachea
Usually requires intubation
May need repeated bronchoscopic toilet
May require tracheotomy

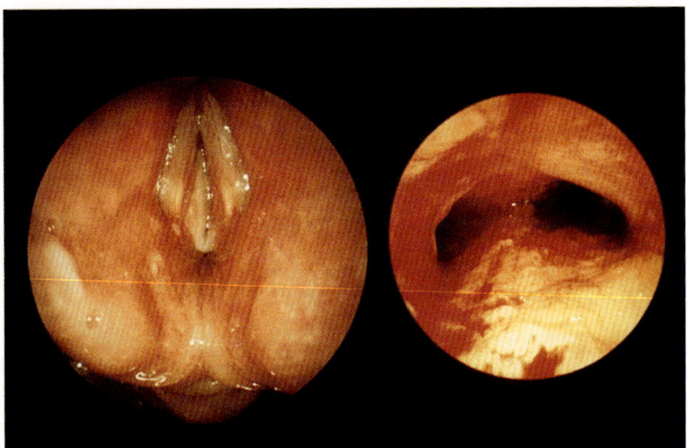

Figure **28.5**
Acute bacterial tracheitis. The severe obstruction in the subglottis is similar to the appearance seen in viral croup. The photograph on the right shows surface ulceration and some bleeding of the mucosa of the trachea after removal of obstructing membranes.

Management

The diagnosis is primarily a clinical one, but sometimes it is not made before examination under the controlled conditions available during general anaesthesia when endoscopy shows the appearance of an airway blocked by mucopus (Fig. 28.5), debris and membranous material extending into the bronchi. This pseudo-membrane usually separates easily from the lining of the airway with little bleeding. Cleaning and suction of the airway results in a striking improvement, but the benefit may be short-lived since the tracheobronchial tree or endotracheal tube often blocks again despite frequent suction. The patient should remain intubated to maintain control of the airway and for repeated tracheobronchial suction. Repeat bronchoscopy should be undertaken without hesitation. Even with meticulous endotracheal toilet difficulty may be experienced in maintaining the airway because of the tendency of thick secretions to form crusts. Management in a paediatric intensive care unit is mandatory with humidification of the airway and frequent suctioning after instillation of saline to loosen the secretions. Tracheostomy may need to be considered particularly if thick crusts are a problem and management of the endotracheal tube is difficult. Tracheostomy has the advantage of ease of suction and the provision of an inner tube which can be cleaned regularly.

Antibiotic coverage must include the broad spectrum of bacteria that have been associated with the disease; a third generation cephalosporin is usually given for 10 days.

Intubation may need to be continued for up to a week and the total hospitalization may be 10–14 days. The decision of when to extubate is difficult but lack of toxicity, absence of fever and decreased secretions are useful guides.

SPASMODIC CROUP

Spasmodic croup is a croup-like illness which is poorly defined and not well understood. It differs from infectious viral acute laryngotracheobronchitis in that clinically it has a more abrupt onset, there is usually no fever, it occurs mostly at night, often after the child has been in bed for some hours, lasts only for a short time and tends to resolve rapidly. Patients have usually improved before they reach hospital.

Spasmodic croup may not differ markedly from acute laryngotracheobronchitis except for being less severe and having a shorter duration. It may be a manifestation of an allergic reaction to viral antigens without the prodromal features of an upper respiratory tract infection, running a milder, shorter course with spontaneous improvement. Sometimes there are frequent recurrences. Spasmodic croup and acute

Spasmodic croup

Poorly defined croup-like illness
Abrupt onset
Resolves quickly
? allergic reaction to viral antigens
Sometimes recurs

laryngotracheobronchitis are therefore possibly different presentations of a similar disease caused by parainfluenza viruses, respiratory syncitial virus and other viral pathogens.

DIPHTHERIA LARYNGOTRACHEITIS

Diphtheria was the true 'croup' of pre-immunization and pre-antimicrobial days. It is a multisystem disease mediated by a powerful exotoxin produced by the causative organism, *Corynebacterium diphtheriae*; the potentially lethal inflammatory process usually starting in the airway. During the nineteenth century almost half the people who contracted diphtheria died. It was a major cause of death in children 2–5 years of age.

Diphtheria

Multisystem disease
Powerful exotoxin
Corynebacterium diphtheriae
Usually commences in URT
Membrane in pharynx
Often fatal if untreated

Clinical features

The incubation period is usually 2–4 days. In most cases infection enters through the respiratory passages causing insidious features such as headache, nausea, vomiting, malaise, nasal congestion, pharyngitis, poor appetite, fever, a hoarse voice, croupy cough, cervical lymphadenopathy and, in some cases, oedematous swelling of the soft tissues of the neck.

Initially the oropharynx is red, in 24–48 hours greyish-white spots appear, then necrosis of the mucosa starts to form a light or dark grey membrane on the tonsils, spreading to the soft palate and uvula. As the membrane becomes thicker and darker it may develop a leather-like appearance and be tightly adherent to the underlying tissues; attempts to remove it cause bleeding. The membrane may be localized to the pharynx or extend deeper to the larynx and tracheobronchial tree. Enlargement, dislodgement or inhalation of the membrane may cause fatal airway obstruction.

The powerful exotoxin causes immediate systemic effects which can include acute myocarditis, acute cardiac failure, acute tubular necrosis of the kidneys and, later, encephalitis, peripheral neuritis and cranial neuropathy.

The clinician must remember the possibility of oropharyngeal and laryngotracheal diphtheria when evaluating a child with acute inflammatory airway obstruction. The circulating toxin causes the patient to be more toxic than would otherwise be expected, there is undue tachycardia, sometimes with a weak pulse, possibly an arrhythmia due to the myocarditis, severe airway obstruction and examination of the oropharynx may be rewarded by visualization of the adherent membrane which is often associated with a fish-like smell.

Less common manifestations include the bull-neck of 'malignant' pharyngeal diphtheria (a variant which runs a more abrupt and aggressive course) or the mucoid or mucopurulent discharge of nasal diphtheria. Laryngeal diphtheria presents with hoarseness, loss of voice and obstructive breathing.

Treatment

Administration of diphtheria antitoxin to neutralize the exotoxin is justified on highly suggestive clinical features of pharyngeal diphtheria. After testing the patient for possible sensitivity to horse serum, the antitoxin is administered intravenously, from 20 000 up to 120 000 units depending upon the severity of the disease. Diphtheria antitoxin is normally prepared with horse serum and should only be administered after an appropriate test-dose. If the patient is sensitive to horse serum then antitoxin prepared from another animal is used. Approximately 10% of the

Treatment

Must be recognized early
Antitoxin
Intubation, usually tracheotomy
Antibiotics

Microbiologic confirmation

Swab membrane or underlying tissues
Selective culture media
Guinea-pig toxigenicity test

population is allergic to the horse serum diphtheria antitoxin.

In addition, antimicrobial therapy to eradicate the organism and prevent spread to other contacts is given using either parenteral penicillin or oral erythromycin for 10–14 days. This antibiotic therapy is mandatory.

Respiratory obstruction due to the membrane may require mechanical intervention to maintain a patent airway, necessitating intubation or tracheotomy.

Toxic complications affect the heart and the nervous system. Myocarditis may occur as early as the first week, but usually develops as the upper respiratory tract improves. Peripheral or cranial nerve neuritis occurs later in the disease, several days to several weeks after onset in about 75% of patients. These toxic complications require supportive therapy.

Microbiology

Antitoxin is given on clinical suspicion without waiting for definitive diagnosis which is based on culture from the membrane or from material beneath it. Selective culture material such as Loeffler's or tellurite medium are used. Positive cultures are evaluated for toxicity using two guinea-pigs, one of which, pre-treated with diphtheria antitoxin will survive, the other will die. This test is necessary to confirm the pathogenic nature of the *Corynebacterium* which has been isolated.

A direct Gram-stain smear of the throat swab from diphtheria may grow a diphtheroid but is unreliable to prove that the patient has a pathogenic *Corynebacterium* diphtheria infection.

Immunization

A diagnosis of diphtheria initiates a search for personal contacts who might require treatment or immunization.

Children and adults are routinely immunized against diphtheria and today the disease is rarely seen except in the unimmunized, incompletely immunized or older members of the population. Unless a high level of immunization is maintained, diphtheria will again become epidemic. The Schick skin test detects the level of immunity in an individual; the absence of immunity is a positive result and indicates the need for active immunization.

Diphtheria is seen much less frequently now that immunization has become almost universal but remains common in communities with a non-immunized population. Active vaccination with diphtheria toxoid is an effective, preventative measure usually given as a component of triple antigen from the age of 2 months.

Prognosis

The prognosis depends on the virulence of the particular organism, the patient's immune status, duration of illness before specific treatment has begun, prompt administration of antitoxin, treatment of airway obstruction and resolution of myocarditis and peripheral neuritis.

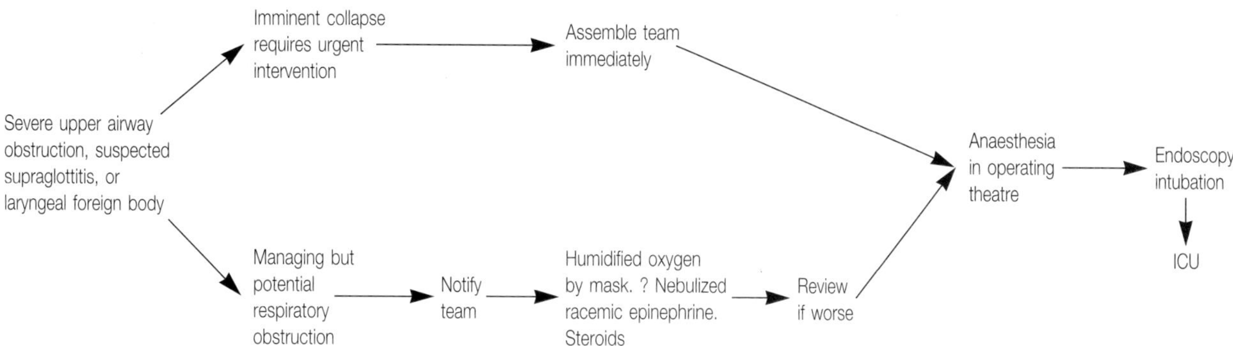

Figure **28.6**
Suggested protocol for management of severe inflammatory airway obstruction.

MANAGEMENT PRINCIPLES IN SEVERE UPPER AIRWAY OBSTRUCTION

General principles

Mortality and morbidity increase when difficulties occur from delayed or erroneous diagnosis, confusion over the need for investigations and inexperience in assessing the need for an artificial airway, especially in infants and children. Each hospital should have a management protocol for the child who presents with acute airway obstruction due to inflammation (Fig. 28.6).

The important principles include:

- provision and maintenance of an airway, preferably by endotracheal intubation; this takes precedence over all other diagnostic or therapeutic procedures;
- avoidance of unnecessary intervention which may increase the child's respiratory distress;
- organization of team skills to optimize patient management; the team involves the resident, paediatrician, laryngologist, anaesthesiologist, intensivist and nurse specialists in intensive care.

When a child presents with severe upper airway obstruction but no clearcut clinical diagnosis the possibilities include acute supraglottitis, bacterial tracheitis, acute viral laryngotracheobronchitis, inhaled laryngeal foreign body, diphtheria and possibly inflammation of enlarged obstructive tonsils. From a practical management viewpoint, the essential distinction is between two groups:

1 those who require immediate examination under anaesthesia for diagnosis and probable intubation;
2 those who require careful observation in intensive care with the option of being taken to theatre for general anaesthesia.

Assessment of severity

A healthy child will tolerate moderately severe airway obstruction but as the obstruction increases, although tidal volume is initially maintained, there is a point of exhaustion when hypoxaemia, hypercapnoea and acidosis progress to cardiorespiratory arrest. The assessment is a clinical one, and reliance should not be placed on blood gases; in fact the disturbance of obtaining blood gases may worsen the situation.

An urgent need to assemble the team to prepare for immediate intervention is indicated by features indicating respiratory failure with imminent collapse:

- decreased respiratory effort, decreased stridor and breath sounds;
- marked restlessness, decreased consciousness and hypotonia;
- extreme pallor or cyanosis.

Intubation should be performed immediately if the following features are present:

- severe obstruction evidenced by intercostal, subcostal and suprasternal retraction on inspiration;
- restlessness, an appearance of anxiety and distress, fatigue and a clinical impression of deterioration;
- increasing tachycardia.

Management in intensive care

Regular observations should be charted to monitor improvement or deterioration as time progresses. Many infants are most comfortable in their parent's arms or older children on their parent's lap. Separation from their parents should be delayed until anaesthesia is actually commenced. Most children should be in a cool, moist atmosphere but the use of a mist tent may be frightening to some children and observation through the mist may be difficult.

Oxygen is given only to those who show signs of hypoxia as the latter is an important indication for airway intervention. Dehydrated patients receive intravenous fluid but placement of an intravenous line is often an unnecessary intervention which may be deferred until the time of anaesthesia.

Although good-quality lateral airway X-rays can distinguish supraglottitis from croup and can demonstrate radio-opaque laryngeal foreign bodies, transfer to the X-ray department may cause undue delay and the actual taking of the film may increase respiratory obstruction. If the film is not interpreted by an experienced radiologist or clinician, misdiagnosis is possible. Antero-posterior chest X-ray in the intensive care unit is performed in selected cases.

Technique of anaesthesia, endoscopy and intubation

When possible, intubation should be performed in a fully equipped operating theatre. In an unexpected emergency, where a laryngoscope and a suitable size endotracheal tube is available, attempted intubation is the preferred technique. If the facilities for intubation are not available or intubation fails, emergency tracheotomy or a cricothyroidotomy should be attempted. A wide-bore needle with a sharpened bevelled tip (Fig. 28.7) can be passed into the upper trachea or the cricothyroid membrane as a temporary measure.

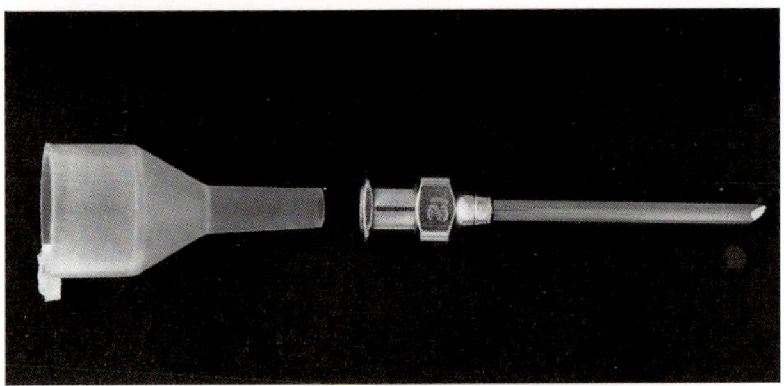

Figure **28.7**
Emergency airway needle. A no. 12 needle has been shortened, the tip bevelled and sharpened. The proximal end of the needle requires a suitable connector for assisted ventilation.

In the operating theatre general anaesthesia is induced by face mask with 100% oxygen and halothane allowing spontaneous respiration with the patient sitting on the parent's lap or resting in the parent's arms until they fall asleep and at this time the parent is excused from the operating suite. All necessary equipment, including an assortment of masks of various sizes, endotracheal tubes, functioning laryngoscopes, several sizes of bronchoscopes and instruments for tracheotomy must be readily available before induction of anaesthesia.

As anaesthesia progresses the patient is placed supine and positive pressure ventilatory assistance is applied via a mask, but an adequate depth which will allow laryngoscopy and intubation to be performed in a controlled fashion takes longer to achieve in the presence of airway obstruction. The application of topical anaesthesia as a spray is optional.

In those patients where the diagnosis is in doubt, laryngoscopy and examination of the subglottic region and upper trachea is performed by an otolaryngologist using slim rigid telescopes to confirm the diagno-

Anaesthesia, endoscopy and intubation

In a fully equipped operating theatre
Induction with 100% oxygen and halothane
Positive pressure assisted mask ventilation
Takes longer to achieve adequate depth
Optional local anaesthesia
Diagnostic endoscopy
Pernasal intubation requires skill
Venipuncture and blood culture
Immediate transfer to ICU

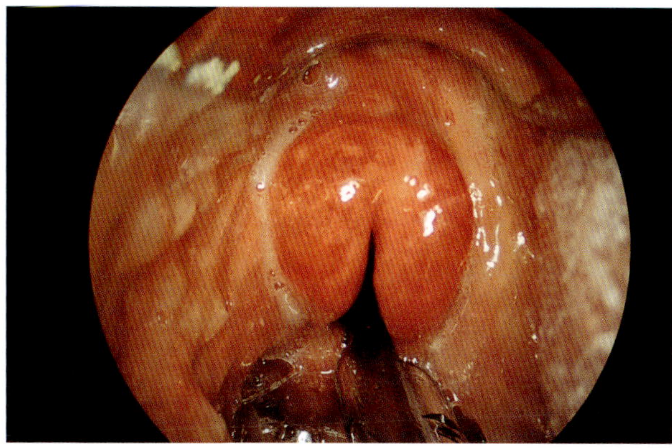

Figure **28.8**
Acute supraglottitis. Swelling of the epiglottis and the surrounding tissues at the base of the tongue. The endotracheal tube has widened the swollen epiglottis so there is an airway beside the tube in addition to the tube lumen.

sis of acute laryngotracheobronchitis, acute supraglottitis or bacterial tracheitis and to exclude the possibility of an inhaled laryngeal foreign body.

Intubation for croup requires considerable experience and skill. Nasotracheal intubation is preferred as the tube can be more firmly secured to the nose than an orotracheal tube can be to the mouth. The size of the endotracheal tube seldom allows a leak when it is first passed through thickened oedematous obstructive supraglottic or subglottic tissues but it must be of an adequate internal diameter for effective suctioning. The presence of a leak around the tube at less than 20 cm water pressure is preferred but not essential.

Skilled nursing care with attention to detail is the best insurance against obstruction of the endotracheal tube or accidental extubation, both of which are a major potential hazard. Arm boards are usually used to keep the arms extended. Restless children who are difficult to control should be suspected of having a possible complication such as tube blockage or hypoxia before sedation is considered. Parents should have as much access to the children as possible.

Postoperative pulmonary oedema is occasionally seen following either intubation or tracheotomy for relief of obstruction caused by acute supraglottitis or acute laryngotracheobronchitis. It is thought that hypoxia causes severe venous constriction in the pulmonary vasculature and increased transcapillary filtration of pulmonary interstitial fluid produces pulmonary oedema. This potentially fatal complication usually responds to intermittent positive pressure ventilation within 24 hours.

In acute supraglottitis, again general anaesthesia is induced by a face mask with 100% oxygen and halothane allowing spontaneous respiration assisted by gentle positive pressure via the face mask. At the appropriate depth of anaesthesia, local anaesthesia solution may be sprayed on the larynx and intubation is attempted. This is made difficult by the distortion and swelling of the supraglottic structures (Fig. 28.4). A relatively small-diameter endotracheal tube, preferably partly stiffened by an introducer, is passed behind the swollen epiglottic tissues but direct laryngoscopy rarely exposes the vocal cords or much of the glottic opening. Air bubbles through a slit-like opening may give a guide to the airway. Once intubation has been achieved the endotracheal tube provides an airway not only through its own lumen but also through the spaces on each side of the tube created by splinting the epiglottis outwards and forward (Fig. 28.8).

When the depth of anaesthesia has been stabilized the orotracheal tube is removed and immediately replaced by a nasotracheal tube which is secured firmly to the nose and face for easier postoperative nursing care.

At this stage, venipuncture allows collection for blood culture and a swab is taken from secretions around the epiglottis for microbiological culture.

Care of the intubated child

The patient is transferred to the intensive care ward and allowed to breathe spontaneously with a continuous flow, humidified, oxygen-enriched atmosphere usually with continuous positive pressure of a few centimetres of water to minimize the chance of pulmonary atelectasis.

Meticulous nursing is necessary in intensive care with 24-hour availability of an intensive care physician. Humidification of inspired gases can be achieved by mist tents, humidifiers connected to the circuit or disposable condensers. Suction must be gentle, frequent and adequate. Antibiotics are given for acute supraglottitis, bacterial tracheitis and complicated acute laryngotracheobronchitis.

BIBLIOGRAPHY

Baum HL (1928) Acute laryngotracheobronchitis. *JAMA* **91**: 1097–102.

Bell LM (1995) Middle respiratory tract infections. In: Jenson HB, Baltimore RS, eds., *Pediatric infectious diseases* (Norwalk: Appleton and Lange); 951–61.

Darrow D, Holinger L (1996) Inflammatory illness of the pediatric airway. In: Fried MP, ed., *The larynx* (St Louis: CV Mosby); 143–54.

Henry RL, Mellis CM, Benjamin B (1983) Pseudomembranous croup. *Arch Dis Child* **58**: 180–3.

Jones R, Santos JK, Overall JC (1979) Bacterial tracheitis. *JAMA* **242**: 721–6.

Kilham H, Gillis J, Benjamin B (1987) Severe upper airway obstruction. *Pediatr Clin North Am* **34**: 1–14.

McEniery J, Gillis J, Kilham H, Benjamin B (1991) Review of intubation in severe laryngotracheobronchitis. *Paediatrics* **87**: 847–53.

Willson D (1995) Inflammatory diseases of the airway. In: Myer CM, Cotton R, Shott S, eds., *The pediatric airway* (Philadelphia: JB Lippincott); 67–99.

Index